EXERCISE PSYCHOLOGY

SECOND EDITION

JANET BUCKWORTH, PhD
Ohio State University

ROD K. DISHMAN, PhD
University of Georgia

PATRICK J. O'CONNOR, PhD
University of Georgia

PHILLIP D. TOMPOROWSKI, PhD
University of Georgia

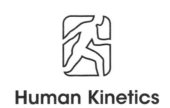

Human Kinetics

Library of Congress Info

Exercise psychology / Janet Buckworth ... [et al.]. -- 2nd ed.
   p. ; cm.
 Rev. ed. of: Exercise psychology / Janet Buckworth, Rod K. Dishman. c2002.
 Includes bibliographical references and index.
 I. Buckworth, Janet, 1953- II. Buckworth, Janet, 1953-. Exercise psychology.
 [DNLM: 1. Exercise--psychology. 2. Exercise Therapy. 3. Physical Fitness--psychology. QT 255]
  613.7'1--dc23

2012037845

ISBN-10: 1-4504-0709-9 (print)
ISBN-13: 978-1-4504-0709-0 (print)

The web addresses cited in this text were current as of August 2012, unless otherwise noted.

Acquisitions Editor: Myles Schrag; **Developmental Editor:** Melissa J. Zavala; **Assistant Editors:** Kali Cox and Jan Feeney; **Copyeditor:** Patsy Fortney; **Indexer:** Nan Badgett; **Permissions Manager:** Dalene Reeder; **Graphic Designer:** Fred Starbird; **Graphic Artist:** Kathleen Boudreau-Fuoss; **Cover Designer:** Keith Blomberg; **Photograph (cover):** Digital Vision; **Photographs (interior):** © Human Kinetics, unless otherwise noted; **Photo Production Manager:** Jason Allen; **Art Manager:** Kelly Hendren; **Associate Art Manager:** Alan L. Wilborn; **Illustrations:** © Human Kinetics, unless otherwise noted; **Printer:** Sheridan Books

Printed in the United States of America   10   9   8   7   6   5   4   3   2   1

The paper in this book is certified under a sustainable forestry program.

Human Kinetics
Website: www.HumanKinetics.com
United States: Human Kinetics
P.O. Box 5076
Champaign, IL 61825-5076
800-747-4457
e-mail: humank@hkusa.com

Canada: Human Kinetics
475 Devonshire Road Unit 100
Windsor, ON N8Y 2L5
800-465-7301 (in Canada only)
e-mail: info@hkcanada.com

Europe: Human Kinetics
107 Bradford Road
Stanningley
Leeds LS28 6AT, United Kingdom
+44 (0) 113 255 5665
e-mail: hk@hkeurope.com

Australia: Human Kinetics
57A Price Avenue
Lower Mitcham, South Australia 5062
08 8372 0999
e-mail: info@hkaustralia.com

New Zealand: Human Kinetics
P.O. Box 80
Torrens Park, South Australia 5062
0800 222 062
e-mail: info@hknewzealand.com

To my husband, Chuck Moody, for his encouragement, support, and love; to the memory of my parents, Sigmund and Lois Buckworth, for nurturing my curiosity and faith; to my students for their questions and challenges; and to the dogs, Bec and Sonya, for their infectious enthusiasm for exercise and for making me laugh.

—*Janet Buckworth*

To serious students and William P. Morgan for the "big picture."

—*Rod Dishman*

Dedicated to two pioneers who touched my life: A.H. Ismail and William P. Morgan.

—*Patrick O'Connor*

Dedicated to two who pushed and pulled me forward: my wife, Regina Smith, and my mentor, Norman Ellis.

—*Phillip Tomporowski*

Contents

PART TWO
Exercise and Mental Health
93

Preface

Exercise psychology is the study of the brain and behavior in physical activity and exercise settings. It is a new field, but it is based on old ideas. The ancient Greek physician Hippocrates, considered the father of medicine, recommended physical activity for the treatment of mental illness. William James, the father of American psychology, stated in 1899 that "muscular vigor will . . . always be needed to furnish the background of sanity, serenity, and cheerfulness to life, to give moral elasticity to our disposition, to round off the wiry edge of our fretfulness, and make us goodhumored and easy of approach" (James, W. 1899).

However, it wasn't until the late 1960s and early 1970s that a systematic body of research related to exercise psychology began to accumulate. The key progenitor of that research was William P. Morgan, who established the ergopsychology (i.e., work psychology) laboratory at the University of Wisconsin in 1970. This happened nearly 100 years after Wilhelm Wundt, the father of psychology, established the first psychology laboratory at the University of Leipzig in 1879, and after William James began conducting experiments at Harvard in 1875. Morgan later founded and served as the first president of Division 47, Exercise and Sport Psychology, of the American Psychological Association in 1986, nearly 100 years after the founding of the APA by G. Stanley Hall in 1892. Division 47 celebrated its 25th anniversary in 2011.

Although subjective experience is the defining feature of psychology that distinguishes it from other disciplines such as physiology and sociology, areas of modern psychology vary in their emphases on physiological, behavioral, cognitive, and social questions and methods. Hence, several subdisciplines exist in psychology. Notable among these are biological psychology, behavioral neuroscience, comparative psychology, evolutionary psychology, behaviorism, and social psychology. Because exercise psychology uses the traditions of each of these subdisciplines

to study physical activity, it is an interdisciplinary field of study rather than a subdiscipline of psychology. Moreover, exercise psychology has roots in exercise science, which itself is an interdisciplinary field of study. Because exercise psychology is concerned with mental health and health-related behaviors within both clinical settings and populations, it also encompasses approaches from the fields of psychiatry, clinical and counseling psychology, health promotion, and epidemiology.

A unique feature of this text is its presentation of the biological foundations of exercise psychology within the broader contexts of cognitive, social, and environmental influences. In our view, social psychology has dominated the early years of exercise psychology. Although the social agency and impact of exercise are very important, it is our view that the biological basis of brain and behavior (e.g., the impact of exercise on the brain and the control of exercise by the brain) is equally important but has been neglected by most researchers in exercise psychology and by most textbooks that have been used in the field. This has been unfortunate given the indisputable fact that physical activity and exercise are uniquely biological in nature; no other behaviors occur for prolonged periods at a metabolic cost several times that of rest. Also, it is instructive to remember that Wilhelm Wundt was trained in physiology and medicine before he established the field of experimental psychology.

The decade of the 1990s was designated by the U.S. Congress as the Decade of the Brain. The years 2000 to 2010 were the Decade of Behavior, an interdisciplinary effort initiated by the American Psychological Association to promote the importance of behavioral and social science research modeled after that of the Decade of the Brain. We have strived in this book to balance the biological foundations of brain and behavior with theory and knowledge derived from the behavioristic, cognitive, and social approaches used to study key topics in the field of exercise psychology.

The social significance of exercise and other forms of physical activity in developed nations has never been greater. Sedentariness is a burden to the public's health in the United States, accounting for more than 250,000 deaths annually from coronary heart disease, type 2 diabetes mellitus, and colon cancer. The combined effect of physical inactivity and excess caloric intake is a key contributor to a doubling of obesity prevalence among U.S. adults and children since the 1960s, most of which occurred since the 1980s. Growing evidence also supports the contention that physical inactivity is a risk factor for poor mental health. The World Health Organization has projected that depression will be second only to cardiovascular disease as the world's leading cause of death and disability by the year 2020 and will be number one by 2030, ahead of cardiovascular disease, with dementia then ranking third.

The promotion of leisure-time physical activity has emerged as an important initiative for public health and enhanced quality of living in many economically developed nations. The U.S. *Surgeon General's Report on Physical Activity and Health,* published in 1996, and the report of the Physical Activity Advisory Committee for the *2008 Physical Activity Guidelines for Americans* each provided a consensus on the benefits of physical activity for reducing the incidence of chronic diseases and improving mental well-being. The *Surgeon General's Report on Mental Health,* published in 2000, acknowledged a role for physical activity in ensuring good mental hygiene. Healthy People 2020, the national health goals of the U.S. Department of Health and Human Services, include several objectives that collectively call for increasing physical activity in all segments of the U.S. population. Similar policy statements about the health importance of physical activity have been issued during the decade in Australia, Canada, and Europe.

Nonetheless, leisure-time physical activity levels have remained below recommendations in nations that keep population statistics about physical activity. In the United States, levels of leisure-time physical activity have not changed appreciably during the past decade. Despite widespread attempts to increase physical activity in the general population, 20 to 25% of U.S. adults aged 18 years or older do not participate in any leisure-time physical activity. Only about one-third say they are active enough to meet current federal recommendations for sufficient physical activity. Even fewer are sufficiently active when an objective measure is used to assess physical activity levels. Less than 15% of American youth participate in the recommended 60 minutes of aerobic physical activity each day.

This book is dedicated to understanding how leisure-time physical activity can enhance people's quality of life. It contains 16 chapters that are organized around key topics that relate to the mental health benefits of physical activity and how to promote them.

Part I contains three chapters that provide an introduction to the field of exercise psychology and its basic concepts. Chapter 1 includes a historical accounting of physical activity in the development of the field of psychology since antiquity; a description of the biological, cognitive, behavioral, and social foundations of modern-day exercise psychology; and brief overviews of the social significance of the promotion of physical activity for mental well-being. Chapter 2 defines the basic concepts and approaches used to measure psychological variables, physical activity, and physical fitness. Chapter 3 provides a rudimentary discussion of behavioral neuroscience. This chapter should be especially helpful to students who have not yet been exposed to the biological bases of psychology.

Part I provides important background information for a fuller understanding of the topics covered in part II, Exercise and Mental Health. We have expanded this part and organized it into two sections; the first covers topics related to stress and affect, including chapters on stress; affect, mood, and emotion; anxiety; and depression. The second section of part II focuses on topics related to exercise and quality of life, including cognition, energy and fatigue, sleep, pain, and self-esteem. Common themes addressed in each chapter are clinical features and treatment, public health burden, the descriptive and experimental evidence that physical activity has benefit, and plausible explanations for that benefit, including possible biological mechanisms.

Part III addresses the correlates of physical activity behavior, theories of behavior change, interventions that can be used to increase leisure-time physical activity, and perceived exertion.

This book is intended to be used as a textbook for upper-level undergraduates and master's degree students who are being introduced to exercise psychology for the first time. We hope that it also might be effective as a companion text in broader-based sport psychology courses that include exercise psychology topics.

A textbook's worth is judged by how well it serves teaching. A good introductory textbook should raise a lot of questions, and answer most of them. It should also instruct beginning students that knowledge is a growing, changing thing. We believe that the key ingredient to effective teaching is up-to-date, logically sequenced content illustrated by clear examples. Keeping this in mind, we have strived to avoid merely presenting annotated outlines of the hot, trendy topics found in research journals or reviews of research literatures rendered uninformative after being watered down for readability by nonresearchers.

We have selected classical and contemporary topics that we believe have a sufficiently large body of knowledge to justify inclusion in a textbook that we feel capable of presenting with a degree of authority. Since the first edition of this book, we have added chapters on exercise and cognition, energy and fatigue, and pain in response to the substantial advances in research in these areas. Undoubtedly, other topics covered in detail would be of interest to many people. Examples include the use of exercise as an adjuvant in the treatment of schizophrenia, bipolar disorder, chronic medical conditions, drug and alcohol abuse, and smoking addiction.

Also new to this edition is an image bank that includes all of the figures and tables from the text, sorted by chapter, that can be used in developing a customized presentation based on specific course requirements or used in creating other learning aids for students. The image bank is available at www.HumanKinetics.com/ExercisePsychology.

Our guiding motive has been to provide a text that has fidelity with the science but translates that science in ways that will engage, inform, and challenge serious students. We hope to dispel the academic myth that researchers don't write textbooks and can't teach.

Acknowledgments

We must accept the blame when the book falls short of its goals. When the book succeeds, credit should be shared with the many people who offered material for the book, ideas about what that material should be or how it would be best presented, and an environment that permitted the book to become a reality. Those people include our mentors, including past and present students, who imparted to us questions and tactics for attacking them; colleagues who motivate us to constantly raise the standard of excellence; and our families, who nurture us and sustain our pursuit of that excellence. Special thanks go to Tim Puetz, Nate Thom, Matt Herring, Cherie Rooks-Peck, Katey Wilson, Derek Monroe, Brett Clementz, Kevin McCully, and Phil Holmes for their contributions to new research included in this edition.

We also gratefully acknowledge the helpful advice given by peer reviewers, and the people of Human Kinetics: Myles Schrag, acquisitions editor; Melissa Zavala, developmental editor; Kali Cox, assistant editor; Dalene Reeder, permissions manager; as well as the copyeditor who valiantly aided our pursuit of mastering the English language.

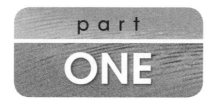

Introduction and Basic Concepts

The psychology of exercise encompasses the psychological and biological consequences of exercise and physical activity and the subsequent effects on mood and mental health. Exercise psychology also entails the study of exercise behavior and the promotion of regular exercise and active lifestyles. Both of these branches are addressed in this text, and have grown in importance since the first edition of *Exercise Psychology* was published. This is an exciting time to be a student of exercise psychology. New technologies are available to help in the study of the brain and neurophysiological responses and adaptations to exercise. We have a better understanding of the effects of the biological and psychosocial mechanisms of exercise on mood and cognitions. Innovative theories have been applied and developed to address exercise adoption and adherence, and there has been an explosion of technologies to aid in physical activity measurement and intervention strategies.

In part I, we place contemporary exercise psychology in perspective with a brief history highlighting notable personalities and studies that made critical linkages between exercise physiology and psychological variables. We discuss tools for a better understanding of exercise psychology research and of subsequent chapters—describing, for example, how psychological variables are measured and analyzed. Definitions and concepts that illustrate the scope and potential of exercise psychology are also presented, and the distinction between physical activity and exercise is discussed. This treatment of exercise psychology differs from others in its emphasis on the biological basis of behavior. A chapter on the physiological structures and functions that link exercise and mental health supports a clearer understanding of subsequent sections on physiological mechanisms, and highlights the importance of biological contributions to behavior and mood.

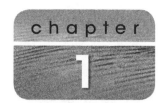

Foundations of Exercise Psychology

Exercise psychology has emerged as a field of study on the basis of a steadily building wave of research conducted during the past 30 years. The ideas underlying the field, however, have been around much longer. Throughout recorded history, philosophers and physicians have written about the connection between mental health and exercise. The relationship between exercise and psychological well-being was recognized as early as the fourth century BC. Herodicus, an early Greek physician who practiced gymnastic medicine (one of the branches of ancient Greek medicine that relied on exercise), based his therapies on vigorous exercise (Kollesch 1989; Phillips 1973). Hippocrates, considered the father of medicine, acknowledged the value of exercise for both physical and mental illness, although he was initially critical of Herodicus for relying on exercise as a treatment (Littre 1842).

Benefits of exercise were noted by early Jewish religious writers. Writings in the old testament of the Bible encouraged purposeful physical activity: "She girdeth her loins with strength, and strengtheneth her arms. She perceiveth that her gain is good. Strength and honour are her clothing; and she shall rejoice in time to come" (Prv. 31: 17-18, 25). "The desire of the slothful killeth him; for his hands refuse to labour" (Prv. 21: 25). "A slothful man is compared to a filthy stone, and every one will hiss him out to his disgrace" (Apocrypha 22: 1). Rabbi Moses ben Maimun (also known as Maimonides), the Jewish philosopher of the 12th century and physician to Saladin, the sultan of Egypt, provided a strong recommendation for physical activity when he wrote in the Mishneh Torah, "Anyone who lives a sedentary life and does not exercise . . . even if he eats good foods and takes care of himself according to proper medical principles—all his days will be painful ones and his strength will wane" (Rosner 1965, 1353). Maimonides also recognized the psychological benefits of physical activity. "The most beneficial of all types of exercise is physical gymnastics to the point that the soul rejoices" (Bar-Sela, Hoff, and Faris 1964, 20).

Robert Burton, British theologian and scholar, warned about the risks of a sedentary lifestyle in *The Anatomy of Melancholy:* "Opposite to Exercise is Idleness or want of exercise, the bane of body and minde, . . . one of the seven deadly sinnes, and a sole cause of Melancholy" (1632, 158). Those early ideas extended into the 20th century. For example, the effects of exercise on depression were reported in 1905 (Franz and Hamilton 1905); and during the 1930s, exercise was included in recreational therapy for psychiatric patients (Campbell and Davis 1939-1940). A psychobiological perspective on mechanisms to explain the effect of exercise was proposed in 1926, when it was suggested that exercise benefits people who are depressed by stimulating nerves and increasing glandular secretion (Vaux 1926).

Philosophers and physicians have acknowledged the connection between mental health and exercise throughout recorded history.

DUALISM VERSUS MONISM

Exercise psychology is defined in part by contemporary questions and approaches toward answering them that have roots in the centuries-old effort by philosophers and early psychologists to explain the nature of the link between mind and body. **Dualism** held that humans have physical bodies and nonphysical souls. Body and mind were viewed as separate, requiring different principles to explain their separate functions. The Greek philosopher Plato was a dualist, asserting a clear distinction between the material world and the soul.

The French philosopher, mathematician, and physiologist René Descartes (1596-1650), shown in figure 1.1, also thought that humans were composed of body and soul, but he held that the two components interacted. In *De homine* (i.e., *Treatise of Man*) (Steele 1972), the first full essay on physiological psychology, completed about 1633, Descartes tried to explain how the soul controlled the body. He believed that the body was a hydraulic machine controlled by a soul that got information from the senses, made

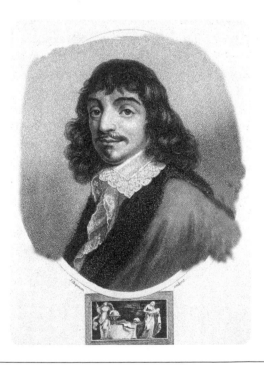

Figure 1.1 Philosopher René Descartes (17th century) conceptualized the human body as a hydraulic machine controlled by a soul.

Provided by the National Library of Medicine.

decisions, and directed the body by using the brain. To explain reflexive behavior, Descartes proposed that the material body was controlled by the flow of animal spirits from the brain to muscles through hollow tubes (the nerves). The nonmaterial soul controlled the body by governing the pineal gland in the brain, which in turn regulated the flow of animal spirits. Descartes' view did not address how a nonmaterial soul could control a material body, or whether the body could affect the soul.

Later, the German philosopher Gottfried von Leibniz (1646-1716) proposed that the body and soul were separate and parallel in function, not interactive. His views laid the philosophical foundation for the emergence of experimental psychology during the mid-to-late 19th century when physicians such as Gustav Fechner (1801-1887), Hermann von Helmholtz (1821-1894), Wilhelm Max Wundt (1832-1920), and William James (1842-1910) broke from the traditions of medicine and physiology to begin the field of experimental psychology. Fechner, shown in figure 1.2, established the basis for the field of psychophysics in 1850 when he reported that one could scientifically study the link between mind and body by comparing changes in the strength of a physical stimulus, such as light, with changes in the subjective experience of the stimulus, such as the sensation of brightness. Helmholtz, pictured in figure 1.3, pioneered the field of physiological psychology with his research on the perception of sound. He was also the first to measure the speed of nerve conduction. Wundt, once an assistant to Helmholtz, is generally considered the founder of scientific psychology as a discipline separate from medicine and physiology. James is acknowledged as the father of American psychology.

Developing about the same time as dualism was the monistic view that a single material principle is adequate to explain reality—that mind and body are the same. **Monism** assumes that the mind exists only by the function of the body and its interaction with the environment. Although Plato's student Aristotle was a dualist, his doctrine of natural dualism held that all matter has form and that the soul and the body constitute a single interdependent entity. The

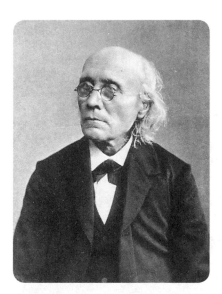

Figure 1.2 Gustav Fechner described research methods for studying the connection between mind and body, providing the foundation for the field of psychophysics in 1850.

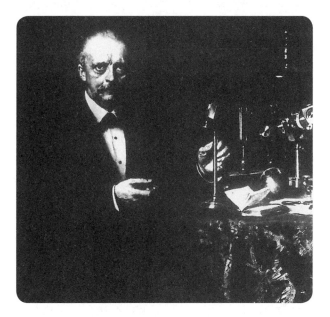

Figure 1.3 German physiologist Hermann von Helmholtz (19th century) pioneered the field of physiological psychology.

Provided by the National Library of Medicine.

English philosopher Thomas Hobbes (1588-1679), a contemporary of Descartes, extended that view and stated, "All that exists is matter; all that occurs is motion." According to Hobbes, the activity of the mind was motion within the nerves and thus would follow the same principles of motion that applied to other matter. Those ideas laid the foundation for regarding the mind and body as the same, to be distinguished from the metaphysical soul.

The father of American psychiatry, Benjamin Rush (1746-1813), a signer of the Declaration of Independence, was a monist. He distinguished between moral action (the mind) and moral opinion or conscience; he argued that physical causes, such as the size of the brain, heredity, disease, fever, climate, diet, drink, and medicines, among other factors, could affect the mind. In 1772, Rush delivered a "Sermon on Exercise" in which he recommended many types of sports and exercises, including dancing, for the young and old to improve the body's strength and health. It is not clear, though, whether Rush appreciated a role for exercise in mental health. Indeed, his "relaxation chair" (see figure 1.4) suggests a rather restrained view of physical activity.

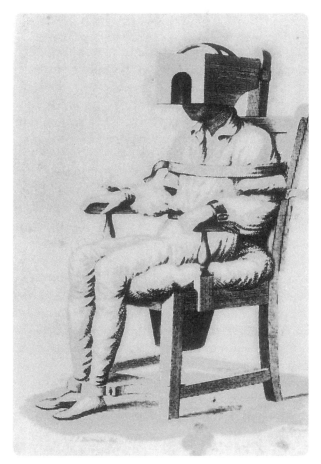

Figure 1.4 Benjamin Rush's relaxation chair.

Provided by the National Library of Medicine.

Early Emphasis on the Biological Basis of Emotions

The brain, and the brain alone, is the source of our pleasures, joys, laughter, and amusement, as well as our sorrow, pain, grief, and tears. It is especially the organ we use to . . . distinguish . . . the bad from the good, and the pleasant from the unpleasant. The brain is also the seat of madness and delirium, of the fears and terrors that assail by night or by day, of sleeplessness . . . of pointless anxieties. (Hippocrates in *Regimen*)

BIOLOGICAL FOUNDATIONS

The study of exercise has a base in physiology, but it may be surprising for beginning students of exercise psychology to discover that the field of psychology also had its origins in physiology. Wundt, the father of psychology, was trained in medicine and physiology before he established the first psychology laboratory at the University of Leipzig in 1879 (see figure 1.5). Before that, in 1875, William James was already conducting psychological experiments at Harvard. The **James-Lange theory** of emotion (co-named for a contemporary Danish physiologist) proposed that bodily responses during emotion are the source of the emotional response. Although unsupported by later research, this theory stemmed from a monistic view and stimulated an empirical debate about the biological basis of emotion that continues today, even in exercise psychology.

Wundt's contemporaries were Emil Kraepelin, Sigmund Freud, and Adolf Meyer, leading psychiatrists who supported the application of neuropathology to advance psychiatry, as research in organic pathology contributed to gains in general medicine (Whybrow, Akiskal, and McKinney 1984). In the early 20th century, mainstream psychiatry shifted away from a neu-

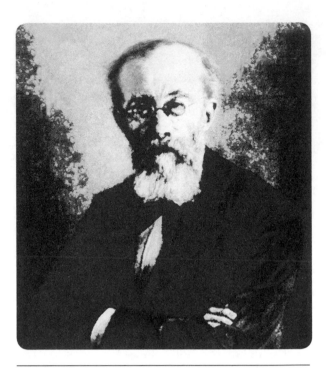

Figure 1.5 Wilhelm Max Wundt, known as the father of psychology.
Provided by the National Library of Medicine.

rophysiological orientation, although Kraepelin continued to pursue the empirical classification of mental diseases based on pathophysiology. Freud and Meyer shifted toward human experience and introspection to explain and treat psychopathology. However, Meyer later criticized Freud for ignoring the biology of mental disease and introduced the concept of psychobiology to the American Medical Association in 1915 (Winters 1951).

> Exercise psychology has roots in physiology through its foundation in exercise science and psychology.

COGNITIVE FOUNDATIONS

Wundt was the first scientist to be recognized as a psychologist, probably because he advocated the use of introspection as his primary method of inquiry in the study of perception and the elements of the mind. Among his 500 published works was *Principles of Physiological Psychology* (2 vols., 1873-1874). He also founded the first psychological journal, *Philosophische Studien (Studies in Philosophy)*, in 1881. Wundt's ideas were brought to America by an English scientist, E.B. Titchener (1867-1927), who came to Cornell University in 1892. However, it was William James (see figure 1.6) who welded the study of consciousness to experimental physiology by expanding the psychophysical methods of Helmholtz and Wundt to link the physiology of perception to symbolic meaning. In 1890, James published the landmark two-volume text *Principles of Psychology,* which advocated that psychology develop as a cognitive study of consciousness. In his doctrine of relations, James stated that a legitimate scientific psychology must account for both the stream of thought and feeling.

The writings of Charles Darwin (1809-1882), the English naturalist who formulated the principle of natural selection (see figure 1.7),

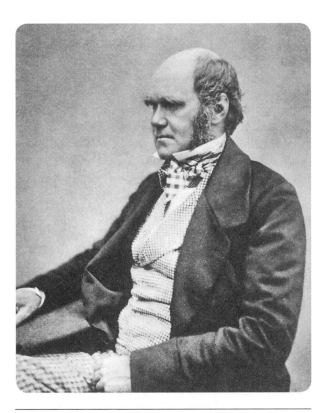

Figure 1.7 Charles Darwin, best known for having developed the principle of natural selection, also wrote about the biological basis of emotional expression.

John van Wyhe, ed. 2002. The Complete Work of Charles Darwin Online (http://darwin-online.org.uk).

facilitated the monistic view of mind and body unity in modern psychology in two ways. First, Darwin's writings emphasized that all of an organism's features have function; and second, his book *The Expression of the Emotions in Man and Animals,* published in 1872, provided a biological view of the basis of emotional expression. Darwin's ideas had a strong impact on the thinking of William James.

BEHAVIORAL AND SOCIAL FOUNDATIONS

William James later focused on the role of attitudes and values in health and disease, and between 1893 and 1896 he taught an advanced graduate seminar on psychopathology at Harvard that influenced the development of scientific psychotherapy. James saw a role for exercise in mental hygiene. In chapter 1, "The Gospel of Relaxation," of his *Talks to Teachers on*

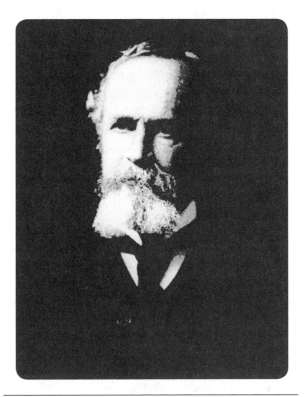

Figure 1.6 William James linked the physiology of perception to symbolic meaning.

Provided by the National Library of Medicine.

Psychology: and to Students on Some of Life's Ideals, he stated the following:

> I wish in the following hour to take certain psychological doctrines and show their practical applications to mental hygiene.... Consider, for example, the effects of a well-toned *motor-apparatus,* nervous and muscular, on our general personal self-consciousness, the sense of elasticity and efficiency that results. They tell us that in Norway the life of the women has lately been entirely revolutionized by the new order of muscular feelings with which the use of the ski, or long snow-shoes, as a sport for both sexes, has made the women acquainted. Fifteen years ago the Norwegian women were even more than the women of other lands votaries of the old-fashioned ideal of femininity, "the domestic angel," the "I gentle and refining influence" sort of thing. Now these sedentary fireside tabby-cats of Norway have been trained, they say, by the snow-shoes into lithe and audacious creatures, for whom no night is too dark or height too giddy, and who are not only saying good-bye to the traditional feminine pallor and delicacy of constitution, but actually taking the lead in every educational and social reform. I cannot but think that the tennis and tramping and skating habits and the bicycle-craze which are so rapidly extending among our dear sisters and daughters in this country are going also to lead to a sounder and heartier moral tone, which will send its tonic breath through all our American life. I hope that here in America more and more the ideal of the well-trained and vigorous body will be maintained neck by neck with that of the well-trained and vigorous mind as the two coequal halves of the higher education for men and women alike. (James 1899, 199-205)

An influential turn-of-the-century force for social psychological thought was Herbert Spencer, who in 1874 extended Darwin's notions from the biological realm into the social. (It was Spencer, not Darwin, who coined the phrase "survival of the fittest.") Social Darwinism influenced the thinking of many early American psychologists, including William James. It is generally agreed that the first experiment in social psychology was reported in 1897 by American psychologist Norman Triplett, who examined social influences on performance in competitive bicycle racing. Although *Introduction to Social Psychology* by British psychologist William McDougall was published in 1908, it wasn't until the 1924 publication of the text *Social Psychology* by Floyd Allport and the *Handbook of Social Psychology* by Carl Murchison in the 1930s that social psychology was distinguished as an experimental discipline separate from the more naturalistic observational techniques used in sociology. Since German-American psychologist Kurt Lewin popularized the idea in the 1930s that behavior is the product of the interaction between a person and the environment, the studies of attitude measurement and change, group dynamics, social learning and personality, social cognition, aggression, and self-perception have been mainstays of social psychology.

By the early to mid-20th century, psychoanalysis was the predominant treatment used in psychology and psychiatry, but other perspectives began to take hold. The conditioned reflex studies by the Russian physiologist Pavlov and by American psychologist John Watson and his colleagues, Robert Yerkes and Karl Lashley, followed by the operant conditioning research of Harvard behaviorist B.F. Skinner, laid a foundation for the emergence of "behavior therapy" in the late 1950s. The development of social learning theory (Bandura 1977, 1986) and cognitive behaviorism (Meichenbaum 1977) followed. Biological psychology became mainly limited to research using animals to model the links between brain and behavior, building on Lashley's pioneering work in neuropsychology. Behaviorism fell out of favor in many sectors of psychology, especially gestalt psychology, because it emphasized behavior and the stimulus–response link to the neglect of the study of consciousness and adaptations by the organism. With the fall of behaviorism, cognitive psychology, which was linked to advances in computer science, language, and biology, emerged as a dominant school of thought.

The 1960s were dominated by various approaches to psychotherapy that included dis-

Behaviorism, also known as learning theory or stimulus–response theory, developed empirical principles of behavior by observing the consequences of environmental manipulation. Later, cognitive behaviorism recognized that people's thoughts and feelings can mediate behavior.

tinct **models** and techniques. The integration of biological, psychological, and social factors in understanding health and disease was introduced by George L. Engel in his seminal work published in 1977. The modern view of multicausal factors in health and disease has been attributed to Engel's **biopsychosocial model of disease**. This perspective benefited mental health research during the 1990s, which was designated by the U.S. Congress as the Decade of the Brain. Such an integrated approach is also reflected in *Mental Health: A Report of the Surgeon General,* published in 2000 (U.S. Department of Health and Human Services), which acknowledged a role for physical activity as part of mental hygiene.

In the new millennium, the American Psychological Association—with endorsement from 50 societies representing the behavioral and social sciences—initiated the Decade of Behavior, an interdisciplinary effort to promote the importance of behavioral and social science research modeled after the 1990s' Decade of the Brain.

Biological psychology is the study of the brain and behavior using methods of natural science. Physiology, anatomy, genetics, endocrinology, immunology, pharmacology, and molecular biology are applied toward understanding behavior. Responses observed at molecular, synaptic, and neural systems levels of observation are related to integrated behavior (Davis et al. 1988).

Health is included as one of the five themes of the initiative.

We need to understand the physiological correlates of behavioral responses to exercise.

Today, theoretical advances around the world have led to a rudimentary understanding of how the brain controls thoughts, emotions, and behaviors within various social and environmental settings. Advances in statistical modeling of relationships among social factors and people's introspections have permitted us to form the ideas of the early psychologists into precise social psychology theories useful for understanding and promoting health. Similarly, technological advances in neuroscience, such as the use of microneurography, electrophysiology, microdialysis, nuclear brain imaging, and molecular biology, now permit closer examinations of the biological mechanisms of mind and behavior.

Social psychology is the study of interpersonal relationships and processes. It deals with the ways people affect and are affected by other people and by their social and physical environments.

The completion of the Human Genome Project in 2003 laid a further foundation for studying the heritability of exercise behavior and the effects of exercise on gene expression related to the neurophysiology of mental health. Thus, the goal of this text is to illustrate the biological foundations of exercise psychology in the study of psychological and behavioral responses to exercise, and to do so within the broader contexts of cognitive, social, and environmental influences.

Areas of modern psychology vary in their relative emphases on physiological, behavioral, cognitive, and social questions and methods. Hence, several subdisciplines exist. Notable

Subdiscipline or a Field of Study

The term *psychology* was apparently first used around 1530 by a German scholar, Phillip Melanchton. Its original meaning, taken from the Greek *psyche* (soul) and *logos* (study), was the "study of the soul." Later *psyche* was translated as "mind" rather than "soul." To William James, psychology was the "science of mental life." Psychology was the description and explanation of states of consciousness . . . such "feelings, desires, cognitions, reasonings, decisions . . . perceptions, emotions" (1890, 1).

During the past 100 years, **psychology** has evolved as a scientific discipline encompassing the study and application of principles of behavior and mental processes. A **discipline** is defined by unique questions and methods. Hence, although psychology addresses physiological and social aspects of behavior, its central focus on introspection and the individual distinguishes it from the disciplines of physiology and sociology.

Health psychology concerns the scientific understanding of how behavioral principles relate to physical health and illness.

among these are biological psychology, behavioral neuroscience and comparative psychology, behaviorism, and social psychology. Because exercise psychology uses the traditions of each of these subdisciplines to study physical activity, it may be more properly regarded as an interdisciplinary field of study rather than a subdiscipline of psychology. This view of exercise psychology is also consistent with its roots in exercise science, which itself is an interdisciplinary field that applies the methods and traditions of other disciplines, including physiology, medicine, and psychology. Moreover, exercise psychology

Behavioral neuroscience and comparative psychology entail the subdisciplines of perception and learning, neuroscience, cognitive psychology, and comparative psychology.

is concerned with mental health and health behaviors within clinical settings and population bases. Thus it has commonly used approaches from clinical psychology and psychiatry, health promotion, and epidemiology.

CONTEMPORARY EXERCISE PSYCHOLOGY

Contemporary exercise psychology emerged as a viable field of study over 50 years ago with the publication of the first modern reviews on exercise and mental health topics by Emma McCloy Layman, who was chief psychologist in the department of psychiatry at Children's Hospital in Washington, D.C. (e.g., Layman 1960). The past 30 years have witnessed tremendous growth in the number of scientists studying the various areas of exercise psychology. There has been a corresponding increase in the volume of research to warrant the creation of new journals (e.g., *Psychology of Sport and Exercise* in 2000, *Mental Health and Physical Activity* in 2008, and *Sport, Exercise, and Performance Psychology* in 2012). Scholars in exercise psychology have roots in psychology, physical education, and sports medicine, but many are second- and even third-generation descendants of the 1960s-era sport psychologists.

A notable "parent" of exercise psychology is William P. Morgan of the University of Wisconsin (see figure 1.8), who expanded the application of psychology to physical performance beyond the study of athletes. The foundation for exercise psychology in the 21st century was laid by Dr. Morgan with seminal studies and writings from 1969 to 1979 on depression (Morgan 1969, 1970; Morgan et al. 1970), anxiety (Morgan, Roberts, and Feinerman 1971), hypnosis and perceived exertion (Morgan et al. 1976), exercise adherence (Morgan 1977), and exercise addiction (Morgan 1979b). In addition to establishing psychology as a viable topic in exercise science and physical education, Dr. Morgan promoted exercise psychology within mainstream psychology in the United States. In 1986, he founded and served as the first president of Division 47, Exercise and Sport Psychology, of the American Psychological Association, nearly 100 years after the founding of the association by G. Stanley Hall in 1892.

Certainly, other key people have been invaluable in the development of the field of exercise psychology. Their contributions are evident throughout this text. Among the early contributors were A.H. Ismail of Purdue University; Herb deVries of the University of Southern California; Robert J. Sonstroem of the University of Rhode Island; Dorothy Harris of Pennsylvania State University; and Daniel M. Landers of Arizona State University, the inaugural editor of the *Journal of Sport and Exercise Psychology*. Especially noteworthy are the seminal contributions of Swedish psychophysicist Gunnar Borg, who pioneered the study of perceived exertion.

The embryonic development of exercise psychology was captured within the inaugural newsletter of Division 47, Exercise and Sport Psychology, of the American Psychological Association. In describing the goals and purposes of the division, founding president William P. Morgan wrote the following:

> Division 47 represents an exciting and quickly developing specialization that cuts across psychology and the sport sciences. Through the Division, scientists and practitioners with a common interest have the opportunity to interact and to further their personal and professional capabilities. . . . The focus of professionals and students in this field of specialization is quite diverse, and scientific inquiry, as well as clinical applications, has historically cut across the interest of many existing divisions. Individuals working in this area come from subspecialties within psychology such as developmental, educational, clinical, counseling, industrial, comparative, physiological, social, personality, hypnosis, motivation, human factors, ergonomics, and health psychology. Although professionals and students in this area represent numerous specialties within psychology, they are bonded together by a common interest in sport and exercise. . . . The term sport can be used as a noun, a verb, or an adjective. For this division, it is used as a noun. This decision follows the European lead where sport can be viewed as competitive athletics; a source of diversion; recreation; or physical activity engaged in for play. In other words, sport involves much more than competitive athletics, and this is the reason why the terms exercise and sport are both included in the Division's title. The terms exercise and sport are intended to broaden the Division's scope. (Morgan 1986, 1–2)

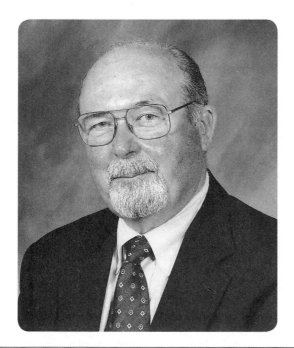

Figure 1.8 Dr. William P. Morgan.

Provided by University of Wisconsin Medical Photography, University of Wisconsin–Madison.

OVERVIEW OF PHYSICAL ACTIVITY AND MENTAL HEALTH

Physical activity can have potent effects on mental health as a function of the exposure (i.e., acute vs. chronic exercise) and the presence and degree of clinical symptoms (i.e., normal psychological health vs. biologically based mood disorders). However, contemporary views of the relationship between physical activity and mental health have been mixed, although support for exercise in the prevention and treatment of mood disorders is growing.

In 1984, a report from a National Institute of Mental Health panel indicated that there were positive effects from acute and chronic exercise on anxiety and depression (Morgan and Goldston 1987). Even so, 5 years later, the U.S. Preventive Services Task Force of the U.S. Office of Disease Prevention and Health Promotion concluded that the quality of the available evidence linking exercise with anxiety and depression was poor and that the role of exercise in the primary prevention of mental health problems was poorly understood (Harris et al. 1989).

The 1994 *Physical Activity, Fitness, and Health* international consensus text edited by Bouchard, Shephard, and Stephens gave more support to the link between mental health and physical activity. However, the controversy over the strength of the scientific basis for the role of exercise in mental health continued with the omission of any reference to physical activity or exercise in *Practice Guidelines for the Treatment of Patients with Major Depressive Disorders (Revision)* (American Psychiatric Association 2000). Many physicians recommend exercise for their depressed and anxious patients, and the third edition of the *Practice Guidelines* published in 2010 supports exercise as a reasonable addition to treatment for major depressive disorder, and as a primary initial treatment for mild depression by patient request (Gelenberg et al. 2010).

In the World Health Organization's *Global Recommendations for Physical Activity* (2011), reduced risk of depression is a stated benefit of regular exercise. Further, the World Health Organization acknowledges reduced symptoms of anxiety and depression in children and adolescents and reduced symptoms of depression in adults and older adults as a result of regular adequate exercise. Improved cognitive function from exercise is also stated as a benefit for older adults.

The U.S. *Surgeon General's Report on Physical Activity and Health* (1996) provided a consensus on the benefits of physical activity for chronic diseases, such as coronary heart disease and diabetes, but also included statements about the effects of physical activity on mental health. Widely distributed research findings from the fields of exercise science, exercise psychology, clinical and counseling psychology, and medicine were reviewed to support the conclusions that regular physical activity reduces feelings of depression and anxiety and promotes psychological well-being. In addition to evidence for the prevention and reduction of mild and moderate depression, several longitudinal studies have indicated that a sedentary lifestyle is also a risk factor for depression. It is not clear whether exercise has an effect on people who are already in good mental health, but there are general reports of improved sense of well-being. Chronic exercise has been found to improve self-concept and self-esteem, with better improvements in self-esteem for those whose self-esteem is initially low and who value fitness.

Acute and Chronic Exercise: Definitions

Acute exercise is a single, relatively short-lived bout of exercise, such as jogging three miles.

Chronic exercise is exercise carried out repeatedly over time, usually thought of as "regular exercise" or "exercise training" and defined by the type of activity, intensity, duration, frequency per week, and period of time over which activity occurs (i.e., weeks, months).

The scientific advisory committee of the *2008 Physical Activity Guidelines for Americans* concluded that there was strong evidence that physically active adults have lower risk of depression, cognitive impairment, and feelings of distress or poor well-being.

The position of the U.S. surgeon general's report and the most recent practice guidelines from the American Psychiatric Association support the use of physical activity as an adjunct treatment for mental health problems. Psychotherapy is expensive and time-consuming and can carry a social stigma in some cultures. Drug treatments are also expensive and can have undesirable aftereffects and side effects, such as weight gain. Physical activity as an alternative form of prevention and treatment does not have the complications associated with psychotherapy or drug treatment, and also offers a decreased risk of physical health concerns.

There are clear health benefits from regular physical activity, and in 2008, the U.S. Department of Health and Human Services published new guidelines for physical activity for children and adolescents, adults, and older adults. For substantial health benefits, adults should exercise for 30 minutes at a moderate intensity 5 days a week, or 20 minutes at a high intensity 3 days a week, or some combination of moderate- and high-intensity exercise, and include at least 2 days a week of strength training involving major muscle groups (Haskell et al. 2007). These recommendations were adopted in 2010 by the World Health Organization in its *Global Recommendations on Physical Activity and Health*. In 2009, half of American adults did not meet these recommendations, and only 18% of adolescents met their corresponding guidelines to be physically active at least 60 minutes each day.

The recently released *Healthy People 2020* (U.S. Department of Health and Human Services 2010) set goals for physical activity that are 10% above the current best estimates of activity rates. These goals are more modest than goals set for 2010 but more realistic considering that most of the 2010 goals for physical activity and fitness were not met. For example, the 2010 goal for the proportion of adults who engage in no leisure-time physical activity was half (20%) of the 1997 baseline estimate of 40%. In 2008, 36.2% of adults engaged in no leisure-time activity, and the goal for 2020 has been set at a 10% decrease (32.6%).

The need to promote exercise and physical activity is not limited to the United States. Exercise is also being promoted globally through the efforts of the World Health Organization and Exercise is Medicine (EIM), a joint program started in 2007 by the American College of Sports Medicine and the American Medical Association. In 2010, the first World Congress on Exercise is Medicine launched a global initiative to make physical activity and exercise a standard part of disease prevention and medical treatment. This is especially important because according to the World Health Organization, 60% of the world's population is not active enough to reduce health risks.

Promoting physical activity is especially important given the role activity plays in weight management and the obesity epidemic in the United States. The United States has the highest mean body mass index (BMI) of high-income countries. Over the past 10 years, rates of obesity have increased by 5% in American adults, doubled for children age 6 through 11, and tripled for adolescents. Although there is some evidence that overweight and obesity are stabilizing (Yanovski and Yanovski 2011), the rates of morbid obesity are increasing in the United States, especially for women (Flegal et al. 2010). Globally, the overall mean BMI has increased since 1980, and rates of obesity have doubled (Finucane et al. 2011).

We have a fairly good idea of exercise dosage for the prevention and treatment of obesity and chronic diseases such as diabetes and heart disease, and more researchers are attempting to quantify the exercise stimulus necessary for finding statistically or clinically significant changes in symptoms of depression. For example, there is some support for the contention that weekly energy expenditure equal to the public health recommendation can reduce depressive symptoms in people with mild to moderate major depressive disorder (e.g., Dunn et al. 2005). However, the relationship between exercise dosage and mental health likely varies based on the diagnosis, characteristics of the person, and application of exercise for promotion, prevention, or treatment.

> **M**ost people do not exercise enough to reap the benefits.

OVERVIEW OF PHYSICAL ACTIVITY BEHAVIOR

The established link between physical and mental health and the level of physical activity has important implications for public health. The realization of this impact, however, hinges on adopting and maintaining regular physical activity. Most Americans do not exercise enough to reap the benefits from exercise, and about one-third are sedentary, a proportion that is similar to those in other industrialized countries. Once people have begun an exercise program, the odds are against their maintaining an active lifestyle. Typically, about 50% of people who begin an exercise program drop out within the first 6 months. Although numerous studies have been conducted to discover interventions that will enhance exercise adherence, this average dropout rate has persisted over the past 30 years. Thus, exercise psychology also encompasses the study of physical activity behavior. Like the psychological benefits of exercise, the problem of motivating people to be physically active is not new.

Near the turn of the 20th century, Robert J. Roberts, director of physical education at the YMCA in Springfield, Massachusetts, from 1887 to 1889, said, "I noticed that when I taught . . . more advanced work in acrobatics, gymnastics, athletics, etc., that I would have a very large membership at the first of the year, but that they would soon drop out . ." (Leonard and McKenzie 1927 p. 315).

In "The Gospel of Relaxation," William James recognized physical inactivity as a challenge to mental hygiene:

> I recollect, years ago, reading a certain work by an American doctor on hygiene and the laws of life and the type of future humanity . . . I remember well an awful prophecy that it contained about the future of our muscular system. Human perfection, the writer said, means ability to cope with the environment; but the environment will more and more require mental power from us, and less and less will ask for bare brute strength. Wars will cease, machines will do all our heavy work, man will become more and more a mere director of nature's energies, and less and less an exerter of energy on his own account. So that, if the *homo sapiens* of the future can only digest his food and think, what need will he have of well-developed muscles at all? . . . I cannot believe that our muscular vigor will ever be a superfluity. Even if the day ever dawns in which it will not be needed for fighting the old heavy battles against Nature, it will still always be needed to furnish the background of sanity, serenity, and cheerfulness to life, to give moral elasticity to our disposition, to round off the wiry edge of our fretfulness, and make us good-humored and easy of approach. (James 1899, 205–207)

The ability to change exercise behavior depends on the identification of factors that mediate or influence the level of activity, assuming that changing characteristics associated with physical activity will cause corresponding changes in behavior. A knowledge of the factors associated with physical *inactivity* can also help to identify high-risk segments of the population and to guide the allocation of resources earmarked to increase **exercise adoption** and adherence. Expanding our knowledge of the characteristics that influence physical activity in specific populations can support the development of personalized interventions and enable more directed marketing of physical activity. Thus, research in exercise behavior must include the identification of exercise determinants as

Benefits of Physical Activity as a Treatment for Mental Health Problems

- Self-administration
- Convenience
- Low cost
- Minimal side effects
- Social acceptability

- Ancillary physical benefits: increased aerobic endurance, altered body composition, increased muscle tone
- Decreased risk of physical health concerns: coronary heart disease, colon cancer, type 2 diabetes mellitus, hypertension, and osteoporosis

well as the development of interventions to foster adoption and **exercise maintenance**.

SUMMARY

Exercise psychology is an interdisciplinary field of study that has a solid foundation in the psychological and biological sciences. Two broad areas of study comprise the psychological effects of acute and chronic exercise and the behavioral dynamics of exercise adoption and maintenance. Physical activity has been shown to affect both physical and mental health, and the mechanisms for psychological effects likely result from an interaction of social, psychological, and biological variables. The examination of exercise behavior and insight into how people adopt and maintain regular physical activity in their leisure time have been grounded in psychological theories of behavior change. The potential impact of exercise interventions on public health is great, considering the low level of activity in most segments of the population and the established links between physical activity and health. While acknowledging the importance of social and environmental context on psychological antecedents and consequences of physical activity, the chapters to follow focus on the inclusion of perspectives from biological psychology on this uniquely biological behavior commonly known as exercise.

WEBSITES

http://serendip.brynmawr.edu/Mind

www.health.gov/paguidelines/guidelines/chapter2.aspx

www.health.gov/paguidelines/committeereport.aspx

Basic Concepts in Exercise Psychology

One of the easiest ways to inject confusion into a conversation is to use terms that mean different things to each person. The terms *exercise* and *physical activity* are often used interchangeably, but their differences have important implications for understanding exercise psychology. Similarly, the term *stress* is one that most people understand, if vaguely, but it often defies a specific definition. Even among psychologists and psychiatrists, there is confusion about terms such as *mood, affect,* and *emotion.* We consider those concepts in detail in later chapters. This chapter clarifies some of the common terms and concepts most relevant to exercise psychology. We pay special attention to the measurement of psychological variables, physical activity, exercise, and fitness. The main goal of the chapter is to create a foundation for a deeper understanding of the material in subsequent chapters. Defining and clarifying terms will also illustrate some of the challenges of conducting high-quality research on the psychology of exercise. To that end, this chapter introduces general issues about research designs, methodology, and analytical approaches as a foundation for understanding the research discussed in the chapters that follow.

GENERAL CONCEPTS

Exercise psychology is the study of the brain and behavior in physical activity and exercise settings. Its main focus has been the psychobiological, behavioral, social, and cognitive antecedents and consequences of acute and chronic exercise (see figure 2.1). It encompasses analyses of changes in affect, emotions, and moods such as anxiety and depression after a single bout of exercise as well as assessments of the long-term psychological consequences of regular exercise. Exercise psychology also entails the study of physical activity behavior, including the psychological, biological, and environmental variables that determine the quality, quantity, and temporal patterns of physical activity.

> **E**xercise psychology includes the study of the psychobiological, behavioral, social, and cognitive antecedents and consequences of acute and chronic exercise.

There is extensive empirical evidence that changes in the brain, including the expression of genes, produce changes in behavior and that changes in behavior in turn produce changes in the brain. Thus, an understanding of exercise psychology would be incomplete without an examination of neurobiological systems along with self-reports of subjective experiences and objective descriptions of observable acts. Physical activity, and especially exercise, are biologically based behaviors and thus are well suited for study using a psychobiological model. Psychobiology encompasses the strengths of cognitive and behavioral psychology and a perspective grounded in neuroscience to provide a model for the biological bases of cognition, mood, and behavior.

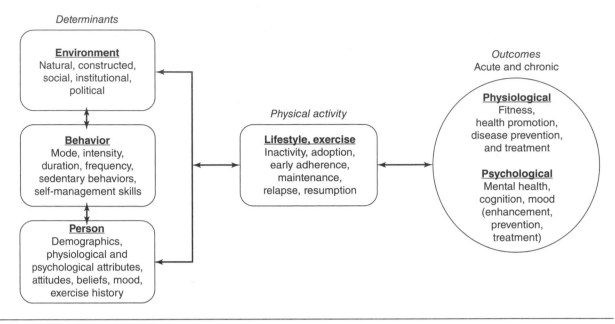

Figure 2.1 The reciprocal relationships among determinants, physical activity, and outcomes.

Changes in the brain produce changes in behavior, and changes in behavior in turn produce changes in the brain.

Nonetheless, a cornerstone of exercise psychology, as with psychology in general, is subjective human experience. So, this chapter begins with a discussion of the definition and measurement of subjective psychological variables, followed by a similar discussion of the measurement of physical activity and fitness. The next chapter addresses such issues in the context of behavioral neuroscience.

PSYCHOLOGICAL CONSTRUCTS

Since its founding by Wundt, Fechner, James, and their contemporaries, psychology has been distinguished from physiology by the measurement of consciousness—for example, of thoughts, judgments, and feelings. Social psychology includes the measurement of judgments people make about themselves and other people. Psychophysics involves measuring judgments people make about their physical environments. Although modern-day psychophysicists have become more interested in comparing people's judgments, the classical approach taken in psychophysics was, and mainly still is, to scale things, not people. This means that the scale of measurement is applied to the thing being judged, not to the person making the judgment; for example, one would measure how foods differ in bitterness and sweetness, not whether people differ in their taste. According to classical psychophysics, differences among people's judgments were error, simply random fluctuations in sensation. Around the 1920s, psychologists L.L. Thurstone of the University of Chicago and Edward L. Thorndike of Columbia University expanded the use of psychophysical methods to measure social judgments—for example, attitudes—and mental aptitude. They began scaling people. Differences among people were viewed not as error in measurement but as real. Concepts such as attitude, personality, and mood were used to describe those differences.

In contrast to psychophysics, which measured consciousness by comparing people's judgments of the characteristic of an object that could also be measured directly (e.g., perceived heaviness versus weight), this new approach, **psychometrics**, was based on the assumption that unobservable (i.e., latent) psychological variables could be measured indirectly by inference. That inference, though, must be constructed by a logical pattern of associations of **phenomenology** (i.e., people's expression of their experiences) with behaviors, physiological responses, and the social and environmental contexts in which they occur. For example, a scale or test used to measure depressed mood should include a representative sample of the adjectives from a language that people commonly use to connote varying degrees of hopelessness and despair. Psychometrics is based on a process called **construct** validation, whereby such patterns are established through the comparison of various constructs, or "traits," using multiple methods of measuring each one (Campbell and Fiske 1959; Cronbach and Meehl 1955; Messick 1989).

Construct Validity

The key steps to measuring a psychological construct involve demonstrating six principal types of validity: content, factorial, concurrent, criterion, logical, and convergent/discriminant.

- Content: The items that make up the test should be representative of the entire known universe of possible items. This ensures that some features of the construct are not omitted and that items better related to other constructs are not included. Researchers usually ensure the completeness of content by canvassing experts on the construct and by using focus groups consisting of the types of people who will be taking the test. Content validity is sometimes confused with **face validity**, which implies that a test is valid because it appears valid on its face to most people. The appearance of validity is an important part of the acceptance of a test by professionals and the public, but it is a weak scientific standard. Nonetheless, for test items to have clear meaning, they must match the experiences of the people who will be taking the test.

- Factorial: Items that correlate more closely with each other than with other items are identified by a statistical technique known as **factor analysis**, which can be

used to determine whether the structure of a test seems consistent with the construct it purports to measure. Exploratory factor analysis (EFA) is strictly empirical; it describes the patterns of correlated responses to items on a test. Confirmatory factor analysis (CFA) ascertains how well the observed pattern of correlated responses fits a predetermined pattern that is based on a theory about what and how many factors are needed to describe the construct. Techniques used to demonstrate factorial validity are discussed later in this chapter because they are a staple of measurement in exercise psychology.

- Concurrent: The test scores should be strongly related to other available measures that estimate the construct. For example, the rankings of people who complete two tests purportedly measuring anxiety should agree.

- Criterion: A person judged to exhibit the key features of a construct according to standardized, expert agreement should score high on a test presumed to measure that construct. For example, someone diagnosed as having a depressive disorder should score higher on a depression scale than a person without a depressive disorder.

- Logical: Scores on the test of the construct should change in response to events believed to be causes of change in the construct. For example, a measure of anger should yield higher scores for most people when they are forced to endure frustration, pain, or insults. Likewise, scores on the anger test should be unchanged by situations known to be joyous.

- Convergent/discriminant: Scores on the measure of the construct should be strongly related to behaviors, contexts, and biological responses theorized to be unique components or elicitors of the construct. For example, convergent evidence for the validity of a test of anger would be shown by correspondence with aggressive behavior, menacing facial expression, and increased blood pressure, especially if they occurred in a combative social confrontation. In contrast, scores on a test of anger would not be expected to correlate highly with scores on valid tests of other emotions or with behaviors and biological responses unique to those emotions. Indicators that scores on the test are specific to the construct being measured provide discriminant evidence for construct validity.

Scaling

The Harvard psychophysicist S.S. Stevens defined **scaling** as the assignment of objects to numbers according to a rule. In most psychometric scaling, the objects are text statements, usually statements of attitude, belief, mood, or emotion. A response scale is the method used to obtain responses from people on an instrument. Common approaches include dichotomous scales such as *agree/disagree, true/false,* or *yes/ no* or ordinal or interval scales ranging, for example, from 1 to 4 or from 1 to 7. However, merely assigning objects or statements to a response scale isn't scaling. Scaling is the development of the measurement instrument. Separately, a response scale is the way responses to each part of the instrument are obtained from respondents.

A controversy that surrounded the emergence of psychometric from classical psychophysical measurement concerned the question of whether subjective judgments can be measured as categories, ranks, intervals, or ratios. This issue is discussed in more detail in chapter 16 as it applies to perceived exertion. For now, it is sufficient to consider whether an unobservable, latent construct based on people's self-ratings can be assumed to exist along some continuum, or whether it is possible only to place people's judgments into categories that are qualitatively different but not quantifiable.

Quantification requires that subjective judgments can at least be ranked according to frequency, size, strength, and so on. If such rankings are equally distant, they can be measured as intervals. If each interval represents the same proportion of the full range of the measurement scale, the scale measures ratios. If it is possible

only to categorize judgments, one could determine that four people held different opinions, but not which person had the strongest or which had the weakest. At least, quantification would permit the people to be ranked 1, 2, 3, and 4 according to the strength of their opinions. However, ranking would not tell us whether person 4 differed from person 3 as much as person 2 differed from person 1. Interval measurement establishes equal differences, but it does not ensure equal proportions unless the scale has a true zero starting point. The feasibility of a true ratio scale that measures attitudes hinges on the plausibility of someone actually having no opinion (true zero starting point) when he or she says so.

Thorndike, the father of educational measurement, made the following observation in 1904:

> If one attempts to measure even so simple a thing as spelling, one is hampered by the fact that there exist no units in which to measure. One may arbitrarily make up a list of words and observe ability by the number spelled correctly. But if one examines such a list one is struck by the inequality of the units. All results based on the equality of any one word with any other are necessarily inaccurate. (Thorndike 1904, 7)

Thurstone Scaling

This conundrum of "inequality of the units" was solved, for most practical purposes, by an electrical engineer and psychologist at the University of Chicago named Louis L. Thurstone. He rejected the stimulus-oriented psychology favored by psychophysics and behaviorism and argued for an approach centered on the person. He believed that the focus of psychology should turn from people's judgments of the features of stimuli to the "satisfaction" that people strive for.

Between 1925 and 1932, Thurstone published 24 articles and a book about solutions to the inequality-of-units problem. He showed that scales for measuring subjective variables, such as attitudes, could be constructed from patterns of variations in people's scores according to the normal distribution (Thurstone 1927)—the very thing that psychophysicists had viewed as error! He devised several methods for developing a unidimensional scale, but the method of equal-appearing intervals was the most practical and influential. Based on people's ratings of separate attitude statements, the approach was to order those items according to their scale values, from highest agreement to highest disagreement, and then select items for the final scale that had equal intervals between their response scale values. These were Thurstone's requirements for useful measures:

- **Unidimensionality**—The measurement of any object or entity describes only one attribute of the object measured. This is a universal characteristic of all measurement (Thurstone 1931, 257).

- **Linearity**—The very idea of measurement implies a linear continuum of some sort, such as length, price, volume, weight, or age. When the idea of measurement is applied to scholastic achievement, for example, it is necessary to force the qualitative variations into a scholastic linear scale of some kind (Thurstone and Chave 1929, 11).

- **Abstraction**—The linear continuum that is implied in all measurement is always an abstraction. "There is a popular fallacy that a unit of measurement is a thing— such as a piece of yardstick. This is not so" (Thurstone 1931, 257).

- **Invariance**—"A unit of measurement is always a process of some kind which can be repeated without modification in the different parts of the measurement continuum" (Thurstone 1931, 257).

- **Sample-free calibration**—The scale must generalize beyond the group measured. "A measuring instrument must not be seriously affected in its measuring function by the object of measurement. . . . Within the range of objects . . . intended, its function must be independent of the object of measurement" (Thurstone 1928, 547).

- **Test-free measurement**—It should be possible to omit several test questions at different levels of the scale without affecting the individual score (measure). "It should not be required to submit every subject to the whole range of the scale. The starting point and the terminal point . . . should not directly affect the individual score (measure)" (Thurstone 1926, 446).

Likert, or Summated, Scaling

Likert scaling was developed in the early 1930s by Rensis Likert (pronounced "lickert"), an industrial and organizational psychologist at the University of Michigan. Like Thurstone scaling, Likert scaling is a unidimensional scaling method. Each respondent is asked to rate each item on a response scale. For instance, respondents could rate each item on a 1-to-5 response scale like this:

1 = *Strongly disagree*

2 = *Disagree*

3 = *Undecided*

4 = *Agree*

5 = *Strongly agree*

Likert's research examined how many ordinal categories are needed to estimate or predict a single underlying variable believed to be continuous and normally distributed. Just adding a response scale like the one shown to a set of items is not Likert scaling. Items must be selected that will yield a normally distributed response (i.e., a mean of zero with a standard deviation of 1 when the raw scores for each item are converted to a standard normal score).

Likert did not consider the number of choices an important issue (Likert 1932); rather, if five alternatives are used, it is necessary to assign values from 1 to 5 with the 3 assigned to the undecided option. There are several other possible response scales (1 to 7; 1 to 9; 0 to 4). All have a middle value that is usually labeled *neutral* or *undecided*. This helps to approximate a normal distribution of responses. Some response scales use a forced-choice (ipsative) format with an even number of responses and no middle *neutral*, or *undecided*, choice. That forces the respondent to choose between the agree end and the disagree end of the scale for each item, and can control response bias. The final score for the respondent on the scale is the sum of his or her ratings for all of the items: a summated scale.

There is no consensus about how many rating categories are best for the scaling of psychological constructs. If there are too few, a test item won't have enough sensitivity to discriminate subtle differences in the true levels of the variable being measured. If there are too many, responding can become overly complex and burdensome. The optimal number would be the number that has good sensitivity, is practical, and approximates a normal distribution of responses. One view has been that rating scales are best when they have about five to nine categories. That view was popularized by Harvard psychologist George Miller in the 1950s (Miller 1956). Miller observed that people's abilities to accurately judge physical stimuli and remember information without errors seemed to be constrained to about seven categories, plus or minus about two. He used binary decisions to illustrate. One bit of information is the amount of information needed to make a decision between two equally likely alternatives. Two bits are needed to decide among four equally likely alternatives. Three bits permit a choice among eight equally likely alternatives. Four bits of information decide among 16 alternatives, and so on. Hence, another bit of information is added each time the number of alternative choices is increased by a factor of two.

Miller reported that people's accuracy at judging tones, taste, colors, and points on a line typically ranged from about 2 to 3 bits, or four to eight categories. He next observed that people's short-term memory capacity averaged about 23 bits. For example, most people can recall about seven decimal digits, approximating 3.3 bits each for a total of 23 bits. On this basis, Miller proposed a theory about how the span of immediate memory should vary as a function of the amount of information per item on a test. That was Miller's number: 7 ± 2. Most of us recognize the increasing challenge of remembering a new telephone number when it includes the area code (10 digits), or a zip code when the plus-four digits are added at the end (9 digits). Today, most psychometric tests offer four to seven response categories, at least in part because of the influence of Miller's ideas.

Guttman, or Cumulative, Scaling

In 1950, sociologist Louis Guttman argued that the meaning of any score from Thurstone or Likert scales was ambiguous unless it was fol-

---

Miller's Number 7 ± 2

"And finally, what about the magical number seven? What about the seven wonders of the world, the seven seas, the seven deadly sins, the seven daughters of Atlas in the Pleiades, the seven ages of man, the seven levels of hell, the seven primary colors, the seven notes of the musical scale, and the seven days of the week? What about the seven-point rating scale, the seven categories for absolute judgment, the seven objects in the span of attention, and the seven digits in the span of immediate memory? Perhaps there is something deep and profound behind all these sevens, something just calling out for us to discover it. But I suspect that it is only a pernicious, Pythagorean coincidence" (Miller 1956, 95).

---

lowed by a hierarchical pattern of endorsement among its items:

> If a person endorses a more extreme statement, he should endorse all less extreme statements if the statements are to be considered a scale. . . . We shall call a set of items of common content a scale if a person with a higher rank than another person is just as high or higher on every item than the other person. (Guttman 1950, 62)

Guttman scaling is also known as cumulative scaling. The purpose is to establish a one-dimensional continuum for the underlying construct to be measured. This means that a person who agrees with any question on the test should also agree with all the questions that preceded it. Said another way, on a 10-item cumulative scale, a score of 5 would indicate that the respondent agreed with the first five items. A score of 7 would indicate agreement on the first seven questions, and so on. The object is to find a set of items that perfectly matches this pattern. That doesn't happen often, but the degree to which it does is an example of the internal consistency of a scale or test, a form of **reliability**.

Reliability

As is the case for all measures, tests of psychological constructs must be reliable; they must be precise, accurate, and stable across the time period that defines their nature. A valid test must first be reliable, although a reliable test is not necessarily valid. Precision means that a test, or its subscales, is internally consistent; the average correlation among the items is high relative to the variation in people's responses to each item. Accuracy means that the test does not overestimate or underestimate the true value of the construct. Stability means that scores on the test do not fluctuate widely without an explainable cause. Reliability of psychological constructs is usually computed using a statistic called intraclass correlation (RI). A common index of RI used to estimate internal consistency is the coefficient α, which is computed as

$$\alpha = \frac{k\bar{r}}{1 + (k-1)\bar{r}}$$

where k is the number of items on the test and $\bar{r}$ is the mean correlation between items. Hence, including more items and including correlated items each increases reliability.

MULTIDIMENSIONAL SCALES

The scales that we have considered up to now are designed to measure a single dimension, such as the length of a line. That's usually sufficient for many constructs, but what about a concept such as self-esteem? Chapter 12 presents overall self-esteem as a concept that is unidimensional but that comprises several dimensions in a hierarchical structure. In chapter 5 we consider various types of moods and emotions. Psychologists who study emotions mostly agree that six basic emotions are experienced in virtually all cultures (love, joy, surprise, anger, sadness, and fear). Moreover, each type of emotional response can be described by an affective dimension (e.g., pleasant versus unpleasant) and an arousal dimension (e.g., low versus high). Separate scales are required to measure these dimensions.

Semantic Differential

In the late 1950s, social psychologist Charles E. Osgood and his colleagues, G. Suci and Percy Tannenbaum, developed a method to graph the differences among individuals' connotations for words and thus measure the "psychological distance" between words (Osgood, Suci, and Tannenbaum 1957). Their method is called the semantic differential. That method advanced the idea of multidimensional scales through the authors' theory that the connotative meaning of any object or term could be essentially described in three dimensions. Osgood and his colleagues named the three dimensions activity, evaluation, and potency. For example, think of the idea of gymnastics. If you like gymnastics, you would probably rate it high on activity, good on evaluation, and powerful on potency. Other adjectives and dimensions can be used to describe the connotative meaning of things to people; but the scaling of several dimensions through the use of antonyms to describe the opposite ends of a continuum was the key and provides an example of what are known as bipolar scales.

Three Dimensions of Connotative Meaning: Osgood and Tannenbaum

Evaluative

Good __:__:__:__:__:__:__ Bad

Potency

Powerful __:__:__:__:__:__:__ Weak

Activity

Active __:__:__:__:__:__:__ Passive

Scales or Measures?

Scores derived directly from a response scale cannot be used as measures of psychological constructs because they will not perfectly fit the true distribution of the variable being scaled. Contrary to the assumptions of a linear normal distribution characterized by Thurstone and Likert scaling, response scores commonly are nonlinear and are peculiar to the group of people sampled. For example, in 1953 a Danish mathematician, Georg Rasch (1960), found that the only way he could compare past performances on various tests of oral reading was to statistically adjust data (i.e., apply the exponential additivity of Poisson's 1837 distribution) that were produced by a new sample of students responding to both tests (Tenenbaum 1999). Nonetheless, it is common to construct measures using factor analysis, which is described next, to determine whether the scale has multiple dimensions.

Exploratory Factor Analysis

A key statistical tool used to determine whether measures of psychological constructs should be unidimensional or multidimensional is factor analysis. Researchers use factor analysis to identify patterns of correlations among items on a test by transforming the correlation matrix of items into a smaller number of dimensions, or factors. Factor analysis is used to estimate the number and nature of factors that may underlie the pattern of correlations among a larger group of variables. Technically, it is used to extract common factor variances from sets of measures. A factor is viewed as a construct that is assumed to explain relationships among items and scales. Factor analysis yields variables that are inferred rather than measured directly, so it is just one

step in the development of valid measures of psychological constructs.

Factor analysis was developed 100 years ago by psychologist Charles Spearman, who thought that all tests of mental abilities such as verbal, mathematical, and analytical skills were explainable by a single underlying factor of intelligence that he called g. Spearman was wrong, but the technique with which he tested his ideas has become one of the fundamental tools used to describe psychological constructs and develop rating scales for their measurement.

The major steps in exploratory factor analysis are (1) selecting a set of variables, (2) generating a correlation matrix from the selected variables, (3) extracting factors from the correlation matrix, (4) rotating the factors to increase clarity, and (5) interpreting the meaning of the factors. An example will help clarify the major steps of exploratory factor analysis.

Suppose a researcher has selected six variables labeled A through F to measure verbal and mathematical ability in a sample of college students. The researcher generates a matrix (i.e., a square array of numbers) containing correlations among scores from the six variables, as shown in figure 2.2. The values, or elements, along the diagonal are 1.0 because any variable is perfectly correlated with itself. The values above and below the diagonals are the same because the matrix is symmetrical. The off-diagonal values indicate the correlations among the six variables, which can range between −1.00 and

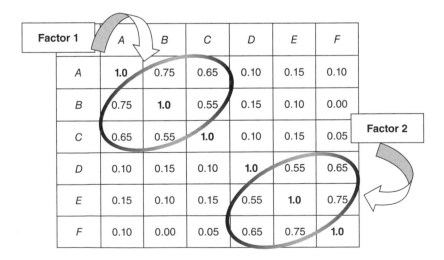

Figure 2.2 Example of a correlation matrix used in exploratory factor analysis.

+1.00. The circled areas in figure 2.2 indicate that two distinct patterns may exist among the correlations. Therefore, the pattern of correlations in the matrix suggests that two dimensions, or factors, underlie the six variables.

The next step is to extract factors from the correlation matrix to determine whether two factors really underlie the relationships among the six variables. The most common method of extraction, labeled principal-axis-factor extraction, uses squared multiple correlations as an initial estimate of the variable communalities. Communalities are the common factor variances of each variable (i.e., the portion of the variable's total variance accounted for by the common factors), and estimates of communalities are a necessary starting point for factor extraction. Exploratory factor analysis extracts n (n = number of variables) minus the number of factors (one or a specified number of factors) from the correlation matrix using an iterative approach such that the first factor accounts for the greatest amount of variance among the items and subsequent factors account for a smaller portion of the variance. The researcher then examines the solution and uses criteria (e.g., the amount of variance explained by the factors or the extent to which the factors reproduce the original correlation matrix) to determine whether the correct number of factors has been extracted. Two factors were extracted from the correlation matrix in the present example.

The extraction of factors yields the factor matrix in table 2.1. The first two columns contain factor loadings, which are weights that express the degrees of relationships between the original six variables and the two factors. Similar to correlation coefficients, the weights range between −1.00 and +1.00. Inspection of the weights indicates that variables A, B, and C load strongly on the first factor, but weakly on the second factor. Conversely, variables D, E, and F load on the second factor, but not the first factor. The values in the third column are the communalities for the variables, which are computed by summing the square of the factor loadings. The communality of variable A is $(.85)^2 + (.05)^2 = .7250$.

The aim in factor analysis is to express each item or scale as the sum of common and unique portions. The common portions of all the variables are by definition fully explained by the common factors, and the unique portions are ideally perfectly uncorrelated with each other. Thus, common factors are linear combinations of the common parts of the original variables. Factor analysis describes components of the common-factor variance. The total variance of a test item includes three parts: (1) common-factor variance (variance attributable to the common factors), or h^2; (2) specific variance (variance not shared with the common factors); and (3) error variance (1.0 minus reliability). Thus, total variance = 1.0 = h^2 + specific variance + error. The sum of a test item's communality plus its specific variance is its reliability. If we use item A to illustrate and assume it has a reliability of .80, its error variance is .20 (.20 = 1.0 − .80), and its specific variance is .075 (1.0 = .7250 + .075 + .20).

Sometimes the matrix of factor loadings is not as clear as that depicted in table 2.1, and it must be rotated. Rotation is a method of reorienting the pattern of factor loadings to a more simplistic or interpretable form. Similar to adjusting the magnification lens of a microscope to clarify the view of the contents of a slide, rotation involves adjusting the pattern of factor loadings to clarify the contents within the factor matrix. The adjustment brings clarity to the factor loadings in the factor matrix. Rotation can be either orthogonal (i.e., independent factors) or oblique (i.e., correlated factors). In our example of two factors, visualize the factors as lines or vectors that intersect. An **orthogonal** rotation would determine factor loadings with the two lines at a right angle to each other. An oblique rotation would reduce that angle to determine whether

Table 2.1　Factor Matrix

Variable	1	2	h^2
A	.85	.05	.7250
B	.75	.10	.5725
C	.65	.10	.4325
D	.10	.65	.4325
E	.10	.75	.5725
F	.05	.85	.7250

the pattern of the loadings would become more distinct.

The final step in exploratory factor analysis involves interpreting the meaning of the factors in table 2.1. The interpretation depends on the size and pattern of the factor loadings for the variables. Variables *A, B,* and *C* load strongly on the first factor, but weakly on the second factor. Inspection of the variable content indicates the common element of the variables and the construct underlying the correlations among the variables (e.g., verbal ability). Variables *D, E,* and *F* load on the second factor, but not the first factor. The common element of the variables and the construct underlying the correlations among the variables may be mathematical ability.

> **E**xploratory factor analysis is a statistical method used to develop rating scales for the measurement of psychological constructs; correlations between variables are used to extract factors or strongly related groups of variables that represent a distinct construct.

In areas of study in which little is known, exploratory factor analysis can be valuable for its ability to suggest patterns underlying the correlations among variables. Unfortunately, the number of factors in the solution is unknown before the exploratory factor analysis, and all of the factors typically influence all of the variables, as shown in figure 2.3. There also is no direct test of the accuracy of the final factor solution (i.e., indeterminacy) or the relationships of items to a specific factor (i.e., factorial validity). Newer techniques that use covariance modeling are more suited for testing hypotheses about the structure underlying the relationships among variables.

COVARIANCE MODELING

Spearman based factor analysis on methods similar to linear regression, whereby regression coefficients and the estimates of error are found by a statistical solution that minimizes the sum

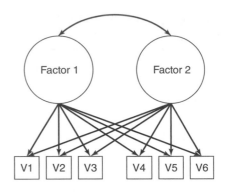

Figure 2.3 Exploratory factor analysis is used to suggest patterns underlying the correlation among variables.

of square differences between a predicted score and an observed score for each person tested. A newer approach called covariance modeling is based on covariances, not each person's scores. Rather than striving to minimize differences between predicted and observed scores, the goal of covariance is to minimize the difference between the covariances observed in a sample of people and the covariances predicted by some theoretical model (Bollen 1989).

Covariance modeling represents a powerful class of analytical tools for directly testing the fit of theoretical models to a variance–covariance matrix underlying a set of variables. Two of the main types of analyses that use covariance modeling are confirmatory factor analysis and structural equation modeling. Confirmatory factor analysis is similar to exploratory factor analysis, but it directly tests the fit of a theoretically derived measurement model to a variance–covariance matrix underlying a set of variables. Structural equation modeling involves testing the fit of a theoretically derived model that describes the measurement of and structural relationships among many latent variables or constructs.

> **C**ovariance modeling uses observed and predicted covariances to determine the fit of theoretical models to a set of variables. Examples include confirmatory factor analysis and structural equation modeling.

Confirmatory Factor Analysis

The major steps in confirmatory factor analysis (CFA) are (1) selecting a set of variables, (2) generating a variance–covariance matrix from the selected variables, (3) prespecifying a theoretically based measurement model that explicitly defines the relationship of each variable to a factor, (4) estimating the model parameters, and (5) testing the adequacy of the model using fit indexes.

The first two steps are very similar to the steps in exploratory factor analysis. The researcher selects a set of variables, collects responses from a sample, and then generates a matrix describing the relationships among the variables. The matrix in confirmatory factor analysis, however, involves variances and covariances rather than correlation coefficients.

The next step, performed after the variance–covariance matrix is generated, illustrates a fundamental difference between exploratory and confirmatory factor analysis. The researcher specifies in advance the measurement model based on a theory that explicitly defines the relationship of each variable to a factor, such as the two-factor, correlated model depicted in figure 2.4. The measurement model defines the number of factors, the relationships between factors, the relationships between factors and variables, and the error terms associated with the measured variables.

The next steps involve estimating the modeled parameters and then determining the degree of fit of the model to the data. Various methods of estimation, such as maximum likelihood (i.e., the "best bet" estimate of a population value based on the prior probability of an observed value occurring in the population), attempt to minimize the discrepancy between the sample variance–covariance matrix and the variance–covariance matrix reproduced by the modeled parameters. The minimization process is iterative, and the final model converges when there is not an appreciable reduction in the discrepancy between the two matrixes.

The model then must be judged for its accuracy, which is based on a number of fit indexes. Most fit indexes are used to judge either the absolute or the relative fit of the model to the sample variance–covariance matrix. Some indexes of fit such as the χ-square statistic (computed as the squared difference between the diagonal and off-diagonal elements of the sample and the reproduced variance–covariance matrixes, multiplied by the sample size minus 1) and the goodness-of-fit index (a measure of the relative amounts of variances and covariances in the sample matrix predicted by the model) test the absolute fit of the model. Relative or incremental fit indexes (e.g., a non-normed fit index, which is a ratio of the χ-squares for the null and the hypothesized models, corrected for the number of parameters in the models) and the root mean square error of approximation (computed as $[(T - d) / d \times n]^{1/2}$, where T = χ-square from maximum likelihood estimation, d = degrees of freedom in the model, and $n = N - 1$) compare the fit of the specified model to a baseline, or null, model, which hypothesizes no relationships among the observed variables. Values of .08, .05, and 0 indicate reasonable, close, and exact fit, respectively. The advantages of CFA include the following:

- It is a direct or relative test of the goodness of fit of an a priori measurement model that is based on theory.

- It estimates correlations among error terms. Ideally, errors are independent, but there are instances when adjusting for correlated errors is justifiable and informative.

- It tests the accuracy of the model and its parameters across distinct groups, such

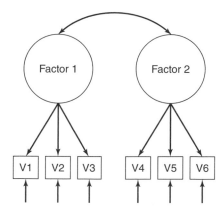

Figure 2.4 A two-factor, correlated model used in confirmatory factor analysis.

as males and females, or across time. If the factor structure underlying a construct is different between groups or times, the summated scores cannot be directly compared; they mean different things, so it is important to demonstrate measurement equivalence or invariance (i.e., equal factor structure, factor loadings, item means, and errors) across groups and time.

• It compares latent means that are constructed from the raw scores of the factors not summated.

Structural Equation Modeling

Many researchers are interested in examining whether theoretical models can accurately describe the exact relationships among multiple latent or hypothetical constructs. Chapter 14 explains theories of physical activity behavior change. Structural equation modeling (SEM), which is an extension of confirmatory factor analysis, can be used to develop and test those theories. For example, a researcher may want to test whether the theory of reasoned action, which postulates that behavior is predicted by intention and that intention is predicted by attitude and societal norms, is a reasonable description of the variables associated with physical activity. Structural equation modeling can determine whether the pattern of relationships among the variables conforms to the theorized pattern.

Structural equation modeling entails several steps. The first is to select a theoretical model to test—for example, the theory of reasoned action—to understand the factors associated with physical activity. An investigator then operationalizes the constructs within the theory using multiple variables or indicators of each hypothetical variable, collects responses from a sample, and generates a variance–covariance matrix.

Next, the researcher specifies in advance the theoretical model to be tested. The model contains two parts: measurement models and a structural model. Figure 2.5 contains the measurement models and a structural model for a hypothetical test of the theory of reasoned action. Measurement models are specified for each latent variable. Similar to what occurs in confirmatory factor analysis, the measurement models define the number of factors, the relationships between factors, the relationships between factors and variables, and the error term associated with each measured variable. One factor is specified for the measurement models for each latent variable in figure 2.5. The structural model specifies the nature of the relationships or paths among the latent variables. For example, the structural model specifies paths from social norms and attitude to intention and from intention to physical activity.

The next steps are to estimate the modeled parameters and then determine the degree of fit of the model to the data. The purpose of the method of estimation is to minimize the discrepancy between the sample variance–

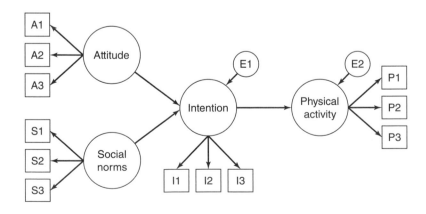

Figure 2.5 Structural model for testing the theory of reasoned action using SEM.

Adapted, by permission, from R.W. Motl, R.K. Dishman et al., 2002, "Examining social-cognitive determinants of intention and physical activity in adolescent girls using structural equation modeling," *Health Psychology* 21(5): 459-467.

covariance matrix and the variance–covariance matrix reproduced by the modeled parameters. Similar to this step in confirmatory factor analysis, the minimization process is iterative, and the model finally converges when there is not a significant reduction in the discrepancy between the sample variance–covariance matrix and the variance–covariance matrix reproduced by the modeled parameters.

The model then must be judged for its accuracy based on the fit indexes as in confirmatory factor analysis. Therefore, an investigator can specify in advance a theoretically derived model and then test the goodness of fit of the model directly using structural equation modeling. The following are some benefits of structural equation modeling:

- It establishes measurement models that partition true and error score variance among the indicators of each latent variable.

- It simultaneously estimates the hypothetical paths among multiple latent variables.

- It provides unbiased estimates of the relationships or paths between latent variables.

- It tests the accuracy of the model and its parameters across distinct groups, such as males and females, as well as across time, and analyzes the effects of experimental interventions on variables (e.g., goals, confidence, mood) that presumably mediate the effects of the intervention on behavior.

Mixed Models for Correlated Measures

Accurately measuring the psychological antecedents and consequences of physical activity is the first step toward understanding the causal relations among theoretical constructs and physical activity. The next step, determining the effects of acute and chronic exercise on psychological outcomes and the effects of various interventions on exercise behavior, often requires complex SEM approaches. These are similar to those described previously, particularly mixed models, which are used when multiple measurements are taken that are correlated with each other. A mixed model is a statistical model containing both fixed effects (e.g., a variation in scores between experimental and control conditions) and random effects (e.g., a variation in scores within a group of randomly selected people or across random samples of time).

In the early 20th century, Sir Ronald Fisher introduced random effects models to study correlated traits among relatives. Then, in the 1950s, Charles Roy Henderson provided unbiased linear estimates of fixed effects and random effects. Today, there are various statistical approaches to estimating these effects and their standard errors, including maximum likelihood (e.g., estimating the population mean, variance, and covariances of scores in a normal distribution based on knowing scores from just a sample of the population) and Bayesian approaches (in which likelihood estimates are based on prior knowledge or probabilities).

Although a simple paired t-test can tell you whether mood was improved for most people after an aerobics class, the full effects of interventions cannot be examined simply because they are influenced by many factors that can affect people differently. The t-test can't be used to understand why some people improved more than others, or even why some got worse after exercise. In contrast, extending SEM to mixed models is useful for describing the growth in variables across time and in determining the patterns of relationships over time among multiple variables, where it can be used to more fully explain the outcomes and antecedents of physical activity by testing **mediation** (i.e., indirect) and **moderation** (i.e., modified) effects. Some examples follow.

Latent Growth Modeling

Determining the rate and shape of change requires at least three sequential measures across time to determine whether change is linear or nonlinear. Latent growth modeling (LGM) estimates the trajectory of change (i.e., the slope) for individuals and for groups by using SEM procedures to estimate two latent variables from longitudinal data: one representing the initial status or starting value, and the other representing the trajectory of change across time (see figure 2.6), which is modeled as a random effect that differs among people (Bollen, Curran, and Wiley 2006). In contrast to analysis of variance for repeated measures (RM-ANOVA) or ordinary least squares (OLS) regression analysis, LGM provides parameter estimates of intra- and interindividual differences in linear or nonlinear trajectories of change and the relation between change and initial status, as well as maximal likelihood techniques for missing data, measures of model fit, and diagnostics for poor fit (Muthén and Muthén 1998-2010). A key advantage of latent growth modeling is the ability to use the initial status and change latent variables as independent or dependent variables in prediction models, such as the SEM models described earlier.

Latent Transition Analysis

Latent transition analysis (LTA) is a special case of latent class analysis (a subset of SEM used to find groups of cases in multivariate categorical data) that provides Bayesian probability estimates of (1) proportions of the population in each latent stage and (2) the conditional probability of membership in stage *b* at time *t*

+ 1 given membership in stage *a* at time *t*. In this case, there are two conditional probability matrixes: (1) time 2 stages given time 1 stages and (2) time 3 stages given time 2 stages. LTA provides Bayesian probability estimates (i.e., posterior estimates that are based on prior probabilities) of participants' movements between discrete latent classes. An example of LTA use was a test of the likelihood that every six months adults would (1) transition positively (i.e., move forward) from being insufficiently active to meeting public health guidelines for physical activity and (2) transition negatively (i.e., backslide) from meeting guidelines to no longer being sufficiently active (Dishman et al. 2009).

Latent class growth modeling has the advantage of determining whether multiple groupings of initial levels and change exist in a group of people. Thus, it is not limited to independent tests of initial status (i.e., baseline levels) and change in the whole group, whereby between-person differences are treated as random error rather than as potentially true individual differences (a fixed effect). Rather, latent class growth modeling provides an opportunity to determine whether discrete classes of the group exist that might have unique relations with classes of change in physical activity that would go otherwise undetected if the entire group were to be evaluated together, as shown in figure 2.7. For example, people who sustain high expectations of personal benefits of being physically active from baseline throughout the observation period should have higher odds of meeting physical activity guidelines at all assessments than people with lower or declining expectations (Dishman, Vandenberg, Motl, and Nigg 2010).

Multilevel Analysis

Although complicated, multilevel analysis is helpful in understanding and predicting levels of physical activity because it takes into account the scope of and relationships among determinants. Physical activity is no doubt determined by individual decisions and motivation, but also by the interaction of those personal determinants with influences exerted on people by their physical and social environments, including homes and families, neighborhoods, places of worship, workplaces, and schools (Duncan et al. 2004;

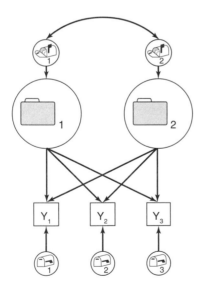

Figure 2.6 A latent growth model. Y_1 to Y_3 represent measures obtained at three equally spaced times, η (intercept, or initial status) and η_2 (slope or change) are latent variables, and the ϵs and ζs represent unexplained variance for the Ys and the ηs, respectively (Singer and Willett 2003). The change trajectories modeled by η and η_2 are random estimates of longitudinal change over time measured without error.

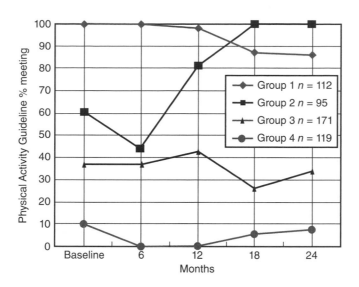

Figure 2.7 Latent class growth modeling showing four patterns of people meeting public health guidelines for physical activity across 2 years.

Reprinted, by permission, from R.K. Dishman et al., 2010, "Using constructs of the transtheoretical model to predict classes of change in regular physical activity: A multi-ethnic longitudinal cohort study," *Annals of Behavioral Medicine* 40(2): 150-163.

King et al. 2008). People can be similarly influenced by shared features of their communities, so they may well choose to be physically active if their family members or friends are active, their schools or workplaces provide for and promote physical activity, and their homes and neighborhoods provide places and opportunities for safe and pleasant physical activities (see figure 2.8). Likewise, a change in physical activity, or its mental health outcomes across time, can be partly determined by genetic traits and physical or social environments that affect people in different ways depending on family traits and their shared and differing environments and cultures (De Moor et al. 2008).

Multilevel modeling (also known as hierarchical linear modeling when observed, rather than latent, variables are used) is a mixed-model case of SEM (i.e., it combines fixed and random effects) that uses regression analysis to estimate how much of the variance among people on a first-level dependent variable (a random effect) is explainable by a second-level factor (a fixed effect) in which people are nested (i.e., share a common influence from only one category of the second-level factor) (Raudenbush and Bryk 2002). For example, students' physical activity (first-level variable) will differ according to their motivation and innate abilities (another first-level

variable) but also according to the school environments they share (physical education teacher ability, friends' habits, and opportunities to be physical activity) but which vary both within and between schools (second-level variable).

Multilevel, or hierarchical, modeling also allows for the analysis of longitudinal data by estimating how much of the change in a first-level dependent variable can be predicted by a second-level variable or its interaction with other first-level variables. For example, the growth in physical activity levels across a school year should be steeper on average for schools with the best physical education teachers and most physical activity opportunities because all students in those schools benefit. However, the growth in physical activity might be even greater for initially sedentary students with lower innate ability who attend schools with the best physical education classes and most opportunities for activity, because those students most need the help and have the most room for improvement.

In multilevel growth modeling, level 1 would model the within-school change over time. For example, schools may have different levels of physical activity in the 9th grade and different forms of change in physical activity between the 9th grade and the 12th grade. The change coefficients are random slopes representing

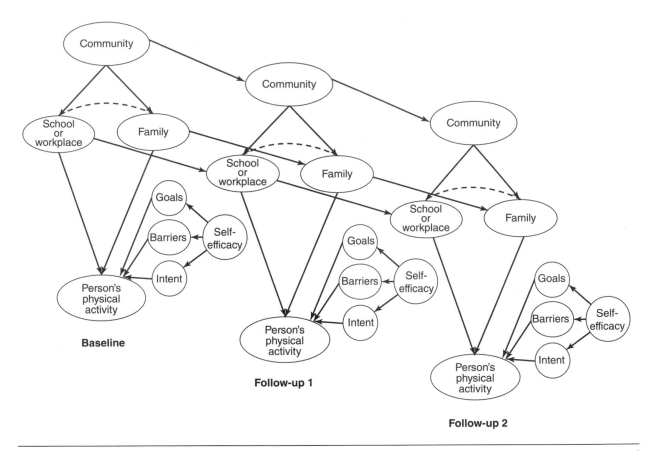

Figure 2.8 Measurement of change using multilevel models. Conceptual models should include variables measured at the individual level (e.g., personal motivation), including the family and home environment, but also at the community level (e.g., neighborhoods, churches, schools).

Adapted, by permission, from Dishman, 2008, "Gene-physical activity interactions in the etiology of obesity: Behavioral considerations," *Obesity* 16 (Suppl. 3): S60-S65.

within-school change across time in physical activity (or any of the primary or secondary outcomes). Level 2 would model the between-school differences in average change over time (a fixed effect) and the variability in changes across schools (a random effect). Predictor variables may be introduced at level 2. For example, both the initial level of physical activity in the 9th grade and the change in physical activity through the 12th grade can be compared between groups of schools classified as having many opportunities for physical activity and schools classified as offering few opportunities.

Multilevel mixed models are based on a theory that specifies direct effects of variables on each other within any one level and cross-level interaction effects between variables at different levels. Thus, a researcher can test hypotheses for mediating mechanisms (i.e., one variable causes the other) or moderating effects (i.e., one vari-

able modifies the causal relations among other variables) for variables at one level that influence variables at another, subordinate level.

Multilevel models require sophisticated statistical methods that can estimate and test variables that operate at the level of the person and at levels higher than the person. This requires conceptual and analytical models that have inherently complex features including (1) multilevel data; (2) the analysis of change across time; (3) hypothesis tests of independent (i.e., direct), mediated (i.e., indirect), and moderated (i.e., interactive) relations; (4) the use of various data forms including self-ratings as well as objective measures of the physical and social environment; and (5) the need to demonstrate the equivalence of the measurement properties of first-level person variables among age, race, and sex and within each of those groups across time (Ployhart and Vandenberg 2010). Given these inherent complexities, traditional analyses such as ordinary regression and repeated measures ANOVA are inadequate (O'Connell and McCoach 2004). Multilevel modeling can accommodate missing data and variability in the time data collected from participants, as well as the time-varying covariates of the variable of interest that are collected at each assessment period (Singer and Willett 2003).

DEFINING PHYSICAL ACTIVITY AND FITNESS

Physical activity is "any bodily movement produced by skeletal muscles that results in energy expenditure," and is usually measured in kilocalories (kcal) per unit of time (Caspersen, Powell, and Christenson 1985). Categories of physical activity include sleep, occupation, transportation, and leisure. Types of leisure-time physical activity are household activities, other chores, recreation and sports, and conditioning activities (i.e., exercise). **Exercise**, a subset of physical activity, is planned, structured, repetitive bodily movements that someone engages in for the purpose of improving or maintaining one or more components of physical fitness or health. Exercise can be acute or chronic. Acute exercise is a single, relatively short bout of exercise; chronic exercise is exercise carried out repeatedly over time, usually several times each week for various durations. Depending on its intensity, frequency, and duration, physical activity can improve physical fitness.

Physical Activity Features

Physical activity occurs at varying intensities spanning a range of energy expenditures from rest to multiples of resting metabolic rate per kilogram of body mass (i.e., **metabolic equivalent [MET]**). Intensity of physical activity can be about 10 to 15 times resting MET in average people or as high as 20 to 25 times resting MET among the very highly aerobically fit. It is important to measure the types, intensities, and durations of physical activity that people engage in because those factors determine physiological responses during exertion that may directly or indirectly influence psychological responses

during or after physical activity. It is not yet known how these features of physical activity affect psychological responses, but, as an example, it is possible that pain occurring at high exercise intensities (e.g., above 60% of aerobic capacity in sedentary people) might negatively influence mood and deter future physical activity. In addition, muscle fiber recruitment and other physiological responses, such as body temperature, breathing rate and depth, hydrogen ions, and hormones (such as catecholamines, cortisol, and β-endorphin) increase linearly or exponentially during moderate to heavy intensities of exercise. Any or all of those responses might influence psychological factors indirectly by influencing perceptions of exertion or brain responses (e.g., regional brain blood flow or metabolism). Some of those possibilities are discussed in some detail in chapters 4 through 6 and chapter 16.

This text focuses on exercise because most of the available literature has used a measure of physical activity that fits the definition of exercise. For example, anxiety usually has been examined before and after 20 to 30 minutes of aerobic exercise (e.g., jogging, cycling, or swimming) at intensities fixed by the investigators, commonly in laboratory conditions. The control of such features of physical exertion is necessary for defining precisely whether a "dose response" exists between exercise and psychological outcomes. However, it is equally or more important to determine whether factors such as the choice of activity type or intensity (e.g., level of preferred exertion, discussed in chapter 16) or the setting where exercise occurs (e.g., indoors or outdoors, on a track or in a park, in solitude or with others) influence the psychological consequences of physical activity. We are only beginning to determine for whom and under what circumstances the anti-anxiety effects of physical activity occur. Such questions require precise definitions and measures of physical activity and exercise. In contrast, more than 30 population-based studies have linked lower levels of physical activity with depression symptoms, and even more studies have shown that people in exercise training programs (e.g., 45-60 min of brisk walking 3-5 days per week) had fewer depression symptoms compared to those in placebo control groups after several weeks or months.

Behavior change interventions directed toward increasing exercise adoption (strategies to recruit new participants) and maintenance (follow-ups to sustain participation) have had better results when the target behavior of the intervention was relatively low-intensity physical activities (e.g., walking) carried out as part of a person's daily lifestyle compared to heavy exercise in a supervised program (Dishman and Buckworth 1996b). There is also evidence for health benefits (e.g., markers of cardiovascular disease) from accumulating higher levels of physical activity (Dunn 2009).

Increasing numbers of interventions target lifestyle physical activity and develop environments that offer opportunities to be more physically active (such as bike paths and attractive, accessible stairs). Lifestyle physical activity has been defined in the context of physical activity recommendations as the "daily accumulation of at least 30 minutes of self-selected activities, which includes all leisure, occupational, or household activities that are at least moderate to vigorous in their intensity and could be planned or unplanned activities that are part of everyday life" (Dunn, Andersen, and Jakicic 1998, 399). Lifestyle physical activities are targets of interventions because they can be alternatives to less active behaviors to achieve a nonfitness goal, such as walking for commuting or carrying groceries instead of using a cart. Thus, lifestyle interventions can promote increased weekly energy expenditure through the accumulation of unstructured physical activity (e.g., taking the stairs instead of the elevator) instead of or in addition to structured exercise.

Physical activity and exercise are behaviors, and the issues in measuring these behaviors are discussed later. Physical fitness is more straightforward to measure (see the next section) and is often used as a behavioral surrogate, under the assumption that the level of physical activity is positively associated with fitness. Changes in fitness may also influence some psychological outcomes of physical activity (e.g., physical self-esteem). Some other positive outcomes of physical activity, such as reduced depression, do not appear to depend on increased fitness. Also, it is possible that different components of fitness may be specifically more relevant for different psychological or behavioral outcomes of physical activity. To find out, fitness components must be defined and measured.

Physical Fitness

Physical fitness is the capacity to meet the present and potential physical challenges of life; it is a set of attributes that people have or achieve that relates to the ability to perform physical activity. Physical fitness components typically associated with health include cardiorespiratory endurance, muscular strength and endurance, flexibility, and body composition (see table 2.2). Blood pressure and metabolic indexes, such as plasma lipids and glucose tolerance, are also affected by the level of physical activity and are related to health. Agility, balance, coordination, speed, power, and reaction time are components of fitness usually associated with sport performance, but can affect activities of daily living and well-being. Poor balance and coordination, for example, are linked to the risk of falls in older adults and can thus play an important role in health.

Aerobic (i.e., cardiorespiratory) **fitness** refers to the maximal capacity of the cardiorespiratory system to take up and use oxygen (i.e., $\dot{V}O_2max$) and is typically expressed in milliliters of oxygen per minute adjusted for total body mass or fat-free mass expressed in kilograms. The use of aerobic fitness to represent physical activity has limitations because 25% to 40% of aerobic capacity is genetically determined and the rate of cardiovascular adaptations to increased activity varies among individuals, even between monozygotic (i.e., identical) twins (Wilmore et al. 1997). It may happen that two people who begin a training program with the same aerobic capacity will achieve the same level of physical activity after a specific period of time, but the person who adapts more rapidly will show a greater increase in aerobic fitness. Nonetheless, it is important to measure fitness to determine the *relative* strain a person experiences during moderate to heavy exertion (i.e., the exertion during standard physical activities expressed as a portion of the person's capacity). Levels of, or changes in, other physical fitness measures,

Table 2.2   Health-Related Physical Fitness

Fitness component	Laboratory	TYPE OF MEASURE	
		Epidemiologic	Self-assessment
Cardiorespiratory	Maximal oxygen uptake	Treadmill time	12 min run/walk
Cycling PWC	Canada Home Fitness Test		
Body composition	Underwater weight; DXA	BMI, BIA, skinfolds	BMI, skinfolds
Muscular strength	Limb/trunk dynamometer	Handgrip dynamometer Trunk/limb lifts	
Flexibility	Goniometer	Goniometer	Sit-and-reach
Muscular endurance	Limb/trunk dynamometer	Isokinetic machines	Pull-ups/sit-ups modified

BMI is body mass index (weight in kg/[height in meters])^2; BIA is bioelectrical impedance analysis; a goniometer measures joint angles; a dynamometer measures force and rate of force; PWC is physical working capacity measured as peak power output during an incremental test; treadmill time is the duration of a grade-incremented test.

Adapted from C.J. Caspersen, K.E. Powell, and G.M. Christenson, 1985, "Physical activities, exercise, and physical fitness: Definitions and distinctions for health-related research," *Public Health Reports* 100: 126-131.

such as muscular strength or endurance, body mass or percentage of body fat, and flexibility, are important to measure because they might influence psychological effects or determinants of physical activity. For example, perceptions of increased muscularity that can result from resistance exercise training may contribute positively to physical self-esteem. Changes in fitness also can be used to document adherence to an exercise program.

Adherence

Adherence means conforming faithfully to a standard of behavior that has been set as part of a negotiated agreement. Research on exercise behavior change has typically defined exercise adherence on the basis of attendance or a specified minimal percentage of attendance, such as 60% to 80%. Although arbitrary, the most widely agreed-upon definition of maintenance of an exercise program is adherence for at least six months. That is so partly because the typical exercise program has about a 50% dropout rate during the first six months. Of course, successful programs exceed that average, and six months of maintenance does not ensure against dropping out later. However, these definitions assume equality among all types of nonattendance, do not take into account

the level of participation, and usually consider only the number of sessions, which precludes the consideration of the equally important features of session intensity and duration.

Exercise **compliance** also refers to how well someone follows an exercise program, but this term is used more often in a medical setting in reference to behaviors related to immediate- and short-term health advice to alleviate symptoms. It has a more authoritative or coercive connotation than does *adherence*, which is a preferred term because of its emphasis on personal control by the participant.

> **E**xercise is a behavior, and fitness is an attribute. Issues related to the valid measurement of both exercise and fitness affect the quality of exercise psychology research.

MEASURING PHYSICAL ACTIVITY

The measurement of exercise behavior and the level of physical activity is fundamental to studying exercise and mental health and in testing interventions aimed at changing exercise behavior. This presents a considerable challenge because there is no single standard for measuring physical activity (Dishman, Washburn, and Schoeller 2001; Prince et al. 2008), and physical activity can be quantified in various ways, such as total time active, hours spent at various intensities expressed in METs or as increased heart rate, units of movement (e.g., number of steps), or energy expenditure expressed in kilocalories. Some of the methods for measuring physical activity are characterized in table 2.3 according to the costs to the study groups; the extent of interference with usual activity level; acceptability by people; and the ability of the method to provide specific information about the type, frequency, duration, and intensity of physical activity (LaPorte, Montoye, and Caspersen 1985). The methods generally can be categorized according to whether they measure a direct or indirect observation of physical activity, motion, a physiological response during physical activity, energy expenditure, or a physiological adaptation to physical activity. Four measurable dimensions of physical activity are type, duration, frequency (e.g., days per week), and **intensity** (rate of energy expenditure), although most methods do not assess all four.

> There are more than 40 methods for measuring physical activity, and the selection of method hinges on the appropriateness for the target population and the level of sensitivity and specificity necessary for answering the research question.

Table 2.3 Free-Living Physical Activity Assessment

Assessment procedure	STUDY COSTS			ACCEPTABILITY		
	Time	Effort	Interference	Person	Social	Activity specifics
Calorimetry						
Direct	VH	VH	H-VH	No	No	Yes
Indirect	H-VH	VH	H-VH	No	No	Yes
Surveys						
Task-specific diary	L-M	L-M	VH	?	Yes	Yes
Recall questionnaire	L-M	L-M	L	Yes	Yes	Yes
Quantitative history	L-M	L-M	L	Yes	Yes	Yes
Physiological markers						
Cardiorespiratory fitness	M-VH	M-H	L	?	?	No
Doubly labeled water	H-VH	M-VH	L-H	Yes	Yes	No
Mechanical and electronic monitors						
Heart rate	H-VH	M-VH	L-M	Yes	Yes	No
Pedometer	L-M	L	L-M	Yes	Yes	No
Accelerometer	L-H	L-M	L-M	Yes	Yes	No
Observation	H-VH	H-VH	L-VH	?	?	Yes

L = low; M = medium; H = high; VH = very high.

Data from LaPorte, Montoye, and Caspersen 1985.

Energy Expended for Various Activities

Activity	Energy expended (METs*/hour)
Sitting and talking	1.5
Driving an automobile	2.5
Pilates (general)	3.0
Yard work (moderate)	4.0
Brisk walk (at 4 mph [6.4 km/h])	5.0
Low-impact aerobic dance	5.0
Weightlifting (vigorous)	6.0
Jogging (general)	7.0
Bicycling (12-13.9 mph [19.3-22.4 km/h])	8.0
Swimming laps (freestyle, vigorous)	9.8
Running (8 min per mile [12 km/h])	11.8

*1 MET = 1.0 kcal/kg body weight

Data from Ainsworth et al. 2011.

Desirable features of physical activity instruments are validity, reliability, practicality (i.e., study costs and acceptability to the target population), nonreactivity or interference (i.e., the method must not alter the population or the behavior it seeks to measure), and specificity (i.e., features of type, intensity, and time are measured). The validation of instruments is a dilemma, and many self-report instruments have not been validated using concurrent measures of energy expenditure such as doubly labeled water, metabolism assessment in a respiratory chamber or using a portable metabolic system, heart rate, or motion counters and accelerometers that estimate the force of motion. And there are limitations in using these methods for validation because they do not tell us either the type of activity or its intensity.

Understandably, all methods that have been used to measure physical activity and exercise have strengths and weaknesses, and different methods will be more or less appropriate based on the research question. For example, a short self-report questionnaire to estimate overall level of activity might be appropriate for classifying a large sample into low-, moderate-, and high-active groups in a descriptive analysis, but more precise and reliable methods should be used in an intervention study designed to measure adherence to a strength training program.

Occupational work potentially accounts for much of someone's total physical activity, and job classification is one method that has been used to categorize people into activity groups. This method is nonreactive and quick and can be used to classify large groups. However, there can be considerable within-job variability, potential misclassifications of intensity, seasonal and secular changes in job requirements, and selection bias. Grouping people into activity categories based on their jobs excludes the contribution of leisure and nonoccupational physical activity; and because people have become less active at work, leisure-time physical activity is generally considered more representative of physical activity in a population (Kriska and Caspersen 1997).

One of the more frequently used methods for assessing physical activity is the survey recall, although surveys fail to explain more than 45% of variance in direct and indirect measures of physical activity (Durante and Ainsworth 1996). People are asked to report various aspects of their physical activity, such as type and duration, for spans of time ranging from a day to a year or even a lifetime. The reliability and validity of self-reports of physical activity depend on the respondent's ability to remember, interviewer or administrator and respondent bias, the day of the week (i.e., weekdays versus weekend), the sequencing of administration of the questionnaire, the saliency of the activity recalled, the social desirability of the response, sociodemographic issues, culture, age, sex, obesity, and education level (Durante and Ainsworth 1996; Kriska and Caspersen 1997). The time frame examined affects the quality of the data such that shorter recall periods are less subject to recall bias and easier to validate, but results are less likely to reflect usual behavior. Correlations between self-report and direct measures are generally low to moderate (Prince et al. 2008).

More objective measures of physical activity include pedometers and accelerometers. Pedometers record unidimensional movement and are used to record steps. They are practical for individual- and population-level applications, and because walking is the most commonly reported physical activity, knowing how many steps people take each day can be used to determine the level necessary for disease prevention and treatment. **Accelerometers** record the force of movement of a body or limb mass in the vertical plane or the vertical and horizontal planes. Accelerometer systems have been widely used to estimate energy expenditure for a range of activities. Devices are usually worn at the waist, legs, or arms and vary in size, reactivity, and the ability to detect features of activity to deduce types of activities. Those data can be translated into caloric expenditure or quantity of movement, such as the number of steps over a period of time. Accelerometers have been validated against a variety of physiological measures, such as graded treadmill maximal workload, treadmill time, submaximal exercise heart rate, body fatness, lung function, and doubly labeled water.

Advances in miniaturization and sensing technology have led to the availability of smaller and less obstructive measurement devices. For example, an ear-worn activity recognition sensor (e-AR) weighing 7.4 grams has been tested for the ability to predict energy expenditure and activity type (Atallah et al. 2011) and has been used to monitor physical activity in clinical populations.

Considering the variety of methods to measure physical activity in adults and youths (LaPorte, Montoye, and Caspersen 1985; Owen et al. 2010; Sallis et al. 1992), the difficulty in comparing results across studies without uniform assessment methods is obvious (Prince et al. 2008). In addition, the fact that physical activity has several definitions as an outcome variable, such as days active per week or total energy expenditure, also makes comparing studies difficult. A collection of popular physical activity questionnaires for various populations, along with descriptions of their use and information about reliability and validity, was published by the American College of Sports Medicine (Kriska and Caspersen 1997). Since then, several questionnaires have been developed and are being used more consistently.

The International Physical Activity Questionnaire (IPAQ; www.ipaq.ki.se/ipaq.htm) was developed to measure physical activity in surveillance studies and has been rigorously tested across the world for reliability and validity. The IPAQ has been used in more than 150 published studies, although in some cases as a measure of change in physical activity after an intervention. The Global Physical Activity Questionnaire (GPAQ) developed by the World Health Organization provides more detail about types of physical activity (www.who.int/chp/steps/GPAQ/en/index.html).

How exercise is implemented as an intervention is another issue in exercise psychology research. Very different types and amounts of activity have been employed as the exercise stimulus for very different types of subjects. Researchers implementing behavioral interventions need to use quantities and qualities of physical activity that match the target group's interests and abilities and meet their goals, such as increased strength or weight loss. Researchers testing the effects of acute exercise on psychological variables need to consider the novelty, the controllability (i.e., forced vs. voluntary, programmed vs. spontaneous), and the social and environmental contexts (e.g., solitary or group, competitive or recreational, indoors on a track or outdoors in a park) of the exercise. Physical activity history must also be considered in administering an acute bout of exercise, as well as in recommending an initial activity mode and dose and in determining the effects of an intervention on exercise adherence. Standardizing exercise intensity based on the percentage of maximal aerobic capacity is probably not adequate unless the researcher controls the effects of other psychobiological variables (e.g., stress hormones, such as catecholamines and β-endorphin) or sensations of force or pain possibly relevant to the mental health variable in question.

BEHAVIORAL GENETICS

Studies show that heritable genetic traits modify how people respond to exercise, both physically (Bouchard and Rankinen 2001; Rankinen, Rice, et al. 2010; Rankinen, Roth, et al. 2010) and mentally (Deeny et al. 2008; De Moor et al. 2008; Rethorst et al. 2010). They also account for variation in leisure-time physical activity (De Moor et al. 2009, 2011; Stubbe et al. 2006).

Studying twins is a common approach used to estimate how much of the differences among people in physical activity, or its outcomes, are accounted for by genetic inheritability (i.e., genotype). For example, comparing the correlation of a physical activity phenotype (i.e., an observable trait) between monozygotic (MZ; identical) twins and dizygotic (DZ; fraternal) twins parses out the influences of twin resemblance on that trait. If physical activity levels are more similar between MZ twins, who share all the same genes, than between DZ twins, who share only half their genes, then there is a genetic component to physical activity or one of its outcomes. If the correlation of physical activity levels between twin pairs is similar for MZ and DZ twins, common environmental factors shared by twin pairs seem to explain variation in this phenotype, regardless of genes. Because MZ twins usually share the same environment and the same genes, a correlation in pairs of MZ twins that is less than perfect (i.e., less than 1.0) indicates that the variation in a physical activity phenotype is explainable by unique environmental experiences not shared by the twins. The extreme example is identical twins separated at birth.

The human genome of *Homo sapiens* is made up of mitochondrial DNA (from the mother) and 23 chromosome pairs (one from each parent) that are composed of 3 billion DNA base pairs (i.e., combinations of the nucleotides adenine [A], guanine [G], cytosine [C], and thymine [T]). About 23,000 genes, less than 2% of the genome, encode proteins. The rest are introns (a nucleotide sequence within a gene that is removed, after transcription but before translation, by RNA splicing to generate the final mature RNA), nucleotide sequences that regulate other genes, and RNA and DNA that do not code for proteins (International Human Genome Sequencing Consortium 2004). The specific location of a gene or DNA sequence on a chromosome is a gene locus. A variant of the DNA sequence at a given locus is called an allele. Gene mapping is the process of identifying gene loci that are associated with phenotypic traits, including diseases and behaviors. This can be done by tracking diseases in big families (genetic linkage studies) or by correlating variations among genes and traits within a population or between population subgroups matched on other traits and environments (association studies). Both approaches have been used in physical activity studies (Bray et al. 2009; Rankinen et al. 2010).

Most genes have more than one effect on a phenotype, which can be either an observable trait or a physiological trait. This is pleiotropism. A trait that itself is unimportant for adaptation can still emerge by natural selection if it is pleiotropically linked to a trait that is important for adaptation to the environment (e.g., physical fitness). Variations in the DNA sequences of genes that occur in more than 1% of the population are called polymorphisms (i.e., multiple forms of a gene). Polymorphisms are heritable and are modified by natural selection. They explain many of the normal differences between people (e.g., eye, hair, or skin color and blood type). However, some polymorphisms influence the risk of developing diseases.

Several thousand diseases are believed to stem from altered genes inherited from one or more parents, but most of them are polygenic. That means they arise from complex, poorly understood interactions between the environment and multiple polygenes, each of which contributes less than 1% to the total effect. For example, at least 22 genes for obesity have been supported by at least five studies (Rankinen et al. 2006), but only about 10 association studies and fewer than a handful of linkage studies have examined candidate genes for variation in people's physical activity levels (Bray et al. 2009; Rankinen et al. 2010), without much replication of results. The U.S. National Institute on Aging, National Institutes of Health, and Centers for Disease Control and Prevention maintain a database of human genetic association studies of diseases, including anxiety, depression, and dementia, as well as physical activity (http://geneticassociationdb.nih.gov).

A gene mutation is a permanent change in its DNA sequence that is not a normal variation among people in a population group. When a gene contains a mutation, the protein encoded by that gene is likely to be abnormal or may not function normally. Mutations range in size from a single DNA building block (DNA base) to a large segment of a chromosome. Gene mutations can be inherited from either one parent (heterozygous) or both parents (homozygous) or acquired. Hereditary or germline mutations are carried in the DNA of the reproductive cells. When reproductive cells containing a mutation combine to produce offspring, the mutation will be in all of the offspring's body cells. The fact that every cell contains the gene change makes it possible to use buccal (i.e., cheek) cells or a blood sample for gene testing.

Mutations that occur only in an egg or sperm cell, or just after fertilization, are called de novo (i.e., new) mutations; these can explain disorders characterized by a mutation in all cells in the absence of a family history of the disorder. Acquired mutations occur in the DNA of individual cells after exposure to environmental factors (e.g., radiation or chemical toxins) or when a mistake is made in DNA replication during mitosis (i.e., cell division). Acquired mutations in cells other than sperm and egg cells are not heritable.

The most common gene change involves a mismatch of a single base nucleotide, which is called a single-nucleotide polymorphism (SNP).

A SNP occurs when a DNA fragment sequence differs within a species by a single nucleotide (e.g., AGCTGGC differs from AGCTGGA by a single nucleotide that has two alleles: C and A). The rarity of SNP alleles can vary between groups of people according to geography, race, and ethnicity. A SNP in which both alleles produce a different protein is a replacement polymorphism, which accounts for about half of disease mutations (Stenson et al. 2009). SNPs that are not in protein-coding regions may still affect gene splicing, transcription factor binding, or the sequence of noncoding RNA. Gene expression affected by this type of SNP is referred to as an eSNP (expression SNP) and may be upstream or downstream from the gene. In the Health, Risk Factors, Exercise Training, and Genetics (HERITAGE) Family Study of 473 sedentary adults from 99 families, the heritability of gains in maximal oxygen uptake ($\dot{V}O_2max$) after a standardized 20-week exercise program was nearly 50%, which was mainly explained by just 21 single-nucleotide polymorphisms (SNPs) out of 324,611 genome-wide (Bouchard et al. 2011).

Claude Bouchard, a pioneer in the genetics of physical activity, has advocated for the expansion of research beyond common DNA variants by combining transcriptomics (or gene expression profiling) with genomics (Bouchard 2011). Unlike the genome, which except for mutations is fixed for a given cell line, the transcriptome varies according to external environmental conditions. Because it includes all mRNA transcripts in the cell, the transcriptome mostly reflects the genes that are being actively expressed at any given time. A common technology to profile gene expression uses a DNA microarray, a thin glass or silicon chip that consists of thousands of single-strand DNA fragments from different genes. Complementary pieces of labeled DNA or RNA are added that will fluoresce when they hybridize (i.e., bind) with activated DNA. DNA microarrays can be used to measure changes in gene expression, detect SNPs, or genotype a mutant genome. When applied to transcriptomics, a DNA copy of RNA is made using the enzyme reverse transcriptase.

Epigenetic events extend beyond the sequence of DNA nucleotides of the human genome. They alter gene transcription, genome replication, and cellular processes without changing the DNA sequence. Epigenetic events include chromatin packaging, histone modifications, and DNA methylation, which are described in chapter 3.

RESEARCH ISSUES

Research in exercise psychology is characterized by many of the issues common to research in cognitive and behavioral psychology, neuroscience, and exercise physiology. The following sections provide definitions of common terms in research, descriptions of research designs that have been used to gain insight into exercise behavior and its consequences, and explanations of experimental artifacts that can confound any scientific study. These topics provide a basis for understanding the discussions of research in subsequent chapters.

Common Terms

Exercise psychology draws from several disciplines, such as epidemiology and clinical medicine; and readers may be unfamiliar with some terms used to describe research in these areas. This section presents selected definitions.

- **bias**—The systematic departure of results from the correct values as a consequence of errors in design or investigational technique.
- **confounder**—An extraneous factor that is not a consequence of exposure or the experimental manipulation. A confounding variable causes a distortion in the study's effects. Confounders are determinants or correlates of the outcome under study and are unequally distributed among the exposed and unexposed individuals.
- **construct**—A term for a concept that exists theoretically but is not directly observable. The existence and level of constructs are inferred from observing and measuring behavior and from indexes, such as scores on a self-report questionnaire. Variables are the operational forms of the constructs, or how a construct is to be measured in a specific

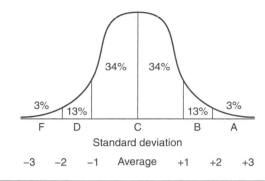

Figure 2.9 Effect size represents the amount of change from the average, or the distance from the mean in a normal curve.

situation. For example, someone's level of self-efficacy to overcome barriers to exercise can be inferred from a score on a self-efficacy scale.

- **effect size**—The magnitude of the outcome of an experimental manipulation, usually expressed as a standard score (e.g., [experimental mean − control mean]/ standard deviation; see figure 2.9). Effect size can be thought of as how much of a change there is from the average, as in the distance from the mean in a normal curve. For example, one standard-deviation effect is the same as raising a letter grade in a course by one letter (from a C to a B) based on a bell-shaped, or normal, grading curve.
- **effectiveness**—The ability of an intervention or method to work in other settings, or its level of ecological validity (i.e., can it be practically applied outside of a laboratory setting? Does it work?).
- **efficacy**—The ability of an intervention or method to do what it is intended to do (e.g., can it work?).
- **epidemiology**—The study of the distribution and determinants of health-related states and events (disease, injury, health behaviors) in a population and the application of this study to the control of health problems. Physical activity epidemiology includes studies of (1) the association of physical activity, as a health-related behavior, with diseases and other health outcomes; (2) the distribution and

determinants of physical activity behaviors; (3) the interrelationships of physical activity with other behaviors; and (4) the application of this knowledge to the prevention and control of disease and the promotion of health.

- **incidence**—The number of new cases of a disease or condition divided by the exposed population over a specified time frame. Incidence is used to measure the effectiveness of treatments or interventions. For example, if there are 150 new cases of depression in a population of 2,000 sedentary postmenopausal women over 5 years, the incidence of depression over 5 years is 7.5%.

- **mediator**—A variable in the causal path between an independent and a dependent variable. It is responsible for or transmits (mediates) the effects of an intervention on the outcome or on the effects of a change in one variable on another variable. For example, many believe that confidence in one's ability to exercise (exercise self-efficacy) mediates the effects of an intervention on exercise participation. Therefore, people adhere after an intervention because of the intervention's effects on self-efficacy. In this way, the intervention has an indirect effect on behavior by operating through self-efficacy.

- **meta-analysis,** or **quantitative review**— A method of synthesizing research literature by cumulating effect sizes or relative risks. This differs from a narrative critique of each study's results based on statistical hypothesis testing, which depends on sample size. A narrative critique of research articles is prone to bias from the subjective perspective of the author. A meta-analysis produces a statistical synthesis with less subjective bias, but it can be biased by the statistical methodology used and the quality of the studies included.

- **moderator**—A variable outside the causal pathway between an independent and dependent variable that modifies how an intervention or a mediator affects the outcome and results in an interaction. For example, age would moderate the effects of rock music on enjoyment in an exercise class if the only participants who liked this music were middle-aged baby boomers.

- **prevalence**—The number of existing cases of a disease or condition divided by the total population at a point in time. Prevalence is used to measure the burden of the disease and to plan for the implementation of services.

- **relative risk**—The ratio of the two rates (i.e., proportions) of the occurrence of disease in two groups. If the disease rates are 20% in an inactive group and 10% in an active group, the relative risk for inactivity is 2.0; or conversely, the relative risk for activity is 0.50.

- **sensitivity**—The ability of a test to detect a disease or attribute. For example, a test that is sensitive for depression will have few false negatives; it will not miss cases of depression when they truly exist.

Sensitivity and Specificity

Imagine that your goal is to discover the prevalence of employees at a local manufacturing plant who are highly physically active in their leisure time. You administer a scale designed to measure level of physical activity. The scale's sensitivity is its ability to identify those who are highly active. With the use of this scale, very few employees who are truly active at high levels are classified as having a low level of physical activity. The scale's specificity is its ability to correctly define those who are not highly active. Very few low-active or moderately active employees are misclassified as highly active. A scale having high sensitivity and specificity will have high predictive validity.

- **specificity**—The ability of a test to discriminate. For example, a test that is specific for depression will detect only symptoms of depression; it will indicate few false positives.

Research Design

Much research in sport psychology has been plagued by studies designed and conducted by psychologists who were unfamiliar with sports medicine, and by exercise physiologists who had a limited background in psychology. The quality of the research in exercise psychology has also been shadowed by this problem. Few researchers have dual degrees in exercise physiology and psychology, and the corresponding gaps in knowledge and experience are reflected in problems in **experimental design** and measurement.

Often, research has not been based on theory, or researchers have not matched the research to the theoretical model of the psychological construct. For example, theoretically, trait anxiety is stable so there is no need to measure trait anxiety both before and after acute exercise. Some researchers who have used theoretical models have applied them only in part, limiting the ability to explain the lack of significant effects. Most applications of social cognitive theories to understanding physical activity typically have not included measures of personal biological influences on physical activity, or have claimed to be based on this theory while only measuring self-efficacy. Only a few studies applying the transtheoretical model to exercise behavior have included all of the model's components.

Several issues relate specifically to research design. Most studies in which the aim is to

Scientific Criteria for Causality

A situation or condition can be considered as causing an event if it is a temporal antecedent to the event and if the event would not have occurred had the situation or condition not been present. There are scientific standards to identify something as a cause. Selected criteria used in epidemiology (Mausner and Kramer 1985) to judge the strength of causal evidence linking exercise with mental health benefits are as follows:

- Strength of association: The lower the disease rate among active people relative to inactive people, the more likely physical activity protects against disease; a halving of the rate of disease is an acceptable standard.

- Temporal sequence: The measurement of physical activity must precede the onset of disease with sufficient time for healthful biological adaptations.

- Consistency: The association of increased activity with reduced disease should appear in different regions and in different

types of people, using different methods of study.

- Independence: The association of reduced disease among physically active people is not explained by disproportionately higher occurrence of other causes of the disease among the physically inactive (e.g., age, smoking, poor social support).

- Dose–response gradient: Increased levels of physical activity should correspond with decreased levels of disease in a linear or curvilinear manner.

- Plausibility: Explanations for reduced disease with increased physical activity are coherent with existing theory or knowledge about the etiology of the disease and about biological adaptations that occur with physical activity.

- Experimental confirmation: Controlled experiments confirm that increasing physical activity prevents or reduces the disease occurrence.

relate exercise and mental health have been cross-sectional (e.g., screening, correlational) or predictive, and therefore cannot provide information about cause and effect.

In **cross-sectional designs**, subjects are identified and classified according to exposure and outcome at the same point in time. These types of studies are also called prevalence studies. Cross-sectional designs are good for general description and for the identification of trends, but there are problems associated with selective survival and with subject recall when questionnaire data are used.

A **case-control design** is a retrospective design commonly used in epidemiology to "reconstruct" the likely causes of health-related events after they have occurred. Ideally, healthy controls are matched with cases (e.g., sick people) on age, sex, and race and are often recruited from the same setting as the cases. Then, a comparison of the two groups is made on the frequency of past exposure to potential risk factors for the disease. Risk factor information is typically obtained by personal interview or from a review of medical records. Disadvantages of the case-control design include difficulty in obtaining a truly representative control group, the inability to study more than one disease outcome at a time, and the potential for recall bias. Case-control studies are useful for the initial development and testing of hypotheses to determine whether there is justification for moving forward to conduct more time-consuming and expensive cohort studies or randomized trials.

Predictive designs and prospective or cohort studies group disease-free subjects according to exposure and then evaluate them over time to determine the disease occurrence in exposed and unexposed groups. The measure of association is expressed as a relative risk. Prospective studies have provided important evidence for the effects of exercise on mental health and have directed attention to potential mediating variables for inclusion in exercise interventions.

Randomized controlled trials (RCTs) are used to determine whether associations uncovered in epidemiological observations or in small laboratory experiments represent cause-and-effect relations that apply to large numbers of people, usually diagnosed with a disease.

The validity of the trial depends on having a representative population sample and on similarities between treatment and control groups with respect to characteristics thought to affect outcome. The random assignment of subjects to treatment or control groups is essential to equally distribute known and unknown confounding variables between groups. **Control groups** should experience all things in common with the treatment group except the critical treatment factor. Some researchers wishing to evaluate the effects of exercise on psychological variables have had the control group sit in a quiet room, attend a lecture, or even receive instructions to imagine exercising. In a clinical population, the effects of exercise on mental health should be compared to a traditional treatment rather than to a no-treatment control. Publishing the results of RCTs with some standardization has been facilitated by the Consolidated Standards of Reporting Trials (CONSORT). In 1996, researchers conducting clinical trials and journal editors created a 25-item checklist for reporting information and a flow diagram to illustrate the passage of participants through the clinical trial. The most recent revision is on the CONSORT statement website, included at the end of this chapter.

Many studies in exercise psychology have used convenient samples and volunteers. This introduces the problem of the self-selection of motivated people into the study. People who volunteer to be in an intervention study are probably already more likely to adhere to a regular exercise program or believe they will benefit. Anxious people are unlikely to volunteer for a study on anxiety and exercise. Many studies of exercise and mental health have thus tested normal subjects, for whom there is little room for improvement regardless of the efficacy of the intervention. Sample size is also an issue in that a large sample may result in a statistically significant effect that has little clinical signifi-

> **C**ontrol groups should experience all things in common with the treatment group except the critical treatment factor.

cance. Likewise, it can happen that the effects from a small sample are clinically important, but a lack of power prevents statistically meaningful differences.

The outcome of interest in mental health research is typically psychological or psychobiological constructs (or both), and the experimental, or independent, variable is exercise behavior. Exercise adoption and adherence research uses interventions and psychosocial variables as experimental, or predictor, variables with the level of physical activity as the dependent, or outcome, variable. Regardless of the focus, there are inconsistencies and limitations in the measurement of the dependent and independent variables in exercise psychology. Often, there is a lack of clarity in the definition of the psychological constructs being tested, as well as an abundance of different instruments that purport to measure the same construct. Sometimes the researcher develops instruments to measure psychological variables but does not report reliability and validity.

Psychological measures of mental health are often inadequate. For example, one should not use self-report alone to assess depression and anxiety; measurements of physiological changes coincident with psychological changes are also needed. Studies in which biological variables are measured can have methodological limitations that restrict the ability to isolate specific mechanisms of action. For example, urinary and plasma levels of metabolites of neurotransmitters involved in mood disorders may be measured in conjunction with acute and chronic exercise. However, absolute levels and increases or decreases cannot be used to estimate adaptations in the central nervous system.

The application of theories, research designs, subjects, and the measurement of independent and dependent variables are issues in exercise psychology research.

Experimental Artifacts

Most often, self-report is used to assess psychological constructs that are treated as outcome variables or as mediators of behavior change. Several behavioral artifacts are known to influence research dealing with psychological outcomes (Morgan 1997), and research in exercise psychology is not immune to these effects. Such effects generally involve an alteration of true responses because of factors related to expectations by the participants (e.g., people respond the way they think the researcher wants them to), expectations by the experimenter (e.g., a subjective rating is biased), or experimenter effects on the participant (e.g., an investigator knowingly or unknowingly tips off the participant about the purpose of the study). Examples of experimental artifacts include the following:

- The **halo effect** is an experimenter expectancy effect in which certain characteristics are ascribed to a subject based on other known characteristics. A tester might assume that someone who scores low on trait anxiety would not be anxious about participating in a graded maximal exercise test, and thus incorrectly interpret signs of anxiety (e.g., high heart rate and high perceived exertion) as indications of low fitness.

- Participants' expectations also influence their responses. Someone who already believes that physical activity helps people sleep better might unwittingly inflate self-reports of how much his or her sleep has been improved after an exercise study.

- Demand characteristics include subtle messages about the experimental hypothesis that permit a motivated participant to guess the hypothesis of the study and strive to confirm or, conversely, sabotage the purpose of the study.

- The **Rosenthal effect**, or the self-fulfilling prophecy, is also known as the Pygmalion effect. This occurs when the participant is motivated to meet the expectations that the investigator has communicated about the participant's attributes or abilities.

- The **Hawthorne effect** is the tendency of the participants to improve after the manipulation of the independent variable simply because of the attention associated with the treatment. This influence is particularly critical to consider in the design of studies of exercise and mental health.

Beneficial psychological changes cannot be fully ascribed to exercise when exercise is compared to a no-treatment condition, because anything might be better than nothing. The researcher should take the Hawthorne effect into account by demonstrating that exercise is better than a placebo treatment condition and that it is as effective as, or more effective than, other traditional treatments.

• **Social desirability responding,** or **motivated response distortion,** must be taken into account because people have a tendency to want to conform to socially desirable images of themselves. People can be consciously motivated to distort answers (i.e., lie) on a test to present a good impression. They also can unconsciously deceive themselves by distorting reality to enhance self-esteem, personal efficacy, and optimism (i.e., self-deception enhancement; Paulhus 1984). This tendency toward socially desirable responses especially threatens the accuracy of scales measuring self-perception constructs that are valued in society, such as self-esteem. People also may overestimate behaviors that are socially valued (e.g., physical activity) or underreport symptoms of disorders that carry a social stigma (e.g., depression).

SUMMARY

The purpose of this chapter is to provide definitions and introduce perspectives on research in exercise psychology. Because an aim of this text is to be accessible to readers with a range of backgrounds, terms familiar to some readers—such as *exercise, physical activity,* and *fitness*—were defined and discussed. Other aspects critical to the definition and measurement of psychological constructs, such as scaling and statistical methods, may be less familiar; these were presented in more depth to help make subsequent discussions clearer and to help the reader become a more critical consumer of research. Issues in research were introduced as a basis for understanding the discussions of methodology in subsequent chapters.

WEBSITES

www.rasch.org/memos.htm (see memo 62)

http://davidmlane.com/hyperstat/index.html

www.consort-statement.org/home

https://sites.google.com/site/theipaq/home

www.afhayes.com/spss-sas-and-mplus-macros-and-code.html

https://sites.google.com/site/compendiumofphysical activities

http://geneticassociationdb.nih.gov

Behavioral Neuroscience

Examining the relationship between exercise and changes in social and cognitive variables, such as self-esteem and personal beliefs, contributes to our understanding of how exercise can affect mental health and how to increase exercise adherence. However, behavior and brain function are also determined by biological factors. Although modern-day muscle biologists may not agree, William James remarked, "It is pretty well understood now that the result of physical training is to train the nervous centers more than the muscles" (James, W., 1899, p. 220).

Thus, readers will need a basic understanding of the central nervous system, the autonomic nervous system, key neurotransmitters, and the cellular and molecular biology of the brain to fully understand subsequent chapters on stress; affect, mood, and emotion; anxiety; depression; cognition; and energy, fatigue, and sleep.

This chapter provides a basic overview of behavioral neuroscience, which is the measurement of neural events applied to the study of brain and behavior. The goal is not to review neuroanatomy and **neurobiology** in depth, but rather to provide a primer for subsequent discussions of physiological mechanisms for effects of exercise on aspects of mental health. For example, when improvements in depression are suggested in light of the relationship between exercise and neurotrophins such as VGF and brain-derived neurotrophic factor (BDNF), or galanin inhibition of the locus coeruleus, or the reduced density of β-receptors in the brain cortex, the reader will be able to refer back to this chapter.

The section The Neural Network presents the basic anatomy of the central nervous system, the autonomic nervous system, and the hypo-

thalamic-pituitary-adrenal axis. Major functions critical to mood and behavior are included. The measurement and interpretation of heart rate variability are also discussed to illustrate the use of noninvasive methods of psychophysiology for understanding how the autonomic nervous system regulates the cardiovascular system during stress or in patients with anxiety disorders.

The section Neurotransmitters reviews the mood-influencing neurotransmitters in terms of their actions in the nervous system. The next section, Cellular and Molecular Biology of the Brain, presents some basic concepts and techniques used to measure gene expression and regulation, including in situ hybridization histochemistry and immunocytochemistry. The use of animal models of human disease and behavior is discussed in the following section. Finally, the section Measuring Brain Activity addresses the methods of electrophysiology, microdialysis, electroencephalography, and neuroimaging as they are applied to measure brain activity during behavior and emotional responses. Most of the material covered in later chapters can be generally understood without this chapter, but this content will help students more fully appreciate these complex phenomena and techniques.

THE NEURAL NETWORK

The anatomical basis for information processing is the extensive network of neural pathways and circuits that serve to connect people with their internal worlds (e.g., memories, tightness in a muscle, hunger) and the external world (see figure 3.1). The neural network is divided

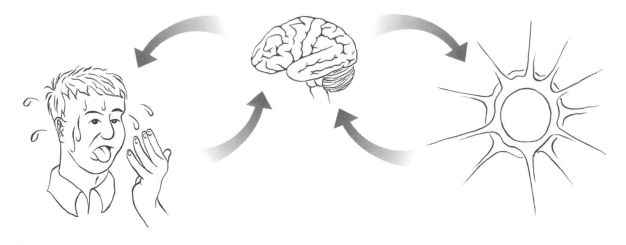

Figure 3.1 The central nervous system processes sensations of heat and light from the environment and orchestrates our physiological, psychological, and behavioral responses.

into the central nervous system and the peripheral nervous system, shown in figure 3.2. The peripheral nervous system is organized into two components: the somatic nervous system (the cranial and spinal nerves), which receives sensory information and controls skeletal muscles, and the autonomic nervous system. Because of their roles in mental health and behavior, the central nervous system and the autonomic nervous system are described in more detail later.

> **T**he central nervous system connects the individual with his or her internal and external world.

Central Nervous System

The central nervous system (CNS) is one of the most intricate and complicated systems in the body (see figure 3.4). It is responsible for sensing, screening, processing, storing, and responding to millions of bits of information 24 hours a day, 7 days a week. This is a dynamic system that has a reciprocal relationship with the rest of the body and the external world. Every time you learn something new, the chemistry of your brain (often including the transcription of genes encoding brain proteins that regulate neural activity) is altered by that process. A biological framework for the etiology of mental disorders

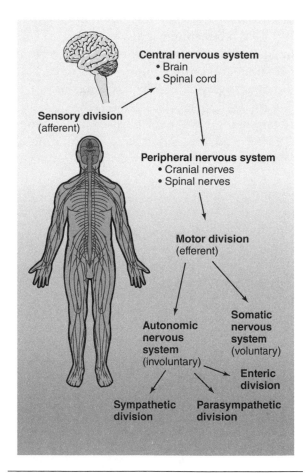

Figure 3.2 The central and peripheral nervous systems in the human body.

Reprinted, by permission, from J.H. Wilmore and D.L. Costill, 1999, *Physiology of sport and exercise,* 2nd ed. (Champaign, IL: Human Kinetics), 64.

The Somatic Nervous System

The **cranial nerves**, connected directly to the brain, include bundles of axons that form 12 pairs. Cranial nerves are sensory (transmit sensory information to the brain, e.g., olfactory, optic), motor (innervate specific muscles, e.g., hypoglossal—moves the tongue), or both sensory and motor (e.g., vagus) (see figure 3.3).

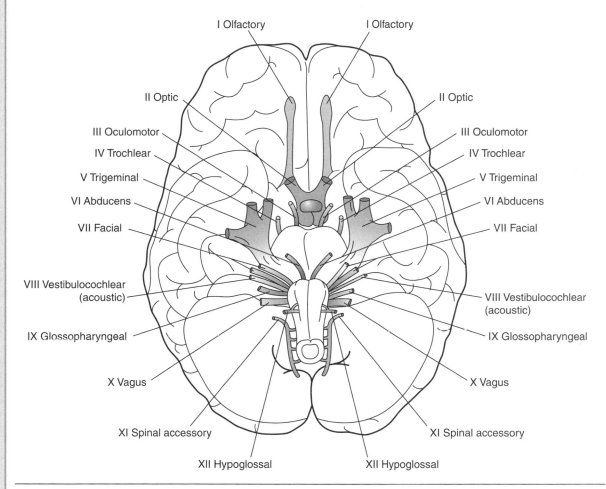

Figure 3.3 Some cranial nerves send sensory information to the brain, some innervate specific muscles, and some do both.

Reprinted, by permission, from S.J. Shultz, P.A. Houglum, and D.H. Perrin, 2000, *Assessment of athletic injuries* (Champaign, IL: Human Kinetics), 348.

There are 31 pairs of **spinal nerves** that join the spinal cord at regularly spaced intervals and are named according to the segment of the spinal cord to which they are attached (i.e., cervical, thoracic, lumbar, or sacral). Each spinal nerve consists of sensory pathways from the periphery to the spinal cord, as well as motor pathways from the spinal cord to the muscles.

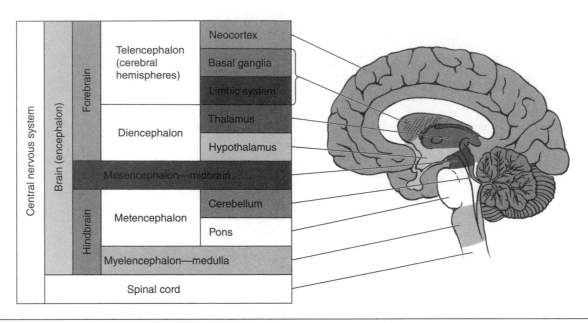

Figure 3.4 The organization of the central nervous system, including the spinal cord and three regions of the brain (forebrain, midbrain, and hindbrain).

that describes the interaction between structure and function was proposed by psychiatrist Eric Kandel (1998). This framework includes five principles:

1. Actions at the brain level are responsible for all mental and psychological processes.
2. Brain functioning is controlled by genes.
3. Social, developmental, and environmental factors can produce alterations in gene expression.
4. Alterations in gene expression induce changes in brain functioning.
5. Treatments for mental illness exert their effects by producing alterations in gene expression resulting in beneficial changes in brain function.

Thus, within this framework, depression and other mood disorders result from disturbances in brain processes; treatments such as psychotherapy, medication, and exercise produce changes in brain function at a genetic level that result in the alleviation of symptoms. How all this happens is not fully understood, but significant progress is being made in describing the structure and function of the nervous system and its interrelationships with behavior and mood.

The structure of the central nervous system consists of the spinal cord, the brain stem, and the brain (forebrain). The **spinal cord** contains neural circuits that control a variety of reflexive functions; it provides the pathway for bringing sensory input from the periphery to the brain and carrying messages or motor signals from the brain to the periphery. The **afferent**, or sensory, signals travel to the brain via the dorsal horn of the spinal cord to send information about internal organs, muscles, body position, and other peripheral sensations. The **efferent**, or motor, neurons travel down the ventral horn to form the motor portion of the spinal nerves and to innervate muscles. Spinal nerves are not like cables that merely conduct a signal. Considerable processing of neural signals occurs in the spinal cord; this can dramatically alter the signal as it passes between organs and the central nervous system. Dorsal (sensory) and ventral (motor) roots from the spinal cord are fused to form the right and left sides of each of the 31 spinal nerve pairs.

Figure 3.5 shows a cross section of a spinal cord with the dorsal and ventral horns labeled. Type III and type IV afferent neural fibers, which primarily transmit nociceptive (pain) signals, innervate mainly both the dorsal and ventral horns of the spinal cord. Dorsal and ventral column pathways are discussed in more detail in chapter 16, which addresses perceived exertion.

Both sensory and motor neurons from the periphery and the brain pass through the brain stem. The **brain stem** is a continuous extension of the spinal cord upward into the cranial cavity; it consists of the **medulla** (mylencephalon), **pons** (metencephalon), and **midbrain** (mesencephalon) (see figure 3.6). Far from being a simple conduit, the brain stem contains several neural centers critical to behavior and mood, in addition to controlling functions basic to life, such as arterial blood pressure and respiration.

The medulla marks the transition from the spinal cord to the brain stem. It contributes to the regulation of cardiorespiratory functions and contains the end of the **reticular formation**, which extends up into the midbrain. The major **nuclei** for serotonin (also known as 5-HT) are the **raphe nuclei**, located mainly in the center line of the brain stem near the locus coeruleus. The raphe cells send projections to parts of the brain that control emotion and behavior (e.g., amygdala, hippocampus, hypothalamus, ventral tegmental area, and frontal cortex), locomotion (e.g., the **striatum** and **cerebellum**),

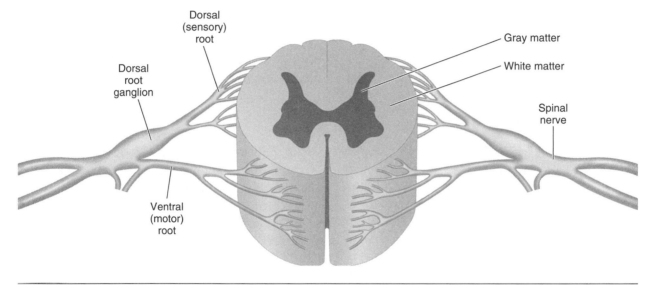

Figure 3.5 Cross section of the spinal cord.

Reprinted, by permission, from J.H. Wilmore and D.L. Costill, 1999, *Physiology of sport and exercise,* 2nd ed. (Champaign, IL: Human Kinetics), 67.

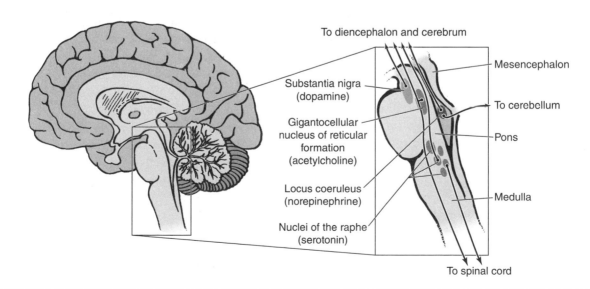

Figure 3.6 Diagram of the brain stem and its primary nuclei and associated neurotransmitters.

blood pressure (e.g., the area postrema in the brain stem just outside the blood–brain barrier, which is sensitive to changes in concentrations of chemicals in the blood), and the processing of other peripheral signals such as pain (spinal cord). Serotonin is a critical neurotransmitter in anxiety and depression and also functions in the regulation of sleep and eating.

> The medulla contains the raphe nucleus, the major nucleus in the brain for the production of the neurotransmitter serotonin.

The pons wraps around the base of the cerebellum and contains nuclei involved in motor control and sensory analysis. The cerebellum is located dorsal to the pons and is a critical component of the motor system, integrating sensory information with information about muscle movement to coordinate movement. The pons contains the **locus coeruleus (LC)**, identified as a bluish area just below the fourth ventricle of the brain (*locus coeruleus* comes from the Latin word *caeruleus,* meaning "blue"). The overall role of the LC is to inhibit spontaneous firing in the areas it innervates, which include the cerebellum, hippocampus, amygdala, thalamic and hypothalamic nuclei, cerebral cortex, mesencephalon (midbrain), and spinal cord. The LC is also involved in rapid eye movement (REM) sleep, attention, and emotional responses, and it is the major nucleus for **norepinephrine (NE)**, a neurotransmitter important in brain activation and mood regulation. About half the cells that make NE in the brain are located in the LC.

The midbrain, or mesencephalon, forms the top of the brain stem. It includes portions of

> The locus coeruleus, which is the primary site for the production of the neurotransmitter norepinephrine in the brain, is located in the pons.

the reticular formation, the substantia nigra, the central gray, and the ventral tegmental area. The reticular formation is a network of neurons running from the upper spinal cord through the medulla, pons, and midbrain to the ventral diencephalon, where we find the reticular nucleus. The reticular activating system is a structure of many diffuse, interconnected networks of nuclei. It plays a role in the sleep–wake cycle, forebrain arousal, attention, temperature regulation, and motor control.

The substantia nigra is a major center for the neurotransmitter dopamine and an important **ganglion** (collection of neurons) in motor control. The central gray (periaqueductal gray; PAG) is a region tightly packed with neural bodies in the center of the brain stem around the aqueduct that connects the third and fourth ventricles. Some of the functions of the central gray are emotional arousal, fighting, mating, and pain. When opioid **receptors** on neurons in the central gray are stimulated by opiates, sensitivity to noxious stimuli decreases.

The ventral tegmental area (VTA) is located below the PAG and medial to the substantia nigra. It is a major source of brain dopamine. Activation of the VTA results in the motivation to engage in appetitive (i.e., seeking) behaviors, and when innervated with opioid neurons in the ventral striatum, these behaviors are rewarding or pleasurable.

Every organ in the body is connected to the brain, which weighs only 1,400 grams (3 lb), or 2% of your body weight (about the weight of this textbook!) (Rosenzweig, Leiman, and Breedlove 1999a). The forebrain is responsible for the ability to read a book, ride a bicycle, and decide whether to enroll in a strength training class. The forebrain, which is the most rostral (anterior) portion of the brain, is divided into the **diencephalon** and the **telencephalon**. The most important structures in the diencephalon are the thalamus and the hypothalamus. The **thalamus** has bidirectional connections with many areas in the cerebral cortex. It is the pathway for all sensory systems except the olfactory. The dorsal thalamus processes, integrates, and relays sensory input into the telencephalon. When you step outside for a walk, the sensations of ambient temperature, light, sound, and feedback from your muscles are all processed in the thalamus before they are received in your higher brain for use in making decisions and taking action. The anterior thalamus projects into the limbic system and is involved in motivation and emotion. The medial and lateral nuclei of the thalamus are involved in the mediation of pain.

The **hypothalamus** projects downward to the brain stem; upward to other areas of the diencephalon, cerebrum, anterior thalamus, and limbic cortex; and into the infundibulum to control secretory functions of the pituitary gland, a critical gland in the control of almost all hormone secretion. The hypothalamus controls vegetative functions such as cardiovascular activity, feeding, sleep, and temperature regulation. It also regulates hormonal balance and plays a major role in many aspects of emotional behavior. The hypothalamus is part of the triumvirate of the hypothalamic-pituitary-adrenal axis, which is central in responding to mental and physical stress, as discussed later in this chapter and in chapter 4.

The telencephalon is composed of the neocortex (cerebral cortex), the basal ganglia, and the limbic system. The **neocortex** surrounds the cerebral hemispheres and is characterized by an elaborate folding of tissue, with small grooves (sulci), large grooves (fissures), and large ridges of tissue (gyri) that triple the area of the neocortex; about two-thirds of the surface is hidden in the depths of these folds. The neocortex is the center of higher brain functions, such as problem solving, creativity, and judgment. Areas of the neocortex, such as the primary visual cortex and the primary motor cortex, have been charted according to their input and function. For example, the medial prefrontal cortex serves to shift affective states on the basis of internal and external stimuli, and is the only cortical region that sends direct projections into the hypothalamus.

The **basal ganglia** are a collection of subcortical nuclei in the forebrain that includes the corpus striatum, consisting of the striatum (caudate, putamen, and nucleus accumbens) and globus pallidus, as well as cell groups associated

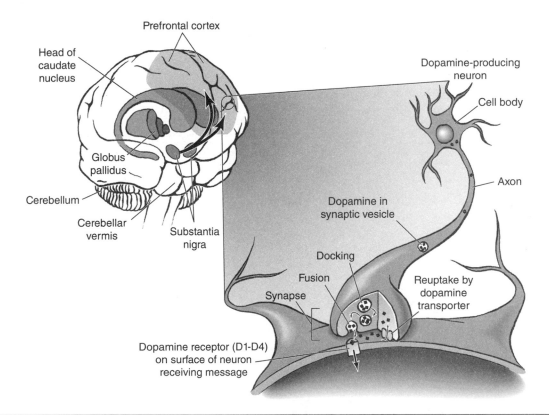

Figure 3.7 Structures of the basal ganglia and the actions of dopamine from production to postsynaptic activation.
Adapted from Barkley 1998.

with the corpus striatum, such as the subthalamic nucleus and substantia nigra. The basal ganglia are critical in the control of movement. The substantia nigra, shown in perspective to the other basal ganglia in figure 3.7, is a major source of dopamine in the brain. Dopamine plays a critical role in motor functions, but it is also associated with motivation and mood, as will be discussed later and in chapter 7.

The **limbic system** is a widespread collection of nuclei that completely surrounds the diencephalon. It has two-way linkages with the neocortex and elicits behavioral functions that are mediated through the reticular nuclei of the brain stem. The limbic system is considered the seat of emotional behavior and motivational drives and has a role in learning. It is involved in the expression of instinct and mood, self-preservation, and the establishment of memory patterns. Thus, the limbic system controls a variety of functions that are of interest if we want to examine the psychobiology of exercise.

Parts of the limbic system that are important in exercise and mental health are the amygdala (Latin for its shape, like that of an almond) and the hippocampus (Latin for its seahorse shape), shown in figure 3.8 in respect to other areas of the limbic system. The **amygdala** is a portion of the limbic system that controls appropriate behavior for social situations and is linked to emotional memory as well as the generation of anger and fear. Its significance in exercise and affect is discussed in chapter 5.

The **hippocampus** functions in labeling changes in the environment as threatening and in declarative memory storage. The hippocampus transfers input that is appraised as important into the cerebral cortex. When the hippocampus is stimulated, the person becomes hypervigilant and apprehensive. Receptors for cortisol on the hippocampus implicate it in physiological responses to depression (chapter 7) and chronic mental stress (chapter 4).

> **T**he limbic system is the area of the central nervous system that is the center of emotional behavior and motivational drives.

Autonomic Nervous System

The **autonomic nervous system** (ANS) is a branch of the peripheral nervous system that spans the central and peripheral nervous systems. It was named autonomic (independent, self-governing) because early anatomists discovered its ganglia outside of the central nervous system. The autonomic nervous system regulates the viscera, some glands, smooth muscle, and cardiac

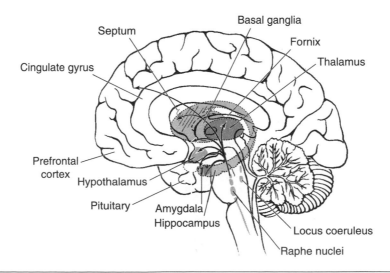

Figure 3.8 Cross section of the central nervous system showing limbic structures (hippocampus, amygdala, cingulate gyrus, fornix). Arrows show the pathways from the raphe nuclei to the central structures.

Adapted from Nemeroff 1998.

muscle primarily by the activity of cranial nerves 3, 7, 9, and 10 and other sympathetic nerves. It is made up of three branches—the sympathetic, parasympathetic, and enteric nervous systems—that send messages via neurotransmitters (NT) from the central nervous system to the ganglia. All preganglionic NT receptors are nicotinic cholinergic (activated by the NT acetylcholine), whereas the postganglionic NT vary as a function of their receptors. The β- and α-adrenoreceptors are activated by NE and epinephrine, and muscarinic cholinergic receptors are activated by acetylcholine. Figure 3.9 shows autonomic nerves and the organs they innervate. Generally, the sympathetic nervous system is involved in energy expenditure, and the parasympathetic is involved in energy conservation. The **enteric system** controls the intestines.

The continuously active basal rates of sympathetic and parasympathetic nerve discharge are known as sympathetic tone and parasympathetic tone. Effects on an organ can be the result of either an increase or a decrease in sympathetic or parasympathetic activation. At one time the accepted view was that these two systems had a linear reciprocal relationship with tightly coupled reciprocal control. However, Berntson, Cacioppo, and Quigley (1991, 1993) provided compelling arguments and experimental evidence for a broader, two-dimensional model of autonomic control. In their doctrine of autonomic space, the activation of the two branches may be coupled or uncoupled. Coupled responses in which both systems are activated simultaneously may be reciprocal or nonreciprocal, the latter entailing concurrent increases or decreases in both parasympathetic and sympathetic activation. For example, an exaggerated stress-related increase in heart rate could be from elevated sympathetic activation alone (uncoupled), potent parasympathetic withdrawal (uncoupled), or both (coupled reciprocal) (Berntson et al. 1993).

The absence of a change in heart rate in response to mental stress does not mean there is no autonomic response, but instead can result from an increase in parasympathetic activity that cancels out sympathetic activation (coupled nonreciprocal). The possibility of a physiological

response that is not manifest in end-organ activity is important to keep in mind when considering the limitations of research on exercise and stress reactivity in chapter 4.

> The autonomic nervous system has two branches that control energy expenditure (sympathetic) and energy conservation (parasympathetic). They can act alone, together with one increasing and the other decreasing activation, or together with both increasing or decreasing activation.

Sympathetic Nervous System

The **sympathetic nervous system** (SNS) is involved in arousal and activities that require energy expenditure, such as exercise. Simply put, the SNS prepares the body for action (such as when you are waiting for the start of a road race) or for the fight-or-flight response to a perceived threat (such as that posed by a large, snarling dog). Preparing the body for action in the face of mental stress when there is no opportunity for physical action is part of the stress response that may contribute to several stress-related illnesses, such as hypertension.

The SNS consists of 22 pairs of ganglia strung together on either side of the spinal cord, connected to each other and to the spinal cord. The preganglionic neurons connected to the spinal cord are short, whereas the postganglionic neurons are long; the latter connect to the effector organs, such as the heart and sweat glands (see figure 3.9). The postganglionic neurons are adrenergic, releasing NE to α- and β-adrenergic receptors on the effector organs to produce a host of effects. The effect from activation and deactivation of the SNS is analogous to turning an electrical current on and off, respectively, to rooms in a house or to the whole house. Depending on the type or severity of circumstances, responses can be specific to a single organ, a few organs, or all the organs innervated by the SNS. Heart rate increases, the person begins to sweat, the eyes dilate, the mouth becomes dry,

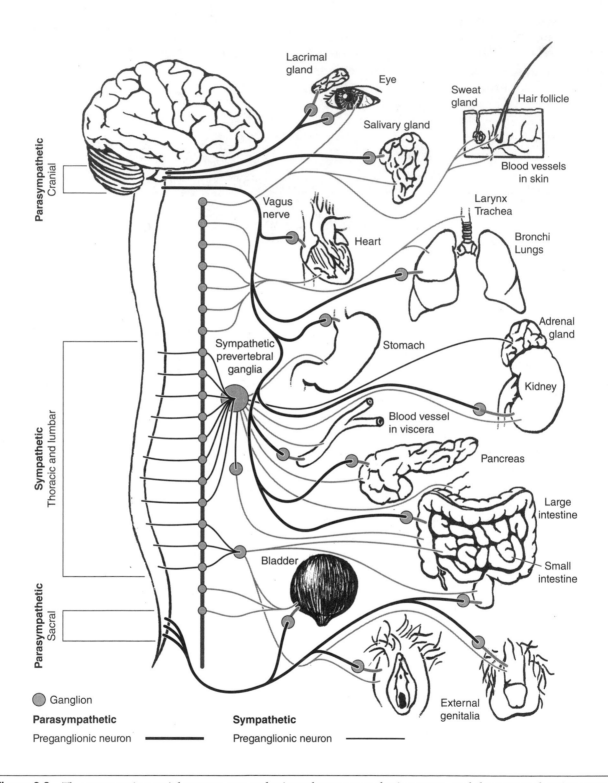

Figure 3.9 The autonomic cranial nerves, sympathetic and parasympathetic nerves, and the organs they innervate.

Carlson, Neil R., *Physiology of Behavior*, 6th Edition, © 1998. Adapted by permission of Pearson Education, Inc., Upper Saddle River, NJ. Copyright 1994 by Allyn & Bacon.

and other less obvious effects of SNS activation occur together.

Parasympathetic Nervous System

The **parasympathetic nervous system** (PNS) is involved in the conservation of energy, such as the slowing of heart rate and the stimulation of digestion. The PNS has long preganglionic neurons that originate in the head and sacral regions (see figure 3.9). The postganglionic neurons are short and are adjacent to the organs they innervate. The NT released postganglionically is **acetylcholine**, and the postsynaptic receptors are muscarinic cholinergic. Activation of the PNS is specific, analogous to turning on a lamp in a house, and so the PNS offers better voluntary control than the SNS. A person can salivate at the sight of a hot piece of pie without a corresponding decrease in heart rate. Acetylcholine results in the release of nitric oxide by endothelial cells in small, resistant blood vessels to relax smooth muscle and lower diastolic blood pressure.

> **T**he sympathetic nervous system is responsible for energy expenditure, and the parasympathetic nervous system contributes to energy conservation.

Autonomic Balance and the Cardiovascular System: Heart Rate Variability

Heart rate variability (HRV) provides information about the modulation of heart rate by the autonomic nervous system in a variety of dynamic circumstances (Task Force of the European Society of Cardiology and the North American Society of Pacing and Electrophysiology 1996), including the experience of emotions and during exercise. Heart rate variability is commonly described by the standard deviation of intervals between successive R waves of the cardiac cycle. Short-term variation (e.g., measured during periods of several minutes) can be decomposed mathematically into components of the frequency spectrum that estimate the autonomic modulation of heart rate. The high-frequency (HF) component (0.15-0.5 hertz; a hertz [Hz] is one complete cycle or period of oscillation per second) is believed to correspond to the modulation of HRV by the vagus nerve during breathing and is also called respiratory sinus arrhythmia (see figure 3.10). These relatively fast fluctuations correspond to the changes in heart rate measured when the vagus nerve is electrically stimulated in animals, and reflect the rapid action of acetylcholine in inhibiting heart cells by directly opening ion channels.

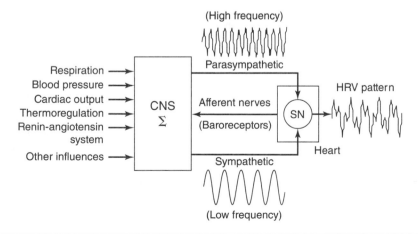

Figure 3.10 The high-frequency parasympathetic and the low-frequency sympathetic contributions to a pattern of heart rate variability.

Reprinted, by permission, from R. McCraty and A. Watkins, 1996, *Autonomic assessment report: A comprehensive heart rate variability analysis. Interpretation guide and instructions* (Boulder Creek, CA: HeartMath Research Center), 7.

The low-frequency (LF) spectrum (0.05-0.15 Hz) corresponds to the baroreflex control of heart rate (i.e., in response to changes in blood pressure) and reflects the mixed sympathetic and parasympathetic modulation of HRV in most circumstances. These slower fluctuations of heart rate result from a slower response by the heart to sympathetic modulation than to vagal modulation, mainly because the action of NE on heart cells depends on a second-messenger system to open ion channels rather than a direct action such as that of acetylcholine. More about the second-messenger system follows later in this chapter. Activity in the very low frequency (VLF) spectrum (0.0033-0.05 Hz) can provide another index of sympathetic influence on heart rate.

To estimate autonomic balance during short-term fluctuations in heart rate, the HF and LF components commonly are normalized to their total power (e.g., [HF / (HF + LF) × 100]) to remove the influences of VLF. Long-term (e.g., 24-hour) monitoring of HRV permits the assessment of the ultra-low-frequency spectrum (<0.0033 Hz), which is strongly correlated with total HRV (i.e., the standard deviation of the RR interval across the 24-hour period).

Low HRV (especially the high-frequency component) is associated with perceived stress and with cardiac arrhythmia, cardiac mortality, and all-cause mortality after myocardial infarction. Low HRV has been reported in people with clinical anxiety disorders, including panic, posttraumatic stress, and generalized anxiety disorders. Because perceived stress is a predictor of transient myocardial ischemia, HRV may be a population risk factor for cardiac events (Tsuji et al. 1996). Several studies have shown that people with high cardiorespiratory fitness have higher HRV, especially in the high-frequency range. Whether fitness can buffer the effects of stress on HRV is not yet known, but one study found that middle-aged adults who report persistent emotional stress have less high-frequency HRV (Dishman, Nakamura et al. 2000), regardless of their age, sex, or level of physical fitness.

Endocrine System

The rich, dynamic interaction between the central nervous system and the autonomic nervous system is illustrated by the sympathetic medullary system and the hypothalamic-pituitary-adrenal axis (HPA), which are both activated by the hypothalamus.

The **sympathetic medullary system** includes the SNS and the **adrenal medulla**, which is activated by the posterior hypothalamus through a direct neural pathway. Norepinephrine is synthesized by the chromaffin cells of the adrenal medulla, and NE and epinephrine (Epi) are secreted by the adrenal medulla as hormones into the bloodstream in a ratio of 1 (NE) to 4 (Epi). The actions of NE and Epi are sympathomimetic; that is, they mimic the effects of SNS activation. However, the effects last 5 to 10 times longer than direct SNS stimulation (1-2 min after the stimulus is over) because of the slow removal of these neurohormones from the blood. The primary effect of plasma NE is to increase blood pressure by increasing peripheral resistance. Epinephrine produces more general sympathetic effects, such as increased heart rate and enhanced cellular metabolism.

The **hypothalamic-pituitary-adrenal axis** includes the hypothalamus, the pituitary, and the adrenal cortex (see figure 3.11). The pituitary gland, which is connected directly to the hypothalamus by the pituitary stalk, consists of two main parts (anterior, or adenohypophysis, and posterior, or neurohypophysis) that are separate in function. The adrenal cortex is the outer covering of the adrenal gland.

The anterior hypothalamus releases two potent hormones (thyroid-stimulating hormone and corticotropin-releasing hormone) that are involved in the response to physical and mental stress. **Thyroid-stimulating hormone** causes the anterior pituitary to release thyrotropic hormone,

> **M**easures of heart rate variability provide information about the modulation of heart rate by the autonomic nervous system and can tell us about the sympathetic and parasympathetic contributions to responses in various situations.

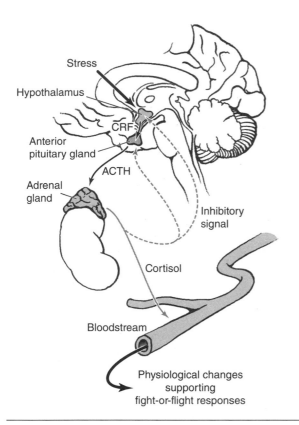

Figure 3.11 Activation of the hypothalamus, pituitary, and adrenal cortex (HPA) in response to stress.

Adapted from Nemeroff 1998.

which stimulates the thyroid gland to release thyroxin. Thyroxin stimulates carbohydrate and fat metabolism and increases metabolic rate. **Corticotropin-releasing hormone** (CRH) is released by the anterior hypothalamus (the parvicellula, or small cell, area of the paraventricular nucleus that lies on each side of the third ventricle of the brain) as part of circadian rhythms and in response to physical and mental stress.

Corticotropin-releasing hormone stimulates the posterior pituitary to release vasopressin (antidiuretic hormone); it also stimulates the anterior pituitary to release prolactin and the co-secretion of **adrenocorticotropic hormone** (ACTH) and β-endorphin into circulation. Adrenocorticotropic hormone activates the **adrenal cortex** to secrete aldosterone and cortisol. It also enhances the response of the adrenal cortex to subsequent stimulation; enhances attention, motivation, learning, and memory retention; and acts as an opiate antagonist.

Cortisol, the major glucocorticoid secreted by the adrenal cortex, plays a role in the stress response and depression. Major effects of cortisol include control over metabolism, such as the stimulation of gluconeogenesis (i.e., the synthesis of new sugars from fat or protein) and the mobilization of fatty acids for fuel during exercise, and the suppression of the immune response. Release of cortisol is controlled by ACTH, but there are receptors for cortisol on the hypothalamus and anterior pituitary that provide feedback to control the secretion of CRH and ACTH, respectively, and thus provide feedback regulation of cortisol secretion.

> **C**ortisol has a role in the response to physical stress (i.e., exercise) and mental stress, as well as in central nervous system dysregulation associated with mood disorders.

Brain and Peripheral Circulation

Later in the chapter we discuss methods used to measure brain blood flow in both cerebral arteries (see figure 3.12) and veins. Here, we consider how to gauge whether chemicals measured in peripheral veins have their origin in the brain.

Cerebral spinal fluid is secreted by the choroid plexus located in the lateral ventricles (see figure 3.13) and is replaced four times a day, about 600 milliliters (20 fl oz) in 24 hours. Cerebrospinal fluid drains into cerebral venus sinuses via arachnoid (i.e., spider-like) granulations in the space between the dura mater and pia mater (see figure 3.14) into the superior sagittal sinus and is returned to venous circulation.

The **superior sagittal sinus** flows under the midline of the cerebral vault (see figure 3.15). It receives the superior cerebral veins from the lateral aspects of the anterior cerebral hemispheres, veins from the spongy bone of the skull and dura mater, and veins from the pericranium, which pass through the parietal foramina. Venus blood drains from the superior sagittal sinus to the confluence of sinuses. From there, two transverse sinuses bifurcate and travel laterally and inferiorly in the sigmoid (S-shaped)

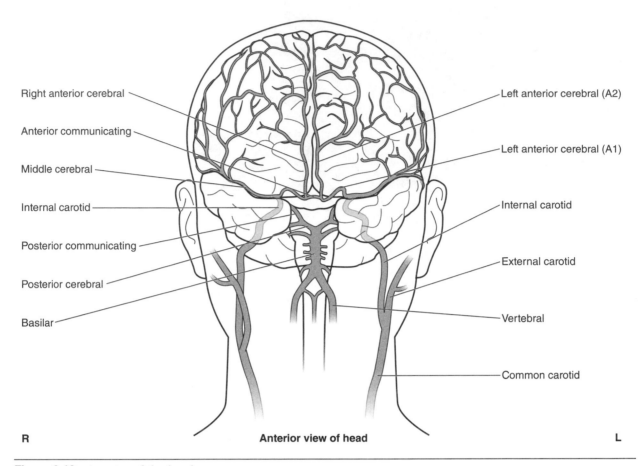

Right anterior cerebral

Anterior communicating

Middle cerebral

Internal carotid

Posterior communicating

Posterior cerebral

Basilar

Left anterior cerebral (A2)

Left anterior cerebral (A1)

Internal carotid

External carotid

Vertebral

Common carotid

R

Anterior view of head

L

Figure 3.12 Arteries of the head.

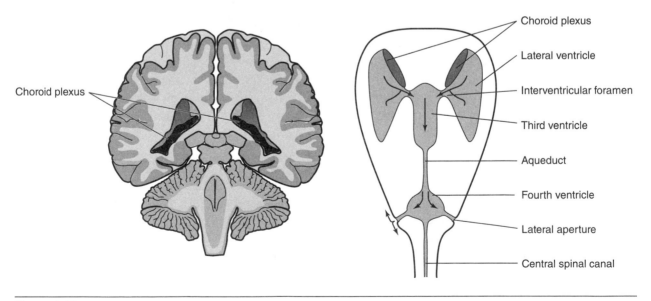

Choroid plexus

Choroid plexus

Lateral ventricle

Interventricular foramen

Third ventricle

Aqueduct

Fourth ventricle

Lateral aperture

Central spinal canal

Figure 3.13 Choroid plexus.

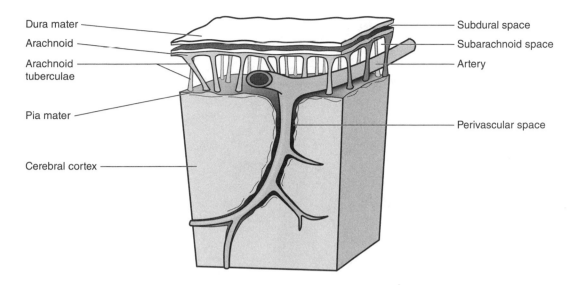

Figure 3.14   Arachnoid space for drainage of CSF into the brain's venous circulation.

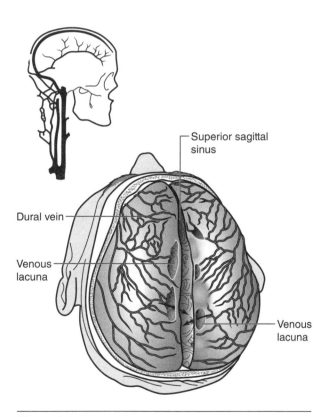

Figure 3.15   The superior sagittal sinus, which drains veins from the anterior cerebral hemispheres.

sinuses that then form the two jugular veins. In the neck, the jugular veins are located parallel to the carotid arteries and drain blood into the superior vena cava.

By measuring the difference between the concentration of proteins in arterial blood and that in blood from the internal jugular vein (cerebrospinal fluid drains into the superior sagittal sinus atop and behind the brain, which then empties into the internal jugular veins), researchers can estimate how much of the increase in proteins in peripheral blood has its origin in the brain (e.g., Rasmussen et al. 2009).

NEUROTRANSMITTERS

The primary way messages are transmitted throughout the nervous system is in the form of nerve impulses carried from one neuron to another (presynaptic to postsynaptic) through interneuronal junctions called synapses (see figure 3.16). Two basic types of synapses are electrical and chemical, but almost all the synapses in the CNS are chemical. The actions on neurons can be excitatory and inhibitory; these actions are produced in the brain primarily through two transmitter substances: glutamate (excitatory) and **γ-aminobutyric acid** (**GABA**; inhibitory). Other neurotransmitters (NT) do not have the information-transmitting effects of glutamate and GABA but produce their effects on the central nervous system by modulating circuits of neurons involved in specific brain functions. They interact with signaling proteins, called G-proteins, that are found in the cell membrane. Brain activity is thus influenced by other NT that alter the way neurons can process

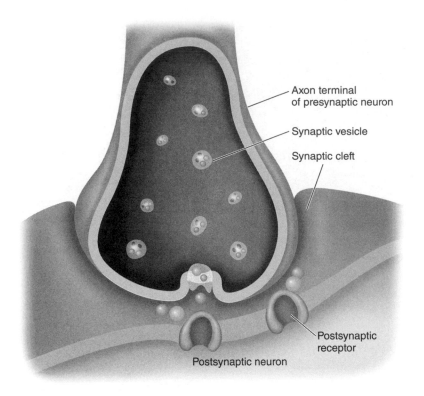

Figure 3.16 A chemical synapse between two neurons.

Reprinted, by permission, from J.H. Wilmore and D.L. Costill, 1999, *Physiology of sport and exercise,* 2nd ed. (Champaign, IL: Human Kinetics), 60.

signals from glutamate and GABA. The basic information provided by the actions of glutamate and GABA is thus modulated by a number of NT so that the outcome has emotional characteristics or significance. These NT, discussed in the sections that follow, have been studied in attempts to uncover biological mechanisms for the effects of exercise on mood, sleep, and pain perception.

Biogenic Amines

There are two classes of biogenic amines, catecholamines and indolamines, which are collectively known as monoamines.

Catecholamines

Catecholamines include the neurotransmitters dopamine, norepinephrine, and epinephrine. They are involved in sleep, reward, feeding, and drinking, as well as in functional illnesses (schizophrenia and depression) and organic diseases (Parkinson's disease, cardiovascular hypertension, paroxysmal tachycardia). Tyrosine is the amino acid precursor of the catecholamines, and

tyrosine hydroxylase is the rate-limiting enzyme under basal conditions. Tyrosine is converted to dopamine via an intermediary step. Dopamine may then be converted to NE or can serve as an NT itself. Norepinephrine may be converted into epinephrine, as shown in figure 3.17.

The **dopamine** (DA) system plays a critical role in motivation and motor functions. It is the key NT in the ventral tegmental area, an area of the brain surrounding the hypothalamus that is involved in the motivational drive to pursue behaviors that are rewarding or pleasurable (i.e., wanting). The pleasure (i.e., liking) occurs, in part, when DA receptor binding alters activity in opioid neurons located in the nucleus accumbens area of the ventral striatum (part of the basal ganglia; see figure 3.18). The VTA-to-nucleus accumbens network is an important brain mechanism involved in the motivation to seek natural rewards experienced from behaviors such as eating and physical movement. It has been established that a brain circuit in humans involving the orbitofrontal region of the prefrontal cortex, the thalamus, and the striatum is pivotally involved in the

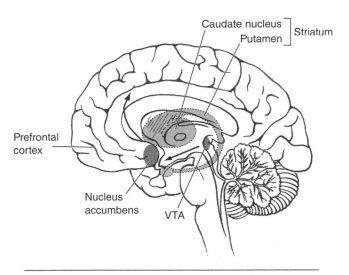

Figure 3.17 The VTA, a major site of brain DA, is shown in respect to the basal ganglia (caudate nucleus, putamen, and nucleus accumbens). Reward pathway extends from the ventral tegmental area (VTA) to the nucleus accumbens to the prefrontal cortex.

maintenance of survival behaviors that require a repetitive pattern, such as eating, mating, and physical activity.

> Important neurotransmitters in mental health and exercise are the biogenic amines, such as norepinephrine and serotonin.

Norepinephrine was the first substance identified (in 1901) as a mediator of peripheral nerve cell activity. Norepinephrine makes up 1% of the brain's NT and is relatively slow acting (seconds) compared to classical NT such as acetylcholine and GABA, which act in milliseconds. Thus, norepinehrine is frequently regarded as a neuromodulator; its slower action helps modulate the rapid actions of other NT on neurons. Norepinephrine is distributed topographically (i.e., in a distinct pattern) in the brain, rather than diffusely. This permits it to affect a wide range of functions in the central nervous system, including behavior during threat, pituitary hormonal release, cardiovascular function, sleep, and analgesic responses.

Norepinephrine is synthesized in neurons from the amino acid tyrosine taken up from

Neurotransmitters

Chemical substances that function as synaptic transmitters are called neurotransmitters (NT). Neurotransmitters are released directly to an adjacent nerve (postsynaptic), which becomes excited, inhibited, or modified in response to the attachment of the NT to specific receptor proteins in the membrane. An NT in the blood is called a neurohormone.

Following are influences on the release of presynaptic NT:

- The amount of transmitter available (depends on the availability of substrates and enzymes; NT reserves)
- The activity of the presynaptic neuron (e.g., chronic activation can deplete presynaptic NT release)
- The activation of receptors on the presynaptic nerve by the NT to inhibit further release (presynaptic inhibition)

Following are influences on the effects of NT on the postsynaptic neuron:

- The type and amount of NT
- The type, density, and sensitivity of the receptor
- The presence of other enhancing or inhibiting chemical substances
- The pH of the surrounding interstitial fluids

blood. The primary central site for the synthesis of NE in the brain is cell bodies in the LC. Axons from the LC project into the periaqueductal gray, thalamic nuclei, and hypothalamus. The LC is the sole source of NE provided to the amygdala, hippocampus, all of the frontal cortex, and the cerebellum. The LC is a major regulatory site for the limbic dysfunction characteristic of both anxiety and depression. It integrates external and internal stimuli to regulate autonomic arousal, attention vigilance, and neuroendocrine responses to behavioral stress. Norepinephrine hyperpolarizes neurons in the LC, enhancing responsiveness to signals from other neurons. A large number of brain NE neurons also lie outside the LC and are located throughout the lateral ventral tegmental fields. Fibers from these neurons intermingle with the LC neurons.

Norepinephrine is also the main nerve chemical of the SNS. Peripherally, it is manufactured in the ganglia of the spinal cord and in the chromaffin cells of the adrenal medulla, but the major source of NE in the autonomic nervous system is SNS free nerve endings. The rate of NE synthesis varies with the degree of sympathetic nerve activity and associated changes in the activity of tyrosine hydroxylase, the rate-limiting enzyme in the conversion of tyrosine to DOPA, and hence DA and NE synthesis. If NE is not taken back into the presynaptic neuron or is taken back into the presynaptic neuron and is not bound in storage vesicles, it is metabolized by the enzymes monoamine oxidase (MAO) and catechol-O-methyltransferase (COMT). The major metabolites of NE are 3,4-dihydroxyphenylglycol (DOPEG), inside the neuron, and 3-methoxy-4-hydroxyphenylglycol (MHPG), outside the neuron. Levels of NE have been estimated by measuring the serum levels of these metabolites, but this method has limitations. An increase in serum MHPG, for example, does not indicate whether the rise is due to increased release or decreased reuptake of NE.

> **N**orepinephrine is an important neuromodulator in the central nervous system and in the autonomic nervous system.

In the adrenal medulla, heart, and some brain regions, NE is further metabolized by the enzyme phenylethanolamine-N-methyltransferase to form the hormone **epinephrine** (Epi), which is also known by the Latin name *adrenaline* (see figure 3.18). The neurohormone was named **adrenaline** because it was thought that the substance was produced solely by the adrenal gland; and indeed, in the adrenal medulla, about 80% of the NE formed is con-

verted into Epi. The adrenal gland is located above the kidney—hence, the alternate name of epinephrine, which is derived from the Greek *epi nephron* ("upon the kidney"). The primary effect of Epi is cardiac stimulation, but it also serves as a minor transmitter in the brain. Functions of NE and Epi vary depending on the receptors (see Adrenergic Receptors).

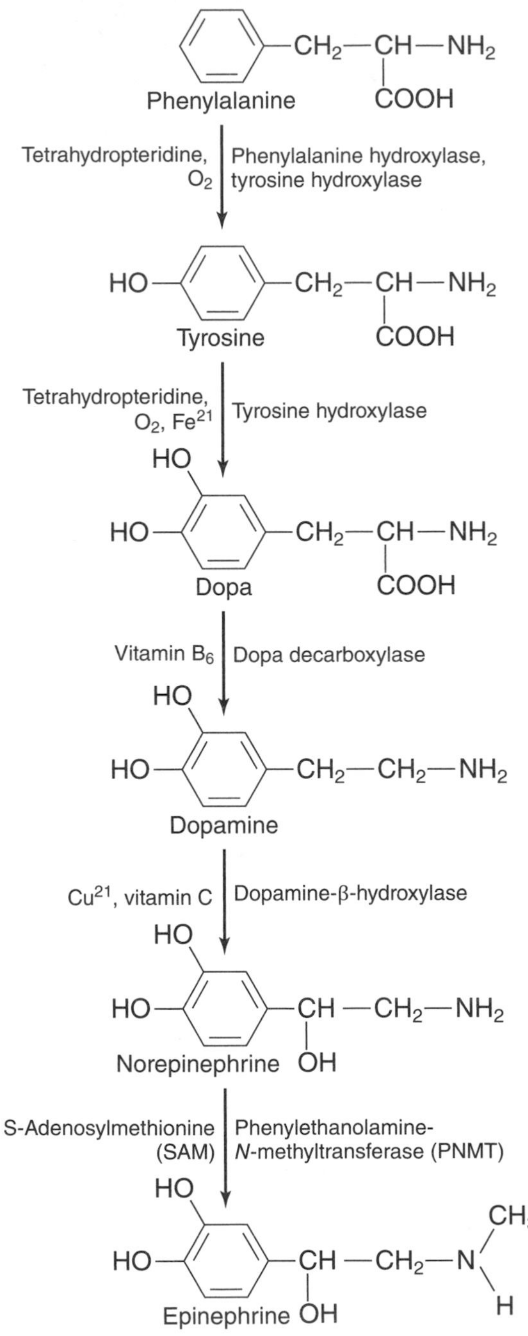

Figure 3.18 Chemical diagram of the synthesis of catecholamines.

Adrenergic Receptors

The effects of neurotransmitters depend on the type of receptors. The actions of norepinephrine (NE) and epinephrine (Epi) are mediated by two types of adrenergic receptors, α-receptors and β-receptors, which are further subdivided into α-1 and α-2 and β-1 and β-2. Generally, NE excites mainly α-receptors and to some extent β-receptors (especially β-1 in the brain), whereas for the most part, Epi excites α-receptors and β-receptors equally.

Alpha-1: Activates second-messenger phosphoinositide system. The phosphorylation of regulatory proteins that control ion channels and neural conductance and resistance consequent to receptor–second-messenger coupling plays a major role in brain NE activity. When α-1 receptors are bound with NE, physiological effects also include vasoconstriction and increased peripheral vascular resistance to blood flow, which increases blood pressure.

Alpha-2: Presynaptic autoreceptors. The binding of presynaptic α-2 receptors with NE is associated with an inhibition of NE release through decreases in both NE neuron activity and the synthesis of NE by a G-protein inhibition of tyrosine hydroxylase. If NE in the locus coeruleus is depleted, the normal inhibition of NE by the α-2 receptors will be reduced, and thus there will be an increased release of NE.

Beta-1: Activates a rise in levels of 3'5'-cyclic adenosine monophosphate (cAMP), which is a second messenger for neural transmissions.

Beta-2: Presynaptic receptors that enhance NE release. They have a higher affinity for Epi in the brain. When β-adrenergic receptors bind with NE or Epi, physiological effects include increased heart rate or stroke volume.

Indolamines

The **indolamines** compose the second class of biogenic amines and include melatonin and serotonin. **Melatonin**, secreted by the pineal gland, influences circadian phases, such as the sleep–wake cycle. **Serotonin**, or 5-hydroxytryptamine (5-HT), is secreted by the raphe nuclei, which have axon projections into the telencephalon, diencephalon, midbrain, and spinal cord. The primary effect of 5-HT is the inhibition of spontaneous activity. It is a general suppressor of the neural gain used to reestablish homeostasis (physiological equilibrium). Serotonin influences sleep and mood and has been the target of numerous antidepressant and anxiolytic drugs. Serotonin is also involved in pain, fatigue, appetitive behavior, periodicity of sleep, blood pressure, and corticosteroid activity. Projections from the raphe nuclei into the spinal cord have the ability to regulate pain by triggering the release of enkephalin, which is an **endogenous** opioid.

The synthesis of 5-HT in the brain depends on the neural concentrations of its precursor, tryptophan, which is an essential amino acid. Neural concentrations hinge on the levels of free tryptophan in the blood and on the transport through the blood–brain barrier. Blood tryptophan is either bound to albumin or in a "free" form. Higher concentrations of free fatty acids result in more free tryptophan because free fatty acids compete for chemical binding to albumin. Levels of free tryptophan also depend on the activity of tryptophan pyrrolase (an enzyme in the liver that metabolizes tryptophan), which is activated by glucocorticoids. Transport through

Levels of serotonin in the brain depend on the neural concentrations of its precursor, tryptophan.

the blood–brain barrier is affected by the competition between free tryptophan and large neutral amino acids (aromatic amino acids and branched-chain amino acids) at the transporter level. If levels of these amino acids increase, the amount of tryptophan that can get into the brain decreases.

There are more than a dozen receptors for 5-HT in the brain (commonly enumerated as 5-HT1 through 5-HT7 and further designated by subclassifications A through D) that mediate a variety of functions related to mood and behavior. For example, postsynaptic 5-HT1A receptors, located primarily in the limbic region, mediate neural inhibition. Presynaptic 5-HT1A autoreceptors in raphe nuclei are desensitized with repeated stimulation, leading to less inhibition and therefore increased serotonergic release, which has an antidepressant effect. Postsynaptic 5-HT2A receptors, highly concentrated in the frontal cortex, mediate neural excitation. Stimulation of these receptors results in the activation of the SNS. The stimulation of 5-HT2C postsynaptic receptors in the choroid plexus (a highly vascular region of the lining of the cerebral ventricles that secretes cerebrospinal fluid) results in anxiety, hypophagia, hypolocomotion, and activation of the HPA. In addition, other substances, such as glucocorticoids, can bind to 5-HT receptors and produce effects independent of 5-HT levels.

Other Neurohormones and Neuropeptides

Other key substances that function as neurotransmitters include glutamate, GABA, **endorphins**, galanin, and NPY. **Glutamate,** or glutamic acid (an amino acid), is a small-molecule, rapidly acting NT that is the major excitatory transmitter in the brain. It is a product of cell metabolism. For example, people who have allergic reactions to monosodium glutamate are responding to the by-product glutamic acid.

Glutamate has three groups of ligand-gated ion channels (ionotropic receptors) and three groups of G-protein coupled (metabotropic) receptors. The metabotropic receptors have multiple roles in synaptic plasticity. The ionotropic receptors are named after the synthetic **ligands** that bind with them. The slowest and more general receptor is NMDA (N-methyl-D-aspartate); it controls a calcium channel, as well as a magnesium channel, and is involved with seizures, learning, and brain damage after anoxia. Another ionotropic receptor is AMPA (α-amino-3-hydroxy-5-methyl-4-isoxazole proprionic acid), which allows sodium and potassium ions, but not calcium, to pass through the channel, leading to very quick excitatory signals. The receptor kainate was named for a nerve poison extracted from seaweed and has a role in the regulation of glutamate release and in excitatory and inhibitory synaptic transmission in the hippocampus.

Gamma-aminobutyric acid (GABA) is an amino acid that is produced from glutamate by the enzyme glutamic acid decarboxylase (GAD). It is the major inhibitory transmitter in the nervous system (see the discussion at the beginning of the section Neurotransmitters). GABA acts as a presynaptic inhibitory transmitter in many cases. It is secreted by nerve terminals in the cerebral cortex, as well as in the spinal cord, cerebellum, and basal ganglia. The two receptors for GABA are rather complex. For example, the key receptor type in the brain, the $GABA_A$ receptor, has five binding sites. Besides a site for GABA binding, there is a site that binds with benzodiazepines, a class of tranquilizers used to reduce anxiety, promote sleep, reduce seizure activity, and promote muscle relaxation. Another $GABA_A$ receptor site binds with barbiturates. Receptors for $GABA_A$ control a chloride channel, and $GABA_B$ receptors control a potassium channel (see figure 6.13).

Endogenous opioids such as β-endorphin, enkephalin, and dynorphin are endogenous opioid peptides whose biochemical actions are similar to exogenous opiates such as heroin and morphine. Endogenous opioids act by binding to mu (μ), kappa (κ) or delta (δ) receptors. Because of the widespread distribution of these receptors throughout the peripheral and central nervous systems, endogenous opioids have diverse effects regarding pleasure, pain, cardiovascular regulation, respiration, appetite and thirst, gastrointestinal activity, renal function, temperature regulation, metabolism, hormonal secretion, reproduction, immunity, learning, and memory (Akil et al. 1998; Evans 1988).

Beta-endorphins are found in the central nervous system in the arcuate nucleus with extensive projections throughout the brain (i.e., hypothalamus, limbic, periaqueductal gray, brain stem) and in the nucleus tractus solitarius with projections to the ventrolateral medulla. Beta-endorphin binds with a strong affinity to μ receptors (named for their high binding affinity for morphine) to produce **analgesia** (pain relief), respiratory depression, bradycardia, contraction of the pupil, hypothermia, and behavioral indifference and dependence. Beta-endorphins also have the capacity to decrease the brain's neuronal excitability via the "disinhibition" of the presynaptic release of GABA. Peripherally, β-endorphin is secreted into the blood from the anterior and intermediate pituitary during vigorous exercise, depending on the intensity of the exercise, and secretion is usually accompanied by increases in ACTH. Hence, peripheral levels of β-endorphin are best viewed as an indication of the stress response to exercise.

The enkephalins (ENK), which include two forms, leu-ENK and met-ENK, are signaling ligands that modulate the neural, endocrine, and immune systems, thereby influencing a wide range of functions including nociception, reward, and stress responses. ENK-expressing neurons are distributed throughout the brain, but ENK is most abundant in the subpopulation of GABAergic medium spiny neurons of the striatum that mainly express dopamine D-2 receptors (Akil et al. 1998; Heimer et al. 1991). ENK neurons of the ventral striatum project extensively to the ventral pallidum, which is a critical neural circuit for the affective functions of endogenous opioids (Smith and Berridge 2007). ENK binds preferentially to δ opioid receptors, but it also binds with μ and κ receptors (Akil et al. 1998). Desensitization of δ opioid receptors in the ventral striatum is accompanied by anxiety and depression-like effects (Perrine et al., 2008; Torregrossa et al. 2006). Other CNS systems in which ENK mediates regulatory functions during affective experience, stress, and nociception include the amygdala, periaqueductal gray, and dorsal horn of the spinal cord (Akil et al. 1998; Jonsdottir 2000). Met-enkephalin and leu-enkephalin are also stored in the adrenal medulla where they are co-released with catecholamines

into the gastrointestinal tract, heart, and blood circulation during stress.

The distribution of dynorphin (DYN) in the CNS overlaps that of ENK, but within the striatum, most DYN is found in medium spiny neurons that express the D-1 receptors (Akil et al. 1998; Jonsdottir 2000). In the ventral striatum, this population of medium spiny neurons projects to the ventral tegmental area. The behavioral functions of DYN are often opposite to functions of ENK. DYN, expressed in A and B forms, binds primarily to κ opioid receptors, which mediate the effects of DYN on stress-induced dysphoria and aversion via projections from the dorsal raphe nuclei to the nucleus accumbens (Land et al. 2009). Furthermore, DYN binding with κ receptors in the VTA inhibits dopamine release by the VTA to the nucleus accumbens, contributing to the rewarding effects of opiates and food, and possibly wheel running in rats and mice (Mansour et al. 1995; Nestler and Carlezon 2006; Shippenberg and Rea 1997). Endomorphins, more recently discovered endogenous substances with a different structure than the endorphins, dynorphins, and enkephalins, bind more tightly to the μ receptor than other opioid peptides do and also have wide-ranging effects, many of which mimic the effects of other opioids (Fichna et al. 2007).

> **P**eripheral levels of β-endorphin are best viewed as an indication of the stress response to exercise.

Met-enkephalin and leu-enkephalin are pentapeptide endorphins that are widely distributed throughout the CNS. They are co-stored with catecholamines in the adrenal medulla, where they are released with the catecholamines into the gastrointestinal tract, heart, and blood vessels. Beta-endorphin, met-enkephalin, and leu-enkephalin bind with opiate receptors in afferent nerves and spinal neurons to produce analgesia. They also bind to opioid receptors in the brain to help regulate behavior. Endorphins play a role in removing the tonic inhibition of

DA release in the parts of the brain involved with pleasure.

These effects, plus increases in plasma levels of β-endorphin and enkephalins with exercise, have led the general public to make the link between enhanced mood with exercise (i.e., "runner's high") and endorphins, even attributing exercise addiction to these endogenous opiates. However, as you will find in subsequent chapters, the evidence for endorphins as a cause of improved mood from exercise is weak (Dishman and O'Connor 2009). Nonetheless, because enkephalin and dynorphin neurons interact with DA release in parts of the brain involved with motivation and pleasure, they could plausibly influence exercise behavior and positive moods (Dishman and Holmes 2012), as discussed in chapter 5.

Neuropeptide Y (NPY) is a 36-amino-acid peptide colocalized with NE in around 40% of LC neurons (Holets et al. 1988). Neuropeptide Y inhibits LC firing **in vitro**. Thus, one of its functions may be to provide feedback inhibition to LC neurons. Most NPY cell bodies in the LC project to the hypothalamus and thus may be important in helping regulate endocrine responses during stress.

Galanin (GAL) is a 29-amino-acid peptide NT that coexists with NE in approximately 80% of LC neurons. Like NPY, galanin hyperpolarizes noradrenergic neurons and inhibits LC firing in vitro. Thus, a possible function of galanin is to provide feedback inhibition to LC neurons. Alterations in gene transcription for tyrosine hydroxylase or galanin (or both) represent plausible mechanisms for noradrenergic adaptations to stress. One study showed that chronic activity-wheel running blunted the release of NE in the brain cortex during stress and was accompanied by higher GAL **messenger ribonucleic acid (mRNA)** levels in the LC compared to those in control animals (Soares et al. 1999). Those findings and a related report of increased GAL mRNA in the LC after treadmill exercise training suggest a neuromodulatory role of GAL in brain noradrenergic adaptation to exercise (O'Neal et al. 2001).

Brain-derived neurotrophic factor (BDNF) is a neurotrophin that exerts widespread effects throughout the central nervous system by supporting neuronal survival, differentiation, connectivity, and neurogenesis, specifically activity-dependent synaptic plasticity (Binder and Scharfman 2004; Zhang and Ko 2009). BDNF is distributed throughout the central nervous system (CNS), and a high expression is found within the hippocampal formation (HF) (Binder and Scharfman 2004). The primary receptor for BDNF is the tyrosine receptor kinase B (trkB), which is responsible for regulating neuronal survival, promoting neurite outgrowth, and maintaining synaptic connectivity within the CNS (Zhang and Ko 2009). BDNF has been linked to learning, memory, and neurological disease (Binder and Scharfman 2004). It promotes the function and sprouting of serotonergic (5-HT) neurons, and effective antidepressants increase BDNF messenger ribonucleic acid (mRNA) (Binder and Scharfman 2004). BDNF protein and mRNA levels in the brain are elevated after both forced treadmill running and voluntary wheel running in rats and mice (Adlard and Cotman 2004; Berchtold et al. 2005; Gomez-Pinilla, Vaynman, and Ying 2008; Neeper et al. 1996; van Hoomissen et al. 2004; van Praag 2009). It is also released from the brain into the peripheral blood system after prolonged exercise in humans (Rasmussen et al. 2009). BDNF is also expressed outside the central nervous system, including in skeletal muscle (Gómez-Pinilla et al. 2001), where it may aid fat oxidation (Matthews et al. 2009). It took 4 hours of moderate-intensity rowing by very fit people for the increase in brain BDNF to show up in peripheral blood (even 2 hours wasn't long enough) (Rasmussen et al. 2009), so it is still not clear whether the exercise people commonly do for recreation or their health increases BDNF in their brains.

Endocannabinoids are endogenous physiological ligands that bind to the same cannabinoid receptors that mediate the psychoactive effects of Cannabis (i.e., marijuana), including the reduction of anxiety and pain, elevation of mood, and impairment of short-term memory. A study that reported increased levels of endocannabinoids in the blood after acute running (Sparling et al. 2003) has been interpreted as a possible explanation for elevated mood after exercise (Dietrich and McDaniel 2004). However, as is the case of endorphins and BDNF in the blood, that conclusion is not yet valid for several reasons. First, their origin and function during exercise are unknown. Second, a link between blood levels of endocannabinoids and psychological responses to exercise has not yet been established. Third, endocannabinoids are also found outside the brain (e.g., in the gastrointestinal tract, pancreas, uterus, liver, adipose tissue, and skeletal muscle, as well as in the spleen and tonsils), and they have many functions that are not psychoactive, including anti-inflammatory effects, the dilation of blood vessels and airways, and the modulation of the HPA axis during stress (Hill and McEwen 2010). Long term, endocannabinoids promote the storage of body fat by increasing appetite and reducing the metabolic rate in brain, adipose, liver, and skeletal muscle (Ginsberg and Woods 2009). Emerging evidence from studies of wheel running in mice suggests that endocannabinoids play a role in the motivation to run, but perhaps not in emotional responses (Dubreucq et al. 2010; Fuss and Gass 2010).

VGF, or **VGF nerve growth factor inducible,** is a neuropeptide (Levi et al. 1985) that helps regulate energy balance, metabolism, and neural plasticity (Alder et al. 2003; Hahm et al. 1999). VGF and VGF-derived peptides are expressed in the central and peripheral nervous systems and endocrine cells in the pituitary (adenohypophysis), adrenal medulla, gastrointestinal tract, and pancreas (Levi et al. 2004). VGF expression is induced by BDNF and regulated by neurotrophin-3 (Bozdagi et al. 2008). Activity wheel running increases hippocampal VGF expression and up-regulates neurotrophin signaling similar to the effects of antidepressants (Hunsberger et al. 2007).

CELLULAR AND MOLECULAR BIOLOGY OF THE BRAIN

To accurately characterize the changes in specific brain regions after acute and chronic physical activity, one must be familiar with some concepts and techniques of cellular and molecular biology. Key concepts are (1) signal transmission by receptor binding and second-messenger regula-

Understanding of changes in specific brain regions after acute and chronic exercise can be enabled by techniques to measure receptor binding, second-messenger regulation, and gene transcription and translation.

tion and (2) gene transcription and translation. Some fundamental techniques include **in situ hybridization histochemistry** and immunocytochemistry.

Receptor Effectors and Second Messengers

The neurotransmitters discussed previously in this chapter cannot directly transmit a chemical signal between neurons. The chemical signal (the first messenger) must be transduced. In transduction, a receptor–effector system activates a second-messenger system that regulates postsynaptic cellular responses. Second messengers were identified by Earl Wilbur Sutherland, Jr., who won the 1971 Nobel Prize in Physiology or Medicine for the discovery. Receptors are cellular proteins that bind endogenous ligands (e.g., neurotransmitters such as NE) and transmit a signal into the cell through the plasma membrane, which results in a structural or metabolic change in an effector cell by the process of phosphorylation. Receptors move from the cytosol (interior of cell) and are embedded in the surface membrane of a cell. Figure 3.19 shows a β-adrenoreceptor for NE that has a serpentine shape and crosses the cell membrane seven times.

Binding causes a receptor like a β-adrenergic receptor molecule to change its three-dimensional shape; its loops protrude into the cytoplasm of the cell. This is called endocytosis. Endocytosis activates another protein known as a G-protein. The 1994 Nobel Prize in Physiology or Medicine was awarded jointly to Americans Alfred G. Gilman and Martin Rodbell for their discovery of G-proteins and their role in signal transduction in cells. A G-protein is formed from three distinct protein subunits, termed α, β,

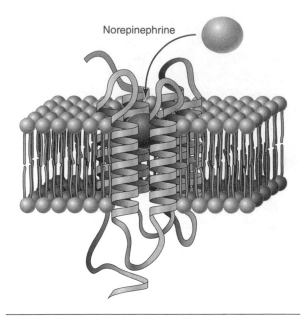

Figure 3.19   Beta-adrenoreceptor for norepinephrine.

and γ. Whether a G-protein is switched on or off depends on whether it binds with guanosine diphosphate (GDP; off) or guanosine triphosphate (GTP; on). In a few seconds or less, the G-protein will then hydrolyze its own GTP down to GDP, which terminates its activity by a down-regulating **negative feedback** system.

A signal cascade is triggered by the active G-protein. When the β-adrenergic receptor activates the G-protein, the α subunit releases GDP, binds GTP, and falls away from the β and γ subunits. The GTP-bound α subunit breaks away from the receptor and activates an enzyme called adenylate cyclase, which promotes the conversion of adenosine triphosphate (ATP) into 3'5'-cyclic adenosine monophosphate (cAMP); cAMP is the second messenger. Other second messengers include phosphoinositol and arachidonic acid systems. Figure 3.20 shows the actions of a receptor that open an ion channel in the cell membrane directly (see figure 3.20a) and indirectly by a second messenger (see figure 3.20b).

High levels of cAMP enable protein kinase A to phosphorylate intracellular proteins that regulate changes in cell structure (e.g., by activating gene expression and protein synthesis) and activity (e.g., by opening ion channels that depolarize cell membrane potentials). Figure 3.21 shows cAMP acting on a calcium channel. A single NE molecule can activate dozens of α subunits of proteins. Each of these will activate the synthesis of an adenylate cyclase, which in turn will synthesize hundreds of cAMP molecules.

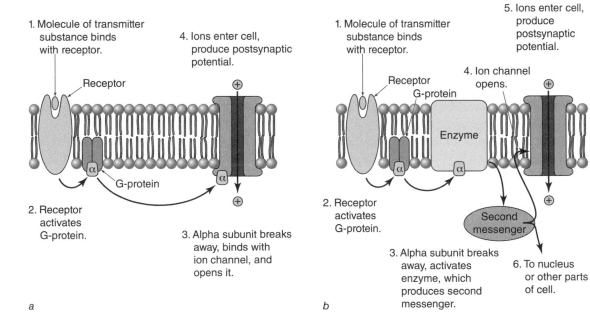

Figure 3.20   Receptors can open an ion channel *(a)* directly or *(b)* indirectly by a second messenger.

Carlson, Neil R., *Physiology of Behavior*, 6th Edition, © 1998. Adapted by permission of Pearson Education, Inc., Upper Saddle River, NJ. Copyright 1994 by Allyn & Bacon.

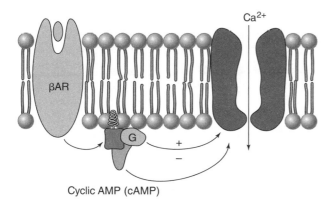

Figure 3.21 Regulation of a calcium channel by the cAMP second messenger.

Gene Transcription and Translation

The example of the receptor–effector system illustrates the importance of changes in cellular protein levels and function in neural transmission. Therefore, some understanding of the role played by gene transcription and translation in the synthesis of proteins is important.

The fundamental, central dogma of molecular biology by Francis Crick (codiscoverer of DNA structure) explains the difference, and the linkage, between DNA (deoxyribonucleic acid) and proteins. It states that genes, encoded in our DNA, are transcribed into **RNA** (ribonucleic acid) and translated into proteins that execute the functions of a living cell. Deoxyribonucleic acid consists of deoxyribose sugar, phosphoric acid, and four nitrogenous bases. The bases can be divided into purines (adenine and guanine) and pyrimidines (cytosine and thymine) based on their chemical structure. These components form what is referred to as a nucleotide. A series of nucleotides joined together creates a single strand of DNA that pairs with a complementary strand (series of nucleotides) to produce the double-stranded helical formation of DNA. The specific sequence of the nitrogenous bases (A, G, C, T) on these strands creates a gene, the information needed to synthesize proteins and other molecules, which ultimately influences the physical and functional characteristics of an organism.

The cascade of information from gene to protein begins with transcription and ends with translation. During **transcription**, one strand of the DNA—called the template or antisense strand—is read by the protein RNA polymerase; an RNA molecule that is complementary to the template strand is synthesized. Ribonucleic acid has four characteristics that distinguish it from DNA: (1) it is single stranded, (2) it contains the sugar ribose instead of deoxyribose, (3) it is smaller, and (4) it contains the nitrogenous base uracil instead of thymine. The remaining strand of DNA that is not read is called the coding strand or sense strand and is considered identical in sequence to the RNA molecule, except for the presence of uracil. The synthesis of RNA, therefore, allows for the transfer of genetic information to a different molecule.

Translation is the process by which the RNA strand is used to create a series of amino acids linked together by peptide bonds. This series of amino acids creates a polypeptide chain that may go through a series of modifications, such as combinations with other polypeptide chains or the addition of carbohydrate groups, lipids, cofactors, and coenzymes to form a functional protein.

Every cell in the human body contains an identical set of genes, yet each type of cell has a different protein expression profile, suggesting that transcription of the various genes is regulated at the cellular level. Regulation of the level of transcription from a gene occurs through the interaction of proteins (transcription factors) and DNA sequences located near the gene (promoters and cis-elements). The binding of transcription factors to the promoter region is important for the recognition of a gene, but the interaction between these factors and other factors bound to cis-elements represents one level of transcription control. For example, some steroid hormones cross the cell's plasma membrane and bind to steroid protein receptors located in the cytoplasm. The bound receptor then enters the nucleus and binds to a region of DNA called the hormone response element. Once bound to the DNA, the steroid and receptor may interact with additional transcription factors located at other regions of the DNA. The interaction of the steroid, receptor, hormone response element, and other transcription factors alters the level of transcription of several genes, thereby influencing gene expression.

> **G**ene regulation allows a cell to respond to the changing environment around it to maintain homeostasis.

Epigenetics

A heritable change in gene expression by causes other than a change in the gene's DNA sequence is an epigenetic event. This occurs naturally when a fertilized egg cell (the zygote) is divided into the pluripotent stem cells that then further differentiate into neurons and muscle cells. During this cell differentiation, the transcription of some genes is activated and that of others is inhibited. Another way that genes are regulated epigenetically is through the remodeling of chromatin, which is the complex of DNA and its associated histones (protein microspheres that DNA is wrapped around). Chromatin remodeling is accomplished through two main mechanisms: DNA methylation and histone deacetylation.

DNA methylation is the addition of a methyl group to DNA, most often at the 5 position of the cytosine pyrimidine ring to convert cytosine to 5-methylcytosine. Like cytosine, 5-methylcytosine pairs with a guanine. Heavily methylated sequences are less active during transcription. Genetic imprinting is when the methylation of cytosines persists from the germ line of one of the parents into the zygote, marking the chromosome as being inherited from that parent.

Histone deacetylation is a posttranslational change in the amino acids that make up histone proteins. This can change the shape of the histone sphere, which is then carried to each new DNA copy during replication. The new histone acts as a template for other nearby histones to also have the new shape. Epigenetic events can produce permanent changes in cells that make them vulnerable to environmental stressors (e.g., hypoxia or chemical toxins that contribute to cancers), or they can lead to virtually permanent changes in how physiological systems are regulated. For example, excessive maternal exertional strain during early fetal development might up-regulate traits linked to exaggerated stress responses during adulthood, whereas moderate physical activity might have the opposite effect.

Gene regulation is an important phenomenon because it allows a cell to respond to the changing environment around it to maintain homeostasis. Thus, altering the in vitro or **in vivo** environment of a cell makes it possible to observe changes in the level of gene transcription and protein production. Techniques designed to measure these changes, such as in situ hybridization histochemistry and immunocytochemistry, provide insight into the mechanisms of the action of specific biological functions and experimental conditions.

In Situ Hybridization Histochemistry

In situ hybridization histochemistry is a technique for examining steady-state levels of mRNA inside a cell that is located in its original, natural setting. Other techniques that measure mRNA require removal of the nucleic acid from the cell and immobilization on a nitrocellulose or nylon membrane. The advantage of in situ hybridization histochemistry is that by taking thin sections of tissue and hybridizing them to a labeled probe (single-stranded complementary nucleic acid), we can examine mRNA without removing it from the cell (see figure 3.22), thereby gaining information about the localization of mRNA within specific regions of the tissue or within specific cells within a region. O'Neal and colleagues (2001) used this technique to observe changes in preprogalanin neuropeptide in the LC (see figure 3.23) after treadmill training in rats. As mentioned previously, galanin is colocalized in 80% of the LC neurons and has been shown to hyperpolarize noradrenergic neurons of the LC. The increase in galanin after treadmill training (see figure 3.24) may explain changes in the function of LC neurons after chronic stress.

Immunocytochemistry

Measurement of mRNA can provide information about the level of gene expression, but ultimately it is the level of functional protein that is of

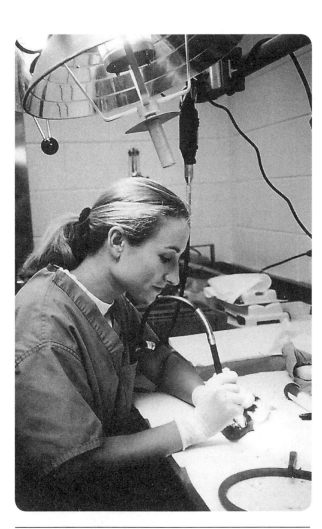

Figure 3.22 Brain surgery conducted on an anesthetized rat.

Provided by the Exercise Psychology Laboratory, Department of Kinesiology, and Department of Psychology, the University of Georgia.

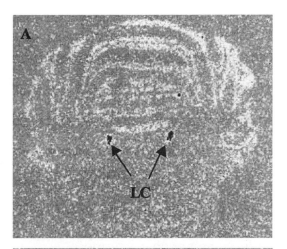

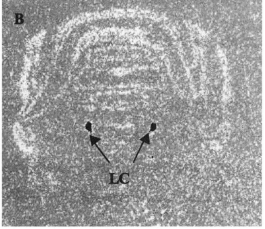

Figure 3.24 Audioradiogram indicating galanin neuropeptide messenger ribonucleic acid in the locus coeruleus after *(a)* treadmill exercise training in rats compared to *(b)* sedentary rats.

Provided by Dr. Heather O'Neal, the Exercise Psychology Laboratory, Department of Kinesiology, and Department of Psychology, the University of Georgia.

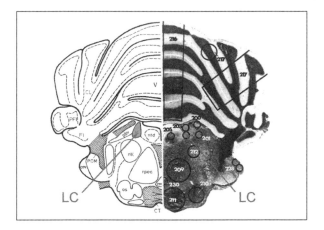

Figure 3.23 Coronal slice through the locus coeruleus.

Adapted from M. Palkovitz and M.H. Brownstein, 1988, *Maps and guide to microdissection of the rat brain* (New York: Elsevier), 175. By permission of Miklós Palkovits.

interest. **Immunocytochemistry**, a technique for measuring protein expression, is similar to in situ hybridization histochemistry in that it is conducted in the cell, permitting us to gain information about the localization of protein. Instead of using labeled complementary strands of nucleic acid to visualize RNA, immunocytochemistry uses antibodies to visualize protein. Antibodies are proteins that recognize regions, or domains, of other proteins called antigens. The binding of the primary antibody to the antigen identifies specific proteins present in a tissue. Additional antibodies that bind to the primary antibody are needed, however, to visualize the protein using chemical reactions. Often, in situ hybridization histochemistry and immunocyto-chemistry are used in conjunction to confirm that changes in mRNA level translate into changes in protein expression.

Early Gene Responses

Specific protein expression among different types of cells can vary, making up what is referred to as the cell's proteome, or the collection of proteins expressed in a cell. However, some proteins are ubiquitous, and the level of expression of these proteins is often used to measure transcriptional activation.

One family of proteins that is often examined after the application of various stimuli is the Fos family of transcription factors, which dimerize (a dimer is a compound of two like molecules) with members of the Jun family to alter transcription of specific genes. A key transcription factor is activator protein-1 (AP-1), which is a dimer composed of combinations of Fos- and Jun-like proteins. AP-1 interacts with AP-1 sites (with a sequence of TGA(G/C)TCA) in the promoter regions of target genes to increase or decrease their rate of transcription. The major members of the Fos family include c-Fos, FosB, Fra-1, and Fra-2; but c-Fos induction is most often examined because it occurs in low levels at baseline and is inducible after a variety of stimuli. In addition, c-Fos is considered an immediate early gene

because of the rapidity of induction following stimuli.

Examples of behavioral neuroscience studies that examined c-Fos after exercise showed that wheel running acutely induces c-Fos expression (Clark et al. 2011; Rhodes, Gammie, and Garland 2005), but chronic wheel running did not alter c-Fos expression in response to foot-shock stress in rats (Soares et al. 1999). Levels of c-Fos are often used as an index of cell activity in response to a stimulus. However, c-Fos responses can be **down-regulated** (decrease in ligand or receptor interactions) after repeated or usual stimulation of the cell, so cells can be activated in the absence of changes in c-Fos (Kovacs 1998).

Delta-FosB is an isoform, or spliced, variant (i.e., truncated) member of the Fos family that lacks the C-terminal 101 amino acids of FosB. In stimulated cells, delta-FosB can limit the transcriptional effects of Fos and Jun proteins (Nakabeppu and Nathans 1991). Studies have found that c-Fos and delta-FosB in the nucleus accumbens are activated during wheel running in rats (Greenwood and Fleshner 2011; Werme et al. 2002), and transgenic mice that overexpress delta-FosB selectively in striatal dynorphin-containing neurons increased their daily running compared with control litter mates (Werme et al. 2002). Delta-FosB could plausibly facilitate wheel running by inhibiting the release of dynorphin by GABA neurons (see figure 3.25), which oth-

Delta FosB inhibits dynorphin?

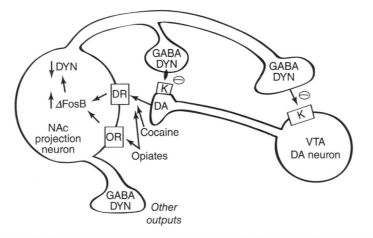

Dynorphin released by GABA neurons binds with kappa opioid receptors to inhibit DA release in VTA or nucleus accumbens

Figure 3.25 The inhibition of opioid modulation of dopamine release in the ventral tegmental area is a hypothetical mechanism of motivation to run (Werme et al. 2002).

Reprinted, by permission, from E.J. Nestler, M. Barrot, and D.W. Self, 2001, "FosB: A sustained molecular switch for addition," *PNAS* 98(20): 11042-11046.

erwise binds with κ opioid receptors to inhibit DA release in the ventral tegmental area (VTA) or accumbens.

Posttranslational Regulation

Not only must changes in gene expression be considered, but changes in protein level as well as posttranslational alterations of protein function are also important. Knowing that the level of gene expression can be tied to protein expression, and that various proteins interact to affect the functional properties of many cellular events, makes exercise a unique and sometimes difficult stimulus to study in the lab. Unlike other experimental conditions, such as those in pharmacological investigations, the "active ingredient" of exercise is difficult to determine and may change depending on a host of factors, including mode, intensity, duration, frequency, and timing. For example, with pharmacological investigation, one can begin by examining the receptors that bind to the drug. With exercise, the point at which to begin characterization can be varied depending on the scientific question of interest. Nonetheless, the use of techniques borrowed from molecular biology to study the effects of exercise on brain function is one of the new frontiers of exercise psychology. Recent advances in neuroimaging techniques that permit the application of molecular biology to the real-time study of the human brain are discussed at the end of this chapter. They are just beginning to be applied during exercise. The application of molecular biology to exercising animals has been taking place for several years.

ANIMAL MODELS

Behavioral neuroscience relies heavily on the use of rats and mice, as well as non-human primates, to study the genetics and molecular biology of the brain in experimental models of human behavior and disease. There has been a steady increase in the study of exercise by behavioral neuroscientists during the past decade, so it is important for students of exercise psychology to be familiar with some basic methods used in animal models.

Transgenic Models

Transgenic rodents are mutants formed when foreign DNA or synthetic genes are introduced so that selected genes are overexpressed, inactivated (i.e., "knocked out"), or activated (i.e., "knocked in").

Transgenic experiments permit the manipulation of genes believed to be keys in the molecular regulation of the brain and behavior. The two widely used methods to produce transgenic rodents are (1) growing transformed embryonic stem cells in a tissue culture with new or altered DNA and (2) injecting a gene into the pronucleus of a fertilized egg, as shown in figure 3.26.

The inserted gene can restore function (i.e., "knock in") in a mutant animal (e.g., by removing a DNA sequence that blocks gene transcription or replacing a gene with a new one) or inactivate (i.e., "knock out") the function of a specific gene locus. If the replacement gene (figure 3.26) is nonfunctional (a null allele), mating of the heterozygous transgenic animal will produce a "knockout" strain homozygous for the nonfunctional gene (both copies of the gene at that locus have been "knocked out"). So-called housekeeping genes (those needed to maintain basic cell functions) are expressed in all types of cells at all stages of development, but other genes are normally expressed in only certain types of cells when they are activated, or turned on, by the appropriate signals (e.g., by a neurotransmitter or a hormone). Newer techniques can knock out a gene in only a single type of cell (e.g., a neuron instead of skeletal muscle).

Selective Breeding

Most mental health disorders and degenerative CNS diseases are noninfectious. They develop over long periods of time, presumably as the results of complex interactions between networks of gene mutations and features of the environment that alter gene expression, translation, and regulation. Transgenic models are an imperfect approach to identifying these polygenic diseases. A gene knockout only shows whether that gene is essential to some function and what

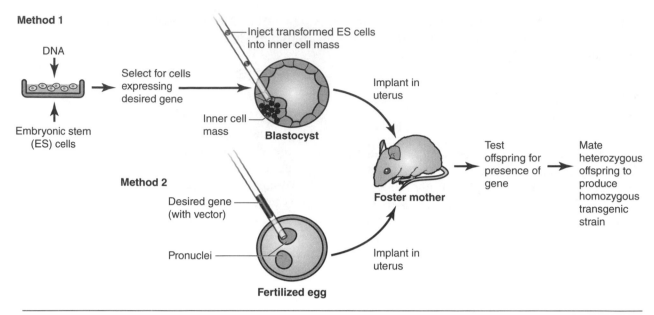

Figure 3.26 Methods used to produce transgenic rodents.

biological adaptation occurs to compensate for its loss. Also, knockout animals are often unaffected by their gene deficiency. Many genes turn out to be dispensable, because the genome has redundancy to compensate for a single missing pair of alleles. Furthermore, most genes are pleiotropic. They are expressed in different tissues in different ways and at different times in development. Finally, transgenic models require the advance knowledge of a DNA sequence that is already recognized as a candidate to be a cause of a disease or a behavioral trait.

Artificial selection for phenotypic traits is a complementary approach to transgenic models because it can produce lines of a species that diverge on clusters of disease-related traits that may share common alleles or their transcripts. Recent selective breeding programs have resulted in high voluntary wheel running in mice (Garland et al. 2011; Swallow, Carter, and Garland 1998) and high treadmill running capacity in rats (Koch and Britton 2001).

The artificial selection for aerobic capacity in rats started in 1996 using a founder population that was developed by the U.S. National Institutes of Health from the intentional crossbreeding of eight inbred strains that represented the widest genetic heterogeneity of laboratory rats available. The goal was to determine which allelic variants from the eight progenitor strains segre-

gate as a result of selection for the running trait (Koch and Britton 2008). For each rat, aerobic capacity was estimated from total distance run on a speed-ramped treadmill test to exhaustion. At each generation, a within-family rotational breeding scheme was applied to 13 families for the low and high lines. The breeding program has retained genetic heterogeneity while keeping the rate of inbreeding at 1% per generation (Koch and Britton 2008). After 21 generations, the selectively bred low-capacity-runners (LCR) and high-capacity-runners differed by 450% in aerobic treadmill running capacity, as well as voluntary wheel running.

HCR males and females run about six times and four times the distance that LCR males and females did. Also, the HCR line runs about twice, and the LCR line runs about half the daily distance run by nonselected albino and hooded strains (Murray et al. 2010). $\dot{V}O_2max$ is about 50% higher in HCR rats than n LCR rats, which is explainable mainly by greater stroke volume and maximal cardiac output, but also by greater oxygen extraction by skeletal muscle associated with better oxygen diffusion in tissues, greater capillary density (the result of smaller fiber size), and higher oxidative enzyme activity. HCR rats are also smaller and have less fat. However, these physiological differences alone are not big enough to fully explain the wide difference in voluntary running. Researchers conducting ongoing studies with these selectively bred mice and rats are searching for other correlated behavioral traits (Geisser et al. 2008; Jónás et al. 2010; Waters et al. 2010) and genetic traits in brain regions (e.g., the locus coeruleus, raphe nuclei, striatum, and ventral tegmentum) and neurotransmitter systems (e.g., norepinephrine, serotonin, dopamine, and enkephalin) involved with the regulation of motivated behavior and adaptability to running wheel exposure (Foley et al. 2006; Mathes et al. 2010; Murray et al. 2010).

Behavioral Models

Animal models permit the experimental manipulation of brain or behavior within a model of a human disease or behavior to help determine whether biological, anatomical, or pharmacological factors can explain some of the psychological effects or determinants of regular physical activity in humans (McCabe et al. 2000). Among humans, however, social determinants of stress interact with differences in how people appraise the meaning of events and how they cope with this appraisal or its consequences. In that way, animal models are inherently limited for drawing inferences about human experience; an animal model is just that, a model. It can guide human studies, but direct inferences about the "human" meaning of animal behaviors are probably more in the eye of the beholder than in the brain of the animal. As Freud is credited with saying, "Sometimes a cigar is just a cigar."

Nonetheless, most researchers in exercise psychology have exclusively used social cognitive models of stress, limiting our understanding of the biology of behavior in physical activity settings and justifying the use of animal models. So, it is important to consider how animals can be used as models to guide human research. Similarities between validating animal models and validating psychological constructs based on human self-reports (outlined early in chapter 2) should be apparent.

A commonly used scheme in pharmacology of judging whether animal models that use stressor tasks are predictive, isomorphic, or homologous is helpful to evaluate the validity of such models for human depression and anxiety. **Predictive models** typically include specific signs or behaviors that can be reliably changed by drugs known to have clinical efficacy in humans. Predictive models must be based on species or strains that respond to drugs in the same ways as humans do. An **isomorphic model** evokes the same features as in the human disease, which abate after the administration of drugs that are clinically useful in humans; but the features generated may not have the same etiology (i.e., course of development) as in the human disease. A **homologous model** meets the standards of predictive validity and isomorphism, and it also has the same etiology as does the human disease. When a homologous model is specific for a single disease, it has construct validity, which is the gold standard, or the ideal test, of validity.

Depression

The escape-deficit model after uncontrollable foot shock is the most highly elaborated animal model of depression, first reported by McCulloch and Bruner in 1939. The hallmark response to uncontrollable, inescapable foot shock is increased latency to escape from controllable shock administered 24 to 72 hours later, presumably resulting from a depletion of NE in the LC. A single session of high-intensity uncontrollable foot shock leads to a large decrease in brain NE with less reliable decreases in the levels of brain serotonin and DA, perhaps due to slower resynthesis of NE. The escape-deficit model is an attempt to simulate the so-called learned helplessness, or behavioral despair, common in human depression. The animal gives up its attempts to escape stressors, such as foot shock, forced swimming, or restraint. The Porsolt swim test has the most widely used measure of behavioral despair in screening the effectiveness of antidepressant drugs, but it has poor construct validity (Yoo et al. 2000).

The escape-deficit model is mostly isomorphic with human depression, featuring weight loss, reduced sexual behavior, sleep disturbances (decreased REM sleep latency), and anhedonia (i.e., loss of pleasure). However, such a model is not homologous with human depression. Although self-reward tasks such as sucrose preference and intracranial self-stimulation are used as surrogate measures in the rat for the phenomenological construct of pleasure experienced by humans, it is not possible to determine whether a rat feels helpless or hopeless. All of these models mimic certain features of human depression, but should not be viewed as synonymous with human disorders (Holmes 2003).

Some types of depression and anxiety in humans appear to be endogenous; they cannot be attributed to an uncontrollable stressor. Relatively new models of endogenous depression in the rat involve injecting neonatal pups with clomipramine, a serotonin reuptake inhibitor, leading to decreased REM sleep latency and other key behavioral signs of depression as the rat reaches adulthood. Another endogenous model disturbs brain NT systems, including NE and serotonin, by surgically removing the olfactory bulbs located below the brain frontal cortex. These models each are isomorphic with human depression, and they are responsive to pharmacotherapy. Because their endogenous etiology differs from animal models that are based on exogenous stress, the clomipramine and the olfactory bulbectomy models have the potential for use in examining the role physical activity plays in preventing depression not arising from chronic stress.

Anxiety

An increase in locomotion can reflect an adaptive motivational state in rats, indicating reduced behavioral inhibition (e.g., less freezing). An increase in open-field locomotion has been reported in rats after forced-exercise swimming and after motorized treadmill running. Locomotion by the rat in an open field is associated inversely with observer ratings of anxiety when the locomotion appears purposeful and the animal exhibits other exploratory behaviors such as approaching the center of the open field. In contrast, low levels of locomotion, few approaches to the center of the open field, freezing, defecation, urination, and shivering have been conventionally regarded as isomorphic with the hypervigilance, hesitancy, fear, and autonomic activation common in human anxiety.

Under certain circumstances of threat, increased locomotion seems to indicate agitation or panic (i.e., the flight response to a predator). Such a dichotomous interpretation of increased locomotion during open-field testing illustrates the importance of environmental context when one is inferring anxiety from locomotion by rats. For example, chronic wheel running has reduced trait anxiety measured by repeated open-field testing (Dishman et al. 1996), but effects on anxiety behaviors in response to a single exposure to a novel open field have yielded mixed results. However, wheel running has consistently reduced anxiety behavior after exposure to acute and chronic stressors, including serotonin agonists, intense light, tail shock, uncontrollable foot shock, social defeat, and maternal separation (Sciolino and Holmes, 2012; Sciolino et al. 2012).

In contrast, other studies have suggested that wheel running increases anxiety by promoting defensive behaviors (e.g., heightened sensory processing, immobility, flight, defensive threat or attack) in exercised rats (Burghardt et al. 2004). However, most studies of the effects of wheel running on anxiety have used tests (i.e., acoustic or fear-potentiated startle, elevated plus or zero maze, hole board, light or dark box, open field, stress-induced hyperthermia) that were not designed to measure defensive behaviors (Sciolino et al. 2012). Structured tests of threat, such as social interaction, marble burying, and the shock probe defensive burying test (Burghardt et al. 2004; Salam et al. 2009; Sciolino and Holmes 2012), permit the detection of defensive behaviors that are useful for understanding the neurobiology of defensive and anxiety behaviors and for screening anti-anxiety drugs.

Learning

Studies have shown that repeated exercise enhances performance in various tests of learning and memory that involve hippocampal functions and memory storage, such as the Morris water maze, the place-learning set-task, the radial arm maze test (Anderson et al. 2000; Fordyce and Farrar 1991a, 1991b; Fordyce and Wehner 1993; Leggio et al. 2005; Van Praag et al. 1999; Vaynman, Ying, and Gomez-Pinilla 2004), and contextual fear conditioning, an aversively motivated form of learning (Greenwood et al. 2009; Van Hoomissen et al. 2004, 2011). For example, rats that have run in wheels for several weeks exhibit an increase in freezing behavior when they are returned to an environment in which they previously experienced a foot shock (Van Hoomissen et al. 2004), but not when they are placed in a novel environment after the shock (Van Hoomissen et al. 2011). This indicates that the strength of the association between learning cues and memory is strengthened by exercise. Exercise also enhanced rodents' learning on the Morris water maze, which measures the time it takes for rodents to locate and swim to a submerged pedestal.

Across several types of tests, exercise training facilitates animals' learning of spatial location (Anderson et al. 2000; Fordyce and Farrar 1991a, 1991b; Fordyce and Wehner 1993; Leggio et al. 2005; Van Praag et al. 1999; Vaynman et al. 2004). Collectively, the evidence suggests that, in rodents, chronic exercise alters the way past experiences are encoded, stored, and then used to solve problems and respond adaptively. Higher-level cognitive functions of planning and goal-directed actions are considered to involve prefrontal neural networks that integrate memories.

A recent study (Rhyu et al. 2010) found that female monkeys aerobically trained by treadmill running for five months had an increase in the density of blood vessels in the primary motor cortex and learned faster to discriminate items associated with food rewards presented by the Wisconsin General Test Apparatus, developed at the world-renowned Psychology Primate Laboratory at the University of Wisconsin in the 1930s (Harlow and Bromer 1938). The degree to which evidence of exercise-related improvements in learning in rodents and monkeys can be generalized to human learning and memory remains to be determined, however. As described in chapter 8, few experiments have reported effects of exercise training on relational learning in humans.

Motivation and Hedonics

Mesolimbic dopamine mediates motivational responses to natural rewards (e.g., feeding, reproductive behaviors, and play) rather than pleasure (Berridge and Robinson 1998; Flagel et al. 2011; Lutter and Nestler 2009; Smith and Berridge 2007; Wise 2004). The incentive salience hypothesis emphasizes the importance of dopamine in the "wanting" that is triggered by

reward-related conditioned stimuli. The "liking," or pleasure, associated with reward involves the activation of other systems parallel to, or downstream of, the mesolimbic dopamine pathways. These other hedonic systems include GABA and opioid peptides in distinct, but integrated, pathways within the ventral striatum and striatal pallidal circuits (Smith and Berridge 2007). The hedonic allostasis theory (Koob and Le Moal 1997) conceptualizes addictive behaviors as a response to hypoactivity in dopamine systems, which are believed to induce compensatory behavioral activation (e.g. drug seeking, sensation seeking, compulsive exercise) to restore normal hedonic tone. In contrast, the incentive salience model of addiction emphasizes the role of dopamine as the driver of the behavioral activation that ultimately leads to the outcomes that induce pleasure. Dopamine thus mediates the motivation that triggers the reward-directed behaviors.

Thus, behavioral measures of the effects of exercise on emotional states in rodent models must dissociate motivational and hedonic variables. For example, reproductive behaviors in rats include both (Holmes 2003). Although some "anhedonia" models, such as diminished preference for dilute sucrose solutions, have some validity, measures of hedonic activation assessed by the increased consumption of palatable food are confounded with variables associated with motivation and energy balance. Measures of affective taste reactions in rats described by Berridge and Robinson (1998) are perhaps the best current option for quantifying hedonic responses.

MEASURING BRAIN ACTIVITY

To determine whether behavior or emotions can be explained by neural activity in the brain, researchers must take measurement during behavior or emotional responses. For example, Wang and colleagues (2000) examined the striatum DA release using positron emission tomography scanning before and after a graded maximal treadmill test in human volunteers. Brain imaging techniques have been applied rarely in the field of exercise psychology, however; neural activity has been mainly estimated by measures of brain electrocortical activity by electroencephalography (EEG). The goal of the following sections is to introduce some of the key techniques in neuroscience that can be used to measure neural activity in the brain of humans and other animals.

Electrophysiology

Electrophysiology uses electrodes positioned in the brain cortex or in specific regions of brain neurons to record electrical potentials during behavior or in response to stress to determine whether those areas play a role in regulating physiology and behavior. Microelectrodes are constructed of metal wires, usually tungsten or stainless steel, or fine glass tubes filled with a conducting electrolyte fluid (e.g., potassium chloride) that can detect the discharge rate of a single neuron. Macroelectrodes, which are bigger, record the activity of thousands of neurons, or more. They can be implanted in the brain or attached to the surface of the brain cortex, or attached as discs to the scalp. The changing electrical potentials (neural discharge rate) are then amplified, displayed, and recorded on an oscilloscope or ink-writing oscillograph or digitized for computer display and storage. Similar electrodes can also be used to stimulate brain neurons.

Electrophysiology has rarely been used to learn about the brain's response to exercise. Two examples are recordings of discharge rates in the LC (Rasmussen, Morilak, and Jacobs 1986) and the raphe nuclei during walking (Veasey et al. 1995) in cats. Investigators at the University of South Carolina also used electrophysiology for the purpose of intracranial self-stimulation: stimulating electrodes were placed in the ventral tegmentum, a pleasure center that surrounds the hypothalamus, and used to operantly reinforce treadmill running by rats (Burgess et al. 1991).

Microdialysis

Although neurons can discharge without a subsequent release of NT (e.g., when NT synthesis has not kept pace with the discharge rate), the normal response to the depolarization of a neuron includes a calcium-regulated migration of vesicles containing stored NT to the cell membrane at the terminal end of an axon, exocytosis of the vesicle (i.e., protrusion into the synapse), and release of the NT into the extracellular, synaptic space between neurons. Other factors can explain increases in the extracellular levels of NT, but under most circumstances NT level is a very good indicator of NT release.

Levels of extracellular NT can be measured by **microdialysis**. Dialysis separates molecules of various sizes using an artificial membrane that is permeable to only some molecules. A microdialysis probe is made of a small metal tube containing inner and outer compartments, or cannulas, that is implanted into the brain through a guide cannula fixed to the skull using dental cement (see figure 3.27). The inner cannula of the probe serves as an inlet through which artificial cerebrospinal fluid can be pumped into the brain at a rate that permits the diffusion of NT molecules from the extracellular brain fluid across the dialysis membrane and into the outer cannula, where it is collected at an outlet (see figure 3.28). The retrieved fluid is then analyzed for the concentration of NT using a chemical analysis technique called high-performance liquid chromatography with electrochemical detection. This technique is based on differing oxidation rates of the proteins that constitute the NT.

As with electrophysiology, microdialysis has been employed rarely in exercise psychology, but it has been used to show that brain serotonin (Wilson et al. 1986), NE (Pagliari and Peyrin 1995), and DA (Meeusen et al. 1997) levels are increased during treadmill running in rats. Another study using microdialysis showed that rats that had run for several weeks in activity wheels had a blunted release of NE in the frontal cortex when they were stressed by electric foot shock (shown in figure 3.29; Soares et al. 1999).

Electroencephalography and Magnetoencephalography

In humans, the main methods of measuring brain activity have been **electroencephalography (EEG)**, **magnetoencephalography (MEG),** and other neuroimaging techniques that measure

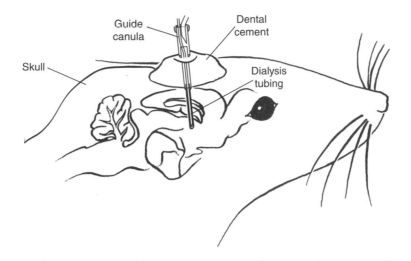

Figure 3.27 Surgically implanted guide cannula for microdialysis of brain neurotransmitters.

Provided by the Exercise Psychology Laboratory, Department of Kinesiology, and Department of Psychology, the University of Georgia.

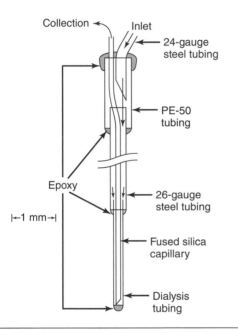

Figure 3.28 Microdialysis probe.

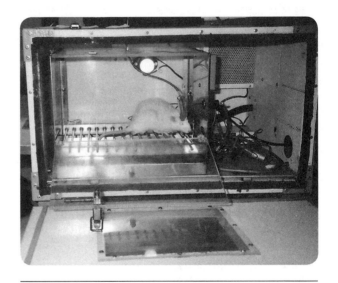

Figure 3.29 Microdialysis during foot-shock stress.

Provided by the Exercise Psychology Laboratory, Department of Kinesiology, and Department of Psychology, the University of Georgia.

nuclear responses by neurons. Several studies of psychophysiological responses to acute exercise have reported the measurement of real-time brain electrical activity via electroencephalographic recording. We will look at these applications in some detail in chapter 5, Affect, Mood, and Emotion; chapter 6, Anxiety; and chapter 10, Sleep.

EEG and MEG measure electromagnetic signals that arise from the summation of excitatory and inhibitory postsynaptic potentials in neuro-

nal assemblies of pyramidal neurons (those that have a triangle-shaped cell body). The measures approximate real-time events but have limited spatial resolution (i.e., the ability to pinpoint the exact source of the signals).

Electrodes are placed on the scalp in standardized locations, and recordings are made of the electrical potentials, or brain waves. The most common locations are based on the international 10-20 system, in which placements are in 10% or 20% increments according to head circumference

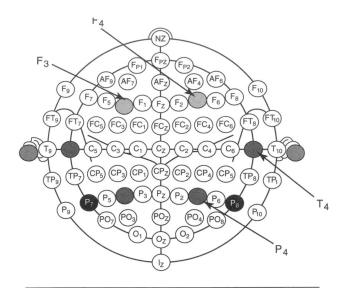

Figure 3.30 Electrode sites and nomenclature for the extended 10-20 system used in electroencephalography.

Adapted from *Electroencephalography and Clinical Neurophysiology*, Vol. (Suppl.) 52, G.H. Klem, H.O. Luders, H.H. Jasper, and C. Elger, "The end-twenty electrode system of the International Federation," p. 6, copyright 1999, with permission from Elsevier Science.

and the distance from the inion (the occipital protuberance, or the bump at the base of the skull) to the nasion (the bridge of the nose; see figure 3.30).

Because the voltage fields generated by the brain are conducted throughout the whole head and some ventral regions of the brain are oriented upward, dense-array sensor network systems nowadays commonly record from 128 or 256 sites, including the face below the ears.

The amplitude of brain waves can reach up to 200 μV, and frequency can range from once every few seconds to 50+ waves per second (Hz). The frequency spectrum is commonly decomposed into ranges, or bandwidths.

In 1875, Richard Caton described brain waves measured directly from the exposed brains of rabbits and monkeys. However, German neurophysiologist Hans Berger is credited with the discovery that electrical potentials could be measured through the scalp. In his 1929 paper, "Ÿber das Elektroen-zephalogramm des Menschen" ("On the Encephalogram of Man"), Berger designated a large regular wave that cycled about 10 times each second as α, and smaller, irregular waves that cycled 20 to 30 times each second as β. Later, H.H. Jasper and H.L. Andrews used γ to designate frequencies above 30 Hz. W.G. Walter used the term δ for all frequencies below the α band, but later designated the 4 to 7.5 Hz range as the θ band because he thought these brain waves were generated by the thalamus.

Brain activation has classically been assumed to be related to the frequency of EEG activity (e.g., δ waves predominate in deep sleep; θ waves are common in drowsiness; α waves reflect relaxed wakefulness; β waves reflect information processing; figure 3.31). However, some research has shown that α waves are most related to attention and that β waves are more active during emotion. Paradoxically, barbiturate sedatives have been shown to increase β waves. Brain wave patterns are reliably associated with neural activity, such as specific phases of sleep (see chapter 10) and epileptic seizures, and EEG readings have also been found to be associated with emotional states in various circumstances (chapters 4 and 5). However, there is very little agreement among psychophysiologists about the meaning of the various bandwidths for the processing of emotions. The character of the waves depends on the activity of the cerebral cortex, but increased electrical activity at one

Electroencephalography Frequency Bands

δ (delta)	0.5-3.5 Hz	20-200 μV
θ (theta)	4-7 Hz	20-100 μV
α (alpha)	8-12 Hz	20-60 μV
β (beta)	13-30 Hz	2-20 μV
γ (gamma)	40-50 Hz	2-10 μV

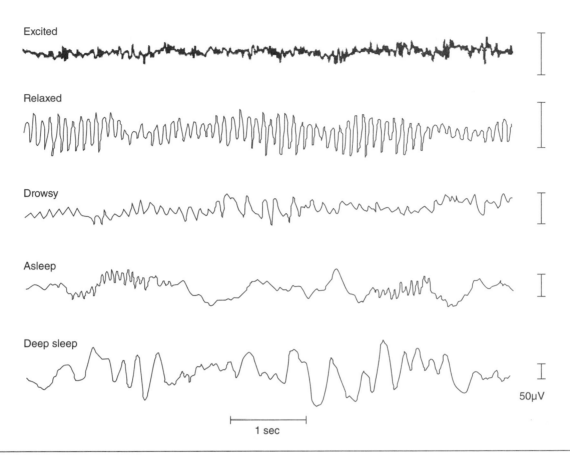

Excited

Relaxed

Drowsy

Asleep

Deep sleep

50μV

1 sec

Figure 3.31 EEG recordings for different mental states.

Reprinted from *Electroencephalography and Clinical Europhysiology* Vol. 4, D.B. Lindsley, "Psychological phenomena and the electroencephalogram," pp. 443-456, copyright 1952, with permission from Elsevier Science.

particular EEG electrode site does not necessarily translate to increased neural transmission from immediately underlying neurons or indicate that brain systems immediately below that particular site are metabolically active.

Recording EEG and MEG activity can be simple: one recording electrode and one reference electrode are needed along with an amplifier and a means to record the amplified signal. However, data acquisition systems used nowadays have become very complicated. To perform mathematical operations on the data, fully digital systems are commonly used. In addition, because of the inverse-solution problem (i.e., an infinite number of electromagnetic sources could account for what is recorded at the scalp), systems with increasing numbers of electrodes (up to 256) have been developed. These so-called dense arrays (see figure 3.32) allow the use of advanced mathematical algorithms to make good inferences about the location of the sources that generate an electromagnetic signal of interest.

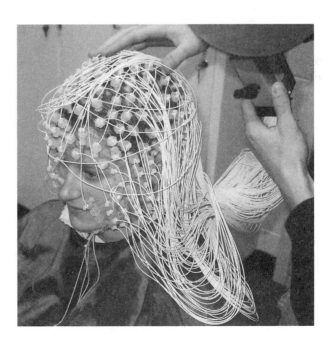

Figure 3.32 Dense electrode array.

Courtesy of Drs. Tim Puetz and Nate Thom, Exercise Psychology Laboratory and Brain Imaging Research Center, the University of Georgia.

Additional considerations, beyond the scope of this chapter, must be dealt with to reduce artifact in the recorded signal. These include correcting for non-brain-related activity (e.g., eye movements, eye blinks, facial muscle movement, and heart signals), filtering the signal appropriately, and selecting the sampling rate.

There are two main ways to evaluate EEG and MEG activity: (1) fast fourier transformation (FFT) and (2) event-related potential (ERP). A fast-fourier transform (FFT) takes time-domain data and translates them into the frequency domain using calculus. The result is estimates of electromotive power in each of multiple frequencies that are typically grouped into bands that can be associated with emotional or cognitive functions such as those described earlier in this section. For example, θ activity (4-8 Hz) is commonly found during sleep or drowsiness, but recent studies have also found frontal midline θ activity that may be generated during focused attention. Traditionally, α activity (8-12 Hz) has been associated with a state of relaxed wakefulness, but recent work has shown that different subbands within the α band are active during varying cognitive operations. Gamma oscillations are thought to reflect processes that support higher-order cognitive operations (e.g., attention and arousal, perceptual binding, or linking various perceptions in memory).

Whereas oscillatory activity can be detected at rest, ERPs can be detected only in the EEG signal when a stimulus is presented. ERPs have a low signal-to-noise ratio, so to detect an ERP, a stimulus must be presented multiple times and an average of the EEG data across each stimulus must be generated. What results is a reduction in amplitude of the random brain activity that is not associated with the stimulus. This allows the ERP to become detectable. The latency or amplitude (or both) of ERP components represents an index of the cortical resources used to process a particular stimulus.

ERP components are typically broken down into two groups, endogenous and exogenous, although some components share characteristics of both. Exogenous components, such as those arising from the brain stem, are considered obligatory (i.e., reflexive) because their properties (e.g., latency and amplitude) are mainly a function of the physical properties of the stimulus. By contrast, the characteristics of endogenous components, such as the P300 (a variation in the EEG that occurs within a window of time that includes 300 ms after the stimulus), are influenced by the interaction between the stimulus and the person.

Many different ERPs can occur across a wide temporal range. For example, some ERPs occur in anticipation of an impending stimulus, whereas others can last up to six seconds. Many of the same technical issues that are present for oscillatory activity also hold for ERP data. Extensive expertise is required to set up an ERP experiment so that the stimulus presentation paradigm results in interpretable ERP parameters.

Determining the source of electromagnetic data is difficult not only because of the inverse solution problem, but also because the signal measured by EEG is distorted as it travels through the brain, CSF, skull, and skin on the head. Neural activity recorded at the scalp at any one sensor and at any single time point contains activity from multiple neural generators. Locations of sources in the brain, therefore, cannot be directly inferred from the spatial distribution of EEG activity without first performing a source–space transformation. The surface Laplacian transformation is proportional to the electrical potential on the brain dura mater and helps reduce the distortion or smearing of the signal through the scalp. It accentuates superficial neural activities that are oriented radially to the sensors. These are the signals best measured with EEG. On the other hand, the surface Laplacian attenuates deep, nonfocal sources that can be either the cause of diffuse noise when examining cortical activity or related to true brain activations (Nunez and Srinivasan 2006).

By contrast, the magnetic potentials associated with the postsynaptic signal are not distorted as they propagate toward the scalp, which can make MEG a more attractive method for measuring electromagnetic activity. However, MEG cannot "see" sources that are oriented in certain directions, which limits its utility. Nonetheless, good estimates of source locations can be made based on well-established assumptions regarding physiology, anatomy, and electromagnetic physics. The details of these assumptions are beyond our scope here, but many source localization techniques are available that generate a source location map. Dipole source modeling (a dipole is a pair of electric charges of equal magnitude but opposite signs, separated by a small distance) assumes that most electromagnetic activity arises from a limited number of dipole sources and allows the user to go through an iterative process of identifying possible sources to arrive at a solution that best fits the scalp data. Other techniques are minimum-norm estimations, low-resolution electromagnetic tomography (LORETA and sLORETA), variable resolution electromagnetic tomography (VARETA), local auto-regressive average (LAURA), and Bayesian methods. Localizing the source of EEG and MEG data is complicated and requires considerable expertise, but with the correct assumptions it is possible and advantageous given the cost and immobility of other techniques that provide superior spatial resolution (e.g., fMRI, PET).

Neuroimaging

The underpinnings of modern-day brain imaging can be traced to Europe in the 1880s after advances in physiological recording established that mental activities led to changes in brain blood flow. Italian physiologist Angelo Mosso, who had already studied brain temperature, developed a recorder for graphing regional changes in cerebral blood flow during cognitive and emotional events in patients who had skull openings because of disease or trauma (Zago et al. 2009). Mosso ingeniously fixed a button to a small wooden dome resting on the exposed dura mater and connected it to a screw on a recording drum. When brain volume changed during the pulse of vessels, the pressure on the button increased, and pressure on the screw increased to compress air inside the drum. Changes in air compression were transmitted to the second recording drum, and then written on the rotating cylinder (a kymograph). Figure 3.33 shows the measurements taken on Michele Bertino, a 37-year-old farmer who had a wide skull fracture. The skull fragments were removed, exposing 2 centimeters (8/10 in.) of the cerebrum's frontal lobe. Mosso's work helped lay the foundation for later research that established the physiological association between increased brain neural activity and cerebral blood flow (Roy and Sherrington 1890).

More sophisticated methods for measuring brain activity in the cortex and areas other than the cortex have been developed with advances in X-ray techniques, spectroscopy, and nuclear magnetic sensing that use complex computer technology, such as seen in figure 3.34.

Computerized axial tomograms (CATs), or **CT** (computerized tomogram) **scans**, use X rays

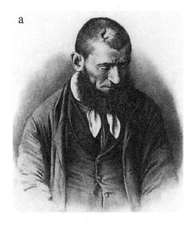
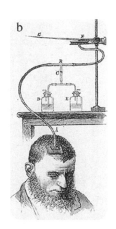
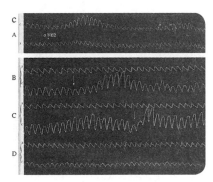

Figure. 3.33 *(a)* Michele Bertino. *(b)* Mosso's device for recording the blood volumes in the brain. *(c)* Brain pulsation recordings when Bertino was requested to multiply 8 times 12. The top trace represents brain pulsation, and the bottom trace represents forearm pulsation. *(d)* Resting state.

Reprinted from *Neuroimage*, Vol. 48(4), S. Zago, R. Ferrucci, S. Marceglia, and A. Priori, "The Mosso method for recording brain pulsation: the forerunner of functional neuroimaging," pg. 652-656, copyright 2009, with permission from Elsevier.

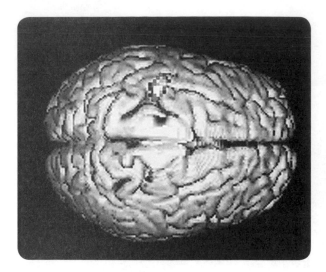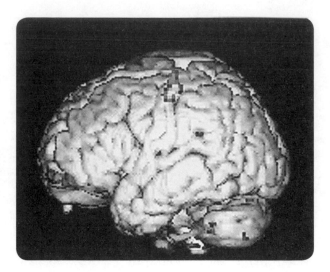

Figure 3.34 Computerized three-dimensional reconstruction of the activation of the motor cortex measured by fMRI.

Provided by Dr. Dane Cook, Department of Kinesiology, University of Wisconsin.

to enhance small differences in brain density. An X-ray source is moved repeatedly in an arc around the subject's head; and the amount of radiation that is absorbed within the brain, which depends on density, is analyzed at each position. The end products are two-dimensional pictures of the skull and its contents. Because different substances absorb different amounts of radiation, it is possible with this technology to identify specific structures of the brain.

The interaction of radio waves and a strong magnetic field is used to produce a more detailed picture of the interior of a living brain. **Magnetic resonance imaging (MRI)** provides images that have more precise resolution than the images CT provides. MRI involves passing a strong magnetic wave through a subject's head. In the presence of a strong magnetic field, the nuclei of some atoms in molecules in the body spin with a particular orientation. These nuclei emit radio waves when a radio-frequency wave is passed through the body. Different frequencies are emitted by different molecules, and the MRI scanner is tuned to pick up those from hydrogen molecules and produce pictures of the brain based on the known concentration of hydrogen in specific tissues. Changes as small as the loss of myelin around a group of axons can be detected with an MRI scan.

CT scans and MRI scans provide useful but static images of the brain. We can view the dynamic activity of the brain using **positron emission tomography (PET)**, which can reveal the glucose uptake of specific nuclei. Radioactive chemicals, most often radioactive glucose, are injected into the blood vessels, and the subject is placed into a device similar to that used for an MRI scan. The device detects the positrons emitted by the radioactive glucose in the brain and can provide a picture of the metabolic activity of various brain regions. The high cost of PET scans is a disadvantage; but newer technology has enabled a modification of the less expensive MRI **(functional MRI: fMRI)** that acquires images rapidly enough to provide a measurement of brain activity, such as oxygen consumption by active brain regions. In the brain, blood perfusion is presumably related to neural activity, so fMRI, like other imaging techniques such as PET, makes it possible to find out what the brain is doing when subjects perform specific tasks or are exposed to specific stimuli.

Advances in scanning technology have enabled scientists to monitor real-time functioning of specific areas of the brain.

Magnetic resonance imaging (MRI): The principles of nuclear magnetic resonance, developed in the 1940s, are based on variations among atomic nuclei in the radio frequencies to which their spinning axes will respond—that is, resonate. All atomic nuclei spin on their axes because they have a positive electronic charge and act as a magnet with north and south poles along the axis of spin. When an object is put in an external magnetic field, the spin axes of all the nuclei in the object line up with the field. Next, a signal with a radio frequency (RF) is broadcast at the object in a line perpendicular to the field, causing the spin axes of the nuclei to tilt from the magnetic field by an angle that is unique to the object and the RF to which it will resonate. About 20 to 300 ms after the RF signal, the spin axis gradually returns to its position parallel to the external magnetic field. This is called the T2 relaxation time, or spin relaxation time. As it relaxes, each nucleus transmits a radio signal. MRI studies of the brain use hydrogen nuclei, which have different T2 relaxation times in fat and water. Hydrogen nuclei transmit at different frequencies in fat than in water, so tissues having different water-to-fat ratios transmit unique radio signals. Those unique radio transmissions are used to form MRI images of the brain's shape and its chemical properties (Horowitz 1995).

Functional magnetic resonance imaging (fMRI): Functional magnetic resonance imaging (fMRI) applies the magnetic resonance principle for the purpose of determining which parts of the brain are activated by different types of physical sensation or motor activity, as shown in figure 3.35. It has better resolution of both space and time than PET (Cohen and Bookheimer 1994). Special software permits an MRI scanner to detect increased blood flow in areas of the brain that have been activated. Oxygenated arterial blood has a small magnetic effect. However, the deoxygenation of hemoglobin has a magnetic effect resulting from the four unpaired iron

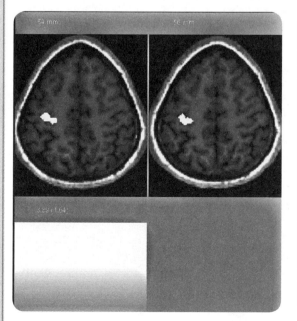 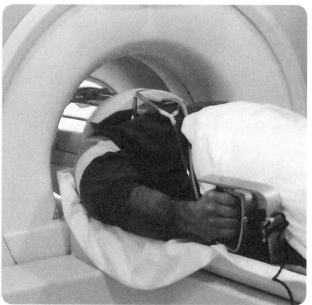

Figure 3.35 Neuroimage of the activation of the motor cortex in the left hemisphere (light area) measured by fMRI *(a)* during handgrip exercise using the right arm *(b)*.

Provided by Dr. Dane Cook, Department of Kinesiology, University of Wisconsin.

(continued)

electrons. This disturbs the local magnetic field in parts of the brain where increased blood flow or increased metabolism occurs. Blood-oxygen-level dependence (BOLD) is the MRI contrast of blood deoxyhemoglobin, which was first reported in 1990 (Ogawa et al. 1990). Blood flow to areas of the brain where neurons are activated is always increased to a greater extent than is the extraction of oxygen by brain tissue. As a result, a surplus of oxyhemoglobin accumulates in the veins of an activated brain area, which can be distinguished as a change of the local ratio of oxyhemoglobin to deoxy-hemoglobin. This provides the BOLD contrast for MRI to estimate the proportionate increase of oxygenated hemoglobin in red blood cells in a brain region, reflecting a longer proton relaxation time that can be visualized as a change in fMRI intensity of about 1% to 10%. The fMRI provides a measure of cerebral oxygenation, as well as other hemodynamic measures (Huppert et al. 2006). However, fMRI requires that the participant remain virtually motionless during data acquisition, which precludes using this technique during dynamic exercise. However, fMRI can be used to determine whether acute exercise or exercise training alters mental responses measured under resting conditions (Colcombe et al. 2004).

Arterial spin labeling (ASL): Arterial spin labeling (ASL) is the only noninvasive magnetic resonance imaging (MRI) technique that allows the absolute, rather than relative, measurement of cerebral blood flow (Williams et al. 1992). It uses radio frequency pulses to invert the spins of water in arterial blood, effectively creating a bolus of magnetically labeled blood that can be imaged as a contrast tracer while it travels along the branching vasculature. In this way, ASL provides cerebral blood perfusion maps without requiring the administration of a contrast agent or the use of radiated isotopes (Buxton, 2009; Brown et al., 2007). ASL fMRI has a lower signal-to-noise ratio, can be less sensitive to weak stimuli, and has poorer temporal resolution than BOLD (Brown et al., 2007). ASL outperforms BOLD for localizing the area of brain activation. The ASL activation signal is believed to be dominated by changes in the capillary bed of the activated area of the cortex, whereas the BOLD signal is likely to be dominated by changes in the oxygenation of nearby veins (Brown et al., 2007; Buxton, 2009). A recent study using pulsed ASL found that global cerebral blood flow was increased by about 20% after 30 minutes of moderate-intensity cycling exercise (Smith, Paulson, et al., 2010).

Diffusion tensor imaging (DTI): Diffusion tensor imaging (DTI) is a related use of MRI to measure the anatomical connectivity between brain areas. It does not measure dynamic changes in brain function. Rather, DTI measures inter-area connectivity between bundles of white matter that carry functional information between brain regions. Because the diffusion of water molecules is impeded along the axes of white matter bundles, measurements of water diffusion can estimate the anatomical location of large white matter pathways. Illnesses that disrupt the normal organization or integrity of cerebral white matter (such as multiple sclerosis) have a quantitative impact on DTI measures. Studies using DTI indicate that cerebral white matter is decreased in neural degenerative diseases such as multiple sclerosis and in the prefrontal region of the brain associated with age-related declines in cognitive function (Madden et al. 2009). A recent cross-sectional study found that aerobic fitness was related to greater white matter integrity in the cingulum (which projects from the cingulate cortex to the entorhinal cortex, the main neural input to the hippocampus), but not the prefrontal brain regions, in both young and old adults who had no neurological impairment (Marks et al. 2007). Aerobically active older adults also have less vessel tortuosity (i.e., fewer twisting curves) and an increased number of small vessels estimated by MRI when compared with less active subjects, which might contribute to cerebral white matter integrity (Bullitt et al. 2009).

Positron emission tomography (PET): Positrons are positively charged electrons.

(continued)

Neuroimaging Techniques (continued)

Molecules such as oxygen15 and carbon11 emit positrons as they decay. When a positron collides with an electron, the annihilation produces two γ rays that travel in opposite directions. A special 360° camera (shown in figure 3.36) can detect those reflected rays and thus determine their position in the brain by their intersecting points of origin. PET can assess glucose uptake, blood flow, and pH in the brain by detecting the point of accumulation of a positron-emitting isotope tracer tagged to a biologically active molecule. If multiple annihilations occur, the point of accumulation of the tracer can be located. For example, deoxyglucose is trapped in brain cells after phosphorylation, so tagging it with carbon11 permits PET to detect its accumulation during increased brain metabolism. The main advantage of PET is that it images metabolic events, not brain structures, as shown in figure 3.37. However, PET can resolve objects about 1 cm apart, whereas fMRI can resolve images in the 1 mm range.

Single-photon emission computed tomography (SPECT): When radiolabeled compounds are injected in tracer amounts, their photon emissions can be detected much like X rays

in computerized tomography. The images that are made represent the accumulation of the labeled compound. The compound may reflect, for example, blood flow, oxygen or glucose metabolism, or DA transporter concentration. Often these images are shown with a color scale. Studies using single-photon emission computerized tomography (SPECT) identified increases in regional cerebral blood flow in the thalamus and several cortical and subcortical regions (insular cortex, anterior cingulate, medial prefrontal), implicating them in the regulation by central command of cardiorespiratory responses during leg cycling and handgrip exercise (Williamson, Fadel, and Mitchell 2006) (see figure 3.38). Because tracer uptake by the brain is proportional to brain blood flow, SPECT allows post hoc estimates of change in blood flow that occurred during dynamic exercise. However, SPECT does not provide direct measures of brain oxygenation.

Near-infrared optical image scanning (iOIS): Brain tissue is opaque; it does not strongly absorb visible light. However, light does not travel in a straight line through brain tissue,

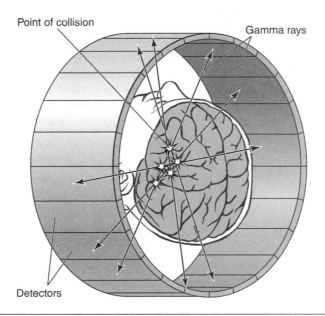

Point of collision

Gamma rays

Detectors

Figure 3.36 Positron emission tomography uses the detection of γ rays emitted from the collision of positron and electrons to provide an image of metabolic activity in the brain.

(continued)

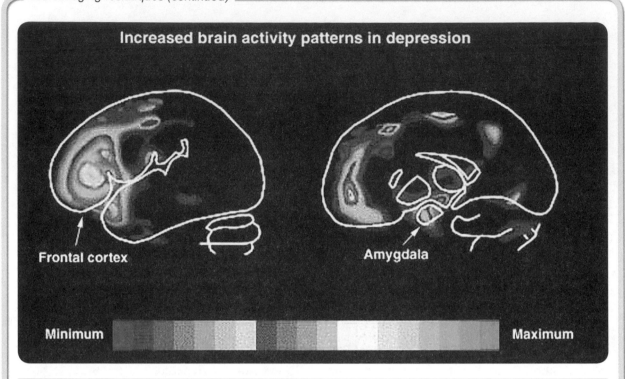

Figure 3.37 PET neuroimage of brain activity in a depressed patient.

Reprinted, by permission, from *Atlas of Brain Perfusion SPECT* at http://brighamrad.Harvard.edu. The official Web site of the Department of Radiology, Brigham and Women's Hospital, Harvard Medical School, Boston. Copyright Brigham and Women's Hospital, Harvard Medical School.

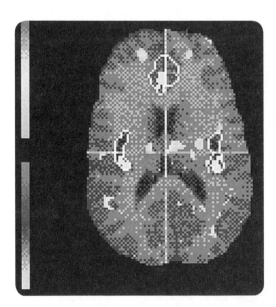

Figure 3.38 Transaxial neuroimage of the activation of the anterior cingulate cortex and insular cortex (outlined in white) in both hemispheres measured by SPECT during cycling exercise.

Provided by Dr. Jon Williamson, Department of Physical Therapy, Southwestern Medical Center, University of Texas, Dallas.

because photons scatter through brain tissue until they pass through or are absorbed. Within the near-infrared light spectrum, the absorption of light by blood and water is small, but the scatter is large. Thus, the transport of near-infrared photons in the brain is very diffuse. Local variations in this diffusion are measured by tissue optical absorption using near-infrared spectroscopy (NIRS). NIRS passes near-infrared (wavelengths of 700-1,000 nm) light through tissue, where it is either absorbed by chromophores such as oxyhemoglobin (O_2Hb), deoxyhemoglobin (dHb), or cytochrome oxidase or is scattered within the tissue. By measuring the returned, scattered light at specific wavelengths, the relative level of O_2Hb and dHb absorbed in the underlying tissue can be determined (Ferrari, Mottola, and Quaresima 2004; see figure 3.39). This technique can resolve changes in brain blood flow and oxygenation within milliseconds. The advantage of NIRS over the other methods mentioned is

(continued)

Neuroimaging Techniques (continued)

that it provides direct, real-time measures of oxygenation in cortical tissue with acceptable spatial resolution (~1 cm, or 4/10 in.) and it is not as sensitive to movement artifact as other measures are. NIRS has been used extensively

to evaluate hemodynamic changes during dynamic exercise in skeletal muscle (Hamaoka et al. 2007) and more recently in the brain (Perrey 2008; Rooks et al. 2010; Wolf, Ferrari, and Quaresima 2007).

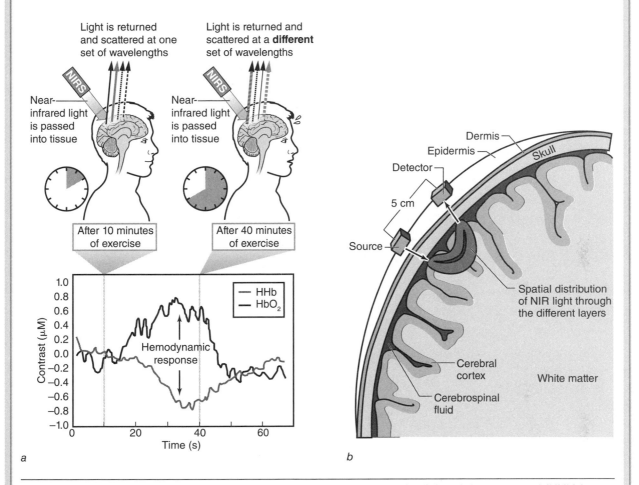

Figure 3.39 Use of near-infrared spectroscopy to measure oxygenated (HbO₂) and deoxygenated (HHb) hemoglobin in the brain cortex during exercise.

(a) Adapted from *Methods*, Vol. 45(4), S. Perrey, "Non-invasive NIR spectroscopy of human brain function during exercise," pgs. 289-299, copyright 2008, with permission from Elsevier. *(b)* Adapted from M. Ferrari, L. Mottola, and V. Quaresima, 2004, "Principles, techniques, and limitations of near infrared spectroscopy," *Canadian Journal of Applied Physiology* 29(4): 463-87. © 2008 Canadian Science Publishing or its licensors. Reproduced with permission.

SUMMARY

Social and cognitive factors, and the methods used to measure and manipulate them, are the cornerstone of exercise psychology, so chapter 2 provided quite a bit of detail on these topics. Nonetheless, neurobiological factors and the methods of behavioral neuroscience are equally

important to understanding exercise psychology. Although it has not yet been used much by exercise psychologists, behavioral neuroscience represents a new frontier in the field of exercise psychology. Thus, this chapter has introduced its key concepts and techniques. Increased use of brain neuroimaging, transgenic rodents, and programs that selectively breed mice and rats for physical activity traits would permit huge advancements in the application of behavioral neuroscience to the study of physical activity and exercise during the next decade. Not only is it important that new students be exposed to this area, but also a rudimentary understanding of this chapter is necessary for a full comprehension of some of the material in later chapters on stress, emotion, anxiety, depression, sleep, energy and fatigue, ratings of perceived exertion, pain, and cognition. Readers can grasp much of what those chapters cover without having read this chapter. But physical activity, especially exercise, is a family of biologically based behaviors, so any serious student of exercise psychology simply must tackle the biological aspects of brain and behavior—as challenging as this may be at times.

WEBSITES

www.loni.ucla.edu

www.neuroguide.com

www.nimh.nih.gov

www.med.harvard.edu/aanlib

www.nlm.nih.gov/research/visible

http://themedicalbiochemistrypage.org

www.egi.com/home

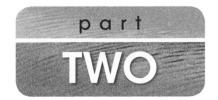

part
TWO

Exercise and Mental Health

The first U.S. surgeon general's report on mental health was published in 2000, bringing attention to the extent to which mental illness affects health and the quality of life in the United States. Mental health is also a serious public health issue on a global level. *The Global Burden of Disease* study, commissioned by the World Health Organization and the World Bank, indicated that, worldwide, more than 98 million people suffer moderate and severe disability from depression, and depression is the leading cause of years lost due to disability for adults (World Health Organization 2008). In developed nations, the direct and indirect cost of mental health disorders is 3% to 4% of the gross national product. The World Health Organization has estimated that by the year 2020, depression will surpass cancer as the second leading worldwide cause of disability and death, behind cardiovascular disease.

The prevalence and cost of affective disorders are high in most nations, although the rates vary among countries (Weissman et al. 1996, 1997). In the United States, the lifetime prevalence of mood disorders is 20.8%, and that of anxiety disorders is 28.8% (Kessler et al. 2005). In 2002 and 2003, the cost of mental illness in the United States was $300 billion, which includes $193 billion from lost earnings and wages (Reeves et al. 2011).

The prevalence and costs of mental illnesses aside, assessing the potential beneficial effects of exercise on the risk and severity of affective disorders is warranted because anxiety and depression are risk factors for other chronic diseases, including coronary heart disease, cancer, obesity, asthma, ulcers, rheumatoid arthritis, and headaches; and mental illness exacerbates the physical effects of these diseases (Friedman and Booth-Kewley 1987; Reeves et al. 2011). We echo UN Secretary-General Ban Ki-moon on World Mental Health Day in 2010 when he said, "There can be no health without mental health." This part addresses the relationship between exercise and mental health by examining the evidence that physical activity can decrease anxiety, prevent and reduce the incidence of mild and moderate depression, improve mood and self-esteem, and enhance quality of life.

Chapters 4 through 7 provide specific information about several mental health concerns and the effects of acute and chronic exercise on their etiology and persistence. Perhaps the cornerstone of exercise psychology is the relationship between exercise and mental health. Early research (e.g., Franz and Hamilton 1905) was conducted to determine the effects of exercise on depressive symptoms, and since then, hundreds of articles have been published on the effects of acute and chronic exercise on stress, affect, anxiety, and depression. Many clinical psychologists and psychiatrists view exercise as a viable adjunct therapy. The relationships among acute and chronic exercise, stress, mood, anxiety, and depression are presented in the context of psychosocial and neurobiological linkages and mechanisms. Each mental health issue is described from a psychobiological perspective.

Chapters 8 through 12 discuss quality of life issues and exercise, focusing on cognition, energy and fatigue, sleep, pain, and self-esteem. The concept of quality of life (QoL) is fully consistent with the 1946 World Health Organization definition of health (i.e., not merely the absence of disease) and the later idea of wellness. The scientific advisory committee of the *2008 Physical Activity Guidelines for Americans* defined health-related QoL as "an individual's overall sense of well-being and includes such factors as pain, mood, energy level, family and social interactions, sexual function, ability to work, and ability to keep up with routine daily activities" (Physical Activity Guidelines Advisory Committee 2008).

Several meta-analyses of mainly randomized controlled trials have reported that overall ratings of QoL and specific psychological states related to QoL are favorably affected by light- to moderate-intensity exercise interventions with both sick and well people, including self-esteem and positive affect (e.g., feelings of energy, happiness, emotional well-being, life satisfaction) (Conn et al. 2009; Netz et al. 2005; Reed and Buck 2009; Schechtman and Ory 2001; Speck et al. 2010). Effects in those trials were generally small (i.e., less than one-third SD), but differed according to whether the interventions were for primary prevention, rehabilitation, or disease management. For example, in people who were well or going through rehabilitation, both psychological and physical QoL showed similar improvements, but people in disease management programs got worse (Gillison et al. 2009).

Sleep is related to levels of physical and mental energy and fatigue, and in part II we address how exercise can affect these contributions to quality of life. There is also evidence that exercise can have positive effects on cognition in specific populations. People often associate exercise, especially high-intensity aerobic and strength training, with pain and fatigue, but this part provides evidence of a more complicated relationship among these variables. Finally, we examine the relationship between physical activity and self-esteem, which is a key indicator of mental health and an important contributor to life adjustment and quality.

Stress

The idea that exercise reduces stress has become a part of folk wisdom, much like views that exercise improves mood, self-esteem, cognition, and sleep—topics of later chapters. The benefits of an enhanced ability to cope with chronic stress are significant, considering the evidence for the role of mental stress in disease risk and recovery. For example, stress is linked to leading causes of death, such as heart disease, cancer, accidents, and suicide. This chapter discusses whether the scientific evidence supports the idea that exercise alters physiological responses during stress. Because other chapters deal with the effects of physical activity on stress emotions related to anxiety and depressive disorders, this chapter addresses whether physical activity or physical fitness blunts physiological responses during types of stress other than exercise, as well as whether it affects people's feelings of distress and well-being.

In the life sciences, stress is viewed as an imbalance in physiological systems that activates both physiological and behavioral responses to restore balance. In this way, a **stressor** is like load, a force that acts on a biological system. Because it is easy to see the analogy between objects resisting or breaking under strain and human tolerance for the burdens of living, it is commonly accepted that stress (imbalance) leads to strain (distortion, tension) in animals as it does in physical objects.

> **S**tress is an imbalance in physiological systems that activates physiological and behavioral responses to restore balance. Stressors are the forces that act on a biological system to cause stress.

BACKGROUND AND DEFINITIONS

The term *stress* appeared in the English language in the 17th century, borrowed from the French words *destresse* and *estrece,* which meant "hardship" and "oppression." The origin is the Latin word *strictia,* from a verb meaning "to draw tight." Since 1660, when the British scientist Robert Hooke reported his law of elasticity (the tension exerted by a stretched string is proportional to the extension), **stress** has been viewed by engineers as the way that load (i.e., external force) impinges on a physical object. Stress is distinguished from **strain**, which is the deformation, distortion, or tension in the object that results from stress.

A Brief History of Stress

In the mid-1800s, the French physiologist Claude Bernard (1867) proposed that life depended on maintaining the *"milieu intérieur"* (i.e., internal environment) in a constant state during changes in the external environment. It is now accepted that mammalian cells can exist only when certain ranges of temperature and acid–base balance are maintained and when water, nutrients, and oxygen are available. Systems of cells also depend on such balances. In the 1920s, Harvard physician-scientist Walter Cannon extended Bernard's views through his research on the roles of adrenaline (i.e., epinephrine) and the autonomic nervous system in regulating and maintaining physiological balance during experiences of

Good and Bad Stress

If chronic stress can increase your risk of conditions such as heart disease, high blood pressure, a suppressed immune system, eating disorders, headaches, sleep disorders, and ulcers, you might be wondering if you should attempt to remove all stress from your life. The answer is no. A certain amount of stress is needed for optimal health and performance—life without stress would be very boring! Stress researcher Hans Selye clearly distinguished between distress ("bad stress") and eustress ("good stress"). Some level of stress (eustress) is desirable for optimal performance and well-being; however, all of us can reach a point where stress can become too much (distress) and it starts to inhibit our mental, emotional, and physiological abilities to function effectively (see figure 4.1).

Excessive stress can blunt positive emotions, such as love, joy, and surprise, and exaggerate negative emotions, such as anger, sadness, and fear. Exercise can contribute to your levels of good stress when it is enjoyable and isn't so intense that it causes strain or so frequent that you don't recuperate. Moderate exercise performed regularly can offset negative stress emotions and possibly enhance positive stress emotions.

Reprinted, by permission, from A. Jackson, J. Morrow, D. Hill, Jr., and R. Dishman, 1999, *Physical activity for health and fitness* (Champaign, IL: Human Kinetics), 282.

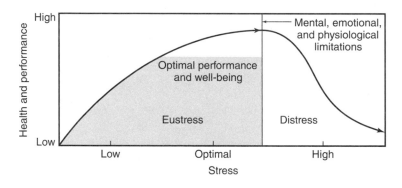

Figure 4.1　A certain amount of stress enhances performance and well-being, but excessive stress can impair mental, emotional, and physiological abilities.

rage and fear. Cannon (1929) introduced the term **homeostasis** to describe this balance, or harmony, of physiological systems. In the early 1930s, Hartman, Brownell, and Lockwood (1932) added to Cannon's ideas by proposing a general tissue hormone theory, which stated that steroids secreted by the cortex of the adrenal gland (e.g., cortisol) are needed by all cells for resisting infection and muscular and nervous fatigue, and for regulating body temperature and body water. Each of these events was credited by the Swiss physician Hans Selye for the formation of his theory of a **general adaptation syndrome (GAS)** and the diseases of adaptation, based on

the activation of the adrenal cortex in response to stress (Selye 1936, 1950).

Homeostasis is the balance, or harmony, of physiological systems.

To Selye, altered homeostasis was not merely a passing response to changes in the environment. He believed that an animal's physiological systems could learn and maintain adaptive defenses against future exposure to stress. Hence, Selye theorized that many diseases result from adaptations to the environment that are either insufficient, excessive, or poorly regulated (Selye 1950). He proposed that "conditioning factors," such as prior exposure and controllability of a stressor, could alter the GAS. Also, Selye believed that stressors, including muscular exercise, might lead to cross-stressor adaptations that would enhance resistance to psychosomatic and neurotic diseases. His research provided a scientific basis for the development of the **cross-stressor adaptation hypothesis** of exercise, which states that exercise training or increased levels of fitness are associated with an attenuation of stress responses in nonexercise situations (Michael 1957; Sothmann et al. 1996).

Bruce S. McEwen (1998), a neuroscientist at Rockefeller University, has used the term **allostatic load** to describe the long-term effects of the physiological response to stress (including the activation of the autonomic nervous system; the hypothalamic-pituitary-adrenal axis; and the metabolic, cardiovascular, and immune systems). **Allostasis** is a term derived from Greek and means the ability to achieve stability through change (i.e., adaptation) (see figure 4.2). Like Selye, McEwen believes that the price paid for such adaptation to stress is allostatic load, the strain that results from the overactivity or underactivity of these allostatic systems.

Some people develop a *hypo*activity or *hyper*activity of the normal stress response. It appears that too small a stress response can be just as harmful as too much of a response, because it may result in other responses that compensate. For example, cortisol stimulates blood glucose for energy, but it also keeps the immune system in check by inhibiting inflammation. If cortisol does not rise during stress, inflammation can result even though there is no infection. On the other hand, too much cortisol can make a person susceptible to infection by overly suppressing the inflammation response; and it can lead to bone loss, muscle atrophy, and elevated insulin levels.

> **A** balanced response to stress is optimal: overresponding or underresponding can be dangerous.

For unknown reasons, the stress response does not subside in some people after a stressful event has ended. For example, public speaking activates the hypothalamic-pituitary-adrenal (HPA) axis and increases blood cortisol in most people, but that response goes away after the person has gained experience. However, about

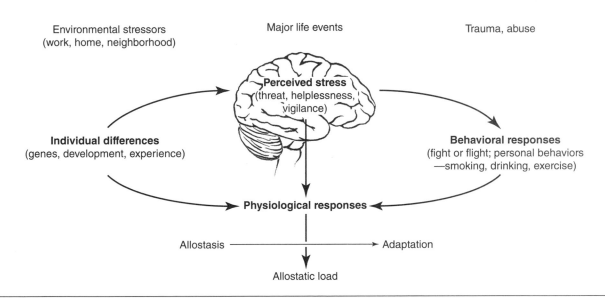

Figure 4.2 Allostasis: the ability to achieve stability through adaptation to stress.

1 in 10 people will continue to have a cortisol response when they speak in public, regardless of their experience. Likewise, it is not understood why some people lose their ability to mount a stress response after chronic exposure to stressful events. Many researchers are convinced that regular exercise of moderate intensity is one of the best ways to offset the allostatic load of chronic stress. That makes sense because we know, for example, that exercise reduces insulin levels that can be raised by high cortisol, and that exercise training lowers blood pressure (BP) and resting heart rate (HR). Before considering evidence for a relationship between exercise and the stress response, we need to define the conditions that elicit stress and the main responses during stress.

Defining Stress

Stress can lead to painful physical symptoms, such as muscle tension, headache, and stomach upset; physiological signs, such as a racing heart, high blood pressure, sweating, flushing, and dry mouth; and behaviors ranging from aggression to hyperactivity to withdrawal. Those signs and symptoms can occur independently

or together with stress emotions, which include the physiological and behavioral responses that are experienced subjectively (e.g., fear, anxiety, anger, despair). Scientists have identified key physiological responses during stress and their patterns of occurrence.

Early studies of humans during the 1950s and 1960s showed that responses by the adrenal glands are largest when stressful tasks are complex and require rapid decision making, or when people are responsible for the welfare of others or have little control over the outcomes of critical events, or both. During the late 1960s and early 1970s, Marianne Frankenhaeuser of the University of Stockholm demonstrated that in novel, unpredictable, and threatening circumstances, levels of epinephrine and its related hormone norepinephrine were increased during muscular exertion or mental challenge in proportion to people's perception of stress. However, the increases, particularly in epinephrine, were blunted as people became familiar with the challenge (Frankenhaeuser 1971). A later study showed that cortisol responded the same way (Mason et al. 1976). Those findings led to additional definitions of stress according to how people appraise (i.e., define and evaluate) events

Table 4.1 Dimensions of Events That Elicit a Stress Response

Dimensions of stressors can interact. For example, frequent daily hassles over which humans have no control that continue for months may have more cumulative ill effects than one short-lived major life event that humans are able to resolve themselves.

Quality	Familiarity	Source
Eustress (positive)	Familiar	Mental (i.e., negative thoughts)
Distress (negative)	Novel	Physiological (e.g., virus)
		Environmental (social, physical)
Quantity	**Coping response**	**Threat level**
Duration	Active	No threat
Frequency	Passive	Life threatening
Intensity	**Sensory focus**	**Types (perceived)**
Minor hassle	Rejection	Challenge (person is confident he or she can overcome the stressor)
Major life event	Intake	Threat (anticipation of harm)
	Intake or rejection	Harm (experienced damage)

as threatening and how they cope with the stress (respond mentally or by their behavior) (Lazarus 1993). People can cope with stress actively by striving to overcome the source of the stress or by trying to avoid it (**active coping**), or passively by accepting it without resistance. Events that result in stress can be described in terms of several other dimensions that are related to the nature of the response (see table 4.1).

Stress can occur during a crisis of high impact and for either a short or long duration, or during the smaller, brief, but nagging hassles of daily living. Positive life events or daily uplifts in spirit can also be stressful, but in a good way, because they reduce boredom and offset negative emotions. Although it is true that some people simply are exposed to more events that cause stress or strain (e.g., family conflicts, money problems, loss of a loved one, too many hard exams), it is also true that personality and coping skills can lessen a person's vulnerability to stress. About 50% of a person's temperament—whether it is usually calm, nervous, or fiery—is explained by heredity and early childhood learning. Nonetheless, people can improve their ability to deal with stress by learning skills to reduce their exposure to stressful events or by changing their outlook

> **Candidates for Chronic Stress**
>
> People may be at risk for chronic stress if they
>
> - feel overwhelmed by responsibilities,
> - think they have too much to do in too little time, or
> - feel uncertain about important consequences that seem out of their personal control.

on life. People who view change as a challenge or an opportunity for success, who feel in control, and who have a strong commitment to a life purpose (e.g., career, other people, spirituality) seem to deal better with misfortune than do people who interpret change as a threat, who feel out of control, and who lack a guiding life purpose.

EFFECTS OF EXERCISE

Most researchers in exercise psychology who have studied stress have looked at whether exercise affects perceived stress. And many studies have confirmed that people generally report reduced or fewer symptoms of stress when they have been physically active. It appears that

> **R**esponses to stress can be active (resistance or avoidance) or passive (accepting it without resistance).

> **Stress Management: Controlling Emotion by Maintaining Rational Thinking**
>
> - Avoid fatalistic thinking *(No matter what I do, I will never be any stronger than I am now).*
> - Avoid all-or-none thinking *(I must get an A in this class, or it will be a waste of my time; I can't have any chocolate or I will blow my whole diet).*
>
> - Avoid catastrophic thinking; that is, making mountains out of molehills *(I couldn't keep up on the runs this week—I must have a metabolic disease that keeps me from adapting to exercise training).*

aerobic types of exercise lasting up to about 30 minutes generally are associated with the largest reductions in perceived stress. Aerobic exercise programs lasting at least a few months seem best for reducing reports of chronic stress. Although exercise usually won't eliminate the source of stress, it could help reduce stress temporarily by providing a short-term distraction from a problem. An exercise program might increase feelings of control or commitment (e.g., success in doing something important for oneself), which could buffer the impact of stressful events.

Relying on people's self-ratings of stress has problems, however. Using self-reports of reduced stress makes it difficult to disentangle the contribution of exercise to stress reduction from a placebo effect. As in research on anxiety and depression, many participants enter the testing environment with expectations that exercise will decrease tension and improve mood. In addition, a self-rating of perceived stress does not adequately determine whether becoming physically active or physically fit indeed reduces behavioral or physiological responses during stressful events.

> **A**cute exercise decreases the behavioral and physiological manifestations of the stress response.

Studies that used objective measures of stress seem to confirm the self-reports, though. A few studies have shown that a single exercise session can reduce tension in the muscles of the face, arms, and legs, as measured by **electromyography (EMG)** after exercise (deVries and Adams 1972; Smith et al. 2001). Other studies have shown that a single session of exercise can increase electrical brain waves (measured from the scalp by electroencephalography; see chapter 3) in the α frequency band (i.e., 8-12 cycles per second) by a half standard deviation when measured during and after exercise (Crabbe and Dishman 2001). Alpha waves are usually believed to reflect a mental state of relaxed wakefulness. However, exercise

also increases smaller, faster β waves (i.e., 13-30 cycles per second) that are increased during brain activation, so it is not yet possible to view the brain wave studies as physiological evidence that exercise reduces stress.

Additionally, these studies did not show that people also *perceived* less tension or stress when the muscle or brain measurements were made. That research is discussed in more detail in chapter 5 on affect, mood, and emotion and in chapter 6 on anxiety. We should note too that most studies of physiological measures related to stress have been in experiments conducted in laboratory conditions and examined whether HR and BP during mildly stressful tasks were lower among young and middle-aged adults who were physically active or fit versus people who were more sedentary and less fit, or examined whether those responses were lessened by a single session of exercise (Jackson and Dishman 2002). Some of the limitations of research on exercise and stress are discussed in later sections of this chapter.

MECHANISMS

Understanding the possible mechanisms for a reduced stress response from exercise requires a basic familiarity with the key physiological responses during stress, how they are controlled by the nervous and **endocrine** systems, and how they differ among types of stressors. (See table 4.2 for types of stressors and associated responses.) Key components of the stress response are neural and endocrine responses that are regulated by the brain and the autonomic nervous system. They include regions of the brain modulated by the neurotransmitters norepinephrine and serotonin, the sympathetic (including the adrenal medulla) and parasympathetic arms of the autonomic nervous system, and the HPA cortical axis.

Brain Norepinephrine and Serotonin

Norepinephrine and serotonin cells in the brain influence attention and vigilance, pituitary hormone release, and cardiovascular function during stress. They also influence pain, fatigue,

Table 4.2 Characteristic Features and Physiological Responses to Common Tasks Used in Human Studies of Stress and the Autonomic Nervous System

Task	Coping (active vs. passive)	Sensory focus (intake vs. rejection)	Response pattern	ANS pattern
Mental arithmetic	Active	Rejection	↑HR, ↑SBP, ↑DBP, ↔SV, ↑CO, ↔TPR	Strong vagal withdrawal, β-adrenergic
Psychomotor reaction time	Active	Intake/rejection	↑HR, ↑SBP, ↑DBP, ↑SV, ↑CO, ↓TPR	Moderate vagal withdrawal, β-adrenergic
Stroop Color and Word Test	Active	Intake/rejection	↑HR, ↑BP, ↑DBP, ↔SV, ↑CO, ↔TPR	Moderate vagal withdrawal, β-adrenergic
Forehead cold	Passive	?	↓HR, ↑SBP, ↑DBP, ↓SV, ↔CO, ↑TPR	Vagal activity, α-adrenergic
Cold pressor	Passive	?	↑HR, ↑SBP, ↑DBP, SV, ↔CO, ↑TPR	Vagal withdrawal, α-adrenergic

ANS = autonomic nervous system; CO = cardiac output; DBP = diastolic blood pressure; HR = heart rate; SBP = systolic blood pressure; SV = stroke volume; TPR = total peripheral resistance; ↑ = increase; ↓ = decrease; ↔ = little change.

Reprinted, by permission, from R.K. Dishman and E.M. Jackson, 2000, "Exercise, fitness, and stress," *International Journal of Sports Physiology* 31: 190.

and sleep. The neural discharge of the locus coeruleus and the raphe nuclei is increased during arousal, decreased during sleep, and absent during rapid eye movement sleep (when motor activity is inhibited). During stress, cells from the locus coeruleus release norepinephrine, and cells from the raphe nuclei release serotonin into the brain's frontal lobe and into the limbic system, including the hippocampus, amygdala, and hypothalamus (see figure 3.8) Norepinephrine regulates other brain cells involved in vigilance against threat, helping to initiate behavioral, cardiovascular, and endocrine responses during stress. Serotonin helps the body return to rest after energy-expending behaviors (e.g., feeling satisfied and full after eating and feeling fatigued after exercise). In these ways, the locus coeruleus and the raphe nuclei operate in the brain similarly to the way the sympathetic and parasympathetic branches of the peripheral autonomic nervous system function to modulate the heart, vessels, and adrenal glands during stress.

> **D**uring stress, norepinephrine helps to initiate behavioral, cardiovascular, and endocrine responses. Serotonin helps the body return to rest after energy-expending behaviors.

Autonomic Nervous System

The features of the autonomic nervous system (ANS) most relevant for understanding cross-stressor adaptations to regular exercise include (1) the innervation of the heart, blood vessels, and adrenal gland by sympathetic nerves and the vagus nerve and (2) hypothalamic-pituitary hormone responses (see chapter 3, figure 3.11). Although there is great specificity in the ANS in response to various types of stressors, common neuroanatomy in the brain also permits the coactivation of ANS responses during intense stress.

Sympathetic and Vagal Effects

Usually, when someone experiences stress, the activation of the sympathetic nervous system (SNS) increases. Sympathetic nerves from the portions of the spinal cord in the areas of the trunk stimulate organs such as the heart, the adrenal glands, and the arteries. Under physical or emotional stress, sympathetic nerves stimulate the heart to beat faster and more forcefully, the adrenal glands to secrete epinephrine and norepinephrine, and the arteries that supply the heart and skeletal muscles to dilate so that blood flow is increased (see figure 4.3).

During exercise, these actions help supply the extra blood needed to carry oxygen to the muscles used in locomotion. While the heart is beating, systolic BP rises to help drive blood to the muscles. While the heart rests between beats, diastolic pressure remains low, so there is little resistance to the flow of blood to the skeletal muscles (see figure 4.3).

During emotional stress, the same responses occur, although usually to a lesser degree, because the nervous, cardiovascular, and endocrine systems are preparing for a threatening situation, the so-called flight-or-fight response to danger. A major difference between the two situations, exercise and emotional stress, is that the responses during exercise are necessary for the large increase in body metabolism (i.e., the need for extra energy). Emotional stress usually occurs at near-resting metabolism while people are anticipating a response such as fighting or fleeing from the danger. It is this elevated sym-

> In emotional stress, the ANS prepares the body for the flight-or-fight response to actual and perceived threat; metabolism is at or near rest with the anticipation of threat. In exercise stress, the ANS supports the increased metabolism of skeletal muscles and regulates breathing and body temperature; metabolism is elevated to perform physical work.

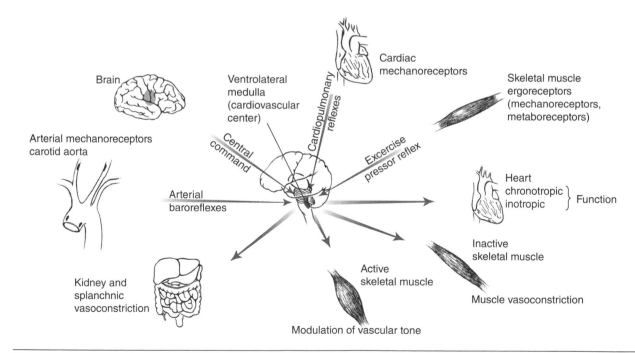

Figure 4.3 Depiction of the control of cardiovascular responses during exercise by central command from the brain and reflexive processing of sensory signals.

Reprinted, by permission, from J.H. Mitchell and P.B. Raven, 1994, Cardiovascular adaptation to physical activity. In *Physical activity, fitness, and health* (Champaign, IL: Human Kinetics), 289.

pathetic response to perceived, not necessarily real, threat that is common among people with depression or anxiety disorders. Chronic elevations in several of the stress hormones when people feel threatened—but do not physically respond by fighting or fleeing—can make tissues in the brain, heart, and vessels vulnerable to injury or death. The physiological effects of chronically elevated stress hormones can contribute to diseases such as coronary heart disease and the suppression of the body's immune system (see figure 4.4).

The main function of the ANS during exercise is to regulate the increases in HR and BP needed to increase cardiac output to support the increased metabolism of skeletal muscle cells. Secondary functions include the regulation of breathing and temperature. The cardiovascular

pressor response, which regulates systolic BP during exercise, is understood to depend on a central command of autonomic efferent neural activity in the region of the temporal sensorimotor cortex. The centrally controlled pressor response is integrated at the ventrolateral medulla of the spinal cord with a pressor reflex arising from mechanoreceptors (e.g., sensitive to muscle tension) and metaboreceptors (e.g., sensitive to hydrogen ions) in exercising muscle (Mitchell and Raven 1994). Cardiopulmonary and arterial baroreflexes modulate the exercise pressor response, apparently by an upward and parallel resetting of the operating (i.e., set) point of the arterial baroreflexes resulting from central command (Rowell 1993). This means that BP is still regulated by changes in HR but at much higher levels than at rest. Increased HR during

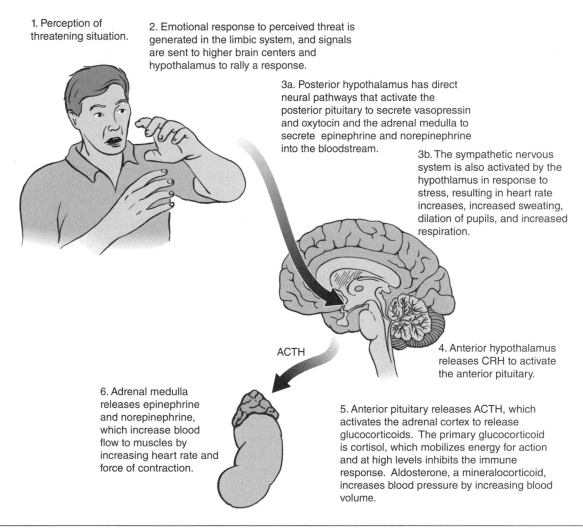

1. Perception of threatening situation.

2. Emotional response to perceived threat is generated in the limbic system, and signals are sent to higher brain centers and hypothalamus to rally a response.

3a. Posterior hypothalamus has direct neural pathways that activate the posterior pituitary to secrete vasopressin and oxytocin and the adrenal medulla to secrete epinephrine and norepinephrine into the bloodstream.

3b. The sympathetic nervous system is also activated by the hypothlamus in response to stress, resulting in heart rate increases, increased sweating, dilation of pupils, and increased respiration.

ACTH

4. Anterior hypothalamus releases CRH to activate the anterior pituitary.

6. Adrenal medulla releases epinephrine and norepinephrine, which increase blood flow to muscles by increasing heart rate and force of contraction.

5. Anterior pituitary releases ACTH, which activates the adrenal cortex to release glucocorticoids. The primary glucocorticoid is cortisol, which mobilizes energy for action and at high levels inhibits the immune response. Aldosterone, a mineralocorticoid, increases blood pressure by increasing blood volume.

Figure 4.4 Several systems are involved in supporting the cardiovascular response to stress.

exercise results from an initial withdrawal of the cardiovagal inhibition of the heart. Vagal withdrawal and the subsequent increase in HR are followed by increased activation of the heart by sympathetic nerve activity and by hormonal stimulation from catecholamines secreted by the adrenal medulla during intense exercise.

During exercise, the increase in blood levels of norepinephrine comes mainly from the sympathetic nerves to the heart. Some of the increase also comes from the exercising skeletal muscles, and some may come from the brain. Exercise training does not usually change the levels of norepinephrine in the blood or sympathetic nerve activity to muscles measured while people rest. However, after exercise training, levels of norepinephrine in the blood are lower at a given **absolute intensity** (standard intensity) of exercise (e.g., running a mile in 6 min) and unchanged when that intensity of exercise is expressed as a percentage of **maximal aerobic capacity** (e.g., running a mile at 80% of top speed), but higher than normal at maximal exercise. This means that exercise training seems to increase the capacity of the sympathetic nerves to respond to maximal exercise, but it does not change their responses to exercise of the same relative strain as before training. Also, there is no evidence that exercise training leads to a reduced sympathetic response to mental stress, when sympathetic response is measured by epinephrine or norepinephrine in the blood or by the activity of sympathetic nerves to skeletal muscle vasculature.

Exercise adaptations for plasma norepinephrine are no change at rest, lower levels at a given absolute intensity, no change at the same **relative intensity**, and increased levels at maximal exercise. Levels of norepinephrine do not change when the person is at rest, rise minimally at a given absolute intensity of exercise, and remain unchanged at the same relative intensity of exercise, and increase in response to maximal exercise.

Studies have shown that fitter people, especially women, have lower HR and BP during active mental stress (e.g., mental arithmetic and public speaking) compared to less fit people (Spalding et al. 2000); but that is mainly explained by their lower resting HR and BP, which are common adaptations to regular exercise. In other words, they have lower levels during stress because they have lower levels to start with, not because they have a smaller reaction to the stressors (Buckworth, Dishman, and Cureton 1994; Graham et al. 1996; Jackson and Dishman 2002).

Physically fit people have lower HR and BP during active mental stress because they typically have lower HR and BP at rest than unfit people have.

Lower HR among fit people could result from the lower intrinsic rate of the heart (i.e., the rate of the heart's internal pacemaker) or lower activity by sympathetic nerves to the heart, but studies mainly show that it results from increased **cardiovagal tone** (see table 4.3 for the measurement of ANS activity). The vagus nerve is part of the parasympathetic branch of the ANS. Its neurotransmitter is acetylcholine. Recall that the sympathetic nervous system stimulates energy expenditure and that the parasympathetic nervous system helps store and conserve energy (see chapter 3). The two systems work together to maintain a balance of the body's energy resources both at rest and during stress. For example, the vagus nerve slows the heart's frequency and force of beating and relaxes, or dilates, arteries that supply blood to skeletal muscle. So, a person who has increased vagal tone after exercise training can better offset the effects of the sympathetic nerves on heart and blood vessels and thus have lower HR and BP at rest and during stress. Increased cardiovagal tone also decreases the risk for irregular heartbeats and sudden death in people who have heart disease.

The high metabolism during exercise produces feedback to the brain and central nervous

Table 4.3 Measurement of Autonomic Nervous System Activity: Heart Rate Variability

It is not feasible to directly measure the firing rates of the sympathetic and vagus nerves that innervate the heart. Thus, their relative activity is commonly estimated by heart rate variability (HRV).

Experiments in nonhuman animals have shown that electrical stimulation of the cardiac sympathetic nerves results in fluctuations in heartbeat that are large but slow (LF), whereas stimulation of the vagus nerve results in rapid changes in heart rate (HF).

Term	Definition
Heartbeat	The period of the heart; the time between the R waves in successive QRS complexes
Hertz (Hz)	Frequency, or the number of cycles per second
Low frequency (LF)	0.05-0.15 Hz
High frequency (HF)	0.15-0.50 Hz
ESTIMATES OF AUTONOMIC BALANCE DURING SHORT-TERM FLUCTUATIONS IN HEART RATE	
Cardiovagal component	HF is normalized to total power: $HF / (HF + LF) \times 100$
Sympathovagal component	LF is expressed relative to HF: (LF / HF)

system from peripheral nerves and hormones in the blood; this feedback is used to regulate physiological homeostasis. It is easy to understand why regular exercise and increased fitness would lead to lower HR, BP, and stress hormones during exercise and to a quicker recovery, because that adaptation would preserve homeostasis and reduce allostatic load. However, it is more difficult to understand why such adaptations to exercise would transfer to other stressors that do not have a high energy cost and do not involve exertion using skeletal muscles. It is not apparent that cardiovascular adaptations to exercise should be expected to generalize to other stressors that do not impose similar psychomotor demands.

In contrast to exercise, most nonexercise stressors elicit little or no sensory afferent activity to regulate cardiovascular responses. Thus, much of any cross-stressor adaptation after exercise must involve central command (i.e., motor nerve discharge to the heart, vessels, or adrenal medulla) or altered organ responses to central command (e.g., decreased number or sensitivity of receptor cells that bind with epinephrine or norepinephrine). Although such propositions are plausible, the studies done to this point do not support the idea that regular exercise or cardiorespiratory fitness results in a blunted physiological response to stress other than exercise.

> **M**uch of any cross-stressor adaptation after exercise must involve central command or altered organ responses to central command.

On the other hand, studies in rats have shown that voluntary running in activity wheels leads to a blunted stress response during foot-shock stress (as measured by less release of norepinephrine in the brain cortex) (Soares et al. 1999) and a protection against the suppression of the innate immune system (Dishman et al. 1995). These actions appear to be modulated by the sympathetic nervous system during stress (Dishman, Hong, et al. 2000).

Hypothalamic-Pituitary-Adrenal Cortex System

The ANS is activated during stress, but the brain also stimulates energy production by activating endocrine organs, including the pituitary gland and the outer part (cortex) of the adrenal gland (see figure 4.5). During stress and exercise, the anterior pituitary gland releases adrenocortico-trophic hormone (ACTH), which stimulates the adrenal cortex to secrete cortisol. The amount of ACTH available for release is regulated by a gene that is activated by corticotropin-releasing hormone (CRH). This gene is located mainly in the arcuate nucleus of the hypothalamus, which expresses a macromolecule, **proopiomelanocor-ticotropin (POMC)**. ACTH and **β-endorphin** are cleaved from POMC and are secreted together from the pituitary during stress. Although nerve cells containing CRH are located throughout the brain, most of the CRH that increases ACTH levels comes from the paraventricular nucleus

(PVN) of the hypothalamus and is released into the portal blood supply to ACTH-secreting cells in the pituitary. During stress, the release of nor-epinephrine and dopamine in the PVN activates CRH to increase ACTH. The secretion of CRH is inhibited by the hippocampus.

Moderate exercise training results in a dimin-ished HPA response during the same absolute exercise intensity compared to that before train-ing. However, heavy exercise training can be associated with abnormal HPA responses under resting conditions (see chapter 5). Generally, fit people have an increased capacity to respond to severe stress, but the effects of fitness on responses to milder mental stresses such as daily hassles is not clear. An early study (Sinyor et al. 1983) indicated that trained men had higher

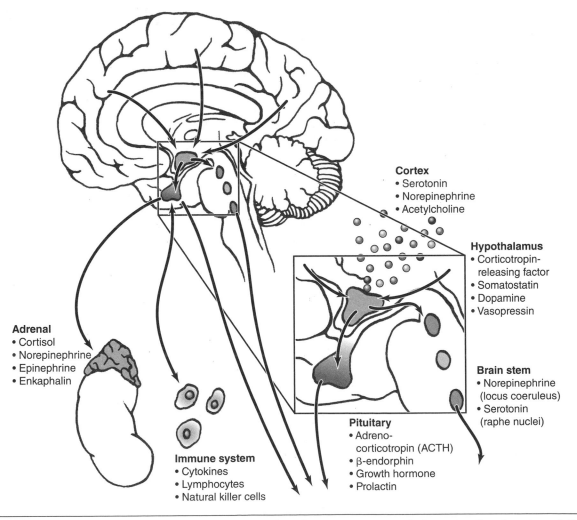

Figure 4.5 Responses of the hypothalamic-pituitary-adrenal cortex system and the sympathoadrenal medullary system during stress.

Adapted from R.H. Black, 1995, Psychoneuroimmunology: Brain and immunity, *Scientific American* 2(6): 17.

levels of cortisol at rest, under mental stress, and during recovery when compared to sedentary men; but the rates of response and recovery were the same for the trained and the untrained men. In other studies, men differing in fitness levels had similar levels of cortisol or ACTH in plasma after mental stress regardless of whether it was novel (Sothmann et al. 1988) or familiar (Blaney et al. 1990). Animal studies have shown no effects of chronic activity-wheel running on plasma levels of ACTH and cortisol after repeated foot shock in female and male rats (Dishman et al. 1995, 1997).

Exercise studies usually have not measured or controlled reproductive hormones known to influence physiological responses to nonexercise stressors, despite evidence of an interaction between the HPA cortical and the HPA gonadal systems in highly trained women. Treadmill exercise training of female rats treated with estrogen was accompanied by an attenuated ACTH response to familiar treadmill running but a hyperresponsiveness of ACTH to novel immobilization or foot shock (White-Welkley et al. 1995, 1996). Whether this hyperresponsiveness of ACTH is a healthful adaptation and whether it is due to increased CRH or other factors that release ACTH is not known. The latter seems likely because treadmill exercise training in male rats is accompanied by reduced ACTH after immobilization stress with no change in brain CRH (White-Welkley et al. 1996). Those findings might indicate that the energy and neuromuscular demands of treadmill running lead to an increased potential for HPA responses to novel stressors.

CONTEMPORARY VIEWS: EXERCISE RESEARCH

The first review of the cumulative evidence from 25 studies of fitness and physiological stress responses concluded, over 25 years ago, that aerobic fitness reduced stress responses by about a half standard deviation, regardless of the type of stressors used or the physiological responses measured (Crews and Landers 1987). Since then, no other scientific consensus has reached that early conclusion. One meta-analysis concluded

that people with higher cardiorespiratory fitness have lower HR and systolic BP responses during mental stress and faster HR recovery (Forcier et al. 2006), but another meta-analysis concluded that fitness was weakly associated with increased physiological reactivity, but quicker recovery, from laboratory stress, and revealed that HR and BP reactivity to stress was unchanged by exercise training (Jackson and Dishman 2006). A recent randomized controlled trial increased and decreased cardiorespiratory fitness by aerobic training and detraining and reported no differences in HR, HR variability, or BP responses during or after active or passive laboratory stressors when compared to a resistance exercise training group that showed no changes in cardiorespiratory fitness (Sloan et al. 2011).

The sustained confusion about exercise, fitness, and stress reactivity is largely the case because research in exercise psychology has done a poor job in building on what is known about the physiology of stress; especially problematic are the absence of a clear characterization of the features of the stressor used and the lack of any consideration of the regulatory mechanisms that govern physiological stress responses. Specifically, the lack of consensus is explainable primarily by the five factors described in the sidebar Factors Limiting Past Research on Exercise and Stress Reactivity (Dishman and Jackson 2000).

The type of stressor used in research on exercise and stress reactivity is a particularly critical issue. Unless a stressor is strong enough to engage a general flight-or-fight response (e.g., life-or-death threat), responses during stress differ widely according to the type of stressor (Allen and Crowell 1989; Dishman, Jackson, and Nakamura 2002) (see table 4.2). Active stressors motivate the person to try to control the challenge (e.g., mental arithmetic, quizzes, reaction-time tasks). Physiological responses include increases in HR, cardiac output, and systolic BP and withdrawal of vagal tone. Passive stressors offer little or no opportunity for the person to control an aversive situation and commonly result in increased HR and increased peripheral resistance to blood flow and diastolic BP. Other responses can also occur such that increased

Factors Limiting Past Research on Exercise and Stress Reactivity

Measurement of Fitness and Exercise

Early studies did a poor job defining or measuring fitness or exercise. Thus, it was hard to determine whether people differed enough to permit a true test of the influence of fitness or exercise habits on stress responses. Also, the use of submaximal HR to estimate peak oxygen uptake ($\dot{V}O_2$peak) confounded the use of HR as both an independent variable (i.e., level of fitness) and dependent variable in several studies. A test-anxious person could show exaggerated HR responses to the exercise test and to the other stressors and be misclassified as unfit because of the effect of emotion on the elevation in HR during exercise.

Measurement of Physiological Variables

The manner of reporting the methods used to measure physiological variables and to compute their change in response to stressors made it difficult to determine whether the procedures in many studies met international standards for psychophysiological research. The accuracy of the measures was questionable in some studies, and the influence of pretest baselines on the stress variables that were measured during stress and recovery was not accounted for in several studies, likely giving a false measure of responsiveness.

Research Design

About two-thirds of the studies used a cross section of time to compare stress responses among groups classified according to levels of fitness or exercise (rather than comparing responses after a change in fitness or exercise) and did not match the groups on other factors known to influence stress responses, such as temperament, behavior patterns, or reproductive hormone status.

Consideration of Integrated Physiological Responses

Investigators gave inadequate consideration to physiological mechanisms that explain variations in integrated responses of variables, such as HR, BP, or circulating stress hormones such as norepinephrine, epinephrine, and cortisol. For example, HR responses to a stressor might be similar in people of different fitness levels, but the reasons might be different. A fit person might have less withdrawal of parasympathetic nerve inhibition of the heart despite a similar or greater sympathetic nerve stimulation of the heart. Although the integrated HR response might not differ from that of an unfit person, the different pattern of cardiac sympathovagal balance would be important, because it is known to have health consequences.

Consideration of the Characteristics of Stressor Tasks

Researchers generally failed to compare standardized stressor tasks of equal novelty or difficulty and did not choose tasks according to common or unique features that induce specific or general stress responses (e.g., different sympathovagal and sympathoadrenal medullary responses). Exercise adaptations might extend to certain types or intensities of stressors but not to others.

vagal tone results in decreased HR and decreased BP (a so-called playing-dead response). One passive test that elicits a cardiovagal response in many people is the application of cold to the forehead. Forehead cold can increase BP because of increased resistance to blood flow even though HR is reduced. This response is similar to the mammalian diving reflex, which involves a vagally mediated bradycardia and α-adrenergic vasoconstriction of the skin and viscera.

Generally, BP responses are greater during hand immersion in cold water (cold pressor) than during mental arithmetic, which in turn elicits greater responses than does a psychomotor reaction-time task. In contrast, cardiac output is greater during a reaction-time task or mental arithmetic than during a cold-pressor test. HR increases the most during mental arithmetic compared to the cold-pressor test or reaction-time task. Increased HR during mental arithmetic is explainable by vagal withdrawal, whereas during a reaction-time task it is more influenced by sympathetic innervation of the heart. Blood flow also differs according to the type of stressor. Increased cardiac output during a reaction-time task is mainly explained by increased stroke volume, whereas during mental arithmetic it is explained by increased HR. Cardiac output during the cold-pressor test is unchanged because the increased HR is offset by decreased stroke volume (Dishman, Jackson, and Nakamura 2002).

Limitations of past research also make it too early to conclude that regular exercise has no effect on responses during stress that are modulated by the sympathetic nervous system. The reason for the absence of effects in past studies might be the narrow range in the increase of plasma catecholamines evoked by the stressors that researchers have used. Most of the stressors used have been mild, eliciting small increases in a range of about 300 to 500 picograms per milliliter (pg/ml) for norepinephrine and 40 to 80 pg/ml for epinephrine. Those levels are below the thresholds for norepinephrine (1,500-2,000 pg/ml) and epinephrine (75-125 pg/ml) that reliably elicit increases in HR and systolic BP (Clutter et al. 1980; Silverberg, Shad, Haymond, and Cryer 1978). A five- to tenfold elevation in norepinephrine and a twofold increase in epinephrine are generally believed necessary for cardiovascular effects, yet the stressors used have seldom resulted in a doubling of catecholamines above basal levels. In contrast, moderate-to-heavy exercise results in a six- to tenfold increase in norepinephrine and a tripling of epinephrine (Clutter et al. 1980).

The types of stressors used in studies of exercise and stress have been milder than many events that are stressful in real life. The experimental stressors usually increase HR by altering the sympathovagal balance of the ANS's innervation of the heart rather than by hormonal response. For example, during mental arithmetic, heart transplant patients—who have had the autonomic nerves to the heart severed—have an increased BP (Sehested et al. 1995) but not the increase in HR (Sehested et al. 1995; Shapiro et al. 1994) that is observed in people with innervated hearts. Thus, tasks such as mental arithmetic do not elicit a stress response by the adrenal gland that is of sufficient magnitude to increase HR.

> **E**vidence for a modification in the response to mental stress after exercise training is equivocal, but there might be beneficial effects from enhanced vagal tone.

Nonetheless, it remains plausible that increased cardiovagal tone after regular exercise might blunt responses to mild stressors that elicit increases in HR and BP mainly by vagal withdrawal (Jackson and Dishman 2006). In contrast, responses by the sympathetic nervous system seem to be unique to particular stress organs during mild stressors. Hence, whether altered regulation of the sympathetic nervous system after regular exercise might lead to a generalizable response seems less clear and could depend on the intensity of exercise and other stressors. Even though responses, such as HR and BP, to laboratory stress have not been affected in exercise training studies that increased cardiorespiratory fitness (Jackson and Dishman 2006; Sloan et al. 2011), vascular and blood flow responses, as well as their modulation by the autonomic nervous system, may be more important to health than gross measures of HR and BP. However, those factors have been understudied (e.g., Dishman et al. 2003; Sloan et al. 2011) especially in people with elevated risk of cardiovascular disease (e.g., Jackson and Dishman 2002).

Similarly, little is understood about the vascular responses to stress after acute exercise

(Hamer, Taylor, and Steptoe 2006), which results in a transient reduction in resting BP (i.e., postexercise hypotension) (MacDonald 2002) that might lead to altered BP and vascular responses to stress after a single session of physical activity. As discussed earlier in this chapter, neurovascular challenges (i.e., those that elicit changes in blood vessels via the autonomic nervous system), such as the Stroop Color and Word test (CWT) (an autonomic vasodilator that acts by sympathetic withdrawal or β adrenoreceptor activation) and forehead cold (an autonomic vasoconstrictor that acts by α-1 adrenoreceptor activation), are commonly used cardiovascular reactivity tests. A typical limitation of many studies of fitness and exercise that employed these tasks is that only BP and HR were measured as cardiovascular responses (Hamer et al., 2006). This limits the conclusions that can be drawn about vascular responses and the underlying mechanisms of the autonomic nervous system that regulate limb blood flow, particularly during stressor tasks that conversely elicit vasodilatory or vasoconstrictive responses.

Endothelial function is commonly assessed by flow-mediated dilation (FMD), which occurs in response to the shear stress or frictional force on the endothelium resulting from increases in blood flow after vessel occlusion (i.e., reactive hyperemia; see figure 4.6). The mechanisms responsible for FMD are primarily mediated by nitric oxide, which is important for the maintenance of vascular health and vascular tone. In a recent study, 30 minutes of moderately intense cycling exercise increased FMD, and decreased arterial velocity and blood flow responses during the Stroop CWT and augmented similar decreases during forehead cold in young women (Rooks, McCully, and Dishman 2011). Overall, acute exercise improved endothelial function despite increasing vascular resistance and reducing limb blood flow during neurovascular stress.

Feelings of Distress and Well-Being

Regardless of whether regular exercise or fitness mitigates the physiological aspects of stress, substantial evidence shows that people who are physically active feel as though they experience less distress and have a higher sense of well-being or positive affect (Netz et al. 2005; Reed and Buck 2009) when compared with people who are physically inactive. Even in people without anxiety or mood disorders, psychological distress is a risk factor for psychiatric disorders and coronary heart disease. Conversely, a positive feeling of well-being can reduce psychiatric risk and is an important feature of high life quality and good health. People frequently experience feelings of distress during the normal course of living and during challenging life events, including chronic medical

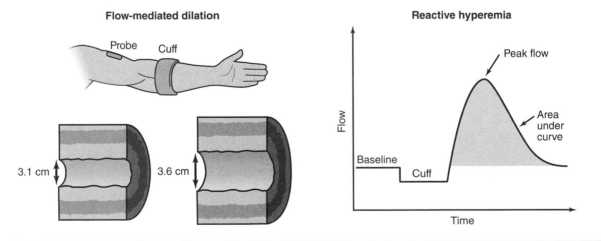

Figure 4.6 Vascular response during flow-mediated dilation.

Courtesy of Dr. Cherie Rooks-Peck, Exercise Psychology Lab, and Dr. Kevin McCully, Exercise Vascular Biology Lab, Department of Kinesiology, the University of Georgia.

The scientific advisory committee of the *2008 Physical Activity Guidelines for Americans* concluded that physically active people have reduced odds of experiencing feelings of distress or poor well-being.

conditions. Thus, it is important to understand the association between physical activity and feelings of distress or well-being as they bear on overall mental health and people's perceptions of their health-related quality of life.

Relevant Studies

Three main types of studies have examined physical activity and feelings of distress or well-being. Cohort studies have measured levels of physical activity and distress or well-being in a population sample, either in a cross section of time, or prospectively by following people for several years to see whether those who are active have lower odds of developing stress-related symptoms. Other studies have been randomized controlled trials that place people in an exercise training program to see whether their feelings of distress are reduced or their feelings of well-being are enhanced. Examples or summaries of each type of study follow.

European Union

A total of 16,230 respondents age 15 years and older reported their physical activity during the prior seven days (in MET-hours) and their feelings of nervousness and depression as well as energy and vitality during the past month using standardized scales administered in a face-to-face interview (Abu-Omar, Rutten, and Lehtinen 2004). Sample sizes were about 1,000 respondents in most nations. Across sociodemographic subgroups of the populations investigated (age, sex, marital status, gross household income, educational status), the researchers found that those who were more physically active had better mental health in general. In some, but not all, of the 15 nations a dose–response relationship existed between physical activity and mental

health regardless of age or sex. (See figures 4.7 and 4.8.)

Prospective Cohort Studies

Thirteen studies of adults in Australia, Canada, Denmark, England, the Netherlands, Scotland, and Wales, and three studies of Americans, used a prospective cohort design. In studies that adjusted for other risk factors such as age, sex, race, education, social class, occupation, income, smoking, alcohol use, substance abuse, chronic health conditions, disability, marital status, life events, job stress, and social support, the average odds of reduced feelings of distress or of enhanced well-being favored active people by nearly 20% (Physical Activity Guidelines Advisory Committee 2008).

Figure 4.9 illustrates 18 crude or adjusted odds ratios and 95% confidence intervals from the 13 prospective cohort studies of physical activity and distress or well-being in more than 100,000 adults from eight countries, including 67,000 American women. Regardless of people's age and sex or adjustment for other risk factors, a linear reduction in odds of about 10% occurred for each level of physical activity (i.e., from low to moderate to high) compared to people who were inactive or had very low activity.

Nurses' Health Study

More than 63,000 women who were 40 to 67 years of age in 1986 reported their physical activity on questionnaires every two years between 1986 and 1996 and were grouped by quartiles of change in activity between those dates (Wolin et al. 2007). In 1996 and 2000, they also rated seven aspects of their health-related quality of life (QoL): physical function, physical roles impairment, emotional roles impairment, pain, vitality, social functioning, and mental health (i.e., low perceived distress, mainly few symptoms of anxiety or depression). The women in the most active quartile had an average activity level of 6 MET-hours per week in 1986, which increased to 30 MET-hours in 1996. After adjustment for age and initial levels of physical activity, QoL, smoking, BMI, and chronic conditions (arthritis, hypertension, diabetes, hypercholerolemia), the most active quartile of women who increased their physical activity

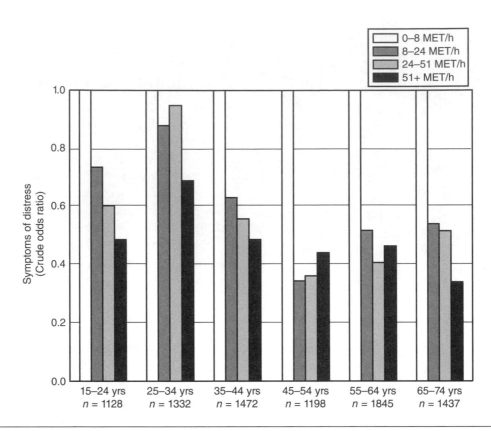

Figure 4.7 Association of physical activity with feelings of well-being in the European Union—females.

Data from Abu-Omar, Rutten, and Lehtinen 2004.

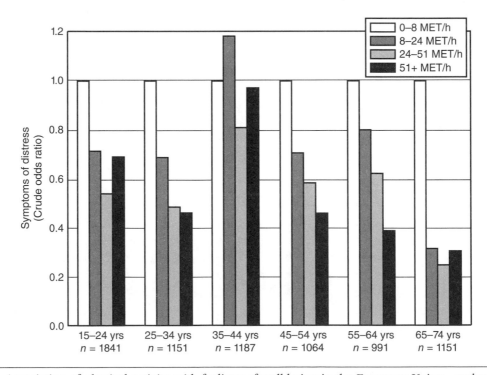

Figure 4.8 Association of physical activity with feelings of well-being in the European Union—males.

Data from Abu-Omar, Rutten, and Lehtinen 2004.

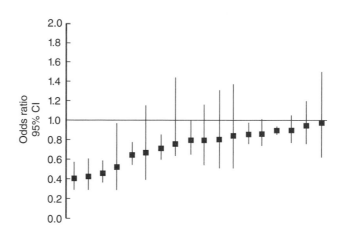

Figure 4.9 Prospective studies of physical activity and reduced odds of distress or feelings of poor well-being.

Data from Physical Activity Guidelines Advisory Committee 2008.

between 1986 and 1996 had higher quality-of-life scores in 1996 and bigger increases from 1996 and 2000 in all seven aspects of QoL than did women whose physical activity stayed about the same during that time. Increases in mental health were the smallest gains, and improvements in perceived physical function and roles were the largest.

Australian Longitudinal Study on Women's Health

The Australian Longitudinal Study on Women's Health examined the cross-sectional and prospective associations between leisure-time physical activity and feelings of distress (anxiety and depression symptoms) in a population-based cohort of 6,663 women ages 73 to 78, who were assessed in 1999, 2002, and 2005 (Heesch et al. 2011). None of the women in 1999 had been told by a physician that they had depression or anxiety disorders. The women completed three mailed surveys about their weekly minutes of walking for leisure or transportation and time spent in other moderate- and vigorous-intensity leisure-time physical activity during the past week (only if each session lasted at least 10 minutes).

About 26% of the women in 1999 and 34% in 2002 reported no leisure-time physical activity. Walking was the only leisure-time physical activity reported by nearly 40% of the women. After adjusting for sociodemographics, marital status,

social networks, life stress, chronic health conditions, smoking, and BMI, feelings of distress were inversely related to leisure-time physical activity averaged across years 1999 and 2002, which also was inversely related to feelings of distress reported three years later in 2005 (see figure 4.10). Although these women did not have depression or anxiety disorders, and the difference in symptoms was small between the least and most active women (fewer than one symptom, when averaged, out of a possible 18), the results still support the idea that physical activity is related to perceived mental health, an important aspect of quality of life in older women.

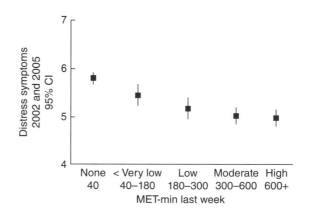

Figure 4.10 Physical activity and feelings of distress among older Australian women.

Data from Heesch et al. 2010.

A Norwegian study of 2,489 adolescents (1,112 boys and 1,377 girls) living in Oslo found an association between hours of physical activity a week at ages 15 and 16 and emotional symptoms (a risk factor for depression and anxiety disorders) 3 years later for boys but not for girls (Sagatun et al. 2007).

Randomized Controlled Trials

Since 1995, at least 26 randomized controlled trials including nearly 3,000 people have examined the effects of exercise on feelings of distress or well-being in healthy adults or adults with medical conditions other than psychiatric disorders or disabling conditions that severely limit physical activity (i.e., spinal cord injury, multiple sclerosis, and stroke or severe head trauma) (Physical Activity Guidelines Advisory Committee 2008). The average effect of exercise compared to a control condition was 0.27 standard deviation (SD) (95% confidence interval [CI] = 0.16-0.38). The outcomes were favorable after exercise in nearly 80% of the comparisons (26 of 33) with control conditions, but only 13 of 33 comparisons reached statistical significance.

When compared to a placebo (usually stretching or health education), the effect of exercise was reduced to 0.10 SD (95% CI: −0.12-0.32) and was significant in just two of nine comparisons.

RENEW (Reach out to ENhanceE Wellness) Study

A large 12-month randomized controlled trial that used home-based telephone counseling targeted changes in both physical activity and diet among 641 overweight or obese survivors of breast, prostate, and colorectal cancers from Canada, the United Kingdom, and the United States (Morey et al. 2009). Recommended targets were 15 minutes of strength training exercise every other day, 30 minutes of endurance exercise each day, the consumption of at least seven servings (for women) or nine servings (for men)

of fruits and vegetables per day, the restriction of saturated fat to less than 10% of energy intake, and a 10% weight loss goal. People in the intervention reported an increase of 18 more minutes of strength exercise and 13 more minutes of endurance exercise each week compared to the control group, as well as better physical function and fewer feelings of distress. Nonetheless, only 15% of the intervention group were meeting the targeted 150 weekly minutes or more of moderate physical activity at the end of the trial (the mean was 70 minutes).

DREW (Dose-Response to Exercise in Postmenopausal Women) Study

In a six-month randomized controlled trial including 430 sedentary, overweight, and obese postmenopausal women, feelings of well-being (mainly reduced symptoms of anxiety and depression) were increased after aerobic exercise training (treadmill or semirecumbent cycling at 50% aerobic capacity three or four times each week) that expended either 4, 8, or 12 kilocalories per kilogram of body weight each week, regardless of whether the women lost weight (Martin et al. 2009; see figure 4.11). Those amounts of physical activity approximated 50%, 100%, and 150% of public health recommendations.

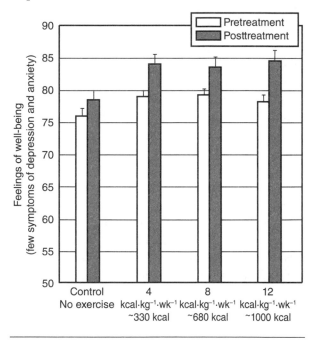

Figure 4.11 Effects of aerobic exercise on feelings of well-being in postmenopausal women.

Data from Martin et al. 2009.

Trials of patients with medical conditions yielded similar outcomes regardless of exercise dose, but most trials used a moderate-to-vigorous exercise intensity of 60% to 80% of people's aerobic capacity or maximal strength, with an average session of 45 minutes, 3 days per week. There is no clear association between fitness increases and changes in feelings of distress or well-being.

Dose–Response Studies?

Large cross-sectional and prospective, observational studies have showed linear dose–response associations. Averaged across a half dozen or so prospective cohort studies, there was a 10% reduction in feelings of distress for each level of physical activity.

SUMMARY

Adults without stress disorders typically say that they feel less stressed after a single exercise session and after a regular exercise program. However, studies have not yet shown convincingly that those findings were uninfluenced by people's expectations of benefits. There has been no research to determine whether exercise reduces stress among people diagnosed with stress disorders. Studies in which physiological responses were measured have shown that cardiorespiratory fitness is associated with a slight blunting of HR and systolic BP reactions during active mental stress, but not during passive stress, such as that caused by placing the hand in ice water. More often, fit people have a lower overall level of HR and, many times, of BP during stress because they have lower resting levels, not because they have smaller reactions to the stress than do unfit people.

Research has not shown that fitness affects catecholamine responses during stress, but the stressors used have been mild and have not led to responses large enough to adequately test whether fitness really alters the sympathetic response by the adrenal gland. There are not enough studies of other hormone responses, such as cortisol, to permit us to conclude that exercise and fitness alter other endocrine responses during stress.

There has been very little use of the traditions and methods of biological psychology and neuroscience in the study of exercise, fitness, and stress. Though many people say that exercise helps them cope with stress, we cannot rely solely on social cognitive models of stress that use people's self-rated perceptions to determine whether, or in what circumstances, cardiorespiratory fitness or regular exercise leads to blunted or augmented physiological responses during stress and enhances recovery from stress. Modern students of exercise psychology should learn the basics of neuroanatomy, neurophysiology, and psychopharmacology as well as the techniques of neuroscience to help them conduct sound research on exercise and stress or to collaborate effectively with physiologists or biological psychologists. Nonetheless, the subjective experience of stress remains a cornerstone of inquiry into the nature of stress emotions such as anxiety and depression, which are discussed in following chapters.

Despite the lack of support from available studies that exercise or fitness reduces physiological responses to other types of stress, current evidence from self-reports is consistent in showing that physically active people say they feel less distress. In a dozen or so observational studies that used a prospective cohort design with follow-ups lasting 9 months to 15 years (mean of 5½ years) and adjusted for other risk factors, the average odds of reduced feelings of distress or of enhanced well-being favored active people by nearly 20%. Studies in Australia, Canada, Denmark, England, Netherlands, Scotland, Wales, and the United States have shown favorable outcomes for physically active adults regardless of age, sex, or race or ethnicity. However, race and ethnicity were poorly represented or not described in most studies in the United States.

In nearly 30 randomized controlled trials, exercise training lasting 6 weeks to 6 months was accompanied by about a quarter of a standard deviation reduction in feelings of distress or improvement in well-being. Those studies included healthy adults or adults with medical conditions other than psychiatric disorders or disabling conditions that severely limit physical activity (i.e., spinal cord injury, multiple sclerosis, and stroke or severe head trauma). Whether those or other medical factors modify associations between physical activity and distress or well-being has not been studied, though. Also, the effects of aerobic or resistance exercise often have not exceeded the effects of placebo control conditions, such as health education or stretching.

Explanations for favorable changes in feelings of distress or well-being are not plausibly explained by reduced physiological reactivity to stress. They more likely include the social, cognitive, and biological mechanisms discussed in chapters 5, 6, and 7 for reducing anxiety and improving mood, which are core features of quality of life in people not diagnosed with anxiety or mood disorders.

WEBSITES

www.nimh.nih.gov/publicat/index.cfm

www.surgeongeneral.gov/library/mentalhealth/index.html

www.nhlbi.nih.gov/health/index.htm

Affect, Mood, and Emotion

Most people say they feel better after they exercise. This chapter is about what that means and why it happens. The focus is on the potential that physical activity and exercise have for improving someone's mood and on whether acute exercise alters emotions. The chapter clarifies distinctions among the concepts of affect, mood, and emotion and presents the neuroanatomy and theories of affect and emotion. It also presents some key factors that likely influence the effects of exercise on negative and positive moods. In addition, we summarize new studies on affect and emotional experiences during and after exercise, and we address some limitations of the research, including questions about proper measurement.

Positive psychological effects from exercise can moderate and perhaps even mediate the determinants of people's participation in physical activity and exercise. Thus, understanding the relationship between affect and exercise fits with studying exercise and mental health, but also has implications for understanding exercise adherence, a topic covered in the last part of this book. This chapter concludes with a description of the mechanisms that may help explain the relationship between exercise and affect, mood, and emotion. The effects of exercise on the specific moods of anxiety and depression, and on feelings of energy or fatigue, are covered in detail in chapters 6, 7, and 9.

OUR MUSCULAR VIGOR will . . . always be needed to furnish the background of sanity, serenity, and cheerfulness to life, to give moral elasticity to our disposition, to round off the wiry edge of our fretfulness, and make us good-humored.

William James (1899, 207)

Physical activity behavior can influence affect, but affect can also have an impact on behavior.

William James, the father of American psychology, extolled the benefits of exercise for positive moods, and that common wisdom holds today. Feeling better and reducing tension are among the most common perceived benefits of exercise endorsed by young and middle-aged adults (Steinhardt and Dishman 1989). In a survey of 10 behaviors that people without clinical disorders use to self-manage their moods, exercise was judged to be the overall winner (Thayer, Newman, and McClain 1994). People rated exercise as the best for improving a bad mood,

Positive Changes With Exercise

Some positive changes with exercise have been described as

- feeling good, relaxed, euphoric, or imaginative;
- having a sense of accomplishment;
- having improved self-worth;
- having a global sense of well-being;
- having improved concentration; and
- experiencing vivid physical sensations.

fourth best for raising energy levels, and third to fourth best for reducing tension.

DEFINITIONS OF TERMS

The idea that people "feel better" after exercise is commonly accepted, but several terms are used to describe the psychological response to exercise, and defining them can be difficult. For example, if someone asks you what kind of mood you're in after you have finished a 3-mile (4.8 km) jog, you might say that you are in a good mood. If, instead, you are asked how you're feeling, your response would be more specific, such as "relaxed," "carefree," or even "relieved" depending on the circumstances.

Feelings are subjective experiences that can be overt or covert. A **feeling state** refers to bodily sensations, cognitive appraisals, actual or potential instrumental responses, or some combination of these responses (Averill et al. 1994) (see table 5.1). **Affect** has been defined as the expression of value given to a feeling state (Batson, Shaw, and Oleson 1992). Wilhelm Wundt, the father of psychology, concluded in 1897 that affect could be described by three dimensions: lust (pleasure), *spannung* (tension or excitement), and *beruhigung* (calm or pacify).

The most widely accepted modern views of affect separate it into two categories: affective experiences and specific emotions. Affective experience varies on two primary orthogonal (independent) dimensions (see figure 5.1): (1) valence, or hedonic tone, which can range from attraction and pleasure to avoidance and displeasure; and (2) intensity, or activation, which can range from calm to aroused. Specific emotions can be described in a circumplex model composed of varying degrees of the primary dimensions of valence and intensity.

Another popular but less supported view, like that of Wundt's, is that there are two dimensions of activation rather than a single continuum (Thayer 1989). From that perspective, the valence of affective experiences depends on the level of activation along two separate dimensions, or continua, of (1) energy (i.e., sleepy to energetic) and (2) tension (i.e., calm to tense). Another theoretical model states that arousal is not a separate dimension but is nested *within* positive and negative affect (e.g., sadness has negative valence and low arousal, whereas joy has positive valence and high arousal) (Tellegen 1985).

The latter two views of affective experience are mainly limited to self-report data, and affect is determined using factor analyses of the patterns of people's ratings of adjectives (see chapter 2). Because the models discussed so far are based strictly on people's feelings, they don't consider that biological arousal can vary both on total-body metabolism and on neural activity in the brain and autonomic nervous system. At this point, most evidence fits best with the view, depicted in figure 5.1, that the bipolar dimension of valence can be associated with, but is not dependent on, the bipolar dimension of arousal (Davidson 1998a; Lang, Bradley, and Cuthbert 1998). The inclusion of arousal as a separate dimension of affect and emotion is important for studies of exercise because physical exertion is a powerful influence on metabolic arousal.

Temperament refers to a mainly stable core component of personality that disposes people to emotional responsiveness and changing moods. We commonly describe someone who has periods of emotional ups and downs as

Table 5.1 Categories and Examples of Feeling States

Categories	Example
Bodily reactions and experiences	Feelings of pain or fatigue
Cognitive appraisals regarding the value ascribed to objects or activities	Positive feelings about finishing a long jog, or negative feelings about the steep hill at the end of a bicycle ride
Actual or potential instrumental responses	Feeling like getting an ice cream cone, or feeling like taking a walk

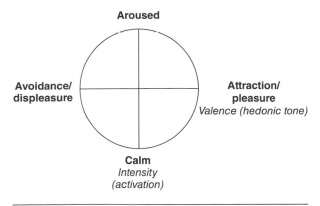

Figure 5.1 A two-dimensional model of affective experience expressed on separate continua of approach–avoidance and level of arousal.

moody. Or, we might describe someone who is often angry as having a fiery temperament. Temperament is based on biological (genetic) factors and learned experiences. **Traits** are narrower features of temperament and indicate the tendency to respond to an internal or external event with a particular mood state. For example, someone with high trait anxiety is more likely than others to be anxious while waiting for the results of a job interview. Traits are relatively consistent over time but are easier to change than temperament.

It is not uncommon to say that someone is in a good or bad humor. That has a basis in antiquity. Second-century Greco-Roman physician Claudius Galenus (aka Galen) believed that humans have four basic temperaments, influenced by the four humors of the body. For example, a melancholic, or sad, patient was said to suffer from excess black bile (*melan chole*); a sanguine, or joyful, person was said to be moved by blood (*sanguis*); a choleric, or angry, person was said to be controlled by yellow bile (*chole*); and a phlegmatic, or unflappable, unemotional person was said to be influenced by excess phlegm (*phlegma*). Later, the *Canon of Medicine,* written by the Persian physician Ibn Sīnā (aka Avicenna) in 1025, spread the Greco-Roman ideas of the four humors throughout the Middle East.

In general, there are four types of proper spirit: One is brutal spirit residing in the heart and it is the origin of all spirits. Another . . . is sensual spirit residing in the brain. The third . . . is natural spirit residing

in the liver. The fourth is generative—i.e. procreative—spirits residing in the gonads.

Although not biologically true, these ancient ideas still influence us today, because the adjectives remain part of the English language. And joy, anger, and sadness are acknowledged by psychologists, along with love, surprise, and fear, as the key emotions. We'll see later in the chapter how these antiquated ideas and questions are still manifest in current approaches in exercise psychology to understand the effects of exercise on affect, mood, and emotions.

> **F**eeling, affect, mood, trait, and temperament are constructs related to emotional responses.

Mood is considered a type of affective state that is accompanied by anticipation, although sometimes unconscious, of pleasure or pain. Moods can last less than a minute or for days. A particular mood state (e.g., positive) is influenced by overall disposition (temperament and traits) and by brief responses (emotions) composed of feelings, distinct autonomic and somatic activation, and behavior. Conditions leading to moods typically occur over a slow time course, and the effect may accumulate from repeated experiences of an emotion. Events evoking an emotion occur quickly: for example, you might achieve a personal best on a leg press and experience a feeling of elation when you realize how much weight you lifted. Then, if you continue to experience events that evoke positive emotions, such as having a good workout, catching all the green lights on your way home from the gym, and finding your favorite supper waiting for you, you are likely to experience a positive mood. You would anticipate a pleasant evening, and the positive expectation and mood might even be sustained for another day. Moods can also develop spontaneously with no apparent specific cause.

Moods might alter the way information is processed, which biases cognitions or thoughts (Smith and Crabbe 2000). A sustained positive mood predisposes a person to access positive thoughts and feelings. It has been suggested that the biological link for this phenomenon is an enhancement of neural pathways linked to pleasant thoughts and feelings, rendering them more accessible than negative thoughts and feelings. The idea of neural pathway facilitation that favors a certain quality or tone of cognitions has also been used to explain the tendency for depressed people to focus on negative thoughts and feelings.

> In his 1878 book *Physiologie de Passions,* Charles Letourneau defined emotions as "passions of a short duration."

Emotions are brief responses of negative or positive feelings evoked by particular situations; as we just saw, they can contribute to mood. It is also possible that a prevailing mood can prime an emotional response. Whereas mood influences the way information is processed, exerting a bias in valence, emotions influence the activity of the autonomic nervous system. The emotional response consists of behavior and the activation of the autonomic and hormonal systems (see table 5.2). Thus, emotion has a physiological component that is essentially lacking in affect, which is the subjective component of emotion. That is not to say that there is no biological basis to affect. As we will see later in the chapter, there is clearly a neurochemical basis to all subjective experience, including affect, mood, and emotion. Indeed, there is good evidence that the integration of overt behavior, autonomic responses, and hormonal responses is controlled by neural systems that consist of some key brain regions. These are discussed later in the chapter.

The terms *feeling, affect, mood,* and *temperament* are all emotion-related expressions and describe constructs that differ from emotional responses. An emotion is narrower in focus than mood and is more short-lived; it is evoked by a specific thought or event, is usually directed toward some goal, and is accompanied by temporary physiological responses. Emotions have been conceptualized as discrete states and paired opposites (see table 5.3). Another view groups emotions into families, which are affective states within a hierarchy from the abstract (basic emotion) to the more concrete. These affective families share common expressions, physiological activities, and cognitive appraisals, or meanings (Lazarus 1991). There is some evidence of specific patterns of autonomic arousal for various emotions (Cacioppo et al. 1993). Specific emotions or moods can also be described in a circumplex model composed of varying degrees of the primary dimensions of valence and intensity, as shown in figure 5.2, *a* and *b*.

Research on positive and negative affect has mainly focused on mood, commonly asking people to report how they have felt during the past 2 weeks including today (Watson and Tellegen 1985). That aspect of affective experience is quite different from the valence and arousal people experience in response to specific emotional events. However, the positive affect (PA)–negative affect (NA) circumplex model has been widely generalized to emotional reactions (Ekkekakis and Petruzzello 2002), and the positive and negative affect schedule (PANAS) is frequently used incorrectly to assess experimental manipulations of specific emotions (Carver and Harmon-Jones 2009a).

Renowned University of California psychologist Richard Lazarus described five ways that

Table 5.2 Components of an Emotional Response

Component	Explanation
Behavior	Muscular movements consistent with a situation that elicits the emotion (e.g., a smile or scowl)
Autonomic	Responses that facilitate the behavior (e.g., sympathetic activation in fear-provoking situations to facilitate the fight-or-flight response)
Hormonal	Reinforcement of the autonomic response (e.g., activation of the hypothalamic-pituitary-adrenal axis to facilitate cardiovascular response and substrate availability)

Table 5.3 Conceptualizations of Emotions

DISCRETE EMOTIONS (EKMAN 1992)	
Happiness, surprise, fear, anger, disgust	
PAIRED OPPOSITES (PLUTCHIK 1994)	
Joy	Sadness
Acceptance	Disgust
Anger	Fear
Expectation	Surprise
EMOTION FAMILIES (SHAVER ET AL. 1987)	
Basic emotion	**Affective states**
Anger	Irritation, annoyance, fury, rage
Fear	Apprehension, anxiety, panic, horror, terror
Love	Affection, attachment, devotion, passion
Joy	Happiness, pleasure, delight, exhilaration
Sadness	Despondency, dejection, depression, grief

emotions are central in people's lives (Lazarus 2006; see table 5.4). First, emotions and other affective states, such as moods, reflect our personal values and gauge how well or poorly we are doing in their pursuit. When we fail to attain our goals, or perceive threat or harm, we feel anxiety, anger, guilt, shame, envy, or jealousy. When goals are attained, or attainable, we experience joy, pride, love, or the exhilaration of a challenge. Second, emotions are among the most prominent features of our social relations with family members, lovers, friends, coworkers, competitors, and chance encounters. Third, emotions facilitate or impair those interpersonal relations. Dealing effectively with interpersonal relations is a basic emotional coping skill. Fourth, the source and personal meaning of an emotion can be hard to grasp or accept. Also, the expression of emotions can be revealing or made deceiving to others. Although some people wear their emotions on their sleeves, others are reluctant to expose their inner selves for fear of social rejection or reprisal. Fifth, emotions are often difficult to control when they are intense. Self-control of emotion is a basic function of emotional coping.

Carver and Connor-Smith (2010) have clarified how the appraisal of events leads to emotions and how they depend on whether circumstances signal approach or avoidance behaviors. For example, a feeling of loss seems specific to approach goals. The death of a loved one ends a valued relationship. Threat and harm are less distinct. In approach settings, they can signal the failure to obtain incentives. In avoidance settings, they indicate a failure to avoid punishers. Threat can indicate that approach behaviors toward a goal will be blocked or that a pleasant circumstance might be interrupted. In either case, harm connotes that the threat of loss has become a reality; damage has been done. Conversely, threat can imply that an aversive, unpleasant event is looming, whereas harm denotes that punishment has already occurred (Lazarus 1993). Threat in an approach setting usually results in frustration and anger, whereas threat in an avoidance setting results in fear or anxiety. Loss is accompanied by sadness and dejection. Thus, when events are appraised as threatening or harmful, the types of negative, unpleasant affect that people experience will depend on whether the appraisals occur in the context of approach behaviors or avoidance behaviors.

In contrast, challenge is a situation that requires strong effort that strains a person's abilities, but is viewed as a likely successful

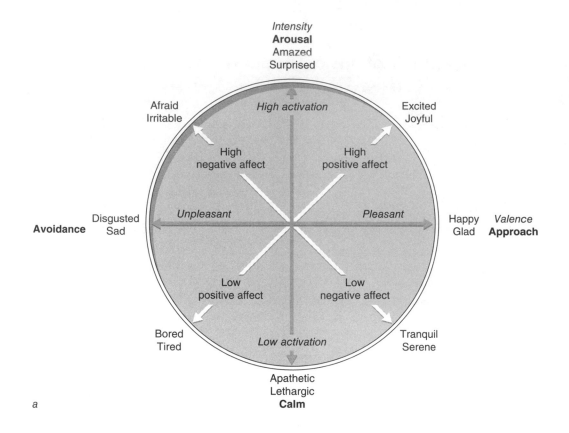

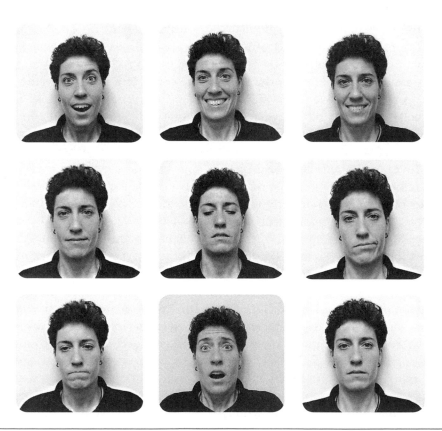

Figure 5.2 Watson and Tellegen's (1985) dimensions of positive and negative affect displayed on Russell's (1980) emotional circumplex *(a)*; facial expressions that correspond to the primary emotions depicted in *(a)*. Facial expressions for surprise, joy, disgust, anger, and fear are common to virtually all cultures *(b)*.

Part *(b)* Provided by the Exercise Psychology Laboratory, Department of Kinesiology, and Department of Psychology, the University of Georgia.

Table 5.4   Core Relational Themes of Fifteen Emotions

Emotion	Core relational theme
Anger	A demeaning offense against me and mine
Anxiety	Facing an uncertain, existential threat
Fright	Confronting an immediate, concrete, and overwhelming physical danger
Guilt	Having transgressed a moral imperative
Shame	Having failed to live up to an ego-ideal
Sadness	Having experienced an irrevocable loss
Envy	Wanting what someone else has and feeling deprived in its absence
Jealousy	Resenting a third party for loss or threat to one's favor or love
Happiness	Making reasonable progress toward the attainment of a goal
Pride	Enhancement of one's ego-identity by taking credit for a valued achievement, one's own or that of a person or group with which one identifies
Relief	A distressing goal-incongruent condition that has changed for the better or gone away
Hope	Fearing the worst but yearning for better and believing the wished-for improvement is possible
Love	Desiring or participating in affection, usually, but not necessarily, reciprocated
Gratitude	Appreciation for an altruistic gift
Compassion	Being moved to offer help by another's suffering

Reprinted, by permission, from R.S. Lazarus, 2006, "Emotions and interpersonal relationships: toward a person-centered conceptualization of emotions and coping," *Journal of Personality* 74(1): 9-46.

opportunity to gain something valuable (Lazarus and Folkman 1984). Pure challenge engages the approach system but not the avoidance system. Affective experiences of challenge include hope, eagerness, and excitement or exhilaration (Lazarus 2006).

Emotions sustain the activation of systems needed to maintain motivated responses (Frijda 1986), and the contribution of emotions to behavior has been explored for decades in theory and research. In the late 1800s, Darwin (1872) proposed that emotions are innate and common in lower species and across cultures. The expression of emotions (i.e., "behavior") takes the form of facial expressions that are a species-specific repertoire of muscle movement. The facial expression of emotion is not learned, but inherited, and serves, along with body language, to communicate our emotions to others and to indicate how we are likely to behave (Zajonc 1985).

The cross-cultural consistency of specific facial expressions and corresponding emotions has been supported by studies by Ekman and his colleagues (e.g., Ekman and Friesen 1971). Facial expressions for joy, surprise, anger, fear, and disgust are recognized in virtually all cultures. This raises the possibility that different brain systems regulate each emotion, not merely positive and negative categories of emotions. If found to be true, that would present a unique challenge for exercise psychology. Why, or perhaps in what circumstances, would exercise be expected to exert an influence on emotions that is independent of the setting where exercise occurs? The biology of exercise mainly depends on the type, intensity, and duration of exertion. To a lesser extent, hostile environmental conditions such as heat or cold, humidity, and altitude affect exercise responses. Is it reasonable that exercise alone would alter specific emotions? Or, might

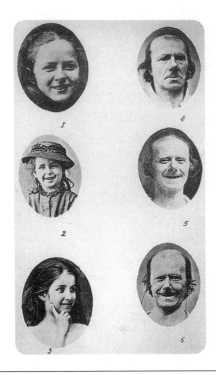

Figure 5.3 Facial expressions of emotion naturally expressed by the young girls and electrically stimulated in the male patient. From Charles Darwin's *The Expression of the Emotions in Man and Animals* (1889).

Provided by the National Library of Medicine.

exercise alter some neural system common to positive or negative moods?

A BRIEF HISTORY

To understand how exercise might alter affect, mood, or emotion, we can examine how views on the origins of those concepts have evolved in history. As noted in chapter 1, the James-Lange theory of emotion proposed that bodily responses during emotion are the source of the affective experience. The following excerpts from the article "What Is an Emotion?" published in the journal *Mind* (James 1884) illustrate the challenge of understanding the precise role of physiological responses in the experience of emotion—a challenge that persists today. James' examples raise the question of whether the modern-day view that physiological and behavioral responses occur only after the person has evaluated events holds true in all circumstances. For example, the unconscious nature of emotions is illustrated by modern-day clinical observations that some brain-injured

patients who have lost vision can nonetheless show emotional reactions to stimuli of which they are not consciously unaware, a phenomenon called affective blindsight (Kunst-Wilson and Zajonc 1980).

Our natural way of thinking about these standard emotions is that the mental perception of some fact excites the mental affection called the emotion, and that this latter state of mind gives rise to the bodily expression. My thesis on the contrary is that the bodily changes follow directly the PERCEPTION of the exciting fact, and that our feeling of the same changes as they occur IS the emotion. Common sense says, we lose our fortune, are sorry and weep; we meet a bear, are frightened and run; we are insulted by a rival, are angry and strike. The hypothesis here to be defended says that this order of sequence is incorrect, that the one mental state is not immediately induced by the other, that the bodily manifestations must first be interposed between, and that the more rational statement is that we feel sorry because we cry, angry because we strike, afraid because we tremble, and not that we cry, strike, or tremble, because we are sorry, angry, or fearful, as the case may be. (James 1884, 189)

Without the bodily states following on the perception, the latter would be purely cognitive in form, pale, colourless, destitute of emotional warmth. We might then see the bear, and judge it best to run, receive the insult and deem it right to strike, but we could not actually feel afraid or angry. (James 1884, 190)

Is there any evidence, it may be asked, for the assumption that particular perceptions do produce widespread bodily effects by a sort of immediate physical influence, antecedent to the arousal of an emotion or emotional idea? The only possible reply is that there is most assuredly such evidence. In listening to poetry, drama, or heroic narrative, we are often surprised at the cutaneous shiver which like a sudden wave flows over us, and at the heart-swelling and the lachrymal effusion that unexpectedly catch us at intervals. In listening to music, the same is even more strikingly true. If we abruptly see a dark moving form in the woods, our heart stops beating, and we catch our breath instantly and before any articulate idea of danger can arise. If our friend goes near to the edge of a precipice, we get the well-known feeling of "all-overishness," and we shrink back, although we positively know him to be safe, and have no distinct imagination of his fall. (James 1884, 196)

James also used psychiatric cases to make his point, describing especially the symptoms of a panic attack, a modern-day anxiety disorder, which is discussed in chapter 6.

In every asylum we find examples of absolutely unmotived fear, anger, melancholy, or conceit; and others of an equally unmotived apathy which persists in spite of the best of outward reasons why it should give way. In the former cases we must suppose the nervous machinery to be so "labile" in some one emotional direction, that almost every stimulus, however inappropriate, will cause it to upset in that way, and as a consequence to engender the particular complex of feelings of which the psychic body of the emotion consists. Thus, to take one special instance, if inability to draw deep breath, fluttering of the heart, and that peculiar epigastric change felt as "precordial anxiety," with an irresistible tendency to take a somewhat crouching attitude and to sit still, and with perhaps other visceral processes not now known, all spontaneously occur together in a certain person; his feeling of their combination is the emotion of dread, and he is the victim of what is known as morbid fear. A friend who has had occasional attacks of this most distressing of all maladies, tells me that in his case the whole drama seems to centre about the region of the heart and respiratory apparatus, that his main effort during the attacks is to get control of his inspirations and to slow his heart, and that the moment he attains to breathing deeply and to holding himself erect, the dread,

ipso facto, seems to depart. (James 1884, 199)

It must be confessed that a crucial test of the truth of the hypothesis is quite as hard to obtain as its decisive refutation. A case of complete internal and external corporeal anaesthesia, without motor alteration or alteration of intelligence except emotional apathy, would afford, if not a crucial test, at least a strong presumption, in favour of the truth of the view we have set forth; whilst the persistence of strong emotional feeling in such a case would completely overthrow our case. Hysterical anaesthesias seem never to be complete enough to cover the ground. Complete anaesthesias from organic disease, on the other hand, are excessively rare. (James 1884, 203)

James next recounts an exchange with a German physician named StrŸmpell who had published a case study of a 15-year-old shoemaker's apprentice. The boy had lost all sensation except in one eye and one ear. He had reportedly shown shame after soiling his bed and grief at the sight of a favorite food that he knew he could no longer taste. James wrote to Professor Strümpell and asked him whether he was sure that the shame and grief were real feelings in the boy's mind, or only reflexes to perceptions that an observer would interpret as an emotion. This was Dr. Strümpell's response (in translation):

I think I can decidedly make the statement, that he was by no means completely lacking in emotional affections. In addition to the feelings of grief and shame mentioned in my paper, I recall distinctly that he showed anger, and frequently quarrelled with the hospital attendants. He also manifested fear lest I should punish him. In short, I do not think that my case speaks exactly in favour of your theory. On the other hand, I will not affirm that it positively refutes your theory. For my case was certainly one of a very centrally conditioned anaesthesia (perception-anaesthesia, like that of hysterics) and therefore the conduction of outward impressions may in him have been undisturbed. (James 1884, 204)

These passages illustrate the difficulty of uncovering laws that govern human behavior in all settings. The interaction among the stimulus, the neural integration of the stimulus, autonomic and hormonal activation, the perception and interpretation of the stimulus and the physiological response, and subsequent emotional and behavioral responses has been the focus of several theories since the introduction of the James-Lange theory (Carlson 1998; Rosenzweig, Leiman, and Breedlove 1999b).

The **Cannon-Bard theory** proposed a different sequence of events. On the basis of physiological studies of animals during fear and rage conducted around the 1920s, Harvard physician Walter Cannon deduced that the brain decided the appropriate response to a stimulus and that the subsequent physiological response and emotion occurred simultaneously. Social psychologist Stanley Schachter followed in the 1960s with a cognitive theory of emotion in which the emotional response is the result of the interaction between nonspecific physiological reactions (i.e., heart rate increase) and the cognitive interpretation of the arousal. Schachter showed that physiological arousal (induced by injections of adrenaline) was perceived by the person as different emotions depending on the social context. For example, you would interpret an increase in heart rate during walking as "I am afraid" if you had just seen a large, growling dog, but as "I am excited" if an attractive runner had just smiled at you. **Schachter's theory of emotion** is based on nonspecific arousal. The level of arousal dictates the intensity of emotion, whereas the interpretation determines the valence.

However, as already mentioned, there is evidence that different emotions exhibit specific patterns of autonomic arousal; and Clore, Schwarz, and Conway (1994) proposed that appraisal determines not only the valence, but also the intensity of emotions. There is also support for stable individual differences for affect intensity and the ways basic emotions are experienced and expressed (Davidson 2000; Gauvin and Spence 1998). Another view is that human emotion is experienced as affect when primitive, reflexive behavioral responses are inhibited (Lang 1995). Contemporary research continues to be influenced by biological-genetic, cogni-

tive, and developmental aspects of emotions (Smith and Crabbe 2000). No single theory has been proven to hold in all circumstances, so it is important to be familiar with the history of the various theories.

The approach–withdrawal model of affect was developed some decades ago when primitive organisms were found to have two primary emotional response dispositions: avoidance and approach. Schneirla (1959) described avoidance as the withdrawal of the organism from noxious stimuli, and approach as attraction and advancement toward appetitive stimuli. This idea was expanded by Konorski (1967) to include the moderating influence of arousal on responses, and by Osgood, Suci, and Tennenbaum (1957) to characterize verbal emotional descriptors in two dimensions: affective valence (aversion to attraction) and biological activation (calm to aroused) (see figure 5.1).

Because the pleasantness or unpleasantness of a mood or emotion commonly connotes approach or avoidance behaviors, a third affective dimension of dominance is included in most theories of affect (Bradley and Lang 1994; Schaefer and Plutchik 1966), especially when applied to social interactions (Leary 1957; Wiggins, Trapnell, and Phillips 1988). Dimensions of pleasantness, arousal, and dominance underlie people's judgments of facial expressions, hand

Aristotle on Emotion

In book two of his classic work, *Rhetoric*, Aristotle recognized the importance of appealing to people's emotions (pathos) in the art of persuasion, including anger, calmness, fear, and shame after submission to dominance.

"We are moreover ashamed of having done to us . . . acts that involve us in dishonour and reproach; as when we surrender our persons, or lend ourselves to vile deeds, e.g. when we submit to outrage. And acts of yielding to the lust of others are shameful . . . ."

William Rhys Roberts (1924)

Approach–Avoidance Behaviors and Positive-Negative Affect: The special Case of Anger

When viewed as a negative mood within the circumplex model, anger is assumed to be linked with aversive or avoidance behaviors (Watson, Clark, and Tellegen 1988). However, growing evidence suggests that both emotional anger and positive affect can be associated with approach motivation. Anger and fear co-occur when impediments to desired conditions (implying the engagement of approach sensitivity) and threats of punishment (implying the engagement of avoidance sensitivity) occur simultaneously (Carver 2004).

Manipulations that cause anger can also increase ratings of other states linked with positive affective experience (e.g., active, alert, attentive, determined, enthusiastic, excited, proud, inspired, interested, strong) (Harmon-Jones et al. 2009). Today, some theorists (Carver and Harmon-Jones 2009a) have proposed, not without controversy (Carver and Harmon-Jones 2009b; Tomarken and Zald 2009; Watson 2009), that anger has a neural basis common with approach behaviors.

Common Adjective Pairs That Describe Affective Dimensions

Pleasure	*Arousal*	*Dominance*
Unhappy–Happy	Relaxed–Stimulated	Controlled–Controlling
Annoyed–Pleased	Calm–Excited	Influenced–Influential
Dissatisfied–Satisfied	Sluggish–Frenzied	Cared for–In control
Melancholic–Contented	Dull–Jittery	Awed–Important
Despairing–Hopeful	Sleepy–Wide awake	Submissive–Dominant
Bored–Relaxed	Unaroused–Aroused	Guided–Autonomous

Reprinted, by permission, from A. Mehrabian and J.A. Russell, 1974, *An approach to environmental psychology* (Cambridge, MA: MIT).

and bodily movements, and postural positions (Mehrabian 1970; Mehrabian and Russell 1974). Whether physical activity and exercise influence emotional arousal, affective valence, and the experience or expression of dominance has yet to be determined; that question is examined later in this chapter. In all the perspectives mentioned, affective experience is broadly defined and is considered more basic than mood and emotion, although the term has been used synonymously with mood (e.g., Tellegen 1985). As we will see, important aspects of mood and emotion involve biological responses as well.

CONTEMPORARY VIEWS OF AFFECT AND EMOTION

The current view of emotions is based on these early perspectives. Affective expression is determined by two basic motivational systems linked to anatomical neural circuits that generate appetitive and defensive behavior for the purpose of survival (Davidson 2000; Lang 2000). Motivation has an intrinsic biphasic organization—that is, approach and avoidance or withdrawal. The approach system engages appetitive behavior and generates types of positive affect (e.g., curiosity, enthusiasm, pride, love) consistent with moving toward goals. The avoidance system engages withdrawal from aversive stimuli and generates types of negative affect (e.g., fear and disgust) consistent with protection from harm.

Lang (2000) explained the motivational basis of emotions through "natural selective attention," in which attention is primarily determined by the salience of the cue, or its intrinsic motivational significance, and the preexisting drive states. Cues that have appetitive or defensive significance are those to which we attend and respond. The intensity of response depends on the level of arousal. For example, if a cyclist has been riding all morning and has forgotten her water bottle, her level of arousal will be high as a consequence of thirst. She will attend to cues that have appetitive value for her, such as a water fountain or soda machine. Her response to seeing a lemonade stand on a side street will be a smile (behavior) accompanied by autonomic and hormonal activation to support her appetitive drive to satisfy her thirst.

> **A**ffect varies as a function of valence (positive versus negative) and intensity.

Although emotions each have unique facial, behavioral, and neural features, they seem to share neural systems in some circumstances (Phan et al. 2002; Vytal and Hamann 2010). It is less clear, though, whether emotional responses can be mapped on the affective dimension of pleasant to unpleasant and the behavioral dimensions of approach or avoidance proposed by the circumplex model that was developed mainly to understand the dimensions of moods (Watson and Tellegen 1985). For example, the classic animal behavior models have concluded that fighting and fleeing are both defensive behaviors regulated by the same punishment system in the brain, which is separate from the neural reward system that regulates approach behaviors.

Similarly, models of human affect have usually assumed that unpleasant moods or emotions are experienced along with avoidance behaviors,

in contrast to pleasant moods or emotions that are associated with approach behaviors. It is not clear that this always holds, though. As discussed in the previous section of the chapter, anger is typically viewed as a negative emotional response and as a defensive, avoidance behavior. Anger can lead to violence, which is socially destructive, or to poor health, depending on how it is expressed or controlled (Chida and Steptoe 2009; Spielberger 1983). In contrast, anger is experienced positively when people stand up for themselves or an ideal rather than shrinking away in fear or despair. As Aristotle noted, anger can lead to resistance against oppression, reducing the shame that can come from being submissive to wrongful acts by others. The subsequent sense of mastery or dominance can result in great satisfaction or pleasure. However, justified or righteous anger, which can feel good, may make a person vulnerable to anxiety about social reprisals or guilt about violating personal morals (Lazarus 2006). In contrast, angry, violent people can derive pleasure from dominating others.

Here, it may help to distinguish the affective experience of an emotion or mood from the behavioral expression of an emotion or mood; each might involve nuanced differences in neural regulation. Common experience shows that a depressed person may be lethargic and show little emotion other than sadness. However, a depressed person who is also anxious (which is very common) will show agitated behavior. In each case, affect is unpleasant, but emotional arousal and behavior are opposite each other.

Anger can be even more complex. People having the same trait for the experience of anger as a mood or an emotional response can express anger very differently. Anger can be expressed outwardly (e.g., outbursts of yelling, cursing, throwing, hitting, or kicking things) or inwardly (e.g., simmering, planning revenge, or even guilt), or it can be controlled by coping (e.g., counting to 10 or blowing off steam by talking or writing about it, or even exercising) (Speilberger et al. 1983). It is very conceivable that the neural basis of various expressions of anger will be somehow different from the neural basis of the experience of anger.

Here it is also helpful to add another dimension to affective experience, dominance. A person who experiences anger in a dominant way would be more likely to exhibit approach behaviors in the form of hostility, aggression, or violence. In contrast, a person who experiences anger in a submissive way would be more prone to avoid confrontation, either by controlling it or keeping it inside.

NEUROANATOMY OF AFFECT AND EMOTION

The evocation and expression of emotion have a strong biological basis. Early Greek philosophers Pythagoras and Alcmaeon believed that the brain was the organ of the mind. Plato agreed, stating that within the head's "spherical body is the divinist part of us and lord over all the rest." But, Plato's student, Aristotle, disagreed, adopting the earlier views of Hebrews, Hindus, and Chinese that the heart was the organ of intelligence and center of nerves. Philosophical debates about the primacy of the brain or heart as the origin of emotions continued throughout antiquity, even extending into Renaissance Europe.

> Tell me where is fancie bred,
> Or in the heart or in the head …
> *The Merchant of Venice* by Shakespeare

As we have seen, theories of discrete emotion (Darwin 1872; Ekman et al., 1972) propose a limited set of basic emotions (e.g., happiness, sadness, anger, fear, and disgust) that have unique physiological and neural profiles. Other theoretical views, such as dimensional theories of emotion, conceptualize emotions using a framework in which affective states can be represented in terms of underlying factors such as emotional arousal (emotion strength) and emotional valence (degree of pleasantness or unpleasantness). Studies measuring EEG or peripheral physiological responses such as heart rate, blood pressures, skin conductance, or stress hormones have for the most part been unable to identify psychophysiological patterns of response that are specific for each basic emotion (Barrett and Wager 2006; Cacioppo et al. 2000; Zajonc and McIntosh 1992). However, the accumulated evidence from studies of the brain, in both lower animals and humans, shows that emotions have unique, and sometimes shared, patterns of activity in structures and circuits in the brain.

In 1937, James Papez (pronounced Papes) suggested that a set of interconnected brain structures is responsible for motivation and emotion. Papez's neural circuit includes the hypothalamus, the mammillary bodies, the anterior thalamus, the amygdala, and the cingulate cortex (see figure 5.4).

The French anatomist Broca described the limbic lobe (meaning border or fringe) of the

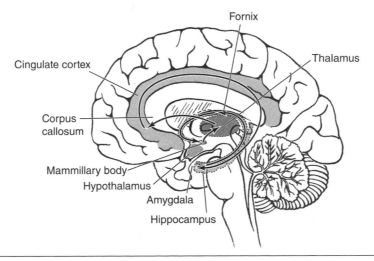

Figure 5.4 Papez (1937) proposed that the experience of emotion was primarily determined by the cingulate cortex, which modulates activity in the hippocampus. The hippocampus projects to the hypothalamus via a bundle of axons named the fornix. Hypothalamic impulses are relayed to the cortex from the anterior thalamus.

brain in 1878. Paul McLean of the National Institute of Mental Health is credited with expanding the circuit of Papez to a "limbic system" as the seat of emotion to include the prefrontal cortex, the hippocampus, the amygdala, and the septum, among others.

The Brain and Emotional Behavior

Later animal studies, mainly using rats as a model to guide human theories, showed that two main neural circuits in the brain activate emotions and behavioral responses to approach or avoid in situations that are potentially rewarding or threatening. The approach, or so-called reward, circuit identified by James Olds and Peter Milner in 1954 is located along the medial forebrain bundle (MFB), and the avoidance, or punishment, circuit identified in 1962 by Antonio Fernandez de Molina and Ralph Hunsperger includes the periventricular system (PVS). Pathways in the MFB motivate "wanting" (i.e., urges, drives, cravings) and approach behaviors (e.g., feeding, mating, playing) and "liking" (i.e., pleasure or satisfaction) that accompany positive, pleasant emotions. They make up a behavioral approach system (BAS). Pathways in the PVS motivate defensive or avoidance behaviors (e.g., fighting or fleeing) that accompany negative, unpleasant emotions. They make up a fight-or-flight system (FFS).

Opposite the BAS, and separate from the FFS, is a behavioral inhibition system (BIS). In the 1970s, English psychologist Jeffrey Gray, who trained at the Institute of Psychiatry in London and succeeded the renowned personality researcher Hans Eysenck as the chair of psychology there in 1983, proposed the BIS as a third emotion system, in addition to the fight-or-flight system (for unlearned punishments or novelty) and the behavioral approach system, in the BAS (Gray 1973, 1994b). The BIS is elicited by threats of punishment or failure, and by novelty or uncertainty (Gray 1987). According to Gray, the primary function of the BIS is to compare actual and expected stimuli. The BIS is activated to focus attention on the environment and inhibit ongoing behavior when a discrepancy exists between the actual and expected stimuli (e.g.,

novelty or uncertainty) or when the predicted stimuli are aversive. The BIS is adaptive when the best decision is to do nothing (e.g., when animals play dead or humans "accept their fate"). In those instances, doing nothing can be adaptive because doing something could make a bad situation worse. The BIS can also be maladaptive when we decide wrongly that our actions will be futile (i.e., give up prematurely or succumb to despair) or when a decision can't be quickly reached about whether it is best to flee or fight a threat (e.g., panic).

In cultures that determine success by competition, people learn to routinely activate the behavioral inhibition system to avoid social reprisals. In the extreme, the inhibition of emotional behaviors can, over time, lead to poor social adjustment and mental disorders such as anxiety, depression, and anger management problems that can contribute to psychosomatic illnesses such as stomach ulcers, high blood pressure, and possibly heart disease and cancer. Because of temperament (e.g., Eysenck's temperament traits of extroversion–introversion or emotional stability–instability) and learning history, people can usually be characterized as having a personality that is more or less dominant on BAS or BIS. People with a dominant BAS are more sensitive to rewards and are likely to be adventurous, outgoing, confident, and impulsive. People with a dominant BIS are more sensitive to punishment and are likely to be timid, withdrawn, shy, apprehensive, and cautious. Present-day applications of these ideas to humans has conceptualized the BAS as a behavioral approach system having three components (drive, fun seeking [e.g., impulsiveness], and reward or incentive sensitivity) and the BIS as a single avoidance system that regulates aversive motives to move away from something unpleasant (Carver and White 1994). The Sensitivity to Punishment and Sensitivity to Reward Questionnaire (SPSRQ) was developed to assess Gray's ideas as they apply to anxiety and impulsiveness (Torrubia et al. 2001).

Neuroanatomy of the BAS

There is not a single pleasure center of the brain but instead a neural system that includes circuits between subcortical areas along the MFB (the ventral tegmental area, nucleus accumbens, and ventral pallidum circuit; the septum; parts of the thalamus; and the amygdala) and cortical regions (orbitofrontal cortex and anterior cingulate cortex).

Pathways in the PVS extend from the medial parts of the hypothalamus (e.g., supraoptic region) along the third ventricle to the thalamus and the visceral and somatic motor neurons of the medulla in the brain stem and include the bed nucleus of the stria terminalis (BNST), the amygdala, and the periaqueductal gray (PAG) matter.

Neuroanatomy of the BIS

To Gray, anticipatory anxiety (especially evidenced by freezing behavior) reflected an emotional state mediated by BIS activation of a brain neural circuit between the hippocampus and the septum, which is modulated by the ascending noradrenergic system from the locus coeruleus in the pons (Gray 1987) and the prefrontal cortex, which appraises complex situations and has ultimate control of most emotional responses (Gray 1994a). Later, the neurobiologist Jan Panksepp argued that the activities of the ascending NA system and Gray's descending BIS prime the brain for emotional responses, but a circuit between the amygdala and the periaqueductal gray (PAG) matter was the key component of emotional states of fear and anxiety (Panksepp 1998).

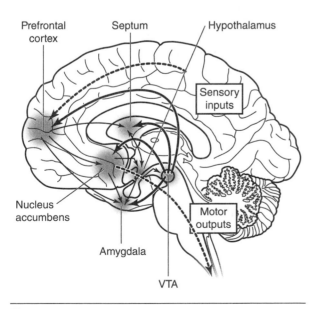

Figure 5.5 Reward circuits in the brain.

The amygdala-hypothalamus-central gray axis and fear. There are three places in the brain where electrical stimulation will elicit responses unique to fear (i.e., fleeing or freezing, increased heart rate, and urination or defecation): the lateral and central areas of the amygdala, the anterior and medial hypothalamus, and parts of the PAG (see figure 5.6; Panksepp 1998).

The amygdala and positive reinforcement and attention. The basolateral amygdala is also involved in the learning and memories of positive reinforcement, likely by its connections with the ventral striatal dopamine systems and the orbitofrontal cortex. Neuroimaging research in humans shows that the amygdala is active during exposure to either pleasant or unpleasant scenes (Garavan et al. 2001). Thus, it is believed that the amygdala helps modulate emotional behavior in ambiguous situations that are perceived as both potentially rewarding and aversive.

The bed nucleus of the stria terminalis (BNST). The BNST, along with the central amygdala and the shell of the nucleus accumbens (NAc), forms what is known as the extended amygdala. The BNST receives neural input from the central and basolateral amygdala, the prefrontal cortex and the hippocampus, as well as from visceral organs, and projects to the paraventricular nucleus of the hypothalamus (PVN) that regulates physiological responses during stress emotions, as well as to the nucleus accumbens and ventral tegmental area, where it modulates the discharge of dopamine neurons (Georges and Aston-Jones 2001). Thus, the BNST is an important relay between perceptions and both the approach–reward (i.e., wanting) and avoidance–punishment circuits.

Human Neuroimaging and Emotion

Early research findings in neuroscience based on lesioning, electrophysiological measures, and **neuroimaging** using positron emission tomography (PET) and functional magnetic resonance imaging (fMRI) identified several key brain regions that seem to be most involved

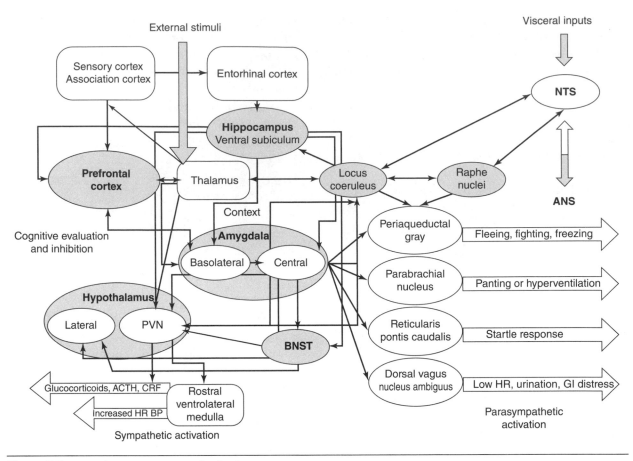

Figure 5.6 Punishment circuits in the brain.

Adapted, by permission, from T. Steimer, 2002, "The biology of fear-and anxiety-related behaviors," *Dialogues in Clinical Neuroscience* 4: 231-249.

in the experience and expression of human emotion (Davidson and Irwin 1999) (see Brain Regions Involved in the Expression of Human Emotion).

Although these brain regions are believed to operate as systems, not alone, they do appear to have some unique functions:

- The prefrontal cortex likely works as a memory of affective consequences, permitting an emotion to be sustained long enough to direct behavior toward the goal appropriate for that emotion.

- The hippocampus appears to process memories of the environment or context in which an emotion occurs. People who have damage to the hippocampus still experience emotion, but often at inappropriate times or places.

- The ventral striatum, especially the nucleus accumbens, is part of the meso-

limbic pathway of dopamine neurons from the ventral tegmental area that express encephalin and dynorphin opioid receptors that are key in what is known as reward-motivated behavior. The infusion of cocaine in addicts or nicotine in smokers, as well as the viewing of positive images, activates the accumbens. Thus, it appears to play a role in regulating approach behaviors associated with positive affect, especially those driven by the ventral pallidum in the basal ganglia.

- The anterior cingulate cortex is part of the primitive cortex common to species lower in evolution than humans. It seems to help regulate attention during the processing of the valence of an emotion. The insular cortex receives sensory inputs from the autonomic nervous system, especially cardiovascular responses, and

Brain Regions Involved in the Expression of Human Emotion

- Three parts of the prefrontal cortex

  1. Dorsolateral (the top, side part of the frontal lobe)
  2. Ventromedial (the middle, bottom part)
  3. Orbitofrontal (the base of the frontal lobe just above the orbits of the eyes)

- Amygdala, especially the central portion
- Hippocampus
- Ventral striatum, especially the nucleus accumbens (below the front of the caudate and putamen)
- Cingulate cortex (a layer of gray matter lying between the cerebrum and the lateral ventricle)
- Insular cortex (an island of involuted cortex near the temporal lobe)

sends signals to the central amygdala and the hypothalamus, which each regulates cardiac and endocrine responses during stress.

- The amygdala plays a key role in integrating overt behavior, autonomic responses, and hormonal responses during stress and emotion. Also, its tonic level of activity is sensitive to negative mood. For example, activity in the amygdala is elevated among patients diagnosed with depression and anxiety disorders. Patients with phobias show increased activity in the amygdala during fear elicited by a phobic object. Even seeing a fearful expression increases blood flow and metabolism in the amygdala. Receptors on the amygdala are also largely responsible for the anxiety-reducing effects of benzodiazepines and opiates (Carlson 1998).

A meta-analysis of 55 neuroimaging studies that used PET or fMRI (see chapter 3) mapped healthy people's responses at 20 brain regions to positive or negative dimensions of affective stimuli or to specific emotions of happiness, fear, anger, sadness, or disgust presented by either visual, auditory, or imagination (Phan et al. 2002). The main findings were as follows: (1) The medial prefrontal cortex had a general role in emotional processing; (2) fear specifically engaged the amygdala; (3) sadness was associated with activity in the inferior anterior cingulate cortex (ACC); (4) emotional induction by visual stimuli activated the occipital cortex and the amygdala; (5) induction by emotional recall or imagery recruited the anterior cingulate and insula; and (6) emotional tasks with cognitive demand also involved the anterior cingulate and insula. However, this analysis did not specifically assess whether each basic emotion could be discriminated from each of the other emotions on the basis of regional activations. A subsequent meta-analysis of 106 PET and fMRI studies (Murphy, Nimmo-Smith, and Lawrence 2003) reported left-sided activity during approach emotions, whereas neural activity associated with negative or withdrawal emotions was symmetrical between the hemispheres. Also, activation sites were different for fear (amygdala), disgust (insular cortex), and anger (globus pallidus and lateral orbitofrontal cortex), but happiness and sadness did not have distinct activation sites.

Neither of those two reviews distinguished between the recognition of emotion (e.g., seeing emotional faces that may not evoke an emotional response) from the experience of emotion (e.g., scenes, smells, or memories that elicit an emotion). A meta-analysis of 83 fMRI or PET studies also analyzed by Murphy and colleagues in 2003 mapped aggregated results onto a whole brain map according to standardized 3-D coordinates (Vytal and Hamann 2010). It concluded that each of five basic emotions (anger, fear, sadness, anger, and disgust) was consistently associated, across studies that used various methods to elicit responses, with unique patterns of regional brain activity. Happiness activated the right superior temporal gyrus (STG) (a gyrus is a ridge on the cerebral cortex usually surrounded by one or more sulci, or fissures; see figure 5.7 and figure 5.8) and the ACC; activity in both of these regions differentiated happiness from sadness, anger, fear, and disgust (ACC only). Sadness activated the medial frontal gyrus (MFG) and the head of the caudate/ACC; activity in both regions differentiated sadness from happiness, anger, fear, and disgust. Anger activated the left inferior gyrus (IFG) and parahippocampal gyrus (PHG); both regions differentiated anger from all other emotion states. Fear activated the amygdala and insular cortex; these regions differentiated fear from happiness, sadness, anger (insula only), and disgust (posterior insular cortex). Disgust activated the IFG and the anterior insular cortex; these regions reliably differentiated disgust from all other emotion states. Facial expressions of emotion were the most frequently used stimulus for studies of all basic emotions (one-half to two-thirds of the studies) except for sadness and disgust, for which emotional pictures were the second most frequent stimulus type. Nonetheless, results of the meta-analysis did not differ substantively when only studies that used faces were evaluated.

A subsequent meta-analysis of 100 studies of emotional face processing and 57 studies of emotional scene processing found that both faces and scenes elicited fMRI BOLD activation (indicative of increased blood flow; see chapter 3) in the amygdala, followed by areas of the medial prefrontal cortex, inferior frontal and orbitofrontal cortex, inferior temporal cortex, and extrastriate occipital cortex (visual neurons there are modulated by attention, working memory, and anticipation of reward). Areas specific to emotional faces were those known to process faces regardless of their emotional expression, including the anterior fusiform gyrus and middle temporal gyrus. Areas specific to emotional scenes were the lateral occipital cortex, as well as the posterior and medial dorsal nuclei of the thalamus (Sabatinelli et al. 2011).

A recent study that measured event-related brain potentials (ERP) showed that viewing emotional faces or emotionally arousing (pleasant and unpleasant) scenes each enhance the N170 potential. The emotional scenes evoked stronger arousal and emotional valence ratings and larger early posterior negativity (EPN) and late positive potential (LPP) responses compared to the emotional faces (Thom et al. 2012). During rewarding behavior, fMRI activation in the meso-

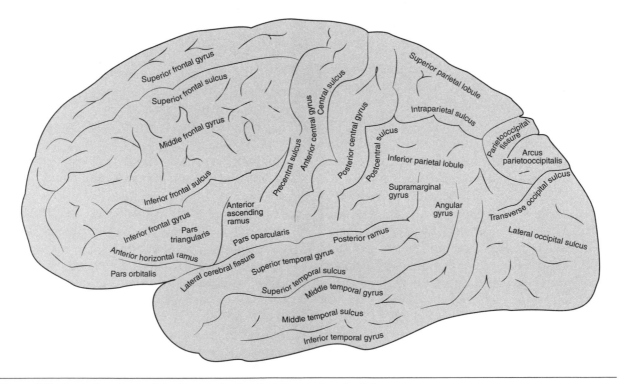

Figure 5.7 Lateral surface of the human brain showing gyri and sulci.

Reprinted, by permission, from H. Gray, 2010, *Gray's anatomy* (London, England: Arcturus Publishing).

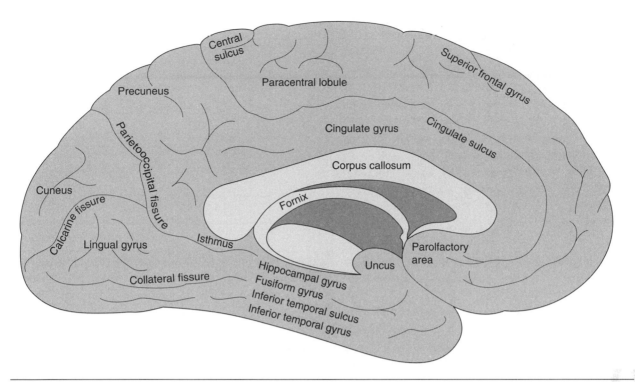

Figure 5.8 Medial sagittal view of the gyri and sulci of the human brain.

Reprinted, by permission, from H. Gray, 2010, *Gray's anatomy* (London, England: Arcturus Publishing).

corticolimbic reward circuit (caudate, amygdala, and orbital frontal cortex) including the ventral striatum and medial prefrontal cortex is positively correlated with the feedback negativity (FN)–evoked EEG potential (which has been source localized to the medial prefrontal cortex and striatum) (Carlson et al. 2011).

The amygdala is especially important for processing neural events associated with the experience of learned fear and anxiety. Lesion studies have shown that the emotion of fear is a primitive, hard-wired reaction to immediate danger, but that learned fear and anxiety also depend on the amygdala (LeDoux 1994). A useful probe for studying brain activity linked with fear, anxiety, and other negative or positive emotional states in humans is the acoustic startle eye-blink response, or ASER (Lang 1995; Lang, Bradley, and Cuthbert 1998). The ASER is elicited by an abrupt noise (e.g., similar to the sound of a starter's pistol), which is processed as an obligatory reflex from the auditory nerve by ventral cochlear root neurons projecting to the nucleus reticularis pontis caudalis and on to the facial nerve innervating the orbicularis occuli (the muscle that blinks the eye) (Davis 1997; Lee

et al. 1996). The ASER is measured by placing surface electrodes beneath and beside the eye to record an integrated electromyographic signal of activity in the orbicularis occuli as the eye blinks. Figure 5.9 shows the placement of the electrodes. A typical electromyographic (EMG) response is shown in figure 5.10.

The nucleus reticularis pontis caudalis is innervated by neurons of the amygdala and the periaqueductal gray (PAG) matter, which provide a neurocircuit enabling the amygdala to modulate the ASER during emotion (see figure 5.11). In humans, the amplitude of the ASER is increased by anticipation of electric shock and by images that evoke fear or are otherwise aversive to the person (Lang 1995). Anti-anxiety drugs such as benzodiazepines reduce the ASER.

Psychophysiologist Peter Lang and his colleagues at the University of Florida believe that the ASER is a defensive reflex elicited mainly in aversive circumstances when the prevailing affect is negative and the motivational state is one of avoidance or withdrawal. By having people view a standard set of pictures that differ in content from highly pleasant to highly unpleasant, these researchers have shown that the ASER

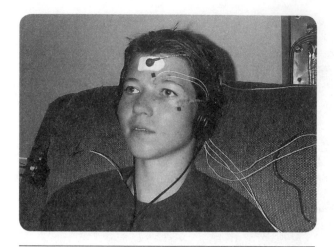

Figure 5.9 Electrode placement for the measurement of the acoustic startle eye-blink response using electromyography.

Provided by the Exercise Psychology Laboratory, Department of Kinesiology, the University of Georgia.

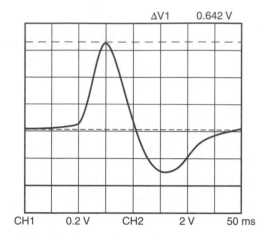

Figure 5.10 A typical startle eye-blink response as measured by electromyography.

Provided by the Exercise Psychology Laboratory, Department of Kinesiology, and Department of Psychology, the University of Georgia.

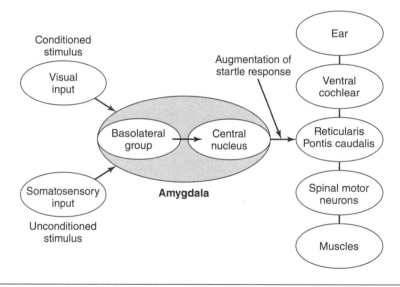

Figure 5.11 Flow diagram of the neurocircuitry of the startle response.

is increased in conditions that elicit attention, aversion, and high emotional arousal (Cuthbert, Bradley, and Lang 1996; Lang 1995; Lang et al. 1998). The ASER tends to be reduced when the emotional content of the pictures is rated by the participant as positive or pleasant.

Hemispheric Asymmetry

The function of the neural circuits of affect can differ between the left and right hemispheres. This difference is called **hemispheric asym-**

metry. For example, people who have lesion damage to the prefrontal cortex, especially the left dorsolateral area, have an increased risk of developing depression (Davidson and Irwin 1999). This is not actually a new finding. The first modern theory of frontal lobe function, proposed by David Ferrier in the 1870s, was in part based on the case of Phineas Gage, who survived massive damage to his left frontal cortex and suffered irreparable loss of mental function. Gage was the foreman of a railway construction gang working for the Rutland and

Burlington Rail Road near Cavendish, Vermont. In September 1848, an accidental explosion of a charge he had set blew a 3.5-foot, 13-pound (1 m, 6 kg) tamping iron point first through his left cheekbone and eye and then completely out of the top of his head, virtually destroying his left frontal cortex (see figure 5.12). He survived, and in the middle of 1849 he went back to work, but his personality had changed dramatically. Before the accident he had been a capable and efficient foreman with a well-balanced mind. Afterward, he was judged as "fitful, impatient and obstinate, yet capricious and vacillating, unable to settle on any of the plans he devised for future action." His friends said he was "no longer Gage." His physician, Dr. John Harlow, reported Gage's case and gave the skull and tamping iron to Harvard Medical School, where they are now displayed at the Countway Library of Medicine

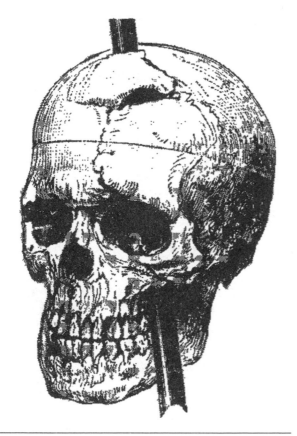

Figure 5.12 Image of a wooden reconstruction from Gage's exhumed skull that appeared in an 1868 report on his case by the attending physician, Dr. Harlow (Harlow 1868). The heavy line approximates the path and thickness of the tamping rod.

Provided by Malcolm Macmillan, School of Psychology, Deakin University, Victoria, Australia. www.hbs.deakin.edu.au/gagepage.

(Macmillan 2000). Modern reconstruction of the brain damage based on measurements of Gage's skull and on neuroimaging data indicated that brain damage occurred in both the left and right prefrontal regions involved with **cognition** and emotion—consistent with reports of Gage's altered personality and temperament (Damasio et al. 1994).

Affective Style

Asymmetry in the activation of the hemispheres of the frontal cortex in people without clinical disorders has been measured by electroencephalography (EEG) during exposure to pictures that elicit positive or negative affect. Not only is left hemisphere activity higher during the viewing of positive images and right hemisphere activity higher during the viewing of negative images; but also some people seem to have what is called an affective style, or disposition, to respond to emotional events in a more positive or negative way. Those who have a characteristically dominant activation of the left frontal cortex tend to view emotional events more positively, whereas those having dominant right frontal activation experience events more negatively. Some recent studies even suggest that people's affective styles also influence how quickly they recover from negative emotions or how long they can savor positive emotions (Davidson 2000).

When negative emotions have been evoked in anxiety disorder patients by phobic images (e.g., snakes or spiders), PET and fMRI images have indicated increased blood flow and metabolism in the right inferior prefrontal cortex. Not much evidence has yet been reported on prefrontal changes during the experience of positive affect. Although early research suggested that greater left than right frontal cortical activity was associated with positive affect, more recent research, primarily on anger, suggests that greater left than right frontal cortical activity is associated with approach motivation, which can be positive (e.g., enthusiasm) or negative in valence (e.g., anger) (Harmon-Jones et al. 2009).

Emotional Coping

We saw earlier in the chapter that people's personalities or temperaments influence and help explain whether they are exposed to approach or avoidance circumstances that elicit emotions (e.g., extroversion or introversion, emotional stability or neuroticism, reward sensitivity or punishment sensitivity). Now we will examine how people differ in the way they appraise the meaning of events as emotionally stressful, and how they deal or cope with them (Lazarus 1966).

At the maladaptive extreme, faulty thinking (e.g., extreme, rigid, unrealistic, illogical, absolute appraisals) can result in self-defeating meanings to emotional encounters that lead to self-blame, self-pity, and cynical anger (Ellis 1957). At the adaptive extreme is effective coping. Coping is classically defined as "constantly changing cognitive and behavioral efforts to manage specific external and internal demands that are appraised as taxing or exceeding the resources of the individual" (Lazarus and Folkman 1985, 141).

As initially conceived, the two broad types of coping are problem-focused and emotion-focused. Problem-focused coping uses an analytical approach to prevent or plan against circumstances that are perceived as harmful, threatening, or challenging. Once the problem is identified, people weigh the costs and benefits of alternative tactics to resolve it. People's tactics can be aimed at themselves, too, such as shifting their goals, reducing the importance of their goals, or switching to other rewarding paths. Emotion-focused coping tries to reduce distress by avoiding, minimizing, tolerating, distancing, selectively attending to, or controlling the circumstances seen as threatening or challenging.

This type of coping by cognitive reappraisal of the situation changes the meaning of a situation to a person rather than the situation itself. For example, selectively attending to or avoiding an emotionally stressful situation can suspend it, but not transform it. Other coping behaviors, such as meditation, prayer, seeking emotional support, compensating with temporarily pleasing behaviors (food, drink, drugs), are not reappraisals but can sometimes lead to reappraisals or problem solving.

Emotion-focused coping ranges from self-soothing (e.g., relaxation, seeking emotional support), to expressing negative emotion (e.g., yelling, crying), to focusing on negative thoughts (e.g., ruminating), to attempting to escape stressful situations (e.g., avoidance, denial, wishful thinking) (Carver and Connor-Smith 2010). Problem- and emotion-focused coping can also facilitate one another. Effective problem-focused coping diminishes the threat, but thereby also diminishes the distress generated by that threat. Effective emotion-focused coping diminishes negative distress, making it possible to consider the problem more calmly, perhaps yielding better problem-focused coping. Hence, problem- and emotion-focused coping can complement each other (Lazarus 2006). People who choose to minimize or avoid situations that elicit emotional distress, rather than deal head-on with the causes of the distress, might find exercise especially helpful. Exercise can also reduce feelings of distress. Some people even say they get insight about solving problems while they exercise.

Albert Ellis proposed the following three core beliefs that lead to emotional disturbance

"I must be thoroughly competent, adequate, achieving, and lovable at all times, or else I am an incompetent worthless person."

"Other significant people in my life must treat me kindly and fairly at all times, or else I can't stand it, and they are bad, rotten, and evil persons who should be severely blamed, demined, and vindictively punished for their horrible treatment of me."

"Things and conditions absolutely must be the way I want them to be and must never be too difficult or frustrating. Otherwise, life is awful, terrible, horrible, catastrophic and unbearable."

Reprinted, by permission, from A. Ellis, 2003, "Early theories and practices of rational emotive behavior therapy and how they have been augmented and revised during the last three decades," *Journal of Rational-Emotive & Cognitive-Behavior Therapy* 21(3): 219-243.

Some Ways of Coping

Confrontive Coping

I stood my ground.

I distanced myself.

I didn't let it get to me.

I tried to forget it.

Self-Controlling

I tried to keep my feelings to myself.

I tried not to act too hastily.

Seeking Social Support

I talked to someone to find out more about the situation.

I accepted responsibility.

I realized I brought the problem on myself.

Escape-Avoidance

I wished that the situation would go away.

I avoided being with people.

Planful Problem Solving

I made a plan of action and followed it.

I changed something so things would turn out all right.

Positive Reappraisal

I changed or grew as a person in a good way.

I found new faith.

Reproduced by special permission of the Publisher, MIND GARDEN, Inc., www.mindgarden.com from the **Ways of Coping Questionnaire** by Susan Folkman & Richard S. Lazarus. Copyright 1988 by Consulting Psychologists Press, Inc. Further reproduction is prohibited without the Publisher's written consent.

Engagement coping: dealing with emotional distress or its causes

Disengagement coping: escaping from dealing with emotional distress (e.g., minimizing negative thoughts) or its causes (e.g., avoidance, denial, wishful thinking)

Figure 5.13 shows some possible ways exercise might directly or indirectly have a positive influence on affect among people with various personalities, stress exposures, and ways of coping with emotional stress.

Personality describes and partly determines how people appraise and cope with emotional experiences. Chapter 4 mentioned that people with a hardy or resilient personality tend to see change as an opportunity rather than a threat and typically believe that they are ultimately in control of their life (Kobasa, Maddi, and Kahn 1982). Similarly, optimism and pessimism reflect confidence rather than doubt about life in general (Carver and Connor-Smith 2010; Tiger 1979). Biological models of personality include approach and avoidance temperaments, such as the so-called five-factor model of personality (extroversion, neuroticism, agreeableness, conscientiousness, and openness to experience; Digman 1990; Goldberg 1981; McCrae and Costa 2003). These researchers hold that approach and avoidance systems are supported partly by distinct brain areas, and that the sensitivity of each system (which varies among people) influences behavior in response to environmental cues signaling impending reward or threat (Carver and Connor-Smith 2010).

Extroversion is an approach temperament. It conveys assertiveness, dominance, spontaneity, energy, sociability, and sometimes happiness. Neuroticism is an avoidance temperament. It conveys sensitivity to emotional distress, anxiety, depression, hostility, and moodiness. People who are agreeable are friendly, helpful, empathetic, and able to inhibit negative feelings; they get less angry at other people than do disagreeable people who use acts of dominance during social conflict.

Conscientious people plan, persist, and strive with purpose toward goals. They also show responsibility and constrain impulsiveness. Openness to experience includes curiosity, flexibility, imagination, readiness to try new things, and possibly intellect. Meta-analyses have concluded that optimism, extroversion, conscientiousness, and openness predict more engagement coping; neuroticism predicts more disengagement coping; and optimism, conscientiousness, and agreeableness predicts less

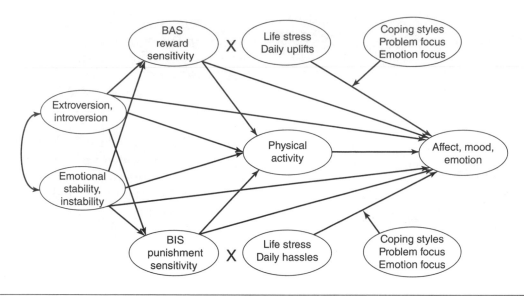

Figure 5.13 Paths by which physical activity could improve affective experience.

disengagement coping (Connor-Smith and Flachsbart 2007; Nes and Segerstrom 2006).

Positive Psychology

The central postulate of so-called positive psychology (Seligman and Csikszentmihalyi 2000) is "if individuals engage in positive thinking and feeling and abandon or minimize their preoccupation with the harsh and tragic—that is, the stressful side of life—they will have found a magic elixir of health and well-being" (Lazarus 2003b, 93). Optimism researcher Martin Seligman, together with Christopher Peterson, developed *Character Strengths and Virtues: A Handbook and Classification*, which they called a positive counterpart to the *Diagnostic and Statistical Manual of Mental Disorders* (*DSM*) of the American Psychiatric Association (Peterson and Seligman 2004). Drawing from their synopsis of cultures during recorded history from Asia, Greece, Rome, and Western civilization, they compiled a list of virtues that includes six character strengths: wisdom or knowledge, courage, humanity, justice, temperance, and transcendence, each of which has several subfactors, in a slight repackaging of the seven virtues of the Christian tradition: temperance (e.g., modesty, self-control), justice (e.g., fairness, citizenship), courage (e.g., fortitude, bravery), practical wisdom, humanity (e.g., charity), and transcen-

dence (e.g., hope, faith) (Cloninger 2005). The scientific basis of positive psychology has been vigorously debated (Lazarus 2003a, 2003b). Nonetheless, applications of positive psychology to the study and promotion of exercise have emerged during the past few years.

FACTORS INFLUENCING THE EFFECTS OF EXERCISE ON AFFECT

Understanding variables that can moderate the influence of exercise on affect begins with understanding factors that influence affect. Affect varies in valence, or hedonic tone, and in intensity, and these two dimensions are influenced by a variety of endogenous and exogenous factors. For example, emotional memory systems contain reciprocal connections such that emotions can activate memories or thoughts about the emotions, and thoughts can activate stored emotional responses (Lang 2000). The key determinants of affect also differ for mood and emotion. Watson and Clark (1994) organized potentially important factors that can influence mood into four broad types: exogenous factors, endogenous rhythms, traits and temperament, and characteristic variability. Exogenous factors can be transient conditions in the environment, such as a series of rainy days or new music in an aerobics class. Endogenous rhythms include innate biological processes that are associated with a natural cyclicity in mood, such as the menstrual cycle. Traits and temperament refer to the general tendency people have for experiencing positive or negative mood states of specific levels of intensity, and characteristic variability describes the stable individual differences in the magnitude of mood fluctuations.

Moods can be altered by intense emotion repeated at a high frequency over time, such as a surprise phone call from an old college friend followed by significant improvements in a negative mood as a result of a long conversation about college football games, parties attended, and the antics of fraternity brothers. Moods are also altered by physiological changes, such as drug effects, lack of sleep, and exercise (Ekman 1994). For example, physical activity was found to influence **diurnal** variation in feeling states in a field study of women: positive engagement, revitalization, and tranquility were higher after exercise than was predicted based on diurnal patterns (Gauvin, Rejeski, and Reboussin 2000). The effects of exercise on mood can be influenced by personal, situational, and task variables, such as exercise mode or intensity.

Affect, emotion, and mood are sensitive to a variety of personal factors, such as health (e.g., negative effects from illness or allergies), hormones, and perceptions. Expectations are personal variables that can influence the effects of exercise training on changes in self-esteem

Example of the Interaction of Factors Influencing Mood

It rained every day for 3 weeks when Jill first moved to the city. Although she enjoyed an occasional rainy day, she was unable to run outside. Jill used exercise to manage menstrual pain during her cycle. Without her workout routine, this typically enthusiastic and cheerful young woman was in a depressed mood for almost a month.

(see chapter 12), but positive changes in mood after acute exercise do not appear to depend on expectations of benefits (Berger et al. 1998; Tieman et al. 2001). There is some evidence that self-efficacy for exercise moderates the effect of exercise on mood, such that higher self-efficacy is associated with positive mood during and after exercise (Bozoian, Rejeski, and McAuley 1994).

Experience with exercise is another personal variable that has been hypothesized as a moderating factor in the effects of exercise on affect, as well as in the importance of mood regulation as a motivator for exercise. A novice exerciser who experiences muscle soreness after the first day of weight training would have a stronger and more negative affective response than an experienced bodybuilder would. The bodybuilder is accustomed to some soreness with exercise, and might even have a positive emotional response if he or she interprets the soreness as a prelude to strength gains from overload based on past training experiences. We should also consider experience with exercise in understanding the effects of exercise on mood. Experienced exercisers rated mood-related reasons for exercising as more important than did inexperienced exercisers in a cross-sectional study of 168 members of fitness centers (Hsiao and Thayer 1998). Advanced members scored higher than beginners on exercising to improve mood and higher than intermediate members and beginners on exercising for socialization.

Situational factors that influence affect include the physical environment (e.g., weather) and the social environment. Laboratory conditions may contribute situational effects that can confound the influence of exercise on mood through the participant's interpretation of the setting. Social environments can interact with a variety of personal and task variables to influence affective responses and mood. For example, a participant in a beginners' aerobics class had felt upbeat and positive with the progress she had been making and the contact with her classmates. She became discouraged and experienced a negative mood after a change in her work schedule caused her to switch to the advanced class, which had a harder routine and more skilled and fit participants.

Characteristics of exercise experience that can influence affective response include intensity,

Interpretation of Arousal
From Exercise Influences Affective Response

Chad and his grandfather Frank, who was recovering from a mild heart attack, both experienced shortness of breath walking up a steep hill together. Frank's emotional reaction was fear, and he was in a depressed mood for the rest of the day. To Chad, the breathlessness was a normal physical response, and it generated minimal emotional response or effect on his mood.

duration, and mode. Recall that affect has valence and arousal dimensions. Exercise itself increases arousal with increasing levels of intensity, and the resulting affect (valence, or hedonic, dimension) hinges on the participant's interpretation of that arousal. The duration of the exercise bout may also influence mood, but this has not been systematically investigated (Yeung 1996). Duration effects should be evaluated for different modes, intensities, and populations. Exercise mode is another task variable that can affect mood. Chapters 6 and 7 present some of the evidence for differences in anxiety and depression as a function of the type of exercise (i.e., aerobic versus strength training).

RESEARCH ON EXERCISE AND AFFECT

Research on affect and exercise has typically involved the measurement of affect with self-report instruments, although human emotion has been estimated using psychophysiological and observational techniques. This section presents a review of self-report instruments that have been used to measure the effects of exercise on affective states and provides examples of studies on the effects of acute exercise and exercise training on affect and mood.

Self-Report Instruments

The most popular instruments used in exercise and affect research have been adjective checklists, particularly the Profile of Mood States (POMS; McNair, Lorr, and Droppleman

1981). Other instruments developed to measure affect include the Positive Affect and Negative Affect Scales (PANAS; Watson, Clark, and Tellegen 1988) and the Affect Grid (Russell, Weiss, and Mendelsohn 1989). Still other scales have been designed specifically to measure affective responses to exercise. These include the Feeling Scale (Hardy and Rejeski 1989), the Exercise-Induced Feeling Inventory (Gauvin and Rejeski 1993), and the Subjective Exercise Experiences Scale (McAuley and Courneya 1994). The development of these three scales was based on concerns that existing, validated mood scales either were not sensitive or were not specific enough to detect true changes in mood during or after physical activity (Gauvin and Spence 1998), or that affective response to physical activity is somehow different from that experienced in other settings. Although the first concern is plausible, it would relate as much to the range of the response scale as to the structure of the scale content. The second concern is harder to understand.

Why would there be a special set of moods or emotions unique to the experience of exercise? Were that found to be true, the results would represent a provocative exception to 100 years of research that supports the invariance of the expression of moods and emotions across situations and even cultures. The logical extension of the exercise-specific argument would be that specific scales are needed for each human behavior. Joy or happiness after a tasty meal would be a different joy than that after sex, or after a big pay raise, and so on. Although the strength of the valence and emotional arousal of joy might vary after each of those experiences, the structure of joy as a distinct affective experience would be the same. This issue is discussed in further detail in chapter 6, Anxiety.

One approach has been to select items from existing general mood or affect scales that seem more sensitive than others to change in response to exercise and to reconfigure those items into a new, specific scale for exercise. Up to now, evidence of the usefulness of this approach (evidence that it yields valid scales measuring affective responses unique to exercise) has not been compelling when judged by the classical standards of construct validation discussed in chapter 2. Nonetheless, exercise-specific scales are discussed in this chapter because it seems likely that this topic will continue to command the attention of exercise psychology researchers for some time (e.g., Ekkekakis and Petruzzello 2000).

The unipolar POMS has 65 items that are rated on a 5-point scale ranging from 0, *not at all,* to 4, *extremely.* It includes six discrete affective states: tension–anxiety, depression–dejection, anger–hostility, vigor, fatigue, and confusion–bewilderment. The respondent is asked to focus on current feelings (i.e., *right now*), but the POMS can also be used to rate daily, weekly, or habitual feelings (i.e., *during the past week, including today*). A shortened 30-item version is also available from Multi-Health Systems, Inc. at www.mhs.com.

The POMS has been used frequently to determine the anti-anxiety and antidepressant effects of acute exercise and in overtraining and staleness studies of endurance athletes. In 1998, LeUnes and Burger published a bibliography of POMS research that included 194 studies using the POMS in exercise or sport since its introduction in 1975. Nonetheless, some investigators have questioned its suitability for use with people without clinical disorders (Gauvin and Spence 1998). The POMS was developed for psychiatric populations for the purpose of detecting the ongoing effects of therapy in outpatients. It is sensitive to these changes, as well as to changes induced by laboratory manipulations. Also, normative data are available according to sex, age, and psychiatric status, including normal youth and young adults. At issue is whether its emphasis on negative affect allows it to be sensitive to changes in positive mood among people who experience few negative moods.

The bipolar POMS was developed to emphasize positive affect and to be more applicable to people without clinical disorders as well as patients experiencing psychiatric disorders. The bipolar POMS has 72 items that are rated on a 4-point scale from 0, *much unlike this,* to 3, *much like this.* It includes six bipolar scales: composed–anxious, agreeable–hostile, elated–depressed, confident–unsure, energetic–tired, and clearheaded–confused.

The PANAS measures positive and negative affect as two relatively independent dimensions using two 10-item mood scales (Watson, Clark, and Tellegen 1988). The scales have high internal consistency and good stability over a 2-month period. The two-factor structure of the PANAS was confirmed in a sample of 645 participants in a sport camp, 10 to 17 years old, immediately after an exercise session; but there were questionable psychometrics with three items from the negative affect scale (irritable, distress, and upset) (Crocker 1997).

The Affect Grid is a one-item instrument that is based on valence, or hedonic tone, and arousal dimensions of affect, defined as pleasure–displeasure and arousal–sleepiness (Russell, Weiss, and Mendelsohn 1989). A circumplex model is applied by placing feeling-related concepts in a circular order in a space formed by the two bipolar dimensions (see figure 5.1). The Affect Grid has been used effectively to describe current mood, the meaning of emotion-related words, and feelings conveyed by facial expressions. It has also been found to be valid across cultures (Russell, Lewicka, and Niit 1989).

The Feeling Scale is another one-item instrument that measures the valence, or hedonic tone, of affect (Hardy and Rejeski 1989). Participants rate their current overall feelings on an 11-point bipolar scale with verbal anchors of *very good* to *very bad.*

The Exercise-Induced Feelings Inventory has 12 adjectives that are rated on a 5-point Likert-type scale ranging from *do not feel* to *feel very strongly* (Gauvin and Rejeski 1993). It was designed to measure four feeling states (enthusiasm, energy, fatigue, and calmness) assumed to be elicited by positive engagement, revitalization, physical exhaustion, and tranquility, which are stimulus properties of acute bouts of exercise.

The Subjective Exercise Experiences Scale was designed to measure global psychological responses that are sensitive to the stimulus properties of exercise (McAuley and Courneya 1994). Two of the three scale factors (positive well-being and psychological distress) correspond to positive and negative poles associated with psychological health. The third factor, fatigue, represents subjective feelings of fatigue. The scale includes 12 items that are rated on a Likert-type scale ranging from *not at all* to *very much so* in terms of the respondent's current feelings.

The validity of the last three scales developed specifically for exercise has been critiqued elsewhere (e.g., Ekkekakis and Petruzzello 2001a, 2001b).

Measurement Considerations

Most questionnaires that have been used to assess emotions are arguably measuring mood because of the time it takes to complete them (Smith and Crabbe 2000). For example, a 65-item questionnaire such as the POMS has several scales to measure specific emotions and has the items for each scale scattered throughout the test. The feeling state or emotion of the respondent when he or she answers the first scale item could change before the other items are answered, which hampers the validity of the scale. Single-item measures (e.g., bipolar line scales) might be better for addressing this limitation of assessing emotional state; these types of instruments are probably less likely to change the variable being measured through the measurement act itself than are longer ones. However, a single-item scale such as the Feeling Scale (Hardy and Rejeski 1989) cannot determine what emotion is being rated, or whether different people are experiencing the

> **M**easures of affect and exercise usually assess mood, not transient emotional responses.

same emotion, without anchoring the rating to a specific emotional stimulus (Lang 1995).

Acute Exercise

There is a general consensus in the literature that exercise improves affect. A meta-analysis of 158 studies published from 1979 to 2005 on the effects of acute exercise on positive affect concluded that exercise increases positive mood (Reed and Ones 2006), and there is evidence that acute exercise at intensities below the ventilatory or lactate thresholds can increase self-reported positive affect (Ekkekakis, Parfitt, and Petruzzello 2011). Mood benefits of acute exercise have been found for clinical populations (e.g., type 2 diabetes: Kopp et al. 2012; spinal cord injury: Martin Ginis and Latimer 2007). In addition, daily positive mood but not negative mood has been associated with objectively measured physical activity (Poole et al. 2011). But as already discussed, it is prudent to be cautious about overgeneralizing the benefits in mood and emotional states without considering some of the moderating variables, such as exercise history, task characteristics, and the environment.

Generally, regular exercisers compared with nonexercisers have greater mood enhancement after a single bout of exercise (e.g., Hoffman and Hoffman 2008). Reed and Ones (2006) showed consistently positive effects of acute exercise at low intensities, durations up to 35 min, for low to moderate exercise doses. In a study comparing objectively measured physical activity with daily mood, light and moderate physical activities were also associated with positive daily affect, but vigorous activity was not (Poole et al. 2011).

Rudolph and Kim (1996) measured mood responses to aerobic dance, soccer, tennis, and bowling in a sample of 108 physical education students at a Korean university. The Subjective Exercise Experiences Scale was administered before and after the activity. Positive mood was enhanced in students participating in aerobic dance and soccer. There were no changes in negative mood or in the moods of tennis players or bowlers. However, participants self-selected into the various exercise modes, and a randomized trial would provide more clarification of the role of exercise task in affective response.

Acute psychological responses to exercise can be affected by factors in the physical and social environment, such as temperature and humidity, odors, and the presence of others. For example, sedentary women exercised on a stationary cycle at moderate intensity based on RPE for 20 min with and without others in a mirrored or nonmirrored setting (Martin Ginis, Burke, and Gauvin 2007). Feeling states were measured by the Exercise-Induced Feeling Inventory before, during, and after exercise. Revitalization increased significantly less and fatigue increased more for women in the mirrored room with others compared to women in the other three conditions when controlling for body mass index (BMI). The responses to exercising with others in front of mirrors indicates the importance of considering environmental factors in analyzing the effects of exercise on mood.

Increases in positive mood have been found in youth sport participants after a game, but the improved mood seemed to be largely determined by the perception of achievement and the matching of skills against a realistic challenge (Wankel and Sefton 1989). One study of college-age participants showed that mood changes after running exercise were not influenced by competition (O'Connor, Carda, and Graf 1991).

A review of studies that used the POMS concluded that the evidence supports associations between acute physical activity and improved mood among nonclinical populations and between chronic exercise and improved mood among clinical populations (Berger and Motl 2000). The POMS has also been employed to identify social or cognitive explanations for mood alteration after exercise. However, currently there is no conclusive evidence identifying a single explanation or clustering of explanations that consistently mediates or moderates the association between exercise and mood change, although researchers are exploring a variety of possible explanations. For example, regular exercisers reported mood before and after 10 min of self-paced jogging, and were also asked after exercise to recall their preexercise mood (Anderson and Brice 2011). Mood as measured by the total mood disturbance (TMD) of the Incredibly Short Profile of Mood States (ISP) increased significantly and compared to the no-exercise control group. In addition, the recalled preexercise mood was favorably distorted to indicate mood enhancement. That is, their recalled preexercise mood was worse than actually reported before exercise, which gave a perceived augmented mood benefit of the acute exercise bout. Additional research is needed to determine the reasons for this memory distortion, such as current mood states and expectations of mood benefits from exercise.

We usually think about how exercise can improve positive mood and affect in the short term, but there is also evidence that exercise can reduce negative moods, such as anxiety and even obsessive-compulsive disorder symptoms (Abrantes et al. 2009), and can have effects beyond the exercise session. For example, 30 minutes of moderate-intensity cycling exercise reduced angry mood in college men who scored high in trait-anger and mitigated the increase in anger that was induced by viewing emotional pictures, but it did not alter the intensity of angry emotional responses during picture viewing (Thom et al. 2012). Thus, even though exercise didn't affect the acute experience of an angry emotion, it provided a prophylaxis against angry feelings elicited up to 45 minutes later. Another study used guided imagery to induce an upset or angry mood and reported a reduction in state anger after a session of resistance exercise, but that change was not greater than seen after quiet rest (Bartholomew 1999).

Training Studies

Bryne and Bryne (1993) reviewed 30 studies published since 1975 on the effects of exercise training on mood adjustment, such as depression, anxiety, and other states of disturbed mood. Ten of the studies evaluated mood changes in nonclinical populations and showed significant improvements in mood that were not related to changes in fitness. Overall, 90% of the studies reviewed supported the contention that exercise improves mood. Reed and Buck (2009) reviewed 105 studies of regular aerobic exercise and positive affect published from 1980 to 2008 and reported a moderate beneficial effect on self-reported affect with the optimal program at a low intensity for 30 to 35 minutes, 3 to

5 days per week for 10 to 12 weeks. Several randomized clinical trials have shown positive effects on mood and quality of life in clinical populations, such as women being treated for breast cancer (e.g., Yang et al. 2011; Mutrie et al. 2007), people with multiple sclerosis (Dalgas et al. 2010), and people with traumatic brain injury (Driver and Ede 2009). There is also some evidence that mood improvements are related to exercise adherence. For example, the Profile of Mood States-Short Form and other psychological measures were administered to 173 obese women at the beginning and end of a 6-month moderate-intensity exercise intervention (Annesi et al. 2011). Mood significantly improved, and changes in mood and body satisfaction but not self-efficacy contributed uniquely to the variance in exercise session attendance, which was significantly related to changes in BMI.

Additional training studies have been generally supportive of positive effects of exercise on mood for various populations, although training intensity has had mixed effects. Mood was improved in initially sedentary older women after a 12-week strength training program (Tsutsumi et al. 1998). Both high-intensity and moderate-intensity strength training groups significantly improved positive mood and demonstrated some decrease in tension and state anxiety, although support for moderate intensity was greater. The greatest improvements in affect were found in young active aerobic exercisers who were randomized to a moderate-intensity resistance training program; those training at high intensity had the greatest decrements in affect, and those training at low intensity experienced no beneficial changes in affect (Etnier et al. 2005).

Mood was monitored before and after each exercise class over a 7-week exercise program in four self-selected exercise groups (Steinberg et al. 1998). Positive mood increased and negative mood decreased during each class, but favorable mood from exercise diminished by the following week. There seemed to be a persistent, acute effect that has also been demonstrated with some of the positive physiological effects of exercise.

PSYCHOPHYSIOLOGICAL AND BEHAVIORAL ASSESSMENT

The evidence from animal research on neurological contributions to appetitive and avoidance behaviors suggests that it is possible to detect emotion in humans with psychophysiological techniques (see figure 5.14). Autonomic activation can be measured with **galvanic skin response** (skin conductance or its inverse, resistance), changes in skin temperature, and cardiovascular responsiveness (see chapter 4). Determining the galvanic skin response involves measuring the autonomic-induced changes in the electrical resistance of the tissue path between two electrodes applied to the skin. Emotional arousal has been associated with these changes; skin conductance has been shown to increase with negative emotions and decrease with positive emotions (e.g., Hughes, Uhlmann, and Pennebaker 1994). Changes in skin temperature indicate reflex vasoconstriction and vasodilation from the sympathetic activation of the vasculature associated with the stress response. Changes in heart rate and blood pressure in the absence of motor activation are also associated with the stress response and concomitant affect. Limitations of these methods include the lack of specificity to particular emotions. For example, heart rate and blood pressure increase both during the stress of reading a letter from the Internal Revenue Service announcing an audit of your tax returns and while reading a letter from a television producer inviting you to be a contestant on a game show. The physiological responses per se do not indicate the different emotional responses to these situations. There are also concerns regarding the consistent application of recommended psychophysiological measurement protocols to assess autonomic activation (Smith and Crabbe 2000).

> **P**ositive changes in mood after exercise training have been found in many but not all sample populations.

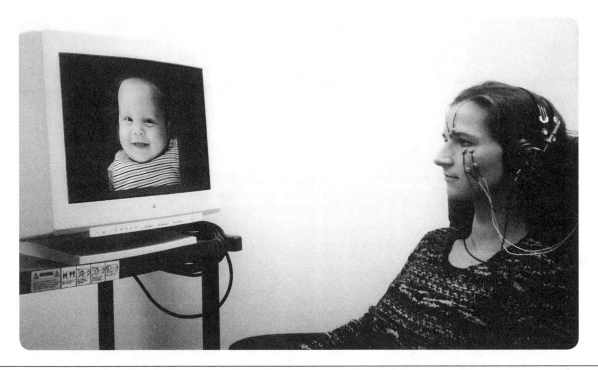

Figure 5.14 Use of emotionally evocative images to elicit the acoustic startle eye-blink response.
Provided by Center for the Study of Emotion and Attention, the University of Florida.

The contraction of muscles involves muscle fiber–generated electrical potentials that can be detected with needle electrodes placed in a muscle or patch electrodes placed on the skin superior to the muscle of interest. Electromyographic measures of distinctive facial muscle activation have been associated with various emotional responses (Cacioppo et al. 1986). For example, zygomatic (smile) muscle activity and corrugator (frown) muscle activity differentiate pleasant and unpleasant emotions (Greenwald, Cook, and Lang 1989). Ekman and colleagues have done considerable work to document facial expressions as a behavioral component of emotions, and it appears that the associations between specific emotions and facial expressions are similar across cultures (Ekman 1989). Ekman and Friesen (1976) developed the Facial Action Coding System (FACS), in which 44 distinct, visually observable facial muscle actions are scored for the duration and frequency of activity in response to emotional stimuli. The original FACS and the updated FACS computer image analysis software have measured facial expressions that have been shown to reliably reflect subjectively felt emotion (Bartlett et al. 1999; Ekman, Davidson, and Friesen 1990).

Methods Used in Exercise Studies

Exercise studies have mainly examined tonic (i.e., unperturbed) or reactive (i.e., in response to a stimulus) neuromuscular activity, including the ASER, skeletal and facial muscle activity, and brain electrocortical activity. The methods used in clinical neurophysiology for measuring biopotentials as emotional probes were described in chapter 3. Commonly measured biopotentials are illustrated in figure 5.15. Their applications to the study of emotions after exercise are described in the following sections along with examples of related research.

Electromyography

The effects of physical exertion, which increases metabolic arousal, on the ASER has not been studied much, but there is reason to think that exertion might directly affect brain biochemistry in a way that could alter the startle response. Although different neurotransmitters have different effects on the startle response depending on the brain region (Davis 1997; Davis et al. 1993), norepinephrine and serotonin generally inhibit

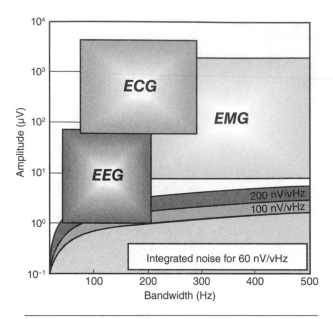

Figure 5.15 Biopotentials in clinical neurophysiology.

startle. Agonists of dopamine D_2 receptors also attenuate the startle response, whereas the augmentation of the startle by a D_1 agonist is partly dependent on the coactivation of D_2 receptors (Meloni and Davis 1999).

Regional effects have not been determined, but studies of rats have shown that brain concentrations of norepinephrine, serotonin, and dopamine (DA) are elevated during running on a treadmill or activity wheel. Treadmill running also increases the turnover of DA (i.e., replacement of used DA with newly synthesized DA) and increases the number of D_2 receptors in the striatum. Chronic activity-wheel running has been reported to increase dopamine levels and decrease D_2 binding in the whole brain (see Tieman et al. 2001 for a review). Thus, in addition to the increase in metabolic arousal during physical exertion, exercise could alter dynamic features of brain biochemistry in ways that plausibly could affect either the reflexive (obligatory) or emotional (modulatory) components of ASER neurocircuitry. Other neurotransmitters (e.g., GABA) corticotropin-releasing factor, and cholecystokinin can alter the startle response depending on their presence in different brain regions (Davis 1997), so the nature of brain responses by those neurotransmitters after exercise needs to be studied.

To date, only three studies have addressed the effects of acute exercise on the ASER. Changes in ASER amplitude and latency were examined in 26 healthy young men after 20 min of cycling at light and hard intensities (40% and 75% $\dot{V}O_2$peak) and after 20 min of quiet rest (Tieman et al. 2001). Neither intensity of exercise affected ASER amplitude or latency in either sedentary or active participants. These findings indicate that we should not expect possible effects of acute exercise on potentiated startle (or startle responses elicited by positive or negative foreground stimuli) to be confounded by an altered baseline ASER when measured in young healthy men having average physical fitness, regardless of their physical activity habits.

Despite that absence of an effect of exercise in healthy young men, it is possible that basal startle responses might be affected among people having disorders that involve altered neurological responses (e.g., anxiety disorders, attention-deficit/hyperactivity disorder [ADHD]). For example, research suggests that brain dopamine systems are disturbed in children who have ADHD. Regional cerebral blood flow studies indicate that children with ADHD have hypoperfusion to the caudate in the striatum, which is largely dopaminergic; and methylphenidate (i.e., Ritalin), the drug of choice for treating ADHD, is a dopamine agonist (Barkley 1998).

The effects of maximal and submaximal treadmill walking (65% to 75% $\dot{V}O_2$peak) on the ASER were studied in 18 boys and girls diagnosed with ADHD and 25 control children equated on several key variables that might affect the startle response (Tantillo et al. 2002).

The main findings were decreased latency of ASER and increased spontaneous eye blinks in boys with ADHD after maximal exercise, and decreased latency of ASER after the submaximal exercise condition in the girls with ADHD. Eye blinks by children without a diagnosis of ADHD were not affected by exercise. The third study (Smith et al. 2002) used the ASER to examine whether exercise alters emotional response.

Measurement of Emotion

Very few studies have examined the effect of sustained exercise (i.e., more than a minute) on emotion. Fillingim, Roth, and Cook (1992) found that self-reports of, and corrugator EMG responses to, sadness and anger imagery were not different 8 min after 15 min of very low-intensity cycle ergometry (50 W) compared to 15 min of rest. However, these researchers used emotional recall (i.e., internally generated imagery), making it difficult to confirm whether an emotion was actually elicited (see emotion research desiderata in Davidson et al. 1990). Also, they did not consider precondition responses in their analyses, nor did they quantify the exercise stimulus relative to an individual's maximal capacity.

In what appears to be the first exercise study to examine emotional responses after exercise according to a contemporary theory of emotion (Lang 1995), the influence of low- and moderate-intensity exercise on self-rated anxiety, ASER amplitude and corrugator muscle activity, and state anxiety was examined in 24 healthy college females who either cycled at low or moderate intensities or rested quietly for 25 min (Smith et al. 2002). Acoustic startle eye-blink and corrugator responses, as well as basal, tonic corrugator EMG activity, were measured immediately before and 20 min after each condition while participants viewed pleasant, neutral, and unpleasant slides. State anxiety was significantly reduced 20 min after each condition, as was startle amplitude to each type of slide. Baseline corrugator EMG activity did not change after seated rest, but decreased after cycling in direct proportion to exercise intensity. The decreases in startle amplitude were correlated with decreases in state anxiety ($r = .44$). Corrugator EMG responses during the slides were not different between or after the conditions. The findings suggest that anxiolytic conditions of low- and moderate-intensity cycling and seated rest are related to decreased startle amplitude but do not lead to changes in appetitive or defensive responses to affective stimuli.

The possible interaction of innate or learned startle reflexes with other spinal reflexes (e.g., myotendinous responses) that are influenced by arousal and emotional stimuli (e.g., Bonnet et al. 1995) might also be interesting. In a series of studies by deVries (deVries et al. 1981; deVries et al. 1982) and others (Bulbulian and Darabos 1986), the spinal H-reflex was reduced after exercise. The H-reflex is a monosynaptic reflex at the level of the S1–S2 sacral spinal roots elicited by electrical stimulation of the mixed tibial nerve at the popliteal space behind the knee and measured by EMG calf twitch (see figures 5.16 and 5.17). Although the H-reflex is mainly viewed as an index of the excitability of the alpha motor neuron, ascending and descending supraspinal tracts exist that would permit it to be modulated by the central nervous system.

Electroencephalography

Several exercise studies have examined EEG-measured brain asymmetry in activation based on reported emotions (e.g., Petruzzello and Tate 1997), but not on stimulus-elicited emotional responses during or after exercise. The subjective appraisal of affective valence has been associated with the frontal region, and the level of arousal has been detected in EEG changes in the parietotemporal area (Smith and Crabbe 2000).

Although the effect of physical activity on mood has been examined extensively, little is known about the effect of altered mood on emotional responsiveness (Ekman 1994) or about whether exercise might modulate such an effect (Smith and Crabbe 2000). Frontal cortical asymmetry, as indexed by EEG, has been shown to be a correlate of emotional responsiveness (Davidson 1998b), possibly more so for motivational engagement (approach versus withdrawal) than for affective valence (Carver and Harmon-Jones 2009a).

There also is evidence that frontal EEG asymmetry may be related to phasic shifts in mood. Petruzzello and colleagues (Petruzzello and Landers 1994; Petruzzello and Tate 1997) showed that resting levels of frontal asymmetry were moderately associated with pre- to postexercise changes in moods such as anxiety and energetic arousal. Their 1994 study also showed that changes in anxiety were related to changes in asymmetry from before to after exercise. It is not known to what extent emotional responsiveness may be altered by phasic mood shifts. Mood is improved after exercise, but emotional responsiveness after exercise has received little attention.

A study of young men and women having moderate levels of cardiorespiratory fitness looked at the effect of 30 min of cycling exercise at 50% peak aerobic power, compared to 30 min

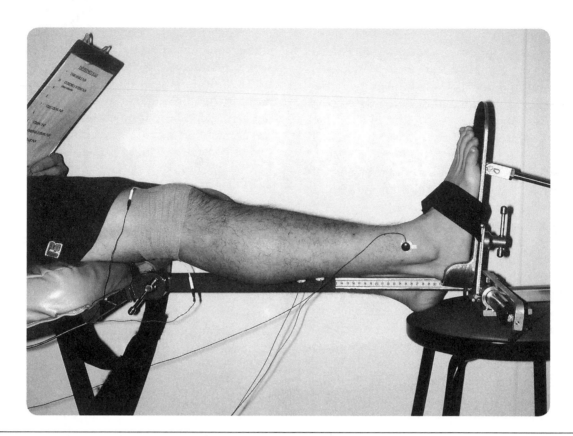

Figure 5.16 Electrode placement for the measurement of the H-reflex in the soleus muscle using electromyography.

Provided by the Exercise Psychology Laboratory, Department of Kinesiology, the University of Georgia.

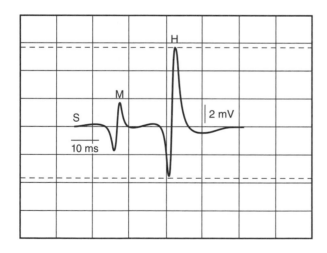

Figure 5.17 An oscillographic record of the H-reflex measured by electromyography.

Provided by the Exercise Psychology Laboratory, Department of Kinesiology, the University of Georgia.

of rest, on changes in emotional responses to standardized slides having negative, neutral, and positive valence (Crabbe, Smith, and Dishman 2007). Emotional responses were measured by

frontal brain electrocortical asymmetry and self-ratings of valence and arousal using a bipolar rating scale called the Self-Assessment Manikin (SAM), shown in figure 5.18.

Consistent with theory (Davidson 2000), frontal brain asymmetry in the α (8-12 Hz) frequency and valence ratings in response to slides were predicted by α asymmetry at rest. However, despite a decrease in state anxiety, the cycling exercise condition did not alter emotional responses or positive and negative affect in response to negative, neutral, and positive slides. Also, although arousal ratings were elevated during exercise, negative or positive affect as measured by the PANAS was not altered by exercise. Hence, the findings did not indicate that moderate-intensity cycling exercise is an emotion-eliciting stimulus or that it affects emotional response by altering mood. Also, the cumulative evidence indicates that EEG activity during or after exercise increases in all frequency bands, not just α, and at all the measured sites, not just frontal or anterior sites,

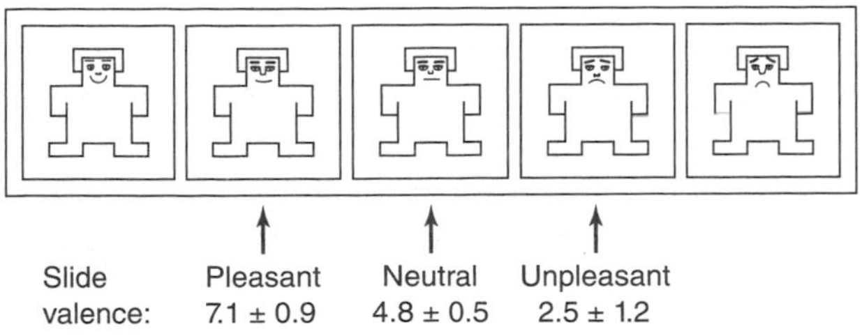

| Slide valence: | Pleasant 7.1 ± 0.9 | Neutral 4.8 ± 0.5 | Unpleasant 2.5 ± 1.2 |

Figure 5.18 Self-Assessment Manikin pleasantness ratings.

Adapted, by permission, from P.J. Lang, M.M. Bradley, and B.N. Cuthbert, 1999, *International affective pictures system (IAPSI): Instruction manual and affective ratings,* Technical Report A-4, (The Center for Research in Psychophysiology, University of Florida). Copyright © Dr. Peter J. Lang.

regardless of hemisphere (Crabbe and Dishman 2004). However, the studies were limited to just a few recording sites and did not use dense-array electrode mapping, as described in chapter 3. Nonetheless, the evidence suggests that acute exercise increases EEG activity in a general way consistent with increased arousal, possibly as a result of increased sensory and cardiovascular neural traffic to the thalamus processed through the brain stem.

Electroencephalography measures relatively few neurons that are superficial. Surface activation does not ensure that underlying brain regions are correspondingly activated. The brain imaging techniques discussed in chapter 3 have enabled researchers to estimate the rate of cellular metabolism in subcortical areas of the brain (e.g., amygdala) during the experience of various emotions; these techniques hold great promise for exploring the relationship between exercise and affect (Irwin et al. 1996; LaBar et al. 1998). To date, neuroimaging studies of affective or emotional responses to acute exercise, or after exercise training, have not been reported. However, at least two studies have correlated EEG responses with feelings of vigor or fatigue after exercise ended (see chapter 9, Energy and Fatigue).

In a recent study of female college students without complaints of energy or fatigue problems, Woo and colleagues (2009) reported that elevated feelings of vigor after 30 min of moderately intense treadmill running was partly explained be EEG activity in δ, θ, and α frequency bands measured at a right, but not left, anterior sensor location. However, only the reduction in

θ activity at the left anterior site was changed by exercise. In a randomized trial of college students who complained of persistent fatigue (Dishman et al. 2010a), posterior θ activity accounted for half the increase in feelings of vigor that college students reported after each of three 20 min sessions of either low- or moderate-intensity exercise during weeks 1, 3, and 6 of training.

More than 20 published experimental and quasi-experimental studies on the effects of acute exercise on mood found that a session of exercise is accompanied by a moderate reduction in state anger. None of those studies was designed for the purpose of evaluating anger outcomes of acute exercise. Most studies involved participants having low levels of trait anger or state anger before exercise, or they did not report trait anger. It is likely that reductions in anger after exercise would be more pronounced after evoking anger, or in high trait-anger individuals, as is the case with anxiety (Motl, O'Connor, and Dishman 2004; O Connor, Raglin, and Martinsen 2000). Also, many of the studies used the Profile of Mood States (POMS) to measure anger. The POMS was designed to measure the intensity of overt anger or hostility (McNair, Lorr, and Droppleman 1981) and does not differentiate between the experience and expression of anger. By contrast, the State Trait Anger Expression Inventory-2 (STAXI-2) was designed to separate anger from hostility and aggression as well as measure the experience and expression of anger. Furthermore, most of the studies evaluated did not attempt to manipulate anger, which precludes causal inferences about reductions in anger after exercise.

Limitations in Research

Acute studies of the effects of exercise on affect share problems with research on emotions and mood in general, such as validity and the appropriateness of measurement methods as well as the possibility of unknown but critical moderating and confounding variables. Unfortunately, most research done in the laboratory to study the effects of a single bout of exercise on mood has limited generalizability (poor **ecological validity**). Although many people choose to exercise in closed environments much like those in laboratories (e.g., walking or running on a treadmill or cycling on a stationary machine), many studies conducted in natural physical activity settings have shown a positive influence on mood.

It is also hard to blind participants to the purpose of the study when they are asked to complete mood questionnaires before and after an exercise bout. Additionally, there has been a failure to standardize the exercise stimulus, which, considering the potential unpleasantness associated with exercising at high intensities (e.g., well above the lactate or ventilatory thresholds), can confound effects on mood. Many studies have not used nonexercise control conditions. The variability in psychophysiological responses between people and within one person over time makes it difficult to gauge the direction and magnitude of change. For example, the use of baseline values for comparison is confounded by the transient nature of feelings, emotions, and mood. The laboratory situation itself could elevate the affect scores at baseline and exaggerate the decrease after acute exercise. On the other hand, research with people without clinical disorders may show no effect from exercise because of ceiling and floor effects (i.e., the range of scores possible on the test doesn't match the full range of the affective experience of the person), or as a consequence of the use of mood instruments designed for clinical populations that may not be sensitive enough to detect changes in people without clinical disorders.

Training studies have been limited by the use of convenience samples, a deficiency in follow-up data, and a lack of replication of findings. Comparisons between exercise and other treatment conditions are often tentative because the conditions have not been equal in terms of exposure so that effects from the amount of attention can be ruled out, and groups have not been randomized. Initial fitness level or physical activity history has often not been considered, and methodologies for measuring fitness and exercise history have been weak. Researchers have analyzed absolute changes before and after acute and chronic exercise without considering the effects of baseline levels or patterns over time on responses (e.g., Gauvin, Rejeski, and Reboussin 2000). Despite these scientific weaknesses, the bulk of the evidence supports the idea that physical activity and exercise have a positive influence on mood for most people in many circumstances.

Sedentary or untrained people can perceive prolonged or short, high-intensity exercise as aversive (Weisser, Kinsman, and Stamper 1973) or less pleasant than lower-intensity exercise (Ekkekakis, Hall, and Petruzzello 2008; Ekkekakis and Petruzzello 2002; Hall, Ekkekakis, and Petruzzello 2002), and frequently frown as perceived exertion increases during intense lifting or cycling exercise (de Morree and Marcora 2010, 2011). However, most people say they feel better after exercise (Morgan 1973, 1985). Of course, for some that might just be because it's over. As Bill Morgan has quipped, "Exercise can be like hitting your thumb with a hammer; it feels good when you stop."

Whether the exercises that people typically do for health or fitness elicit an affective response during the exercise hasn't been studied much. Smith and colleagues (2002) found that ratings of pleasantness by college women were elevated during moderate-intensity cycling exercise and lowered during high-intensity exercise. Very low-intensity cycling was rated as even more pleasant (Smith and O'Connor 2003). Some research shows that people rate their affective experience as more positive during low-intensity, as compared to high-intensity, cycling exercise (Bixby and Lochbaum 2006), whereas other research found that 30 min of moderate-intensity cycling (i.e., below the ventilatory or lactate thresholds) is viewed as mildly arousing but not more or less pleasant than quietly resting (Crabbe, Smith, Dishman 2007). Good feelings can increase slightly in some people and lessen slightly in others during 20 min of moderately hard exercise but remain positive nonetheless (Van Landuyt et al. 2000).

Taken together, the emerging evidence shows that most healthy, normally active young adults report feelings of moderate pleasure during the intensities of exercise typically recommended for fitness and health, even when they report high ratings of emotional arousal and mild to moderate leg muscle pain (Smith and O'Connor 2003; Smith et al. 2002). We'll revisit these subjective responses during exercise in chapter 16, Perceived Exertion.

Whether emotional responding or attention to an environmental threat or potential reward might be altered during exercise has only recently been studied. People's facial muscle reactions to emotional pictures are not altered during low-intensity cycling exercise (Smith and O'Connor 2003), but people are quicker to accurately detect both threatening and neutral, nonthreatening images while exercising at either moderate or hard intensities (Shields et al. 2011). In a study of college students with high trait anxiety, moderate cycling exercise for 30 min did not lower their negative affect or change their attention to positive scenes after the exercise ended, even though ratings of positive affect were increased (Barnes et al. 2010). In contrast, college students' attention to pleasant-looking faces was increased and attention to unpleasant faces was decreased while they cycled for about 10 min at a moderate intensity, but not a hard intensity (Tian and Smith 2011).

Collectively, findings show that people's attention to external stimuli is enhanced during exercise, which is contrary to the hypothesis that emotional circuits are inhibited during exercise (Dietrich and Audiffren 2011). However, it is not yet known the extent to which typical exercises, and their settings, selectively activate the brain circuits dedicated to motor control, body awareness, and vigilance for threats or rewards in ways that affect emotions or mood either during or after exercise.

MECHANISMS

Berger and Motl have proposed that to optimize mood enhancement after physical activity, the activity should be enjoyable, aerobic, and noncompetitive and should be performed regularly in a closed environment that is predictable in place and time, at moderate intensities for at least 20 min (Berger and Motl 2000). However, very few studies of humans have manipulated social, psychological, or biological factors to determine mechanisms that might explain the mood-altering effects of physical activity or exercise. Most of the human studies, as well as those conducted on nonhuman animals to test plausible mechanisms, have been directed toward understanding the effects on the specific moods of anxiety and depression. Those moods and mechanisms are discussed in detail in chapters 6 and 7, but they are introduced here.

Biological

The **thermogenic hypothesis** proposes that increased body temperature is responsible for positive changes in mood with exercise, but the effects are mixed, and there is little support for this as a valid mechanism (e.g., Koltyn 1997; Koltyn et al. 1992; Koltyn and Morgan 1997; Youngstedt et al. 1993).

Brain blood flow is increased by various stressors, but the effects of exercise seem mainly limited to regions involved with motor, sensory, and cardiovascular regulation, rather than emotional responses (Nybo and Secher 2004; Secher, Seifert, and Van Lieshout 2008). Although both acute and chronic exercise has influenced blood flow in the anterior cingulate and insular cortexes (areas that are involved with emotional processing and cardiovascular control) (Colcombe et al. 2004; Williamson, McColl, and Mathews 2003), it remains to be determined whether such responses to exercise reflect emotional responding to exercise or sensory and cardiovascular responses to increased arousal.

The **transient hypofrontality hypothesis** speculates that during submaximal exercise, neural activity is down-regulated in the brain areas not directly involved in motor control, such as the prefrontal cortex (Dietrich 2003). According to Dietrich, "Studies on cerebral blood flow and metabolism have provided the strongest support for the hypothesis that exercise decreases neural activity in the prefrontal cortex" (Dietrich 2006, 81). However, the results of a recent systematic review and meta-analysis of studies of exercise on brain hemodynamics measured by near-infrared spectroscopy (NIRS) (see chapter 3) are inconsistent with that interpretation (Rooks et al. 2010). The pattern of cerebral oxygenation, deoxygenation, and blood volume in the studies reviewed suggested responses opposite to the transient hypofrontality hypothesis. Figure 5.19 shows that only during highly intense, exhaustive exercise were cerebral oxygen values lowered. In contrast, moderate-to-hard submaximal exercise was

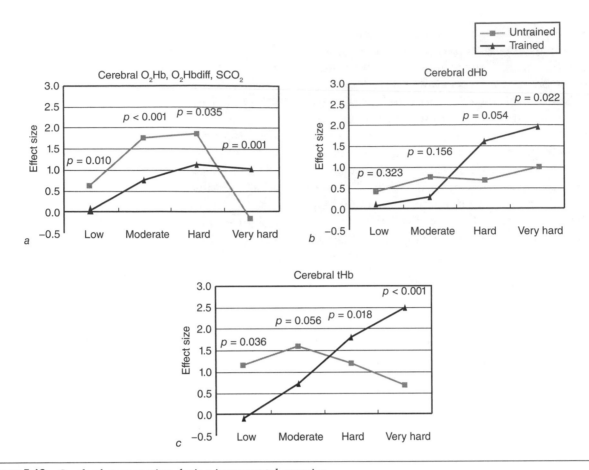

Figure 5.19 Cerebral oxygenation during incremental exercise.

Reprinted *Progress in Neurobiology,* Vol. 92(2), C.R. Rooks, N.J. Thom, K.K. McCully, and R.K. Dishman, "Effects of incremental exercise on cerebral oxygenation measured by near-infrared spectroscopy: a systematic review," pgs.134-50, copyright 2010, with permission from Elsevier.

accompanied by increases in cerebral oxygen and blood volume (Rooks et al. 2010).

The **endorphin hypothesis** continues to percolate through the lay population. Because plasma endorphins, which are natural opioids, increase with exercise, they are thought of as the "cause" of the enhanced mood and euphoria accompanying exercise. However, there has been little success in finding associations between mood changes and levels of endorphins in well-controlled empirical studies (e.g., Hatfield et al. 1987; see Other Biologically Based Hypotheses in chapter 7).

The popular hypothesis that endorphins are responsible for changes in mood or anxiety after exercise remains plausible, but it has been perpetuated without much consideration of available evidence. Plasma β-endorphin is elevated after release from the pituitary gland during intense exercise (Boecker et al. 2010; Goldfarb and Jamurtas, 1997). A plausible link between peripheral β-endorphin or enkephalins and mood or analgesic responses to acute exercise has not been established. The bulk of the research has shown that opioid antagonists do not block mood changes after exercise. The ability of increased β-endorphin in the blood to have an influence on the brain is blocked by the blood–brain barrier to peptides at the body temperatures characteristic of typical exercise.

There is no consensus on brain changes in opioid activity after exercise. Although opioid-mediated analgesia could indirectly influence mood, exercise-induced analgesia has not yet been shown to explain improved mood in humans (Cook and Koltyn 2000). Peripheral opioid responses to acute exercise apparently inhibit catecholamine influences on cardiovascular, respiratory, and endocrine responses during exercise, but their direct influence on mood is implausible based on current evidence. Notwithstanding the limitations of past evidence, a recent uncontrolled study reported a correlation between self-reports of euphoria and brain opioid binding measured by positron emission tomography in 10 experienced distance runners (Boecker et al. 2008). This is the first and only evidence that brain opioids are influenced by exercise in humans in a way that may help explain mood changes associated with running, if confirmed by experimental studies. As for the peripheral opioids, caution is advised when interpreting new discoveries of blood-borne responses to exercise (Sparling et al. 2003; Szabo, Billett, and Turner 2001; White and Castellano 2008a) as surrogate measures of the brain or as putative explanations for mental outcomes of physical activity (Morgan and O'Connor 1988).

Brain Dopamine and Opioids

The modulation of brain opioid systems by the mesolimbic dopamine system has recently been reviewed (Dishman and Holmes 2012). The hedonic allostasis theory (Koob and Le Moal 1997) conceptualizes addictive behaviors as a response to hypoactivity in dopamine systems. This hypodopaminergic state is purported to induce compensatory behavioral activation (e.g., drug seeking, sensation seeking, compulsive exercise) as a means to restore normal hedonic tone. In contrast, the incentive salience hypothesis emphasizes the importance of dopamine in the "wanting" that is triggered by reward-related conditioned stimuli. According to this model, the "liking," or pleasure, associated with reward involves the activation of other systems parallel to or downstream of the mesolimbic dopamine pathways. These other, hedonic-based systems involve GABA and opioid peptides in distinct yet integrated pathways within the ventral striatum and striatal-pallidal circuits, among others (Smith and Berridge 2007).

In the incentive salience model, dopamine is the driver of the behavioral activation that ultimately leads to the outcomes that induce pleasure. Dopamine thus mediates the motivation that triggers the relevant behaviors, such as drug seeking, sensation seeking, and exercise. These two models make opposite predictions about the roles of dopamine and opioid peptides

in the motivation to exercise and the pleasure, or "high," that may be derived from this activity. The anhedonia model predicts that dysphoria, presumably mediated by deficits in dopamine transmission, drives the need to reexperience the euphoria that is a consequence of the relevant behavior. Thus, in some people the desire to exercise would be linked to low baseline dopaminergic tone, and engaging in exercise might restore dopaminergic transmission to the levels necessary for achieving euphoria.

In this model, compulsive exercise, or "addiction" to exercise, would depend on normalizing a dysphoric state caused by low dopaminergic (and presumably also opioid) tone. (See figure 5.20.)

Alternatively, the incentive salience model predicts that higher dopaminergic transmission drives appetitively motivated behaviors such as exercise because the mesolimbic dopamine system has this adaptive role, within the neural system, to increase attention to environmental cues associated with enhanced survival, adjust motivational levels, and execute the appropriate approach or avoidance behaviors. Whether this coordinated activation leads to a subjective

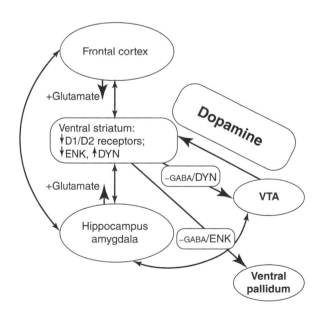

Figure 5.20 Hypothetical model of dopamine modulation of opioids in the brain.

Reprinted, by permission, from R.K. Dishman and P.V. Holmes, 2012, Opioids and exercise: Animal models. In *Functional neuroimaging in exercise and sport sciences,* edited by H. Boecker et al. (New York: Springer), 51. With kind permission of Springer Science and Business Media.

experience in humans related to pleasure or dysphoria may depend on the constellation of cues predicting the outcome that was learned to be associated with that event (whether it is running toward a potential mate or running away from a potential predator). In either case, the primary cognitive state is motivation (i.e., craving, desire, impulse), the related behavioral state is activation, and dopamine mediates both of these functions. In the example of behavioral activation that leads to positive outcomes, such as feeding or mating, the consummatory cues, such as ingesting or copulating, may trigger the GABAergic or opioid hedonic circuits (or both) (Smith and Berridge 2007). In the case of fleeing from or fighting off an enemy, the activation of the hedonic opioid circuits may depend on cues that signal successful escape or avoidance of the threat (Dishman and Holmes 2012).

No single neurotransmitter or neuromodulator system will solely explain human mood, which depends on complex interactions of many neural circuits that are regulated by many excitatory and inhibitory neurotransmitters (e.g., acetylcholine, GABA, and glutamate); neuromodulators (e.g., dopamine, norepinephrine, and serotonin); neurotrophic factors (e.g., brain derived neurotrophic factor [BDNF] and nerve growth factor [NGF]); neuropeptides besides opioids such as β-endorphin, enkephalin, and dynorphin (e.g., cholecystokinin, corticotrophin releasing factor [CRF], galanin, neuropeptide Y [NPY], and VGF); membrane lipids (e.g., endocannabinoids); gases (e.g., nitric oxide); and intracellular signaling

that controls gene transcription and translation, as well as the posttranslational regulation of neurons. Drugs such as opiates, amphetamines, benzodiazepines, and tetrahydrocannabinol have strong, direct effects on mood. However, equally strong effects by endogenous systems during exercise that mimic those drug effects would not be biologically adaptive in most cases. Why and how physical exertion alters brain neural systems in mentally healthy and unhealthy ways among most people, or in special populations, remain key questions (Dishman and O'Connor 2009).

Psychosocial

Although more support exists for psychosocial explanations of mood enhancement from exercise, the effects are likely generated by an interaction among physiological and psychological influences on mood that are altered with exercise.

According to the **mastery hypothesis**, mood is improved after completing an important and effortful task. Self-efficacy may interact to influence the effects of exercise on mood such that higher efficacy is associated with more positive effects on mood, as found in the study by Bozoian, Rejeski, and McAuley (1994).

The **distraction hypothesis** proposes that the time out from worrisome thoughts and daily stressors during exercise produces the mood-enhancing effects. The increasing trend of multitasking, in which people negotiate business

---

Psychological Benefits From Exercise That May Be Related to Enhanced Mood

- Improved emotional stability, self-sufficiency, and conscientiousness from intense, persistent involvement in meaningful activity
- Heightened sense of well-being, euphoric high, enhanced sense of self, greater appreciation of the surrounding world

- Decreased awareness of feelings of fear, tension, irritability
- Distraction from worry and dejection
- A countering effect on inertia, fatigue, depression, and confusion

Adapted from Casper 1993.

transactions and organize reports on treadmills and stair climbers, may counter the psychological benefits of exercise if distraction is the primary mechanism for effects. In fact, increases in vigor measured by the POMS were correlated with the tendency to engage in nonassociative thought in 150 experienced runners who completed the POMS before and after a typical run (Goode and Roth 1993). Thoughts about interpersonal relationships as measured by the Thoughts During Exercise Scale were also associated with decreases in tension and anxiety.

HAZARDS OF EXERCISE?

This chapter has focused on positive affect and mood enhancement with exercise. An exception to the benefits of physical activity is the risk of disturbed mood sometimes seen among highly trained endurance athletes who have become stale as a result of overtraining (i.e., exceeding a physical and psychological optimal volume and intensity over time) (Morgan et al. 1987). Staleness is a syndrome typically characterized by increased tension and depression, chronic fatigue, appetite loss, insomnia, decreased libido, decreased functional capacity or performance, and endocrine abnormalities and the suppression of the immune system (Dishman 1992).

Excessive exercise that is problematic has also been observed in nonathletes (Morgan 1979b). *Compulsive exercise, compulsive athleticism,* and *exercise dependence* are some of the terms that have been used in connection with an exercise routine that takes on greater priority than work, family, friends, and social functions. The person continues exercise despite serious injury and experiences symptoms of withdrawal, such as mood disturbances, anxiety, guilt, and depression when prevented from exercising (Mondin et al. 1996; Cockerill and Riddington 1996).

Some studies have indicated that the rate of staleness among nonelite runners and age-group swimmers is about 33% (Raglin and Moger 1999; Raglin and Wilson 2000). However, no epidemiological studies have been done to identify the prevalence or risk factors associated with athletic staleness or abusive exercise in the population. At this time, it appears that each represents a clinical medicine problem among select groups of athletes and fitness fanatics, but neither seems to be a problem for public health. As will be seen in the last part of the book, very few adults in developed nations are physically active at a level that would put them at risk for overtraining or exercise abuse. This topic is addressed in more detail in the section Exercise Abuse in chapter 12 as it pertains to problems of emotional adjustment and an imbalanced self-concept.

SUMMARY

Affect is typically measured with self-report via paper-and-pencil instruments, but other ways to measure feeling states, affect, mood, and emotions include techniques that measure physiological indicators (such as skin conductance, EMG, EEG, and neuroimaging) and behavioral indicators, such as facial expressions. Up to now, the research evidence, although not all scientifically strong, supports the folk wisdom passed down from antiquity that exercise enhances mood. Social, cognitive, and biological explanations for that observation have not yet been identified, but attributing the positive effects of exercise on mood merely to people's self-fulfilling expectations of benefits appears inadequate. Very few studies of physical activity and exercise have examined mood or emotion within a contemporary theory of affect. Also, studies have yet to show that acute exercise of the type commonly practiced for leisure or fitness alters emotional responses. Especially interesting is the question of whether a reduction in neuromuscular tension after exercise, as reported in a few studies, may play a role in the direct effects of exercise on mood or emotional response.

The reasons many people decide to adopt exercise include weight loss and health benefits. Adoption involves considerable time and effort in the short run, and noticeable results do not occur for a long time. Short-term rewards of mood regulation may prove to be more significant in helping people sustain regular exercise. Exercise motivational inventories have included mood as a factor, and mood continues to be conceptually meaningful as a reason people exercise. Positive mood effects from exercise may be subtle, however, and may not readily surface among novices. Mood enhancement from exercise is hypothesized to be more of a motivator for those who have exercised in the past (Hsiao and Thayer 1998). The influence of intrapersonal factors on exercise adoption and maintenance is covered in chapters 13 and 15.

WEBSITES

www.deakin.edu.au/health/psychology/gagepage/
   pgstory.htm

www.personalityresearch.org/basicemotions.html

chapter

6

Anxiety

Many people who exercise during their leisure time have noticed a calming effect from a hard workout, reporting that they use exercise to "forget worries" or as an outlet for "nervous energy." Others say they feel more relaxed after moderate physical activity such as a brisk walk. The research literature supports the ability of exercise to reduce anxiety in nonclinical populations. Recent study suggests that clinical populations also benefit, although there was a time when exercise was believed to *induce* anxiety in patients who have panic disorder. This chapter provides statistics on the social and financial impact of anxiety and gives definitions of anxiety and anxiety disorders. It presents research connections between anxiety and exercise, including a discussion of the mechanisms for beneficial effects.

PREVALENCE AND SOCIAL IMPACT

About 18% of adults aged 18 years or older in the United States—about 23 million people—experience anxiety disorders each year (Kessler et al. 2005b), and 29% will have some type of anxiety disorder during their lifetimes (Kessler et al. 2005a). In fact, anxiety disorders are more prevalent than all other types of mental disorders except substance abuse. Compared to men, women are more likely to have experienced an anxiety disorder in their lifetimes. Women's lifetime odds (about 30%) are 60% higher than men's odds (about 20%) for any anxiety disorder (Kessler et al. 2005c). The prevalence of various anxiety disorders over 12 months and over a lifetime are compared for males and females in figure 6.1.

Young-to-middle-aged people tend to have more anxiety than do older people. Figure 6.2 shows that the prevalence of all anxiety disorders increases with age until age 60. Nonetheless, people 15 to 24 years old experience episodes of anxiety about 40% more often than do people 25 to 54 years old, regardless of race. Data on 5,424 Hispanics, non-Hispanic blacks, and non-Hispanic whites from the National Comorbidity Survey Replication (Breslau et al. 2006) found that both minority groups had lower risk for generalized anxiety disorder and social phobia. Non-Hispanic blacks had lower risk for panic disorder. Lower risk among minorities was more pronounced at lower levels of education (see figure 6.2).

Social phobia is the most common anxiety disorder, with reported prevalence rates of up to 18.7%. The onset of social phobia typically occurs in childhood or adolescence, and the clinical course, if left untreated, is usually chronic, unremitting, and associated with significant functional impairment. Social phobia exhibits a high degree of comorbidity with other psychiatric disorders, including mood disorders, anxiety disorders, and substance abuse or dependence. Few people with social phobia seek professional help despite the existence of beneficial treatment approaches (Van Ameringen et al. 2003)

One of the most commonly encountered anxiety disorders in the primary care setting, panic disorder is a chronic and debilitating illness. Patients with panic disorder have medically unexplained symptoms that lead to the overuse of health care services (Pollack et al. 2003). Panic disorder is often comorbid with agoraphobia and major depression, and patients may be at increased risk of cardiovascular disease and, possibly, suicide.

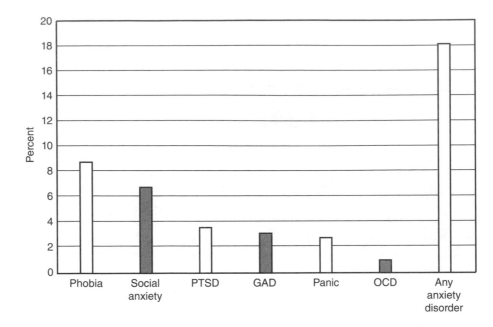

a

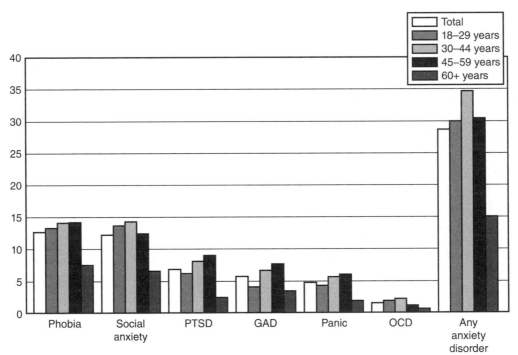

b

Figure 6.1 *(a)* Twelve-month prevalence of anxiety disorders in U.S. adults. *(b)* Lifetime prevalence estimates of anxiety disorders in U.S. adults according to age.

Based on Kessler et al. 2005.

Generalized anxiety disorder (GAD; defined later) is a common disorder with a lifetime prevalence of 4% to 7% in the general population. The onset of GAD symptoms usually occurs during the early 20s; however, high rates of GAD have also been seen in children and adolescents. The clinical course of GAD is often chronic, with 40% of patients reporting illness lasting more than five years. GAD is associated with pronounced functional impairment, resulting in decreased vocational function and reduced quality of life. Patients with GAD tend to be high users of outpatient medical care, which contributes significantly to health care costs (Allgulander et al. 2003).

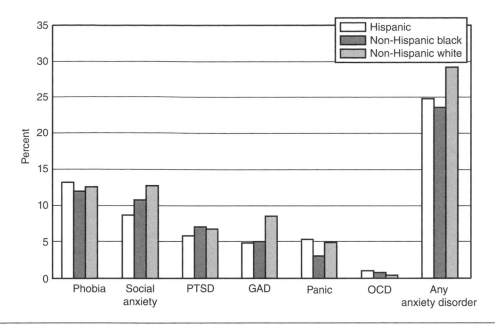

Figure 6.2 Lifetime prevalence estimates of anxiety disorders in U.S. adults according to race and ethnicity.
Data from Breslau et al. 2006.

Anxiety disorders are frequently complicated by depression, eating disorders, or substance abuse, and patients with panic disorder are also at greater risk for cardiovascular morbidity (Kessler et al. 2005b; Weissman et al. 1990). Quality of life is impaired in various ways because of anxiety, such as lost productivity at work (Greenberg et al. 1999). In addition to the personal suffering, results from the National Comorbidity Survey indicate that anxiety disorders in the United States probably cost about $85 billion each year, mainly for health care, drugs, and lost productivity (DuPont et al. 1996; Greenberg et al. 1999). Anxiety costs haven't been updated for the United States since an annual estimate of $45 to $46.6 billion in 1990, which was 31.5% of total mental health costs at that time (Greenberg et al. 1999; Rice and Miller 1998). However, anxiety costs have surely kept pace with the costs of depression. For example, in 2009, antidepressant drugs, mainly prescribed to depression and anxiety patients, were the fourth leading prescription drug class in the United States, accounting for $9.9 billion in sales (www.imshealth.com/portal/site/imshealth).

DEFINITIONS

Anxiety is a state of worry, apprehension, or tension that often occurs in the absence of real or obvious danger. Although it is a normal response to real or imagined danger, anxiety is distinguished from fear, which usually is regarded as a brief emotional reaction to a threatening stimulus. Except in the case of most phobias, anxiety is longer lasting and more abstract than is fear. Anxiety is considered a disorder when its symptoms or behaviors are so frequent or severe that they cause pain or impair normal physical or social functioning.

Anxiety is not a new problem. For example, six subtypes of anxiety are found in the writings of the ancient Greeks: death, mutilation, separation, guilt, shame, and diffuse, or nonspecific, anxiety, denoted by words such as *agitated, danger, desperate, frightened, nervous, panic, threatened, timid,* and *troubled* (Newbold 1990). A century ago, Freud noted that chronic, free-floating anxiety occurred frequently in the general population.

> **A**nxiety disorders are more prevalent than any other type of mental disorder except substance abuse.

TYPES OF COMMON ANXIETY DISORDERS

There are several types of anxiety disorders: phobias, panic disorder, obsessive-compulsive disorder, posttraumatic stress disorder, and generalized anxiety disorder. Each type has specific psychological and behavioral characteristics.

• The most common type of **anxiety disorder** comprises social and specific **phobias**. Social phobia, or social anxiety disorder, is the fear (anxiety) of being judged, criticized, and evaluated by others. People with social phobia have an overwhelming fear of scrutiny and embarrassment in social situations that causes them to avoid many potentially enjoyable and rewarding experiences. Social phobias are equally common in men and women. They may be discrete (e.g., restricted to eating in public, to public speaking, or to encounters with the opposite sex) or diffuse, involving almost all social situations outside the family. Direct eye-to-eye confrontation may be particularly stressful in some cultures. Social phobias are usually associated with low self-esteem and fear of criticism. Symptoms often involve flushing, hand tremor, nausea, or an urgent need to urinate; a person with social phobia is sometimes sure that one of these secondary symptoms of anxiety is the primary problem. Symptoms may progress to panic attacks.

• *Agoraphobia* translated from Greek means "fear of an open market place," but it refers specifically to the fear of being in situations from which escape might be difficult, or the avoidance of situations such as being alone outside of the home; traveling in a car, bus, or airplane; or being in a crowded area. People with agoraphobia commonly are afraid to leave their houses or specific rooms in their houses and confine themselves to reduce their anxiety. Simple phobia is the irrational fear and avoidance of specific things (e.g., spiders) or places (e.g., heights). Specific phobias generally do not result from exposure to a single traumatic event (i.e., being bitten by a dog or nearly drowning). These phobias are more likely to run in the family or to be learned vicariously through the observation of the experiences of others.

• **Panic disorder** involves repeated episodes of intense fear that strike without warning and without an obvious source. Physical symptoms include chest pain; heart palpitations; choking sensations or shortness of breath; dizziness; abdominal distress; feelings of unreality; and fear of dying, losing control, or going crazy. A panic attack usually lasts for minutes, during which a crescendo of fear and autonomic symptoms builds to a maximum within 10 to 15 minutes. Attacks usually lead the person to flee and subsequently avoid the situation in which the attack occurred, often producing fear of being alone or going into public places and persistent fear of another attack.

• **Obsessive-compulsive disorder** involves repeated, intrusive unwanted thoughts, impulses, or images or compulsive behaviors that seem impossible to stop, and is typified by repetitive acts or rituals to relieve anxiety. Obsessive-compulsive disorder has more of a familial origin than most other anxiety disorders.

• **Posttraumatic stress disorder** comprises anxiety and behavioral disturbances that are a delayed or prolonged response to a stressful event or situation (either brief or long lasting) that was especially threatening or catastrophic (e.g., natural disaster; combat; a serious accident; witnessing the violent death of others; or being the victim of torture, terrorism, rape, or other crime). Symptoms commonly include flashbacks or dreams of the original trauma, a state of autonomic hyperarousal with hypervigilance, an enhanced startle reaction, and insomnia. About 50% of cases of posttraumatic stress disorder improve within 6 months. For the rest, the disorder typically persists for years and can be overwhelming.

• **Generalized anxiety disorder (GAD)** is defined by recurrent or persistent excessive, uncontrollable worry about multiple concerns on more days than not for at least 6 months. As already mentioned, Freud noted that chronic, free-floating anxiety occurred frequently in the general population. Generalized anxiety disorder is accompanied by exaggerated **vigilance** and somatic symptoms of stress and anxiety, such as muscular tension. Among the anxiety disorders, GAD has the highest rate of comorbidity with

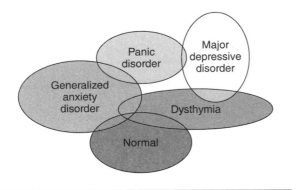

Figure 6.3 Comorbidity of generalized anxiety disorder.

Reprinted, by permission, from Medscape Mental Health (www.medscape.com/medscape/psychiatry/journal/1997/v02.n05/mh3070.woodman/mh3070.woodman.html), © 1997, Medscape Inc.

State anxiety is the immediate psychological and physiological response to a perceived threat, whereas trait anxiety is the predisposition to label events as threatening.

other disorders (see figure 6.3). The diagnostic criteria for GAD are still being refined. It is still controversial whether excessive worry is a necessary criterion (e.g., excessive worry is not required by the *International Classification of Diseases* [World Health Organization 1992]; Weisberg 2009).

Components of anxiety include cognitions, emotional responses, and physiological changes, such as increased motor tension and autonomic nervous hyperactivity. The cognitive and emotional dimensions distinguish anxiety from **arousal**, which is a nonspecific physiological response characterized by muscle tension, increased heart rate, and heightened alertness. Someone who is highly aroused is not necessarily anxious, but an anxious person typically demonstrates the physiological characteristics of arousal along with apprehensive expectations, agitation, vigilance for danger signals, and decreases in effective cognitive coping.

Anxiety is commonly described as transient or temporary (state anxiety) and as an expression of personality (trait anxiety). **State anxiety** refers to the immediate psychological and physiological response to a conscious or unconscious perceived threat (i.e., are you anxious now?). State anxiety involves subjective feelings and objective manifestations (e.g., increased heart rate). **Trait anxiety** is a personality characteristic that refers to how prone someone is to appraising events as threatening (i.e., are you an anxious person?). In general, people characterized by

high trait anxiety perceive a greater number of situations as threatening, more frequently exhibit periods of elevated state anxiety, and have a stronger anxiety reaction to a given situation than people characterized by average or low trait anxiety (Spielberger et al. 1983) (see figure 6.4). Trait anxiety is related to personality, but it is more amenable to change than is a person's core temperament, which is very resistant to change. Although anxiety is a common reaction, a distinction is usually made between normal levels of anxiety and clinical anxiety disorders based on the number and intensity of symptoms, the degree of personal suffering, and the extent to which normal function is impaired (see figure 6.5).

EFFECTS OF EXERCISE

The 1996 *U.S. Surgeon General's Report on Physical Activity and Health* (U.S. Department of Health and Human Services 1996) concluded that regular physical activity reduces feelings of anxiety. However, the scientific advisory committee for the *2008 Physical Activity Guidelines for Americans* concluded that the amount of evidence supporting that physical activity or exercise reduces symptoms in anxiety patients or protects against developing an anxiety disorder was minimal (Physical Activity Guidelines Advisory Committee 2008). Unlike the study of physical activity and depression, few population-based prospective cohort studies have examined whether regular physical activity protects against developing anxiety symptoms, and less than a handful of randomized controlled trials have tested whether an exercise program can reduce anxiety symptoms in people diagnosed with an anxiety disorder. Most studies have been experimental studies of the effects of acute

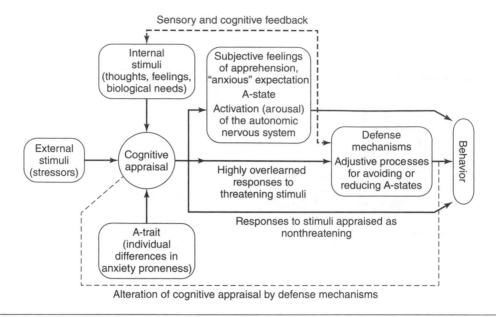

Figure 6.4 A trait-state conception of anxiety.

Reprinted, by permission, from C.D. Spielberger, 1966, Theory and research on anxiety. In *Anxiety and behavior* (New York: Academic Press), 17.

exercise on state anxiety or chronic exercise on trait anxiety among people without anxiety disorders or patients with medical conditions other than anxiety who were enrolled in randomized controlled trials of exercise mainly to improve their fitness and primary medical condition.

Bill Morgan at the University of Wisconsin surmised that this lack of research attention on the use of exercise to manage anxiety stems from medical attitudes in the late 1960s and early 1970s, when physical activity was thought to be a predicating factor in inducing panic attacks in people with anxiety neurosis and in some people without anxiety neurosis (Morgan 1979a). This negative attitude toward exercise as a potential treatment for anxiety was based on evidence from one study showing increased anxiety with infusions of lactate. Pitts and McClure (1967) measured the anxiety response to intravenous infusions of lactate, sodium DL-lactate with calcium, and a placebo (glucose) in 10 controls and 14 people with anxiety neurosis at rest. They found increased anxiety in the people with anxiety neurosis after infusion of the sodium DL-lactate that raised blood levels of lactate to about 40 mg/dl. All but one patient experienced an anxiety attack. In some cases, anxiety persisted for 2 to 5 days. Pitts and McClure also

documented anxiety reactions in some of the control subjects, and concluded that lactate could produce anxiety symptoms. Thus, it appeared that physical activity could cause anxiety symptoms because intense exercise increases muscle and blood lactate; maximal exercise typically increases blood lactate two to three times higher than does sodium DL-lactate infusion.

However, Grosz and Farmer (1972) and Morgan (1979a) presented numerous reasons infused lactate *would,* and increased lactate from exercise *would not,* induce anxiety symptoms. For example, infused lactate is quickly converted to bicarbonate and carbon dioxide, which has been shown to be associated with anxiety attacks as a function of the metabolic alkalosis and subsequent hyperventilation (Maddock, Carter, and Gietzen 1991). Exercise-induced elevations in lactate result in metabolic acidosis. Empirical evidence from 15 studies conducted since 1987 also refutes the association between exercise and panic attacks; only five panic attacks were reported during exercise involving 444 exercise bouts performed by 420 panic disorder patients (O'Connor, Smith, and Morgan 2000). Research has also shown that just one of 35 panic patients had a panic attack during supramaximal treadmill testing that elicited blood lactate levels (8 to 14 mmol/L) that were much higher than

Social Phobias

All of the following criteria should be fulfilled for a diagnosis of social phobia:

- The psychological, behavioral, or autonomic symptoms must be primarily manifestations of anxiety and not secondary to other symptoms such as delusions or obsessional thoughts.
- The anxiety must be restricted to or predominate in particular social situations.
- Avoidance of the phobic situations must be a prominent feature.

Panic Disorder

Panic disorder should be the main diagnosis only in the absence of any of the phobias. For a definite diagnosis, several severe attacks of autonomic anxiety should have occurred within a period of about 1 month

- in circumstances in which there is no objective danger,
- without being confined to known or predictable situations, and
- with comparative freedom from anxiety symptoms between attacks (although anticipatory anxiety is common).

Obsessive-Compulsive Disorder

Obsessional symptoms or compulsive acts, or both, must be present on most days for at least two successive weeks and must be a source of distress or interference with activities. The obsessional symptoms should have the following characteristics:

- They must be recognized as the person's own thoughts or impulses.
- There must be at least one thought or act that is resisted unsuccessfully, even though others may be present that the sufferer no longer tries to resist.

- The thought of carrying out the act must not in itself be pleasurable (simple relief of tension or anxiety is not regarded as pleasure in this sense).
- The thoughts, images, or impulses must be unpleasantly repetitive.

Posttraumatic Stress Disorder

Posttraumatic stress disorder should not generally be diagnosed unless there is evidence that it arose within 6 months of a traumatic event of exceptional severity. In addition to evidence of trauma, there must be a repetitive, intrusive recollection or reenactment of the event in memories, daytime imagery, or dreams. Conspicuous emotional detachment, numbing of feeling, and avoidance of stimuli that might arouse the recollection of the trauma are often present but are not essential for the diagnosis. Autonomic disturbances, mood disorder (e.g., depression, dramatic bursts of fear or panic), and behavioral abnormalities (aggression disorder, alcohol abuse) all contribute to the diagnosis but are not key.

Generalized Anxiety Disorder

Primary symptoms of anxiety must be present most days for at least several weeks at a time and usually for several months. These symptoms usually involve elements of the following:

- Apprehension (worries about future misfortunes, feeling "on edge," difficulty concentrating)
- Motor tension (e.g., restless fidgeting, tension headaches, trembling, inability to relax)
- Autonomic overactivity (e.g., lightheadedness, sweating, tachycardia or tachypnea, epigastric discomfort, dizziness, dry mouth)

In children, a frequent need for reassurance and recurrent somatic complaints may be prominent.

Reprinted, by permission, from WHO, 1992, *International classification of diseases-10* (Geneva: World Health Organization).

typically achieved by infusion (5 to 6 mmol/L), which provokes attacks in about two-thirds of panic patients (Martinsen et al. 1998a). Also, lactate accumulation resulting from exercise is not related to postexercise anxiety in people without clinical disorders (e.g., Garvin, Koltyn, and Morgan 1997). Acute submaximal exercise also reduces the frequency of panic and severity of anxiety symptoms after the administration of the panic-inducing drug cholecystokinin in both panic patients and healthy people (Strohle et al. 2005; Strohle et al. 2009). Moreover, small randomized clinical trials showed that 10 weeks of aerobic exercise training was effective in reducing symptoms of anxiety among patients with panic disorder and agoraphobia, although not as effective as drug therapy (Broocks et al. 1998) and was superior to relaxation treatment alone or when combined with the SSRI anti-anxiety drug Paroxetine (Wedekind et al. 2010). Just two weeks of moderate-intensity aerobic exercise reduced fears of anxiety symptoms among young adults who scored high on a test of anxiety sensitivity, a feature of panic disorder (Smits et al. 2008).

The study of physical activity as a treatment for anxiety was impeded in the late 1960s and 1970s by the lactate–anxiety controversy, but the effects of acute and chronic exercise on anxiety have been the topic of numerous studies over the past 40 years. Seminal studies on the effects of acute physical activity on state anxiety conducted by Morgan (1973, 1979a) laid the foundation for a large body of research showing reductions in self-rated anxiety after aerobic exercise. For example, Morgan (1973) measured state anxiety in 40 men before vigorous exercise, shortly after vigorous exercise, and 20 to 30 min after 45 min of vigorous exercise. There was a slight increase in anxiety immediately after exercise, but a significant decrease below preexercise anxiety 20 to 30 min later. In a subsequent study, state anxiety reduction after 20 min of exercise

> **E**arly research erroneously attributed panic attacks to participation in vigorous exercise.

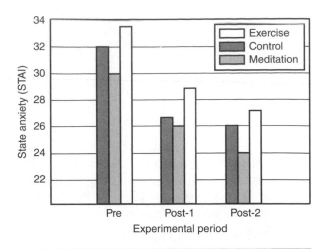

Figure 6.5 State anxiety before and after exercise, meditation, and control treatments.

Data from Bahrke and Morgan 1978.

at 70% of aerobic capacity was comparable to reductions after meditation or quiet rest in a group of 75 middle-aged men, shown in figure 6.5 (Bahrke and Morgan 1978). That study was especially important because it generated the hypothesis that the key feature common to the conditions was "time-out," or diversion from the source or symptoms of anxiety—and that distraction might be a plausible explanation for anxiety reduction after exercise, a view that has been subsequently supported (Breus and O'Connor 1998).

Preventing Anxiety: Observational Studies

An early cross-sectional population study suggested that active people had lower anxiety symptoms than inactive people did (Stephens 1988). The Canada Health Survey asked nearly 11,000 Canadians aged 15 years and older questions about anxiety and their physical activity during the past two weeks. Women over 40 years of age and men, both under and over 40, who said they expended the equivalent of 5 or more kilocalories per kilogram of their body weight each day in leisure-time physical activity also reported fewer anxiety-like symptoms than those who expended fewer than 2 kilocalories per kilogram of body weight each day.

At least five large, population-based cross-sectional studies published during the past

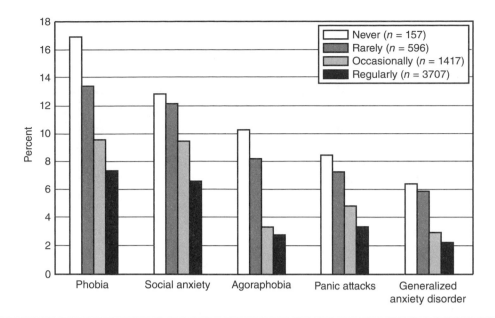

Figure 6.6 Twelve-month prevalence rates of anxiety disorders according to the frequency of physical activity in the U.S. National Comorbidity Survey.

Data from Goodwin 2003.

decade, including data from nationally representative samples of nearly 350,000 Americans, show that regular physical activity is associated with lower odds of anxiety symptoms.

U.S. National Comorbidity Survey

Goodwin (2003) analyzed data from the U.S. National Comorbidity Survey (n = 5,877), a nationally representative sample of adults ages 15 to 54 in the United States. After adjustment for age, sex, race, marital status, education, income, physical illnesses, and other mental disorders, people who said they regularly got physical exercise for recreation or at work had 25% to 35% lower odds of being diagnosed with anxiety disorders during the past year as follows: agoraphobia (OR = 0.64; 95% CI = 0.43-0.94), social anxiety (OR = 0.65; 95% CI = 0.53-0.80), specific phobias (OR = 0.78; 95% CI = 0.63-0.97), and panic attacks (OR = 0.73; 95% CI = 0.56-0.96). A nearly 40% reduction in the odds of generalized anxiety disorder (OR = 0. 61; 95% CI = 0.42-0.88) was no longer significant after adjustment for other mental disorders (OR = 0.76; 95% CI = 0.52-1.11), likely reflecting the high comorbidity between GAD with depression and other anxiety disorders. There was a dose–response reduction in the odds of each anxiety disorder

with higher frequency of physical activity. See figure 6.7.

2006 Behavioral Risk Factor Surveillance Survey

The 2006 Behavioral Risk Factor Surveillance Survey was a random-digit-dialed telephone survey of 217,379 participants in 38 states, the District of Columbia, Puerto Rico, and the U.S. Virgin Islands (Strine et al. 2008). About 11% of people (14.3% of women and 8.2% of men)

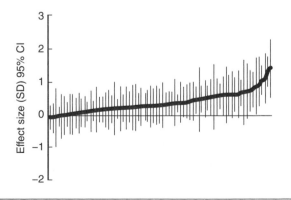

Figure 6.7 Randomized controlled trials of exercise training and anxiety symptoms among patients with medical conditions other than anxiety.

Data from Herring, Matthew, O'Connor, and Dishman 2010.

said they had at least once been told by a physician or health provider that they had an anxiety disorder (including acute stress disorder, generalized anxiety disorder, obsessive-compulsive disorder, panic attacks, panic disorder, phobia, posttraumatic stress disorder, or social anxiety disorder). About 24% of participants said they had not participated in any leisure-time physical activity or exercise during the past 30 days. Regardless of age, inactive people were 40% more likely to have a lifetime anxiety disorder (OR= 1.4; 95% CI = 1.3-1.5). After adjustment for age, sex, race and ethnicity, education, marital and job status, chronic medical conditions (CVD, diabetes, asthma), smoking, obesity (BMI ≥ 30 kg/m^2), and alcohol use (drinks per day: >2 men; >1 women), that risk remained elevated by 10%.

Health Study of North Trøndelag County, Norway

A total of 1,260 survivors of testicular cancer and 20,207 men from the general population completed a mailed questionnaire that assessed leisure-time physical activity (including walking to work) and symptoms of anxiety (Thorsen et al. 2005). People who said they spent less than 1 hour each week during the past year in low-intensity physical activity (i.e., not hard enough to be sweaty or breathless) and no time in high-intensity physical activity were classified as physically inactive (18% of the people). The prevalence of elevated anxiety symptoms was higher among those who were physically inactive (17%) than among those who were active (13%), regardless of cancer diagnosis (OR = 1.36; 95% CI = 1.23-1.51). After adjustment for age, BMI, education, living alone, smoking, and elevated depression symptoms, the odds of elevated anxiety symptoms were no longer higher among physically inactive people.

The Netherlands Twin Registry

In the Netherlands Twin Registry, 12,450 adolescents (at least 10 years old) and adults participated in a study on lifestyle and health from 1991 to 2002 (De Moor et al. 2006). The prevalence of exercise participation (at least an hour each week in activities rated at 4 METs or more) was

51.4%. After adjustment for sex and age, the odds of general feelings of anxiety were approximately 16% lower among exercisers (OR = 0.84; 95% CI = 0.81-0.87). However, that association was likely confounded by personality because the exercisers also were more extraverted and emotionally stable, traits that reduce the risks of anxiety disorders. Among pairs of identical twins (479 males and 943 females) aged 18 to 50, the twin who exercised more did not report less anxiety than the twin who exercised less (De Moor et al. 2008). Also, longitudinal analysis (follow-up ranged from 2 to 11 years) showed that increases in exercise participation did not predict decreases in anxiety.

Prospective Cohort Studies

At least three population-based studies that used a prospective cohort design have shown that physical activity is associated with 25% to 40% reductions in the risk of an anxiety disorder

Northern Rivers Mental Health Study, Australia

A cohort of community residents living in the Richmond Valley of New South Wales was followed for a two-year period to identify the factors that were predictive of changes in their mental health status regardless of their history (Beard et al. 2007). After random telephone screening to recruit a cohort at risk of mental disorders, 1,407 invited subjects completed baseline face-to-face interviews using the Mini WHO CIDI diagnostic interview (ICD-10 criteria). There were 859 likely cases (51.4%) and 548 likely noncases (56.9%). After two years, 968 adults ages 18 to 85 were reinterviewed. Those who reported more than 3 hours per week of vigorous physical activity at baseline had 43% lower odds of developing any anxiety disorder compared to those who said they got no activity (OR = 0.57; 95% CI = 0.31-1.05), but the odds reduction was extinguished after adjustment for sex, stressful life events, emotional stability, and symptoms of distress measured at baseline.

SUN (Sequimiento Universidad de Navarra) Study

A reduction in the incidence of anxiety was observed in a cohort of 1,0381 graduates (mean age ~43 ± 12) of the University of Navarra, Spain, who were followed up for four to six years (Sanchez-Villegas et al. 2008). There were 731 incident cases of anxiety disorder defined as self-reported physician-diagnosed anxiety or habitual tranquilizer use. After adjustment for age, sex, caloric intake, smoking, marital status, arthritis, ulcers, and cancer at baseline, the odds of incident anxiety were reduced by one-third in the 20% of the people who expended 19 to 33 MET-hours per week in leisure-time physical (OR = 0.67; 95% CI = 0.52-0.85) and by 25% in the 20% who expended 33 MET-hours per week or more (OR = 0.74; 95% CI = 0.58-0.94) compared to the 20% least active people.

Swedish Health Professionals Cohort data collected in 2004 and 2006 from health care professionals and social insurance workers in western Sweden (2,694 women; 420 men) were analyzed (Jonsdottir et al. 2010). Compared to those who were sedentary, people who said they engaged in either light physical activity (gardening, walking, bicycling to work at least 2 hours each week) or moderate-to-vigorous physical activity (aerobics, dancing, swimming, soccer, or heavy gardening at least 2 hours each week, or 5 hours at high intensity) during the past 3 months in 2004 were less likely than sedentary people to report elevated symptoms of anxiety at follow-up in 2006 (OR = 0.64; 95% CI = 0.42-1.02 and OR = 0.56; 95% CI = 0.34-0.94, respectively).

State Anxiety

A temporary reduction in state anxiety after acute exercise has been reported widely in quantitative (i.e., meta-analysis) reviews of studies conducted on adults without anxiety disorders (e.g., Landers and Petruzzello 1994; Petruzzello et al. 1991). Studies published from 1960 to 1993 indicated an average reduction ranging from 1/4 (McDonald and Hodgdon 1991; Petruzzello et al. 1991) to 1/2 (Landers and Petruzzello 1994) SD, with larger changes typically occurring 5 to 30 min after exercise that had lasted about 20 to 30 min. Several studies have suggested that acute exercise is as effective as meditation (Bahrke and Morgan 1978), biofeedback, and drugs (Broocks et al. 1998), but no more effective than quiet rest or distraction in decreasing state anxiety (Bahrke and Morgan 1978; Breus and O'Connor 1998). However, the **anxiolytic**

> **A**cute exercise can decrease state anxiety as effectively as other traditional treatments, such as meditation.

effects of exercise apparently last longer than those of rest or distraction, and short periods of exercise have been associated with decreases in state anxiety that have persisted up to several hours after exercise. For example, Raglin and Wilson (1996) reported that state anxiety was decreased up to 2 hours after 20 minutes of cycling at either 40%, 60%, or 70% of $\dot{V}O_2$peak.

Changes in anxiety after exercise reported in studies that were published before 1993 did not differ significantly among exercise intensities expressed as a percentage of $\dot{V}O_2$peak (Landers and Petruzzello 1994; Petruzzello et al. 1991), but most of those studies did not quantify relative exercise intensity according to various levels of cardiorespiratory fitness or compare intensities within the same participants. Often, aerobic capacity was estimated based on submaximal fitness tests or heart rate, which can be up to 20% off from actual aerobic capacity. The accurate assessment of exercise intensities is critical for determining the levels of exercise intensity necessary or optimal for reducing anxiety after acute exercise and for prescribing a training program. Studies published since 1993 typically have used standard methods for quantifying exercise intensity. These studies show decreased or unchanged anxiety after intensities ranging from 40% to 70% of $\dot{V}O_2$peak (Breus and O'Connor 1998; Dishman, Farquhar, and Cureton 1994; Garvin, Koltyn, and Morgan 1997; Koltyn and Morgan 1992; O'Connor and Davis 1992; Raglin and Wilson 1996) and increased, decreased, or unchanged anxiety after maximal exercise testing with different samples of participants (Koltyn, Lynch, and Hill 1998; O'Connor et al. 1995).

The fitness levels of participants varied among those studies, but physical activity history was usually described poorly or not measured. A common limitation of the literature on anxiety reduction after acute exercise is the failure of studies to directly compare participants who differ in fitness and physical activity histories. Also, the common approach of expressing relative exercise intensity as a percentage of $\dot{V}O_2$peak does not fully equate intensity among people who differ in exercise training. Inactive people experience more metabolic strain than active people when exercising at the same percentage of $\dot{V}O_2$peak (Wilmore and Costill 1994), and this difference could affect anxiety responses after exercise. Moreover, physically active adults, compared with less active adults, have higher expectancies of psychological benefits from exercise (Hsiao and Thayer 1998; Steinhardt and Dishman 1989), and this might bias their self-reports of anxiety reduction after acute exercise.

The bulk of the evidence about anxiety after exercise comes from studies that measured anxiety via self-ratings (Morgan 1997; Petruzzello et al. 1991), which are transparent in their content. Hence, the researchers did not discount the possibility that the reduction in anxiety after exercise was confounded by subject expectancy about the psychological effects of exercise (Morgan 1997). Investigations that addressed an effect of expectancy on reduced anxiety after cycling (Youngstedt et al. 1993) and reduced tension after jogging (Berger et al. 1998) showed mixed evidence of such an effect. A study that controlled for physical activity history, fitness, and expectancy of psychological benefits of exercise indicated that young men with low fitness, but not those with high fitness, had reduced state anxiety after 20 min of cycling at a light intensity (40% of $\dot{V}O_2$peak), despite having higher anxiety than the fit men shortly after maximal exercise (Tieman et al. 2002). Thus, in that study, lower fitness and a recent history of physical inactivity did not prevent the young men from experiencing reduced anxiety after submaximal exercise.

Most research on anxiety and exercise has examined the effects of aerobic, low-resistance exercise, such as swimming, cycling, or running at moderate or high intensities. Anxiety reductions after high-resistance exercise, such as weightlifting, have been examined less frequently. In 1993, Raglin, Turner, and Eksten found no decrease in state anxiety after weight training but significant decreases after leg cycle exercise. Focht and Koltyn (1999) found a reduction in state anxiety after 50% but not 80% of resistance exercise at 1-repetition maximum (1RM), although this effect was delayed by more than 60 min after exercise. In another study, anxiety reductions after resistance exercise were delayed until 1.5 to 2 hours after exercise (O'Connor et al. 1993). Bartholomew and Linder (1998) found decreased state anxiety after 20 minutes of resistance exercise at 40% to 50% of 1RM, and this effect occurred 15 and 30 minutes after exercise. They also found that anxiety was increased at 5 and 15 minutes after 20 minutes of high-intensity resistance exercise (75% to 85% of 1RM).

Trait Anxiety

A large number of studies have supported the contention that regular exercise can reduce people's general feelings of anxiety. Two early meta-analyses agreed that exercise training reduced trait anxiety in people without an anxiety disorder or other medical conditions. A more recent review found similarly beneficial reductions in anxiety symptoms among patients with chronic disorders other than anxiety.

Petruzzello and colleagues (1991) concluded from their early meta-analysis of exercise and anxiety research that the typical reduction in trait anxiety after exercise training was about 0.33 SD, a change of about 3 points on the most common rating scale used in the studies (Spielberger's State-Trait Anxiety Inventory, which ranges from 20 [*almost never anxious*] to 80 [*almost always anxious*]). Despite the fact that virtually all the people studied did not have diagnosed anxiety disorders, greater reductions were seen among those people who had higher trait anxiety. The effects for exercise were as good as those for other active treatments and better than those for control conditions.

Long and van Stavel (1995) subsequently reported a mean effect of 0.40 SD for decreases in trait anxiety after exercise training averaged across 40 quasi-experimental and experimental studies of healthy adults. Since 1995, about 50 randomized controlled trials of exercise training have been reported.

A recent meta-analysis of 40 randomized controlled trials including 2,914 patients with chronic medical conditions other than anxiety disorders found that compared with no treatment conditions, exercise training significantly reduced anxiety symptoms by a small amount (0.29 SD; 95% CI = 0.23-0.36) when compared to control groups that did not exercise (Herring, O'Connor, and Dishman 2010). (See figure 6.7.) Anxiety reductions were greatest in trials lasting no more than 3 months, when sessions lasted at least 30 minutes, and when people reported their experience of anxiety symptoms for more than the past week.

Dose–Response Studies?

No exercise training studies have manipulated exercise program length or exercise type to see whether the size of anxiety reductions differ. About half the studies used aerobic exercise alone (walking, jogging, or cycling), and a fourth of the studies used resistance exercise alone or combined aerobics with resistance training, usually low-intensity strength training. The magnitude of anxiety reduction has been similar regardless of the type of exercise, the duration (usually 25-60 min), or whether it was continuous or intermittent (i.e., with rest breaks). However, most studies were imprecise in describing how much time was actually spent in active exercise compared to warming up, resting, and cooling down. It is not known whether the intensity of aerobic or resistance exercise affects anxiety reduction in clinical trials. More than half the trials used moderate-to-vigorous exercise intensity (i.e., 60% to 80% of aerobic capacity, or maximal strength) with a weekly frequency of 3 or more days per week. Reductions in anxiety symptoms were similar across those variations in exercise intensity.

It is unlikely that chronic exercise will have a large effect on trait anxiety among people without anxiety disorders, but it can decrease state anxiety in nonpatients who have relatively high trait anxiety.

Exercise Training Among Patients With Anxiety

Few training studies have been conducted with clinical populations, but generally, such people show reductions in anxiety regardless of training intensity or changes in aerobic capacity. Martinsen, Hoffart, and Solberg (1989) examined the effects of aerobic (walking and jogging) and nonaerobic (strength, flexibility, and relaxation) exercise on 79 inpatients with various anxiety disorders. Patients, randomly assigned to the groups, exercised for 1 hour, 3 days per week. After 8 weeks of training, patients in the two groups showed similar and significant reductions in anxiety regardless of changes in aerobic capacity. The benefits of exercise training were also documented in another study of 44 inpatients with a variety of anxiety disorders (Martinsen, Sandvik, and Kolbjornsrud 1989). Inpatients performed 1 hour of aerobic exercise 5 times a week for 8 weeks. All exhibited improvements in anxiety symptoms during the study except those diagnosed with social phobia. Patients with GAD and those with agoraphobia without panic attacks maintained their improvements at 1-year follow-up. Sexton, Maere, and Dahl (1989) also reported persistence in reduction in anxiety 6 months after hospitalized patients had participated in 8 weeks of moderate- or low-intensity aerobic exercise training. In addition, improvements in psychological symptoms were similar for the two intensities.

At least three randomized controlled trials have shown a reduction in anxiety after exercise training among people who have an anxiety disorder (e.g., Broocks et al. 1998; Herring et al. 2012; Merom, et al. 2008).

Aerobic Exercise Versus SSRI for Panic Disorder and Agoraphobia

A randomized clinical trial showed that 10 weeks of aerobic exercise training was effective in reducing symptoms of anxiety among patients with panic disorder and agoraphobia, though not as effective as drug therapy (Broocks et al. 1998). In that study, 46 outpatients suffering from moderate to severe panic disorder with agoraphobia (4 did not have agoraphobia) were randomly assigned to a 10-week treatment consisting of regular aerobic exercise (running), the serotonin reuptake inhibitor clomipramine (112.5 mg/day), or placebo pills. The dropout rate was 31% for the exercise group, 27% for the placebo group, and 0% for the clomipramine treatment group. Compared with placebo, both exercise and clomipramine were accompanied by a significant decrease in symptoms, but clomipramine treatment improved anxiety symptoms sooner and more effectively than exercise did (see figure 6.8). Although some evidence has suggested that people with panic disorders are physically inactive and actually avoid exercise (Broocks et al. 1997), there is no scientific consensus that patients diagnosed with panic disorder avoid physical activity because of fear (O'Connor, Smith, and Morgan 2000).

Walking Plus Group Cognitive Behavioral Therapy

A group randomized trial in an outpatient clinic for people diagnosed with panic disorder, generalized anxiety disorder, or social phobia compared a group receiving a home-based walking program along with group cognitive behavioral therapy (GCBT plus walking) (21 people) with a group receiving GCBT and educational sessions (GCBT plus education) (20 people) (Merom et al. 2008). After adjusting for self-ratings of depression, anxiety, and stress at the study outset and the type of anxiety disorder, the GCBT-plus-walking group reported fewer symptoms of depression, anxiety, and stress than did the GCBT-plus-education group.

Generalized Anxiety Disorder

Thirty sedentary women 18 to 37 years of age at the University of Georgia who had a primary *DSM-IV* diagnosis of generalized anxiety disorder were randomly assigned to six weeks of resistance exercise training or aerobic exercise training, or to a wait-list control group in which they had the opportunity to get an exercise program after the trial ended (Herring et al. 2012). About 70% of the women had a comorbidity with another anxiety or mood disorder, and one-third of the women were being treated with antide-

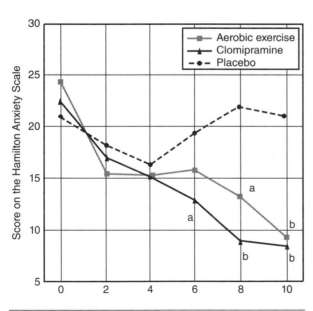

Figure 6.8 Aerobic exercise or drug therapy for panic disorder.

Data from Broocks et al. 1998.

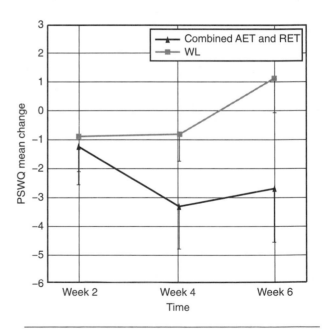

Figure 6.9 Feasibility of Exercise Training for the Short-Term Treatment of Generalized Anxiety Disorder: A Randomized Controlled Trial.

Reprinted, by permission, from M.P. Herring, M.L. Jacob, C. Suveg, R.K. Dishman, R.J. O'Connor, 2012, "Feasibility of exercise training for the short-term treatment of generalized anxiety disorder: A randomized controlled trial," *Psychotherapy & Psychosomatics* 81: 21-28.

pressants. Women exercised twice a week under supervision by either lower-body weightlifting or leg cycling matched between conditions according to body region, positive work load progression, and time actively engaged in exercise. There were no adverse events. Remission rates were 60%, 40%, and 30% for resistance exercise, aerobic exercise, and the control condition, respectively. Figure 6.9 shows that worry symptoms were reduced by the exercise conditions compared to the control condition.

Issues in Research

It is important to know whether physical activity and exercise can relax people even though they don't have anxiety disorders. The stress of daily living is routinely accompanied by anxieties that don't lead to a disorder but still negatively affect the quality of the day by causing discomfort or impairing people's work or leisure activities. This is one reason most studies of exercise and anxiety have involved people who had average or even low levels of anxiety. However, that approach has led to four problems. The first is the problem of generalizability. Obviously, the study of people who are not clinically anxious does not tell us whether exercise will be an effective treatment for any of the several anxiety disorders. Considering the high prevalence of the various anxiety disorders, it is important for public health that we learn more about the potential benefits and any hazards of physical activity and exercise among patients diagnosed with anxiety disorders.

The second problem is one of initial levels of low anxiety, which leave little room for anxiety to improve. In other words, exercise would not be expected to make people who aren't anxious less anxious. A few recent researchers studying nonclinical populations were able to examine elevated anxiety by screening large numbers of people to find those who had elevated trait anxiety scores (e.g., Breus and O'Connor 1998), or by provoking higher anxiety pharmacologically by using caffeine (Youngstedt et al. 1998).

The third problem is whether the rating scales used to measure anxiety in most exercise studies have been sensitive enough to detect true reductions in anxiety after exercise. This concern is amplified when the participants are people who have low initial anxiety. Most rating scales that have been used in exercise studies give a single score for anxiety. Some psychologists argue that, at the least, worry and physiological symptoms should be measured separately. A special concern has been voiced that the scales used in exercise studies have not been sensitive or specific enough to measure anxiety in response to exercise. Self-report of anxiety usually has been assessed with the State-Trait Anxiety Inventory (STAI; Spielberger et al. 1983), the tension/anxiety scale of the Profile of Mood States (POMS; McNair, Lorr, and Droppleman 1981), or other similar scales that use adjectives to assess an anxious or tense mood. The STAI is the most strongly validated measure of anxiety

Physical Activity and Anxiety in Youth

No randomized controlled trials of children or adolescents diagnosed with anxiety disorders have been reported. A meta-analysis located six poorly controlled trials including youths aged 11 to 19 from the general population that compared exercise training with a no-treatment condition or with an intervention other than drugs or psychotherapy (Larun et al. 2006). The exercise group experienced a moderately large but statistically nonsignificant effect of exercise on the reduction of anxiety scores (−0.48 SD; 95% CI = −0.97-0.01) regardless of exercise intensity. Whether that apparent effect is generalizable to a reduction in the primary risk of developing depression among adolescents is not yet established. A four-year longitudinal study of 2,548 adolescents and young adults aged 14 to 24 in Munich, Germany, found that those who said they regularly exercised or played sports at baseline had a lower overall incidence of any mental disorder and anxiety (Andreas Strohle et al. 2007).

in the world. However, some researchers have become concerned that the STAI and POMS do not measure anxiety or tension during or after exercise (see Ekkekakis and Petruzzello 1999 for a discussion). One concern is that the questions on the scales might be artificially affected by people's perceptions of physical arousal during exercise. Another is that anxiety during or after exercise is experienced differently than anxiety in response to other situations or settings—that the structure of anxiety might be changed by exercise. Some researchers even believe that measures of anxiety designed specifically for exercise are required. Research has yet to show that this is the case. It's hard to imagine why or how anxiety during or after exercise could be a unique phenomenon. Nonetheless, some people experience symptoms related to anxiety, such as muscle tension or pain, without reporting worry. So, it is possible that people having nonclinical anxiety before exercise still might feel calmer and more relaxed after exercise, but that the scales used to measure anxiety don't have enough of the right questions to measure a change in a person's feelings of relaxation. It is an unresolved issue in psychology whether feelings of relaxation are merely the absence of anxiety, whether relaxation and anxiety are opposite extremes of the same feeling (i.e., arousal, activation), or whether they are different feelings.

The fourth problem is the virtual absence of physiological evidence of reduced anxiety. That absence is important for three reasons. The first is related to the problem of sensitivity and specificity of measurement just explained. A few early studies (e.g., deVries et al. 1981), and a more recent one (Smith et al. 2002), have shown that acute and chronic exercise can reduce muscle reflexes and tension. It is not yet clear, though, whether reduced muscle tension after exercise is part of anxiety reduction or is a biological response to exercise that is independent of anxiety. Similarly, moderate to large increases in the α brain wave band frequency measured by electroencephalography (EEG) are common during and after exercise (Crabbe and Dishman 2001; Kubitz and Mott 1996; Petruzzello et al. 1991; see figure 6.10). Increased α activity is traditionally viewed as an index of relaxed wakefulness, but this is not a universal view

among EEG experts, and the exercise studies did not show that the increased α activity was caused by the exercise or related to reduced anxiety; other brain wave frequencies presumably unrelated to anxiety also are increased after exercise (Crabbe and Dishman 2001). In addition, reductions in blood pressure after exercise have been interpreted by some investigators as indirect evidence of an anxiolytic effect of exercise (e.g., Petruzzello et al. 1991; Raglin, Turner, and Eksten 1993). However, postexercise hypotension (lowered blood pressure for up to 2 hours after exercise) is a well-known physiological phenomenon that occurs even when anxiety is not lowered after exercise (e.g., Youngstedt et al. 1993).

The second reason physiological measures of anxiety are desirable is the need to corroborate the validity of self-rating of anxiety as a true measure of mood or emotional response. Although physiological measures cannot serve as a substitute for self-report, which is the only way to directly measure a person's feelings, they are more objective than self-reports of anxiety. Hence, they are not as affected by experimental artifacts, such as demand characteristics, experimenter influences on participants' ratings, social desirability, or other participant expectancies about exercise that can artificially bias self-ratings.

Finally, and third, the absence of physiological evidence of reduced anxiety is a problem because physiological variables have been a part of most theories of negative emotions, including anxiety, since the time of Hip-

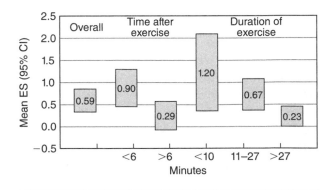

Figure 6.10 Results for encephalogram α brain wave band frequency after exercise.

Data from Crabbe and Dishman 2004.

pocrates, through the era of Charles Darwin and William James, until today (see chapters 1 and 7). Several modern theories propose that electromyographic measures of startle (Lang, Bradley, and Cuthbert 1998) and EEG measures of asymmetry in brain waves (Davidson 1992) provide indexes of people's predisposition to interpret environmental events as negative or threatening. Recently, asymmetry as indicated by EEG (Petruzzello, Hall, and Ekkekakis 2001; Petruzzello and Landers 1994; Petruzzello and Tate 1997) and an electromyogram measure of startle (Smith et al. 2002) have been shown to be related to self-ratings of anxiety, but not to overall emotional responses (Crabbe, Smith, and Dishman 2007; Smith et al. 2002). The cumulative evidence on studies of acute exercise and EEG activity indicates that activity in all frequency bands increases in response to exercise regardless of hemispheric site (Crabbe and Dishman 2004). However, the studies were limited to just a few recording sites and did not use dense-array electrode mapping. The evidence suggests that acute exercise increases EEG activity in a general way consistent with increased arousal, possibly from increased sensory and cardiovascular neural traffic to the thalamus processed through the brain stem.

The spinal Hoffmann reflex (H-reflex) has been studied in respect to exercise to locate evidence for effects of exercise on central nervous system aspects of self-reported anxiety. The H-reflex is a monosynaptic reflex, but, ascending and descending nerve tracts from the spinal cord to and from the brain exist that would permit it to be modulated by the central nervous system. A series of studies conducted by deVries and others (deVries et al. 1982; Bulbulian and Darabos 1986) showed a reduction in the H-reflex after exercise and hypothesized that the reduction was indicative of a tranquilizing effect of exercise. Recent research, however, has found that changes in the H-reflex are not correlated with changes in self-reports of anxiety after exercise (Motl and Dishman 2004; Motl, O'Connor, and Dishman 2004), and it appears that the reduction of the H-reflex after exercise does not extend beyond the specific spinal segments involved with the limbs involved in the exercise (Motl and Dishman 2003).

A final concern is that the influence of the setting in which physical activity occurs is poorly understood. Thayer (1987) reported that 10 to 15 min of walking outdoors reduced self-rated tension, but earlier research showed no effect on anxiety after acute treadmill walking (Morgan 1973). McAuley, Mihalko, and Bane (1996) found a reduction in anxiety after exercise of self-selected intensity, despite small increases during exercise, in both laboratory and natural settings.

PSYCHOTHERAPY

The two most effective forms of psychotherapy used to treat anxiety disorders are behavioral and cognitive behavioral therapy. Behavioral therapy helps patients change their actions through breathing techniques or through gradual exposure to what is frightening them. Cognitive behavioral therapy, in addition to these techniques, teaches patients to understand their thinking patterns so that they can react differently to the situations that cause them anxiety.

PHARMACOTHERAPY

Although nearly two of three anxiety patients in the United States were treated long term with antidepressant drugs in 2005 (Olfson and Marcus 2009), a classification of drugs called the benzodiazepines (BDZs) provides the most effective short-term treatment of several anxiety disorders, especially generalized anxiety (Ballenger 2001). Benzodiazepines have a quick, short-lived effect by binding to the $GABA_A$ receptor, which inhibits neurons by opening chloride channels that hyperpolarize the cell and make it less sensitive to firing. Benzodiazepines are central nervous system depressants that are in a class of drugs known as sedative-hypnotics. Sedative drugs reduce anxiety (anxiolytic) and have a calming effect. Hypnotic drugs produce a state of drowsiness that helps people go to sleep and stay asleep.

In 2009, an estimated 88 million prescriptions were filled in the United States for benzodiazepines, making them the 10th most prescribed class of drugs (IMS Health 2010; www.imshealth.

Common Drugs Used to Treat Anxiety

Benzodiazepines

Ativan (lorazepam)

Centrax (prazepam)

Halcion (triazolam)

Klonopin (clonazepam)

Paxipam (halazepam)

Restoril (temazepam)

Serax (oxazepam)

Valium (diazepam)

Versed (midazolam); intravenous injection in hospital only

Xanax (alprazolam)

Barbiturates

Librium (chlordiazepoxide)

Tranxene (clorazepate)

Tricyclics

Surmontil (trimipramine) for panic disorder and OCD

Serotonin antagonist

Buspar (buspirone)

Selective Serotonin Reuptake Inhibitors

Celexa (citalopram)

Luvox (fluvoxamine)

Paxil (paroxetine)

Selfemra (fluoxetine); for panic attacks and OCD

Zoloft (sertraline)

Selective Serotonin and Noradrenaline Reuptake Inhibitors

Cymbalta (duloxetine); for generalized anxiety disorder

Effexor (venlafaxine); for generalized anxiety disorder

Luvox (fluvoxamine); for OCD, social anxiety, panic disorder, PTSD, GAD

Dopamine Agonists

Wellbutrin (bupropion); for panic disorder

Side effects: sedation, low muscle tone, anticonvulsant effects; tolerance or dependence and withdrawal may develop.

com). Xanax (alprazolam) is by far the most prescribed benzodiazepine in the United States (44.4 million prescriptions filled in 2009). High-potency benzodiazepines (e.g., alprazolam, clonazepam, and lorazepam) are effective in treating panic disorder and panic attacks with or without agoraphobia, as add-on therapy to selective serotonin reuptake inhibitors in the treatment of obsessive-compulsive disorder, and panic disorders (Chouinard 2004). Drugs that block receptors for noradrenaline, called β-blockers (e.g., propranolol), help reduce panic symptoms, especially rapid heartbeat and palpitations. Selective serotonin reuptake inhibitors (SSRIs) are front-line treatments for social anxiety and panic disorder. The benzodiazepine clonazepam and certain monoamine oxidase inhibitors may also be of benefit.

The treatment of social phobia may need to be continued for several months to consolidate a response and achieve full remission. In light of the chronicity and disability associated with social phobia, as well as the high relapse rate after short-term therapy, it is recommended that effective treatment be continued for at least 12 months (Van Ameringen et al. 2003).

An integrated treatment approach that combines pharmacotherapy with cognitive behavioral therapy may provide the best treatment for panic disorder. Long-term efficacy and ease of use are important considerations in treatment selection, because maintenance treatment is recommended for at least 12 months, and in some cases, indefinitely (Pollack et al. 2003).

Currently, benzodiazepines and buspirone are prescribed frequently to treat GAD. Benzodiazepines are not recommended for the long-term treatment of GAD, because of the associated development of tolerance, psychomotor impairment, cognitive and memory changes, physical dependence, and a withdrawal reaction on discontinuation. SSRIs (e.g., paroxetine) and serotonin and noradrenaline reuptake inhibitors (e.g., extended-release venlafaxine) appear to be effective in treating GAD. Of the psychological therapies, cognitive behavioral therapy (CBT) shows the greatest benefit in treating GAD patients. Treatment gains after a 12-week course of CBT may be maintained for up to one year. Currently, no guidelines exist for the long-term treatment of GAD (Allgulander et al. 2003). Drug actions provide models of psychopharmacology that can help guide research into the biological mechanisms that account for the anti-anxiety effects of exercise.

MECHANISMS

It is important to determine whether reduced anxiety after acute exercise or an exercise training program can be explained by a direct effect of exercise or merely by other aspects of the exercise setting. It is unlikely that exercise would directly decrease the occurrence of some forms of anxiety, but it might help a person cope with the experience of anxiety. For example, there is no reason to expect that exercise would reduce simple phobias. A person who is afraid of spiders will experience anxiety when exposed to a spider whether that person is active and fit or sedentary.

Similarly, people who have social phobias usually recognize that their anxiety is irrational, but their self-consciousness and fear of judgment in social situations persist. As a result, they try to avoid people in social situations as much as possible. There is no reason to expect that physically active people would somehow be protected against developing social anxiety disorder, because it is mainly a learned response. Indeed, cognitive behavioral therapy has proven the most effective treatment for social phobia. In a cognitive behavior group, patients might work on their anxieties in a progressive hierarchy, learning to engage in social introductions, small talk with others, presentations to the group, mock job interviews, sitting in front of the stare of others,

performing drama with others, and so on. The idea is to desensitize their anxiety in social situations through the experience of social evaluation without negative consequences. Exercise could not do that directly. Indeed, social phobia could well keep someone from exercising in public. However, cognitive behavioral therapy could be carried out in a group exercise setting, such as in a fitness club. In that case, although exercise would not be the treatment, a person with social phobia might find exercise a way to reduce the symptoms of anxiety caused by a social encounter. A few case studies have even indicated that exercise could help patients who have situational phobia, perhaps by helping them learn to cope with feelings of arousal such as those produced by heavy exertion (e.g., Orwin 1974).

On the other hand, exercise might hold more promise for helping people cope with the symptoms of GAD. If shown to be effective, exercise could offer an important public health benefit for people with GAD; one survey has indicated that only about 25% of people with GAD ever receive treatment (Uhlenhuth et al. 1983).

Clarifying the exercise intensity, mode, and duration that make the greatest impact on anxiety symptoms, and identifying the effects on psychological and physiological markers of anxiety, can provide insight into the mechanisms for the anxiolytic effects of exercise. There is consensus that exercise reduces anxiety, but there is no consensus on how this happens. The first step in understanding the relationship between exercise and anxiety reduction is to understand something about the etiology of anxiety. There is evidence for a moderate genetic contribution to an individual's susceptibility to developing an anxiety disorder, but the genesis of anxiety disorders is likely a function of biological, behavioral, and environmental factors (O'Connor, Raglin, and Martinsen 2000). Theories that have been used to explain the genesis of anxiety disorders include genetic, as well as cognitive behavior, psychodynamic, sociogenic, and neurobiological theories. No single theory can adequately explain the etiology of anxiety, and the effects of exercise on anxiety are likely also multifaceted. The most active areas of research have been in cognitive and neurobiological aspects of anxiety (O'Connor, Raglin, and Martinsen 2000).

Cognitive Theories

Cognitive theories, as noted in chapter 14, explain behavior and feelings by focusing on cognition. For example, the development of trait anxiety is characterized as cognitively learned through personal or observed exposures to physical threats or negative evaluations of failures. From this perspective, pathological anxiety develops as a result of cognitive appraisals, such as overestimating the intensity of a feared event, underestimating one's ability to cope, or catastrophically misinterpreting physiological symptoms associated with anxiety (e.g., interpreting an increased heart rate as a possible heart attack) (O'Connor, Raglin, and Martinsen 2000). Support for a cognitive component in anxiety disorders is provided by McNally, Foa, and Donnell (1989), who found that patients with anxiety disorders exhibited a recall bias for anxiety-related information compared to nonclinical controls. The patients with anxiety were more likely to attend to and remember stimuli that were either threatening or perceived as threatening.

Cognitive explanations of the effects of exercise on anxiety have also been proposed. Physiological sensations from exercise can help redefine the subjective meaning of arousal and can compete with the perception of anxiety symptoms. Sensations of the heart pounding during exercise can be "reframed" from being a symptom of anxiety to being a sign of a good workout. Exercise can also distract attention from anxiety-provoking thoughts and produces a "time-out" from cares and worries (distraction hypothesis). Breus and O'Connor (1998) tested the time-out, or distraction, hypothesis (Bahrke and Morgan 1978) by measuring state anxiety (STAI) in 18 high-trait-anxious college females before and after exercise at moderate intensity (40% of aerobic capacity) while studying, study-

ing only, and quiet rest. There was no change in anxiety after exercise while studying, studying only, or quiet rest. There was a significant decrease in anxiety after the exercise-only condition, which indicates that the anxiolytic effect of exercise (exercise as time-out from worries and concerns) was blocked by studying.

Neurobiological Theories

Neurobiological explanations of the etiology and manifestation of anxiety have been enhanced by the increased sophistication of measurement techniques in human research, such as brain imaging technology. Neurobiological theories on the development of anxiety have been intertwined with those for depression because there is evidence that anxiety and depression are linked to the dysregulation of some of the same neural systems (e.g., noradrenergic and serotonergic systems). Patients with major affective disorders usually have anxiety as a prominent symptom, and many anxious patients have a history of depression.

A neurobiological perspective on anxiety supports the integration of cognitive and neurological theories. For example, neural circuits involved in anxiety must include afferent nerve fibers that allow potentially threatening stimuli to be sensed so they can be interpreted as threatening by higher brain areas. These brain areas must appraise the input and integrate it with relevant memories. If the stimuli are then interpreted as representing a threat, the response depends on efferent nerves that generate a coordinated endocrine, autonomic, and muscular response. The effects of these neural systems are dependent on several neurotransmitters, which have been targets for the pharmacological treatment of anxiety disorders.

There is evidence from human and animal research that the amygdala, locus coeruleus (LC), midbrain, thalamus, right hippocampus, anterior cingulate cortex, insular cortex, and right prefrontal cortex are involved in the genesis and expression of anxiety (Goddard and Charney 1997; Reiman 1997). The amygdala seems to be the critical central neural structure involved in the psychophysiological components of fear and anxiety responses (see chapter 3) (Goddard

> The time-out hypothesis states that exercise distracts attention from anxiety-provoking thoughts and produces a time-out from cares and worries.

and Charney 1997). The amygdala receives input from the thalamus and LC and from sensations that have been integrated with higher cortical areas. Anxiety from direct experiences (state anxiety when a dog growls), unconscious processing (spontaneous panic attack), and prior experiences (posttraumatic stress) can thus be mediated through the amygdala. Efferent projections to a variety of centers controlling cognitive, affective, neuroendocrine, cardiorespiratory, and musculoskeletal functions allow the amygdala to play a key role in the manifestation of anxiety symptoms (Goddard and Charney 1997). For example, the amygdala and the LC have projections into the hypothalamus, which contributes to the activation of the sympathetic nervous system.

Much of our understanding of the neurobiological mechanisms involved in anxiety has built on studies of animal behavior. For example, as noted in chapter 3, increased locomotion in the rat usually reflects an adaptive motivational state of low behavioral inhibition (e.g., less freezing), especially when the locomotion appears purposeful and the animal exhibits other exploratory behaviors such as rearing or approaching the center of the open field. In contrast, low levels of locomotion, few approaches to the center of the open field, freezing, defecation, urination, and shivering in rats are conventionally regarded as indexes of hypervigilance, hesitancy, fear, and autonomic activation, which are responses that are common in human anxiety. Under some circumstances of threat, increased locomotion in rats indicates panic (i.e., the flight response to a predator).

Neurobiological mechanisms for the antianxiety effects of exercise have not been well studied with an established animal model of anxiety. The limbic–motor integration model of anxiety elaborated by Mogenson (1987) is relevant for the study of physical activity and anxiety behaviors in the rat. In this model, fearful locomotion is controlled by the limbic system's modulation of the tegmental pedunculopontine nucleus of the mesencephalic locomotor system by reciprocal inhibition between γ-aminobutyric acid (GABA) and dopamine transmission within the **corpus striatum**. GABA efferents from the nucleus accumbens to the ventral pallidum apparently inhibit locomotion.

Important inputs to the amygdala, which coordinates freezing or flight behaviors during perceived threat, come from the hippocampus, which helps regulate the checking of the environment against memories of danger; the ventral tegmental area (VTA), a pleasure center that surrounds the hypothalamus and helps regulate approach behaviors (see figure 6.11); and the periaqueductal gray (PAG), a pain-processing area that surrounds the duct between the third and fourth brain ventricles, as well as the dorsal raphe nuclei, which each influence locomotion during threat.

Insight into the mechanisms for anxiety disorders and potential explanations for the effects of exercise come from the psychopharmacology literature, studies on the effects of drugs on neurotransmitter systems, and research on the effects of exercise on these systems. The serotonergic and noradrenergic systems have been implicated in anxiety, and there is good evidence for contributions from specific neurotransmitters, such as GABA.

Serotonin

Numerous antidepressant and anxiolytic drugs affect serotonergic systems—for example, by blocking serotonin reuptake (see figure 6.12)

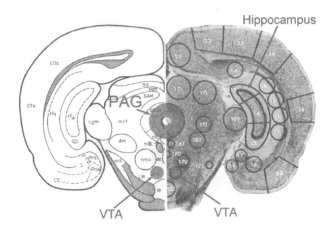

Figure 6.11 Anxiety-associated locomotion; periaqueductal gray matter (PAG) surrounding the aqueduct between the third and fourth brain ventricles, the hippocampus, and the ventral tegmental area (VTA) surrounding the hypothalamus regulate fear behaviors during threat in the rat.

Reprinted from *Maps and guide to microdissection of the rat brain*, M. Palkovits and M.H. Brownstein, pg. 152, copyright 1988. By permission of M. Palkovits.

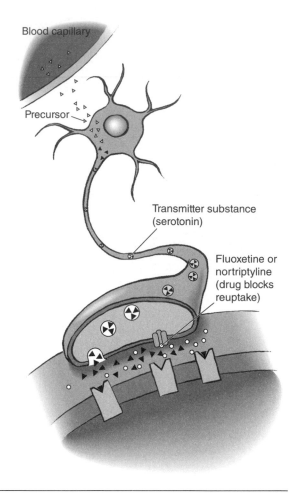

Figure 6.12 Serotonin reuptake inhibition at the level of the receptor.

or acting on serotonergic receptors as agonists or antagonists. The serotonin reuptake–inhibiting drugs, such as clomipramine and fluoxetine, are often used to treat several anxiety disorders (Goddard and Charney 1998). Anxiety can be induced in a majority of panic patients, but in a minority of controls, by blocking the binding of serotonin at the receptor level with serotonin receptor agonists, such as the nonselective serotonin agonist m-chlorophenylpiperazine (Charney et al. 1987), which implies a dysregulation in the serotonergic system in these patients. Activation of 5-HT2 serotonin receptors induces anxiety-like behaviors in mice (Fox, Hammack, and Falls 2008; Salam et al. 2009), and transgenic mice that lack 5-HT2 receptors are resistant to fearful environments (Heisler et al. 2007). Animal studies have shown increased activity of the raphe nuclei and serotonin synthesis

with exercise training (Dishman 1998). There is also indirect evidence for effects from exercise on central serotonergic systems based on measures of tryptophan disposition in the blood and concentrations of **5-HIAA** (serotonin [5-HT] metabolite) in cerebrospinal fluid (Chaouloff 1997). Mechanisms for increased brain levels of serotonin with exercise involve the effects of exercise on the substrate tryptophan (see chapter 3). Exercise induces increased lipolysis, or the breakdown of triglycerides into free fatty acids, which are used to fuel increased levels of muscular contraction. Increased serum levels of free fatty acids compete with tryptophan for binding with albumin, leading to increases in free tryptophan. This increase in free tryptophan stimulates an influx of tryptophan into the brain, and thus the potential for the increased synthesis of serotonin. The increase in free fatty acids has the best support as a mechanism for increased serotonin with exercise (Chaouloff 1997). Exercise also may result in decreased levels of large neutral amino acids (aromatic amino acids and branched-chain amino acids), which compete with free tryptophan at the transporter level of the blood–brain barrier. However, there is mixed evidence for changes in branched-chain amino acids with acute exercise (Chaouloff 1997).

Studies at the University of Colorado (Greenwood et al. 2005; Greenwood et al. 2008) have provided more evidence that voluntary exercise alters central 5-HT function. Six weeks of voluntary exercise in rats was associated with an up-regulation of mRNA for 5-HT1A autoreceptors in the dorsal raphe nucleus (DRN), which could decrease DRN activity by enhancing the autoinhibition of DRN cell firing and subsequently decrease 5-HT release in DRN projection areas that help elicit anxiety-related behaviors (Greenwood and Fleshner 2011). Consistent with this,

> **E**xercise may affect anxiety by altering the substrate use that facilitates the uptake of tryptophan into the brain and the subsequent increased synthesis of serotonin.

Dishman and colleagues (1997) found that six weeks of activity-wheel running led to decreased levels of the 5-HT metabolite 5-hydroxyindole acetic acid in the hippocampus and amygdala that was accompanied by less anxiety-like behavior after uncontrollable foot-shock stress. Just two weeks of voluntary exercise mitigated the startle-enhancing effect of an anxiogenic 5-HT2B/C agonist (Fox et al. 2008).

Norepinephrine

Several lines of evidence implicate the noradrenergic system in anxiety (O'Connor, Raglin, and Martinsen 2000). Suppressing the effects of norepinephrine (NE) with β-adrenergic blockers, which down-regulate the NE receptor–effector system, have shown efficacy in the treatment of social phobia (Gorman and Gorman 1987). The function of the LC and the release of NE have also been implicated in anxiety disorders. There is a general association between spontaneous LC activity and vigilance and arousal. The LC increases the signal-to-noise ratio by decreasing the background rate of spontaneous firing in the hippocampus, thalamic, and cortical areas and enhancing evoked responses in the lateral geniculate nucleus and visual cortex. It has been hypothesized that patients with panic disorder have an abnormally regulated α-2 noradrenergic receptor system, which is involved in the regulation of NE release from the LC. Panic patients have been found to exhibit both a blunted growth hormone response to the α-2 receptor agonist clonidine (Tancer, Stein, and Uhde 1993) and an exaggerated anxiety and physiological response to the α-2 receptor antagonist yohimbine (Charney et al. 1992). Alpha-2 receptor agonists, such as clonidine, decrease LC activity (i.e., decrease NE release); and antagonists, such as yohimbine, increase LC activity. In animals, stimulation of the LC results in anxiety-like behaviors and produces behavioral and physiological changes commonly associated with anxiety. Ablation of the LC eliminates these anxiety responses.

Differences in adrenergic receptors can serve as an indication of SNS and NE or EPI activity. Researchers interested in the effects of exercise on these systems have examined adrenergic receptor density in humans. Endurance-trained athletes have higher-than-normal β-adrenoreceptor density on lymphocytes (a type of white blood cell), and a session of prolonged physical activity at high intensity is accompanied by increased β-adrenoreceptor density on lymphocytes. However, lymphocyte adrenoreceptors are β_2 types with high affinity for epinephrine, like those found in skeletal and smooth muscle, the liver, and peripheral sympathetic tissue. It is unclear whether they provide an index of peripheral SNS receptors, but they do not provide a measure of brain NE activity (Dishman 1998).

> The effects of exercise on NE to benefit people with anxiety disorders may be at the level of the LC, but research with humans to prove this has been limited.

In rats, exercise training has been found to increase levels of NE in the LC, amygdala, hippocampus, and hypothalamus (Dishman et al. 2000) and to decrease the release of NE in the brain frontal cortex (Soares et al. 1999) after stress. In humans, changes in brain NE activity after acute physical activity have been estimated via measurement of 3-methoxy-4-hydroxyphenylglycol (**MHPG**), an NE metabolite) levels in urine, plasma, or cerebral spinal fluid. Studies of urinary MHPG after a single session of physical activity showed increased MHPG excretion or no change. At rest, 20% to 60% of MHPG in peripheral blood or urine comes from the metabolism of brain NE. However, the increase in blood levels of NE during exercise comes mainly from sympathetic nerves innervating the heart, with some coming from the exercising skeletal muscles; thus the relevance for anxiety of increased MHPG in the blood after acute exercise is unclear (Dishman 1998).

Gamma-Aminobutyric Acid (GABA)

The function of GABA as the major neural inhibitory neurotransmitter implies a role in moderating arousal level, and a substantial body of evidence implicates GABA in anxiety disorders. Gamma-aminobutyric acid neurons and receptors are widely distributed in brain areas thought to be important for the expression of anxiety, including the hypothalamus, periaqueductal gray, septum, hippocampus, and amygdala (Menard and Treit 1999). Gamma-aminobutyric acid and benzodiazepines, such as diazepam, or Valium, bind to the GABA_A receptor and inhibit activity of neurons in the brain by opening a chloride channel and hyperpolarizing the cell (see figure 6.13). The benzodiazepines are effective in treating GAD, and the benzodiazepine receptor inverse agonists (e.g., the β-carbolines) produce strong anxiety reactions (Dorow 1987).

Another proposed hypothesis has linked the biological and cognitive processes characterizing anxiety (Sarter and Bruno 1999). Benzodiazepines inhibit cholinergic neurons originating in the basal forebrain. These basal forebrain neurons innervate all cortical areas and are known to be involved in modulating cortical information processing. Basal forebrain neurons also receive afferent input from the LC and amygdala. Sarter and Bruno (1999) hypothesized that increases in the excitability of cortical cholinergic inputs from the basal forebrain play a role in the cognitive aspects of anxiety and promote an increased processing of anxiety-related stimuli. The inhibition of these cholinergic neurons by benzodiazepine would be a mechanism for decreasing the cognitive processing of stimuli that promote anxiety.

Dishman and colleagues (1996) studied the effects of chronic activity-wheel running and treadmill exercise training on central nervous system neurotransmitter systems in rats. They found increased levels of GABA and a decreased number of GABA_A receptors in the corpus striatum and increased open-field locomotion among the activity-wheel runners, consistent with an anxiolytic effect according to the limbic–motor integration model of Mogenson (1987). The explanation for an anxiolytic effect of exercise based on GABA may be through the exercise effects on the central cholinergic function, which is inhibited by benzodiazepine receptor agonists. Exercise training can induce alterations in peripheral cholinergic function (Zhao et al. 1997), which presents the possibility that improvements in anxiety after exercise training may accrue as a result of adaptations in central nervous system cholinergic neural circuits (see O'Connor, Raglin, and Martinsen 2000 for a discussion).

> Improvements in anxiety after exercise training may be through adaptations in central nervous system cholinergic or GABAergic neural circuits.

SUMMARY

Anxiety is a response to a real or perceived threat that has cognitive, behavioral, emotional, and physiological components. Acute anxiety is experienced by most people at some time or another with minor effects, but an anxiety disorder can be incapacitating. Millions of people in the United States and worldwide have anxiety disorders, and the financial and emotional costs are considerable. Pharmacological treatment has some risks and disadvantages, and the potential use of exercise as a means of prevention and treatment is appealing in view of its additional health benefits.

Little research has been conducted with clinical populations besides people with panic disorder, and most studies have tested participants with nonclinical initial levels of anxiety. However, anxiety reductions after acute exercise have been consistently observed in people with nonclinical levels of anxiety, even with little room for anxi-

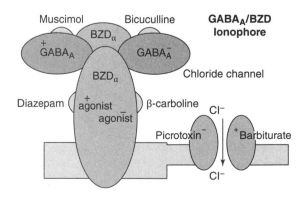

Figure 6.13 Gamma-aminobutyric acid receptor A/benzodiazepineionophore receptor complex.

ety scores to improve, and the bulk of the initial research on the effects of exercise training on clinical populations has been promising. Aerobic exercise seems to decrease acute anxiety, but the effects of intensity and duration need more study. There are also mixed results on the effects of resistance exercise on acute anxiety.

Several plausible mechanisms have been examined in attempts to explain how acute and chronic exercise might bring about reductions in anxiety. Plausible mechanisms linking anxiety improvements with exercise are being developed with an increased understanding of relevant neurobiology. This mechanistic work needs to be conducted in patients who have clinical anxiety disorders and in people without clinical anxiety disorders who are experiencing above-average anxiety. Multiple approaches are recommended, including the use of noninvasive brain imaging, neurotransmitter-blocking agents, and psychophysiological methods (e.g., correlating brain cortical EEG or electromyographic measures of neuromuscular reflexes with self-reported anxiety responses to exercise). Animal models of anxiety also have a potentially important role to play in generating useful new knowledge about neurobiological mechanisms that might explain anxiety reduction after exercise and physical activity.

WEBSITES

www.nimh.nih.gov/health/topics/anxiety-disorders/index.shtml

www.mentalhealth.com/p.html

www.medscape.com/psychiatry

Depression

Most people have experienced transient feelings of sadness or depressed mood. The depression passes after minutes or hours, but they remember how much effort routine activities, even doing the laundry, seemed to require. Many people report that periods of physical inactivity make them vulnerable to feeling depressed, whereas exercise seems to lighten their mood. However, the relationship between exercise and depression is like the chicken-and-egg dilemma: are people depressed because they are sedentary, or are they sedentary because they are depressed? Longitudinal studies have offered some evidence that physical inactivity increases the risk of depression, and exercise training studies with clinically depressed patients have demonstrated improvements in depressive symptoms. We may find an explanation for this by examining the extensive research on the psychobiological mechanisms of depression. This chapter provides a foundation for understanding the relationship between exercise and depression by reviewing the scope of the problem; offering clinical definitions; describing the research literature on exercise and depression; and explaining the current social, cognitive, and psychobiological mechanisms for effects.

depression in the United States increased steadily between the 1940s and 1990s. A decade or so ago, one-third of all Americans were expected to experience at least one bout of depression in their lifetimes (Ernst, Rand, and Stevinson 1998). In 1996, 12.6 million annual office visits to physicians were for major depression or other types of depressive disorders (Schappert 1998), and depression is one of the most common complaints of all adults who seek psychotherapy.

Feeling depressed, however, is only part of clinical depression, which is a severe condition with persistent emotional, physiological, and cognitive components. Estimates from epidemiological research in England, Finland, Australia, and the United States suggested that 8% of women and 4% of men have some form of clinical depression at any point in time (Lehtinen and Joukamaa 1994). In the United States, 4.5% to 9.3% of all women and 2.3% to 3.2% of all men have a major depressive disorder.

The National Comorbidity Survey indicated a lifetime rate of 17% for major depression (21% among women and 13% among men) and a rate of 9.5% when people were asked whether they had been depressed in the previous 12 months (Kessler et al. 1994). With the exception of manic episodes in bipolar disorder, women have nearly

PREVALENCE AND SOCIAL IMPACT

Depression was among the 10 leading risk factors of disability-adjusted life expectancy in high-income nations during 2001 (Lopez et al. 2006). It is projected to rank second worldwide by the year 2020 and then first by 2030 (Mathers and Loncar 2006). The annual prevalence of major

> The World Health Organization has projected that depression will be second only to cardiovascular disease as the world's leading cause of death and disability by the year 2020 and first by 2030.

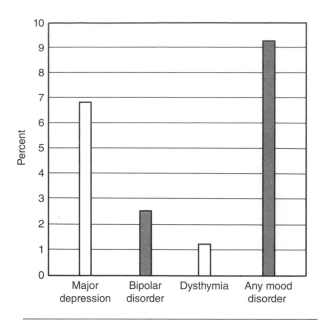

Figure 7.1 Twelve-month prevalence estimates of mood disorder in U.S. adults.

Data from Kessler et al. 2005

twice the rate of depression that men do. As shown in figure 7.1, the National Comorbidity Survey Replication conducted a decade later estimated that 9.5% of U.S. adults have a depressive mood disorder each year (Kessler et al. 2005b), and 21% have a mood disorder during their lifetime (Kessler et al. 2005a). The most recent estimate of lifetime prevalence of major depression among U.S. adults is 16% (Kessler et al. 2003).

Rates of mood disorders in the United States differ according to sex, age, and race. Women's lifetime odds are 50% higher than men's for any mood disorder. Figure 7.2 shows that the prevalence of major depressive disorder and dysthymia increases with age until age 60. The median age of onset of mood disorders is 30 years, which is later than most other mental disorders (Kessler et al. 2005a). However, depression affects about 8% to 9% of early adolescents annually (Rushton, Forcier, and Schectman 2002). The annual rate of depression among teenagers and young adults is about twice that of adults 25 to 44 years of age and four times the rate among people over age 65 (Kessler et al. 1994).

African Americans tend to experience less depression than white Americans, and nonwhites of Hispanic ancestry have more depression than whites. Results of the National Comorbidity Survey Replication (Breslau et al. 2006) found that both Hispanic blacks and non-Hispanic blacks had lower risk for depression. Hispanics had lower risk for dysthymia. (See figure 7.3.)

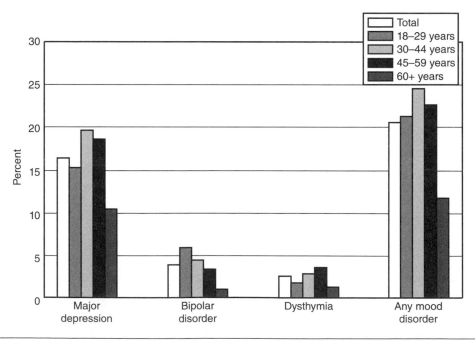

Figure 7.2 Lifetime prevalence estimates of anxiety disorders in U.S. adults according to age.

Data from Kessler et al. 2005

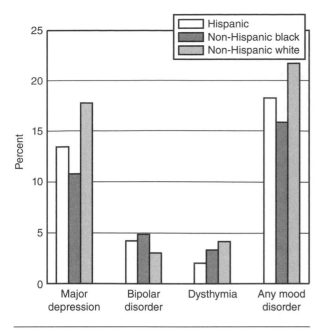

Figure 7.3 Lifetime prevalence estimates of mood disorders in U.S. adults according to race and ethnicity.

Data from Breslau et al. 2006.

Results from the National Comorbidity Survey Replication in the United States and the World Health Organization's World Mental Health Surveys found that people who have had major depression are two to three times more likely to attempt suicide. The odds of suicidal thoughts are elevated in people who are depressed, but people who have severe anxiety or agitation (e.g., posttraumatic stress disorder) and poor impulse control (e.g., conduct disorder or substance use disorders) are most likely to make a plan to commit or attempt to commit suicide (Nock et al. 2009; Nock et al. 2010).

In addition, the rate of suicide attributable to depressive disorders increases dramatically from age 10 through young adulthood (Greenberg et al. 1993). Suicide is the third leading cause of death among teenagers and young adults. Depression is especially prevalent among girls and women under age 25, who have twice the rate of depression as boys and men of the same age and six times the rate of women ages 25 to 54 (Regier et al. 1988).

Worldwide, 12-month prevalence estimates of suicidal thoughts, plans, and attempts are about 2.0%, 0.6%, and 0.3% of the populations, respectively, in developed nations and are similar in developing nations (Borges et al. 2010).

Risk Factors for Suicidal Behaviors

- Female sex
- Younger ages (<50)
- Less education
- Low income or unemployed
- Unmarried
- Parental psychopathology
- Childhood adversities
- Presence of 12-month *DSM-IV* mental disorders

Reprinted from Borges et al. 2010.

About 80% of Americans who attempt suicide have a prior mental disorder (especially mood disorders comorbid with anxiety and impulse-control and substance use disorders) (Nock et al. 2010). There are nearly a million suicide deaths each year worldwide. In the United States, more than 30,000 people commit suicide each year, making suicide the 11th leading cause of death.

In 2008, suicide was the seventh leading cause of death for males and the fifteenth leading cause of death for females in the United States. Suicide is the second leading cause of death among American Indians and Alaska Natives ages 15 to 34. Almost four times as many males as females die by suicide, but women are two to three times more likely to attempt suicide. For every suicide in the United States, there are 24 nonfatal suicide attempts (Centers for Disease Control and Prevention [CDC] 2010a).

Clinical depression has high personal, social, and economic costs. People with depression experience loss of pleasure, feelings of hopelessness, and difficulty with interpersonal relationships. Someone who is depressed has an increased risk of suicide. Clinical depression is the strongest mental disorder risk factor for suicide in youth and adults (Petronis et al. 1990).

If you, or someone you know, are at risk, call the National Suicide Prevention Lifeline at 800-273-TALK (800-273-8255).

Suicide in the United States

According to the CDC (2010a, 2010b):

- Suicide is the second leading cause of death among 25- to 34-year-olds.

- It is the third leading cause of death among 15- to 24-year-olds.

- Among 15- to 24-year-olds, suicide accounts for 12.2% of all deaths annually.

- 13.8% of students in grades 9 through 12 seriously considered suicide in the previous 12 months (17.4% of females and 10.5% of males).

- 6.3% of students reported making at least one suicide attempt in the previous 12 months (8.1% of females and 4.6% of males).

- Suicide death rates are highest among elderly men.

Estimated costs of depression in the United States in 2000 were $26.1 billion (31%) in direct medical costs, $5.4 billion (7%) in suicide-related mortality costs, and $51.5 billion (62%) in lost productivity at the workplace (Greenberg et al. 2003). In 2009, an estimated 169 million prescriptions for antidepressants were filled in the United States, making them the third most prescribed class of drugs behind only lipid drugs and codeine-based medicines. Sales, mainly to depression and anxiety patients, were the fourth highest among prescribed medications during 2009, accounting for $9.9 billion (www.imshealth.com/portal/site/imshealth).

The total annual cost of depression in Europe was estimated at 118 billion euros in 2004, which corresponds to a cost of 253 euros per capita (Sobocki et al. 2006). Direct costs were 42 billion euros, which broke down as follows: outpatient care (22 billion euros), drug cost (9 billion euros), and hospitalization (10 billion euros). Indirect costs from morbidity and mortality were estimated at 76 billion euros. Depression was the most costly brain disorder in Europe, accounting for 33% of the total mental health care costs and 1% of the gross domestic product (GDP), or total economy, of Europe.

There is evidence for some long-term physical consequences of depression, such as decreases in bone mineral density and increased rates of coronary disease and hypertension (Gold and Chrousos 1999; Jonas, Franks, and Ingram 1997). Depression and obesity have a complicated bidirectional relationship (Stunkard, Faith, and Allison 2003), which is especially important considering the high rates of obesity and overweight among all age groups. There is some evidence that depression increases the risk of obesity (Luppino et al. 2010), especially for adolescent females (Herva et al. 2006), although the relationship between obesity and people being treated for depression must be weighed against the weight gain associated with some antidepressants.

Although 8% of women and 4% of men have clinical depression at any point in time, only 30% of people with depression seek professional help and less than half get adequate treatment.

CLINICAL DESCRIPTION

Defining depression can be difficult because it includes several types of mood disorders with opposite symptoms (e.g., increase *or* decrease in sleep; increase *or* decrease in appetite) (see table 7.1). The *Diagnostic and Statistical Manual of Mental Disorders* (American Psychiatric Association 2000) places mood disorders into four categories: (1) depression; (2) bipolar, or manic-depressive, disorder; (3) mood disorders due to a medical condition; and (4) substance-induced mood disorders. The first category includes **major depression** and the milder chronic form, **dysthymia**. The two principal subtypes of major depression are melancholic and atypical depression, although 53% of patients who meet the criteria for major depression do not meet the

Table 7.1 Subtypes of Unipolar Affective Disorder (Major Depression)

Melancholia	Atypical depression
Physiological hyperarousal	Physiological hypoarousal
Insomnia	Hypersomnia
Loss of appetite	Increased appetite
Early-morning awakening	Fatigue
Profound sense of unworthiness	Blunted affect
Diminished libido	Diminished libido
Endocrine dysregulation	Endocrine dysregulation
Pessimism	Profound inertia
Loss of pleasure	
Decreased slow-wave sleep	
Fear	
Preferential access to painful memories	

criteria for either subtype. The second category, bipolar, or **manic-depressive**, **disorder**, is characterized by periods of depression alternating with periods of elevated, expansive, or irritable mood; exaggerated self-confidence; risky or asocial behavior; or even paranoia.

In Europe, the International Classification of Diseases (ICD-10), endorsed in 1992 by the World Health Organization (WHO) in Geneva, Switzerland, defines a depressive episode as depressed mood, loss of interest and enjoyment, and reduced energy leading to increased fatigability (often after only slight effort) and diminished activity (WHO 1992). The depressive episode is classed as mild, moderate, or severe.

During a depressive episode, the lowered mood is usually persistent from day to day for at least 2 weeks, regardless of circumstances, yet tends to improve during the day. A depressive episode may be diagnosed when symptoms have not lasted for 2 weeks but are very severe and appeared very rapidly. In some cases, anxiety and motor agitation can be more prominent symptoms than depressed mood. Also, mood disturbance can be less apparent than other features such as irritability; abuse of alcohol; and the worsening of existing comorbid phobias, obsessions, or a preoccupation with physical symptoms.

Some symptoms included in the ICD-10 classification system have special clinical significance for defining typical somatic depression and are similar to the U.S. *DSM-IV* system for the diagnosis of **melancholia**.

At least four of the following are required for a diagnosis of somatic depression:

- Loss of interest or pleasure in activities that are normally enjoyable
- Lack of emotional reactivity to normally pleasurable surroundings and events

Manic-Depressive Disorders

- Bipolar I: Major depression alternates with mania, or uncontrollable elation.
- Bipolar II: Major depression alternates with hypomania, a milder form of elation.
- Cyclothymia: Milder depression alternates with hypomania.

Common Symptoms of a Depressive Episode According to the International Classification of Diseases (ICD-10)

- Reduced concentration and attention
- Reduced self-esteem and self-confidence
- Ideas of guilt and unworthiness (even in a mild type of episode)

- Bleak and pessimistic views of the future
- Ideas or acts of self-harm or suicide
- Disturbed sleep
- Diminished appetite

Reprinted, by permission, from WHO, 1992, *International classification of diseases-10* (Geneva: World Health Organization), 100.

- Waking in the morning 2 hours or more before the usual time
- Depression worse in the morning
- Objective evidence of definite psychomotor retardation or agitation (remarked on or reported by other people)

When a person has a major depressive episode, these symptoms cause significant distress and impairment in social and occupational settings as well as in other areas of the person's life. Depression is not considered a major depressive episode if it is caused by drug abuse or medication or a medical condition such as hyperthyroidism, heart disease, diabetes, multiple sclerosis, hepatitis, or rheumatoid arthritis. Also, many people have these symptoms within the first 2 months after a loved one has died, but it is not considered major depression unless the symptoms are associated with marked functional impairment, a preoccupation with worthlessness, ideas of suicide, psychotic symptoms, or psychomotor retardation.

Nearly twice as many women as men are depressed. Reasons for this difference are unknown, but they likely relate to genetics, endocrine effects, and social learning. For example, risk factors for bipolar depression include being female, especially aged 35 to 45, having a family history of depression or alcoholism, parturition in the previous 6 months, recent negative life events, lack of a confiding relationship, and having a negative home environment. The etiology of depression in general involves stress emotions linked by neurobiological processes.

Depression can be caused by catastrophic events, such as the death of a loved one, a loss of self-esteem (e.g., feeling unworthy because a valued goal was not met), or chronic anxiety or stress. It can also occur for no apparent reason.

In a landmark national study in the United States, about half of depressed patients treated with antidepressant drugs, psychotherapy, or both still have residual symptoms after 2 or more months of treatment. In the Sequenced Treatment Alternatives to Relieve Depression (STAR*D) study, only 47% of nearly 2,900 depressed patients had a favorable response (i.e., a 50% drop in symptoms) after 6 weeks or more of antidepressant treatment with the SSRI citalopram. Only 27% remitted (i.e., no longer had symptoms). Then, nonremitters who still had symptoms were switched to either sertraline (another SSRI), venlafaxine (a combination SSRI and NSRI), or bupropion-SR (a norepinephrine and dopamine reuptake inhibitor). About 25% of those patients subsequently remitted (Rush et al. 2006; Trivedi et al. 2006a). Another group of nonremitters were switched to cognitive therapy and had a similar remission rate (31%) during the second round of treatment. Psychotherapy was better tolerated than drug therapy, but the augmentation of citalopram with another drug was quicker acting than the augmentation with cognitive therapy (40 days compared with 55 days, on average) (Gaynes et al. 2009).

These facts indicate the potential importance of self-help behaviors, such as exercise, which can enhance mental health (Freeman et al. 2010). Many studies agree that regular physical activity can reduce symptoms after a person is depressed and can reduce the odds that a person will experience depression. As discussed later, exercise may have effects on the brain monoamine systems similar to the effects of antidepressant drugs, or the exercise setting may have cognitive effects that are beneficial, such as increasing physical self-esteem. Exercise can also help offset residual symptoms of ineffective drug therapy by increasing feelings of energy and by promoting better sleep and improved sexual function. Exercise training has even been successful as an augmentation therapy among patients who have not responded to pharmacotherapy (Trivedi et al. 2006b).

EFFECTS OF EXERCISE

Physical activity has been recommended by physicians since ancient times to combat depression. About 2,500 years ago, Hippocrates prescribed exercise for his patients who experienced *melancholia*—a term still used today by psychiatrists to describe deep depression. A report from the beginning of the 20th century appears to have been the first modern study of exercise and depressed patients. The mood and reaction times of two depressed males were improved on days when they exercised for about 2 hours compared to days when they rested (Franz and Hamilton 1905). About 65 years later, the first experimental study showed that self-ratings of depressive symptoms could be reduced in men after an exercise training program (Morgan et al. 1970). That finding was extended to a small randomized clinical trial of psychiatric outpatients showing that the reduction in depressive symptoms after 12 weeks of running therapy was equivalent to or greater than that after two forms of group psychotherapy (Greist et al. 1979). Moreover, 9 of the 10 patients treated with running therapy were still running and not depressed 9 months later, whereas depressive symptoms had returned in the other patients.

About a decade later, three early population-based surveys suggested that regular participation in leisure-time physical activity might reduce the odds of developing depression during adulthood:

- The National Health and Nutrition Examination Survey I (NHANES I), a 1975 survey of nearly 7,000 Americans aged 25 to 74, found that people who said they got little or no exercise in their leisure time also reported more symptoms of depression (Stephens 1988).

- The Canada Health Survey of 24,000 Canadians aged 15 and older in 1978-1979 and the Canada Fitness Survey of 22,000 Canadians aged 10 and older in 1981 yielded similar findings (Stephens 1988). In these surveys, people who said they were moderately or very active in their leisure time also were more likely to report feelings related to positive moods.

- A study conducted in Upper Bavaria, Germany, between 1975 and 1984 of 1,500 people aged 15 and older noted the prevalence of several types of depressive disorders for those who stated that they currently did not exercise for sports, as compared with those who stated that they did regularly engage in sports (Weyerer 1992).

In all three studies, higher rates of depression occurred among inactive people regardless of physical illness, sex, age, and social class. However, the studies presented only cross-sectional comparisons of active and inactive people; that is, the studies merely took a "snapshot" of physical activity and health measured at the same time. They didn't determine whether it was inactivity or depression that occurred first. It's possible that people became less active after becoming depressed rather than becoming depressed as a consequence of inactivity. As shown in figure 7.4, physical inactivity did not predict higher depression 5 years later in the Upper Bavaria study.

Results from the NHANES study were more encouraging. About 1,500 of the people originally interviewed in NHANES I were interviewed again 8 years later (Farmer et al. 1988). That follow-up survey first measured physical activity and then looked for the later occurrence of the

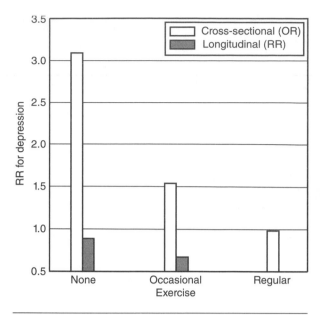

Figure 7.4 The Upper Bavarian field study measured the level of physical activity and assessed depression by clinical interview in 1,536 community residents. The odds ratio (OR) for depression for inactive people was 3.15, but physical inactivity did not significantly increase the risk of depression at 5-year follow-up.

Based on Weyerer 1992.

symptoms of depression. Among the findings of the NHANES I follow-up were these:

- The rate of depression among sedentary Caucasian women who were *not* depressed in 1975 and who remained inactive was twice that of women who said they participated in a moderate amount of physical activity and who remained active over the 8 years.
- Caucasian men who were depressed and inactive in 1975 and who remained inactive were 12 times more likely to be depressed after 8 years than those who were initially depressed but who had become physically active.

These findings were observed regardless of age, education level, and socioeconomic status.

Two other important prospective studies followed depression over time and compared people's risk according to their physical activity:

- In the Alameda County Study conducted near Oakland, California, about 5,000 nondepressed adult men and women

completed surveys on physical activity and depression in 1965, 1974, and 1983 (Camacho et al. 1991). Participants were classified as low active, medium active, and high active based on the frequency and intensity of self-reported physical activity. Inactive people who were not depressed in 1965 had a 70% increase in risk of depression in 1974 compared to those who were initially highly active. Associations between changes in activity from 1965 to 1983 and symptoms of depression in 1983 suggested that the risk of depression was alterable by increasing exercise, but this association was not independent of the other risk factors for depression.

- In a study of about 10,000 Harvard male alumni from the mid-1960s through 1977, physical activity was shown to reduce the likelihood of developing physician-diagnosed depression (Paffenbarger, Lee, and Leung 1994). Men who expended 1,000 to 2,500 kilocalories per week by walking, climbing stairs, or playing sports had 17% less risk of developing depression than their less active peers. Those who expended more than 2,500 kilocalories per week had a 28% lower risk.

Since those early studies, there have been more than 30 prospective observational studies of reduced risks of the development of elevated depression symptoms among physically active people and at least 25 randomized controlled trials testing whether exercise training can reduce symptoms in adults diagnosed with a mood disorder, mainly major depression. In 1984, the National Institute of Mental Health Workshop on Exercise and Mental Health concluded that exercise was associated with a decreased level of mild to moderate depression (Morgan and Goldston 1987). That conclusion was upheld at the Second International Consensus Symposium on Physical Activity, Fitness, and Health held in Toronto in 1992 (Bouchard, Shephard, and Stephens 1994), the 1996 U.S. surgeon general's report, *Physical Activity and Health*, and the scientific advisory committee of the 2008 *Physical Activity Guide-*

Diagnostic and Statistical Manual of Mental Disorders (DSM-IV) Criteria for Major Depression

At least five of the following symptoms are present during the same 2-week period, one of which must be either depressed mood or loss of interest or pleasure:

1. Depressed mood most of the day, nearly every day (can be irritable mood in adolescents or children)

2. Markedly diminished interest or pleasure in all, or almost all, activities most of the day, nearly every day

3. Significant weight loss or gain without dieting

4. Insomnia or hypersomnia

5. Psychomotor agitation or retardation

6. Fatigue or loss of energy

7. Feelings of lethargy or restlessness

8. Feelings of worthlessness or excessive guilt

9. Impaired concentration or indecisiveness

10. Recurrent thoughts of death or suicide

To be diagnosed as major depression, the symptoms should not meet criteria for mania, should not be due to direct physiological effects of a substance (e.g., alcohol) or to a general medical condition (e.g., hypothyroidism), and cannot be better accounted for by bereavement.

Based on American Psychiatric Association.

lines for Americans. The documentation of an association between exercise and the reduction in symptoms of mild to moderate depression has come from population studies, narrative and quantitative reviews (i.e., meta-analyses) of the research literature, and exercise training studies conducted with clinical and nonclinical populations.

Most studies of exercise and depression have involved young to middle-aged adults. Too few studies have been done with children to permit a conclusion. Among people over age 65 (O'Connor, Aenchbacher, and Dishman 1993), the evidence suggests that the benefits of exercise for *reducing* symptoms of depression may diminish as people age; however, despite more

> The benefits of physical activity for helping prevent depression apparently occur regardless of people's age, sex, race, or socioeconomic status.

age-related symptoms of depression among older people (e.g., sleep and cognitive disorders), older adults have a lower prevalence of clinically diagnosed depression than young and middle-aged adults do. The benefits of physical activity for helping *prevent* depression usually occur regardless of people's age, sex, race, or socioeconomic status.

Preventing Depression: Population Studies

Two main types of study designs have been used to examine the protective association between physical activity and depression symptoms. Most studies, especially early ones, have sampled a cross section of time, measuring physical activity and depression simultaneously. Those studies can't determine whether physical activity reduced depression or depression reduced people's physical activity levels. During the past decade or so, many studies have used prospective cohort designs that measure physical activity first and then track depression symptoms that appear years later. When these longitudinal studies control for confounders that are associated with both low physical activity and depression symptoms, they provide much stronger evidence that physical activity reduces depression.

Cross-Sectional Studies

An association between leisure-time physical activity and reduced symptoms of depression among adults has been generally supported in more than 100 population-based, cross-sectional observational studies from many countries published since 2000, including nationally representative samples of nearly 200,000 Americans. Active people on average had nearly 45% lower odds of depression symptoms than did inactive people. In the national samples of Americans, active people had approximately 30% lower odds of depression. The studies did not have the temporal sequencing needed to infer that lower depression resulted from more physical activity and often failed to adjust for other risk factors of depression that might have also been less prevalent among more active people. Nonetheless, these studies provide some evidence for dose–response associations and consistency across population subgroups (Physical Activity Guidelines Advisory Committee 2008).

U.S. National Comorbidity Survey Goodwin (2003) analyzed data from the U.S. National Comorbidity Survey (n = 5,877), a nationally representative sample of adults ages 15 through 54 in the United States. People who said they regularly participated in physical exercise for recreation or at work had 25% lower odds of being diagnosed with major depression during the past year after adjustment for age, sex, race, marital status, education, income, physical illnesses, and other mental disorders. A 14% reduction in the odds of dysthymia and a 6% reduction in the odds of bipolar disorder did not reach statistical significance. However, there was a dose–response reduction in the odds of major depression, dysthymia, and bipolar disorder with higher frequencies of physical activity (see figure 7.5).

CARDIA A history of elevated depression symptoms was measured by the CES-D scale (the number of times scores were 16 or more from three assessments, years 5, 10, and 15 of follow-up) in black (1,157 men and 1,480 women) and

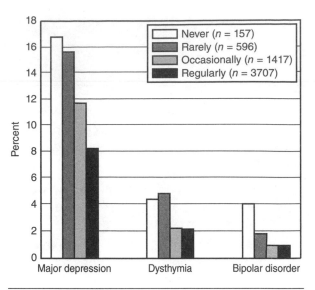

Figure 7.5 Twelve-month prevalence rates of mood disorders according to the frequency of physical activity in the U.S. National Comorbidity Survey.

Data from Goodwin 2003.

white (1,171 men and 1,307 women) Americans enrolled in the Coronary Artery Risk Development in Young Adults study (CARDIA; Knox et al. 2006). After adjustment for age, education, alcohol use, smoking, and body mass index (BMI), there was an inverse association (about 28 fewer METs during the past year for each episode of elevated depression symptoms) between a history of depression symptoms and physical activity at year 15 that was consistent across race.

Medical Expenditure Panel Survey A nationally representative survey of the U.S. population in 2003 asked 23,283 adults whether they engaged in moderate or vigorous activity 30 minutes or more, three times per week (Morrato et al. 2007). Information on sociodemographic characteristics and medical conditions, including depressive disorder or major depression diagnosed according to the International Classification of Diseases-version 9, was obtained. Odds of depression were 40% lower in people who were physically active. Lower odds of depression in active people were attenuated but remained significant after adjustment for sex, age, race and ethnicity, education, income, BMI, cardiovascular disease, hypertension, hyperlipidemia, and physical disability.

2006 Behavioral Risk Factor Surveillance Survey The 2006 Behavioral Risk Factor

Surveillance Survey was a random-digit-dialed telephone survey of 217,379 participants in 38 states, the District of Columbia, Puerto Rico, and the U.S. Virgin Islands (Strine et al. 2008). Current symptoms of moderate depression (except thoughts of suicide) were assessed with the Patient Health Questionnaire, which is based on *DSM-IV* diagnostic criteria. People reported whether they had ever been told by a physician or health provider that they had a depressive disorder (including depression, major depression, dysthymia, or minor depression). Regardless of age, inactive people (24% of those sampled) were three times more likely to have current depression symptoms and 50% more likely to have a lifetime diagnosis of depression. After adjustment for age, sex, race and ethnicity, education, marital and job status, chronic medical conditions (CVD, diabetes, asthma), smoking, obesity (BMI ≥ 30 kg/m^2), and heavy alcohol use (drinks per day: >2 men; >1 women), those risks remained elevated at 100% and 20%, respectively.

Netherlands Twin Registry The Netherlands Twin Registry sample consisted of 12,450 adolescents (at least 10 years old) and adults who participated in a study on lifestyle and health from 1991 to 2002 (De Moor et al. 2006). Exercise participation was defined as at least an hour each week in activities rated at 4 METs or more. After adjustment for sex and age, the odds of symptoms of depression were approximately 17% lower among exercisers. However, that association was likely confounded by personality because the exercisers also were more extroverted and emotionally stable, traits that reduce the risks of anxiety (see chapter 6) and depression disorders. In fact, among pairs of identical twins (479 males and 943 females) aged 18 to 50, the twin who exercised more did not report fewer symptoms of depression than the one who exercised less (De Moor et al. 2008). Also, longitudinal analysis (follow-up ranged from 2 to 11 years) showed that increases in exercise participation did not predict decreases in symptoms of depression.

Prospective Cohort Studies

More than 30 population-based prospective studies of exercise and depression have been

---

Examples of Methods to Assess Depression

Self-Report Population or Community Screening

Center for Epidemiological Studies (CES-D: 21 items; CES-D 10: 10-items; CED-DC for adolescents aged 12-18: 20-items)

Geriatric Depression Scale (GDS: 30-items; shortened versions of 15, 12, and 10 items)

Self-Report of Clinical Symptoms

Beck Depression Inventory (BDI-II: 21 items)

Hospital Anxiety and Depression Scale (HADS: 7 depression items; also used as physician interview)

Interview by Trained Raters to Assess Clinical Symptoms and Diagnose

Montgomery-Asberg Depression Rating Scale (MADRS: 10 items for symptom severity)

Hamilton Rating Scale for Depression (HRSD: 21 items for symptom severity)

Structured Clinical Interview for Depression (SCID: semistructured interview for diagnosis)

---

reported around the world since the first one in 1988. They have included about 50,000 adults from studies from the United States and 11 other countries (Australia, Canada, China, Denmark, England, Finland, Germany, Israel, Italy, Netherlands, and Japan). Nearly all of them showed that symptoms of depression are more likely to appear among people who report little or no leisure-time physical activity. However, about half the results did not reach a high level of statistical significance, often because the sample sizes were too small (a fourth of the comparisons included 500 or fewer people) given relatively small and varying reductions in risk. Because the studies are prospective and satisfy temporal sequencing, the associations seen in cross-sectional studies were less likely to be explainable by people becoming less active after they experienced depression symptoms. The average follow-up was about 4 years (ranging from 9 months to 37 years).

When averaged across the studies, the odds of elevated symptoms were about 33% lower among active compared with inactive people, without adjustments for depression risk factors that might have differed between the active and inactive groups. After adjustment for risk factors, such as age, sex, race, education, income, smoking, alcohol use, chronic health conditions, and other social and psychological risk factors, the odds remained about 20% lower among active people (see figure 7.6).

The apparent protective effect of physical activity against depression is not limited to self-rated symptoms measured by questionnaires. At least 10 studies have reported lower rates of physician-diagnosed incident depression among people who were active at baseline. After adjustment for risk factors, such as age, sex, race, education, income, smoking, alcohol use, and medical conditions (but not psychiatric comorbidities), the average odds were about 25% lower among active people.

Alameda County Study
Participants in the Alameda County Study were 1,947 adults aged 50 to 94 living near Oakland and Berkeley, California, and were assessed in 1994 and then followed for 5 years (Strawbridge et al. 2002). The incident rate of depression measured using *DSM-IV* diagnostic criteria was 5.4% of the cohort. Physical activity was measured using an eight-point questionnaire assessing whether people never, sometimes, or often participated in four aspects of physical activity: physical exercise, active sports, long walks, and swimming. After adjustment for age, sex, ethnicity, financial strain, chronic health conditions, disability, BMI, alcohol use, smoking, and social relations, there was a 17% reduction in the risk of incident depression over 5 years for each point scored on the physical activity measure in 1994 (OR = 0.83; 95% CI: 0.73-0.96).

Australian Longitudinal Study on Women's Health
The Australian Longitudinal Study on Women's Health examined the dose–response relations between physical activity and depressive symptoms, using cross-sectional and prospective data from a population-based cohort of 9,207 middle-aged women who were assessed in 1996, 1998, and 2001 (Brown et al. 2005). Depression symptoms were lower with increasing levels of previous, current, and habitual activity. After adjustment for nation of birth, education, marital status, occupation, smoking,

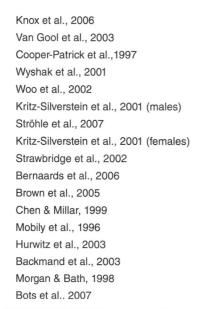

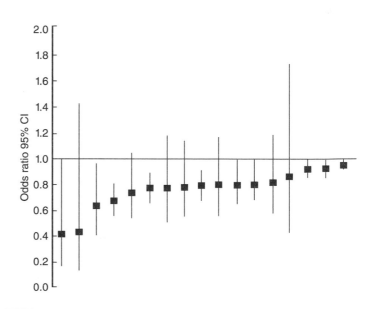

Figure 7.6 Adjusted odds ratios and 95% confidence intervals from prospective cohort studies published between 1995 and 2008.

Data from Physical Activity Guidelines Advisory Committee 2008.

BMI, menopause, health conditions, and scores on another measure of feelings of depression and anxiety, odds ratios for elevated CES-D scores in 2001 were 30% to 40% lower among women who reported an hour or more of moderate-intensity physical activity per week currently or in the preceding years, compared with those who reported less than an hour.

In another cohort of 6,677 young women (22 to 27 years old in 2000), depressive symptoms were reported in 2000 and at follow-up in 2003 (Ball, Burton, and Brown 2009). Moderate physical activity was equivalent to 150 min of moderate-intensity activity per week. Women who were sedentary in 2000 (i.e., participated in no physical activity or very low levels) had a 25% reduction in adjusted odds of elevated depression symptoms in 2003 if they increased their activity to a moderate level and a 50% reduction if they became highly active by 2003 (see figure 7.7).

U.S. Black Women's Health Study A sample of 35,224 African American women ages 21 to 69 answered mailed questions on past and current exercise levels at baseline (1995) and follow-up (1997) (Wise et al. 2006). The Center for Epidemiologic Studies Depression Scale (CES-D) was used to measure elevated depressive symptoms in 1999. After adjustment for age, education,

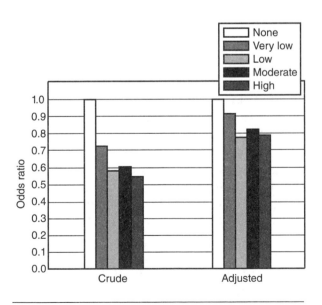

Figure 7.7 Dose–response of physical activity and incident reports of depression symptoms in the Australian Longitudinal Study on Women's Health.

Data from Ball, Burton, and Brown 2008.

occupation, marital status, BMI, heath conditions, smoking, alcohol use, and child care, the odds of elevated depressive symptoms were inversely related to weekly vigorous physical activity during adulthood up to 4 hours each week but not more. Women who said they got vigorous exercise both in high school (5 or more hours per week) and adulthood (2 or more hours per week) had a 25% reduction in the odds of depressive symptoms compared to women who said they were never active. Walking for exercise was not associated with a risk of depressive symptoms.

Copenhagen City Heart Study Leisure-time physical activity and potential confounders were measured in 18,146 residents of Copenhagen, Denmark, at baseline in 1976-1978 and again in 1981-1983 and 1991-1994 (Mikkelsen et al. 2010). Depression incident cases through 2002 were obtained from two Danish hospital registers according to ICD-8 or ICD-10 diagnostic criteria. Depression risk at each of the two follow-up assessments was predicted by physical activity and confounders measured at the preceding assessment (i.e., approximately 5 to 10 years earlier). Adjustments were made for age, education, and chronic diseases. Compared to women with a high physical activity level, women with a moderate level of physical activity had a 7% elevated risk of incident depression, whereas women with a low level of physical activity had an 80% higher risk. Compared with men with a high physical activity level, men with a moderate level of physical activity had an 11% higher risk of incident depression, whereas men with a low level of physical activity had a 39% higher risk (see figure 7.8).

Honolulu-Asia Aging Study A total of 1,282 elderly men 71 to 93 years of age reported their daily walking distance (12 city blocks = 1 mile, or 1.6 km) in 1991-1993 and their symptoms of depression 8 years later in 1999-2000 (Smith, Masaki, et al. 2010). Age-adjusted 8-year incidence rates of depression symptoms were 13.6%, 7.6%, and 8.5% for low (<0.25 miles, or 0.4 km, per day), moderate (0.25-1.5 miles, or 0-4-2.4 km, per day), and high (>1.5 miles, or 2.4 km, per day) walking groups. After adjustment for age, education, marital status, BMI, diabetes, alcohol use, smoking, cancer, Parkinson's disease,

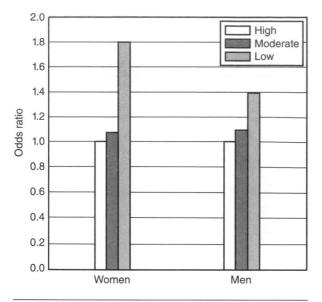

Figure 7.8 Copenhagen City Heart Study of incident depression in inactive women and men

Data from Mikkelsen et al. 2010.

cognitive impairment or dementia, and disability, men in the lowest walking group had 60% to 90% higher odds of incident depression symptoms than did the men in the moderate and high walking groups, respectively.

Taiwan's Health and Living Status of the Elderly Survey

A nationally representative cohort of 3,778 adults aged 50 and older in 1996 was followed in 1999 and 2003 (Ku, Fox, and Chen 2009). Adjustments were made for age, sex, education, marital status, living alone, satisfaction with income and social support, alcohol use, chronic diseases, and limitations in activities of daily living. People classified as low active (n = 1,139) in 1996 (they reported fewer than three sessions of physical activity each week in their leisure time) had 34% higher odds than active people (three sessions or more per week) of developing elevated depression symptoms in 2003. Participants who were low in leisure-time activity in both 1996 and 1999 (n = 818) had 40% higher odds of incident elevation in depression symptoms in 2003 than people who said they were active each time (n = 714).

Dose-Response Studies?

Fewer than 10 prospective cohort studies included the three or more levels of physical activity necessary for determining whether the odds of depression symptoms had a dose-gradient reduction with increased levels of exposure to physical activity (Physical Activity Guidelines Advisory Committee 2008). After adjustment for age, sex, and other risk factors, the reduction of odds was smaller for the lowest level of physical activity (OR = 0.86; 95% CI = 0.79-0.94) compared with the next two levels of physical activity, which did not differ (OR = 0.77; 95% CI = 0.72-0.82). Also, about half the prospective cohort studies provided enough information to determine whether active people were meeting public health recommendations for participation in moderate or vigorous physical activity (i.e., moderate-intensity aerobic physical activity for a minimum of 30 minutes on 5 days per week, or vigorous-intensity aerobic physical activity for a minimum of 20 minutes on 3 days per week). After adjustment for other risk factors, there was a protective benefit of moderate or vigorous physical activity (OR = 0.77; 95% CI = 0.72- 0.82) compared with people who were active but did not reach the recommended levels (OR = 0.84; 95% CI = 0.78-0.90). So, the evidence, although incomplete, supports a dose–response relationship between physical activity level and reduced depression scores that needs testing in randomized clinical trials.

Causality in Prospective Cohort Studies?

Longitudinal studies satisfy temporal sequence, but they cannot confirm that incident depression resulted in physical inactivity (De Moor et al. 2008). Even adjustment for confounders at baseline does not rule out that there could be residual confounding from other traits common to both physical activity and depression proneness. Results from the Canadian National Population Health Survey found that major depressive episodes were associated with a 60% increased risk of becoming physically inactive but not more active (Patten et al. 2009).

Findings from a cohort (n = 424) of adults diagnosed with major or minor depressive disorder (Research Diagnostic Criteria) found that physical activity counteracted the effects of medical conditions and negative life events on depression, but physical activity was not associated with subsequent depression (Harris,

Other research supports that physical activity and depression can influence each other. Annual assessments of 496 adolescent girls for 6 years found that physical activity reduced the risk of depressive symptoms and the onset of major or minor depression, but depressive symptoms and major or minor depression subsequently reduced future physical activity (Jerstad et al. 2010).

Cronkite, and Moos 2006). Measures of physical activity during the past month (swimming, tennis, and long hikes or walks), depression, and other demographic and psychosocial constructs were measured at baseline and 1 year, 4 years, and 10 years later. More physical activity was associated with less concurrent depression, even after controlling for sex, age, medical problems, and negative life events.

With few exceptions, past cohort studies were limited to just one or two estimates of physical activity exposure, despite follow-up periods lasting many years. Depression incidence rates were often not related to the dose of physical activity. However, previous studies relied on self-reports of physical activity (most without any corroborating evidence of validity) and used various criteria and methods to classify people into activity groups that were not equivalent across studies. None of the studies assessed change in physical activity exposure or sequential measures of outcome. This is necessary to estimate trajectories of change and judge misclassification errors resulting from people who over- or underreport their physical activity and to discount residual confounding by fluctuating traits common to physical inactivity and depression risk, including psychiatric comorbidities of depression such as anxiety and alcohol abuse or sleep disorders, which were not assessed in past studies. Cardiorespiratory fitness (CRF) provides an objective, surrogate measure of physical activity exposure. The decline in CRF seen in healthy adults during ages 40 through 60 is best explained by reduced moderate-to-vigorous

physical activity, after accounting for age, BMI, and smoking (Jackson et al. 2009).

The Aerobics Center Longitudinal Study was a prospect cohort study that included measures of fitness as well as depression symptoms. Cardiorespiratory fitness was assessed at four clinic visits, each separated by 2 or 3 years, to objectively measure cumulative physical activity exposure in 7,936 men and 1,261 women who had not complained of depression at their first clinic visit (Dishman et al. 2012). Across subsequent visits, there were 446 incident cases of depression in men and 153 cases in women. After adjustment for age, time between visits, BMI, and fitness at visit 1, each minute decline in treadmill endurance (i.e., a decline in fitness of one-half MET) between ages 51 and 55 in men and between ages 53 and 56 in women increased the odds of incident depression by approximately 2% and 9.5%, respectively. The increased odds remained significant but were attenuated to 1.3% and 5.4% after further adjustment for smoking, alcohol use, medical conditions, anxiety, and sleep problems. (See figure 7.9.) The results support

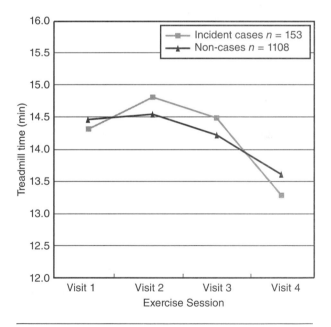

Figure 7.9 Decline in cardiorespiratory fitness and incident depression in women adjusted for age, time between visits, BMI, smoking, alcohol use, number of medical conditions, and complaints of anxiety or sleep problems.

Reprinted from *American Journal of Preventive Medicine*, Vol. 43(4), R.K. Dishman et al., 2012, "Decline in cardiorespiratory fitness and odds of incident depression," pgs. 361-368, copyright 2012, with permission from Elsevier.

Other Risk Factors for Depression Often Controlled Statistically in Population Studies

- Age
- Education
- Chronic conditions
- Social isolation
- Perceived health

- Physical disability
- Physical symptoms
- Autonomy
- Stressful life events (moving, job loss, separation or divorce, death of a spouse, and financial difficulties)

that the maintenance of cardiorespiratory fitness during late middle age, when decline in fitness typically accelerates, helps protect against the onset of depression complaints made to a physician.

Treating Depression: Experimental Studies

Most of the experimental research showing that exercise improves self-ratings of depressive mood has been done with mentally and physically healthy people, but some experiments involving people diagnosed with mild to moderate unipolar depression have shown improvements in mood after several weeks of moderately intense exercise. When the exercise program lasted several months, the improvements in people's self-ratings of depression were as large as those usually seen after psychotherapy. The best results for fighting depression occurred when outpatients were in an exercise program and also received psychotherapy. A few studies of exercise programs lasting 4 to 6 months showed improvements comparable to those typically seen after drug treatment. Although exercise appears comparable to drug therapy for treating mild to moderate depression, its clinical effects on reducing symptoms occur later than they do with drug therapy. The minimal or optimal type or amount of exercise for reducing depression is not yet known; but it appears that an increase in physical fitness is not required, and resistance exercise has been effective in a few studies.

Reviews and Meta-Analyses

Meta-analyses published in the past few years support earlier reviews of exercise and depression research, which concluded that exercise reduces depression symptoms in patients diagnosed as being depressed (Craft and Landers 1998; Martinsen 1990, 1993, 1994; Morgan 1994b; North, McCullagh, and Tran 1990). In addition, exercise training also reduces symptoms in patients who have a medical condition other than depression (see Recent Meta-Analyses of Randomized Controlled Trials of Depressed Patients sidebar for summaries of results). Evidence for improvements from limited research on acute exercise (Bartholomew, Morrison, and Ciccolo 2005) and substantial evidence at follow-up in exercise training studies suggests that the antidepressant effects of exercise are both immediate and long term. Exercise also compares well with traditional forms of treatment in these studies. In 40 studies that included 2,408 people without a clinical diagnosis of depression, those assigned to exercise training had nearly 0.60 SD lower depression scores than those allocated to a control treatment (Rethorst, Wipfli, and Landers 2009). A meta-analysis of 14 trials of chronic exercise among people diagnosed with depression (Lawlor and Hopker 2001) showed that exercisers had a 1.1 SD (95% CI = –1.5 to –0.60) reduction in depression symptoms measured using the Beck Depression Inventory compared with people who were not treated, which is equivalent to a 7-point reduction in symptoms (95% CI = –10.0 to –4.6) on a scale that ranges up to 61. People who score at least 10 are judged to be mildly depressed, and higher scores indicate increasingly severe depression. The effects of exercise were similar to the effects of cognitive psychotherapy.

A recent systematic review of 90 randomized controlled trials involving 10,534 sedentary adults with a chronic illness other than depression found that exercise training reduced depressive symptoms by a mean effect approximating 0.30 SD (95% CI = 0.25-0.36) (Herring et al. 2012). Larger antidepressant effects were obtained when (1) baseline depressive symptom scores were higher; (2) patients met recommended physical activity levels; and (3) the trial's primary outcome, predominantly function related, was significantly improved among patients with baseline depressive symptoms indicative of mild-to-moderate depression.

By comparison, psychotherapy trials show similarly sized effects when compared to a wait-list control group (0.88 SD), a usual-care control group (0.52 SD), or a pill placebo control group (0.36 SD) (Cuijpers et al. 2008a) and about 0.30 SD smaller effects (–0.28; 95% CI = –0.47 to –0.10) when compared to pharmacotherapy for the treatment of depression or dysthymia (Cuijpers et al. 2008b).

Nonetheless, exercise trials of depressed patients have had several scientific weaknesses that made it difficult to conclude that the reduced depression symptoms were the independent result of exercise (Krogh et al. 2010; Lawlor and Hopker 2001).

A clinical response in a treatment for depression is usually judged as favorable when the symptom reduction is 50% or more of the initial number, or strength, of symptoms. However, about half of patients who respond to treatment do not have remission of their symptoms, which is the desired end point of treatment. Remission is generally defined as a score of 7 or less on the 17-item HAM-D (HAM-D-17) physician rating scale, minimal or no symptoms of depression, loss of the diagnosis (i.e., the patient no longer meets the criteria for major depressive disorder listed in the *DSM-IV*), and the return of normal social and occupational function. Very few exercise trials have reported whether the reductions in symptoms were sufficient to indicate a favorable response or remission (e.g., Dunn et al. 2005; Singh et al. 2005).

Although the quality of the methods used in future randomized trials of aerobic and resistance exercise training for the treatment of depression symptoms should be improved (Physical Activity Guidelines Advisory Committee 2008), the limitations of research methods used in past exercise studies are also common in psychotherapy trials (Cuijpers et al. 2008b, 2010).

Exercise Training Studies

Most studies involving chronic exercise and depression have used an aerobic exercise intervention

> **B**oth aerobic exercise training and resistance exercise training have a positive effect on patients with clinical depression.

Some Method Flaws of Exercise Trials of Depressed Patients

- Use of volunteers
- Use of symptom ratings rather than clinical diagnoses as the measure of treatment response

- Failure to conceal group assignment
- Exclusion of dropouts from the treatment response tally

Adapted from Lawlor and Hopker 2001.

Recent Meta-Analyses of Randomized Controlled Trials of Depressed Patients

Mead and colleagues (2009): An update of the Lawlor and Hopker 2001 review located 23 randomized controlled trials of 907 adult patients diagnosed with depression, excluding women with postpartum depression.

- On average, exercise reduced symptoms by −0.82 SD (95% CI = −0.51 to −1.12).

- The effect was half that size, though, in the three trials judged by the authors to have the best quality control (e.g., treatments were concealed from the patients and dropouts were included in outcome assessments).

Rethorst and colleagues 2009: Seventeen studies that included 574 participants examined the effect of exercise on people clinically diagnosed as depressed.

- Clinically depressed participants in the exercise treatment had significantly lower depression scores than those receiving the control treatment (ES = −1.03 SD).

- The average change in BDI was 10.60, and the average change in HRSD was 8.11.

- Interventions lasting 10 to 16 weeks resulted in larger effects compared with interventions of 4 to 9 weeks in length (95% CI = 0.102-0.870), but effects were smaller in 13 trials lasting more than 16 weeks.

- The effects of studies that used adequate concealment were significantly larger than the effects of studies that did not use adequate concealment (95% CI = 0.106-0.893).

- Studies that used adequate intent to treat resulted in significantly larger effects than those that did not (95% CI = 0.357-1.340).

Krogh and colleagues 2011: Identified 8 of 13 trials that had adequate concealment of patient allocation to experimental groups.

- Six studies blinded raters of symptoms from knowing those group assignments.

- Six studies used intention-to-treat analyses (i.e., included dropouts in the average effect of exercise and control conditions).

- The mean effect of exercise was a 0.40 SD reduction in symptoms (95% CI = −0.66 to −0.14).

- Effects varied across studies and were inversely related to the length of the intervention, which ranged from 4 to 16 weeks.

- However, adherence ranged from 100% to 42%, and some of the longest trials had the lowest adherence and smallest effect on depression.

- The three studies judged to have the best research design (adequately concealed random assignment to groups, blinded outcome assessment, and intention-to-treat analysis) had a smaller effect that was not statistically significant (−0.19 SD; 95% CI = −0.70-0.31).

- Each of those three studies compared exercise to another group that might have been an active treatment without aerobic or resistance exercise (e.g., stretching or relaxation exercises or biweekly visits with a psychiatrist) rather than to a control that received no treatment (e.g., a group that was untreated but was offered the exercise program after the control period passed).

- Placebo comparisons judge whether exercise is better than some other minimally effective treatment, but they underestimate the efficacy of exercise alone, which is also important to know given the high number of people with depression who do not seek treatment from a health professional.

such as walking or jogging. However, the types of people studied, degree of initial depression, use of comparison groups, measurement of depression, and implementation of the exercise program have varied among studies.

Martinsen, Medhus, and Sandvik (1985) and Martinsen, Hoffart, and Solberg (1989) examined the effects of exercise training on depression in hospitalized psychiatric patients diagnosed with major depression. In the first study, 43 patients were randomly assigned to either exercise or an occupational therapy control group in addition to their standard treatment, which included psychotherapy and medication. After 9 weeks of training, patients in the exercise group exhibited significantly larger reductions in self-reported symptoms of depression relative to the control group. In the second study, 99 inpatients diagnosed with unipolar depressive disorders (major depression, dysthymic disorder, and atypical depression) were randomly assigned to either aerobic or nonaerobic exercise. After 8 weeks of training, both groups exhibited significant reductions in depression scores. However, the change in depression scores did not differ between the two conditions, although the aerobic group exhibited significant increases in maximal oxygen uptake ($\dot{V}O_2$max) compared to no change in $\dot{V}O_2$max for the nonaerobic group. Thus, both forms of exercise were effective in reducing depressive symptoms.

Doyne and colleagues (1987) compared the effectiveness of aerobic exercise and resistance exercise in decreasing depression. Forty females aged 18 to 35 who were diagnosed according to Research Diagnostic Criteria for depression were assigned to aerobic exercise (running) or weightlifting groups. After 8 weeks of exercise training, both exercise groups exhibited significant reductions in depression scores while the wait-list control group exhibited no changes. The reduction in depression scores was similar for the two forms of exercise. Results from these two studies imply that changes in aerobic capacity are not necessary to realize antidepressant effects of physical activity.

Singh, Clements, and Fiatarone (1997) conducted a 10-week progressive resistance exercise training study among elderly subjects who met *DSM-IV* criteria for major or minor depression

or dysthymia. Compared to a health education comparison group, the resistance exercisers had larger reductions (about 4-5 SD) in depressive symptoms on both Beck Depression Inventory self-ratings and diagnostic interview ratings by clinicians.

Fremont and Craighead (1987) compared aerobic exercise to traditional psychotherapy for depression in a sample of 49 men and women 19 to 62 years of age with self-reported symptoms of mild-to-moderate depression. Participants were randomly assigned to a supervised running group, individual cognitive psychotherapy, or combined running and psychotherapy. After 10 weeks of treatment, all groups exhibited significant reductions in depression scores, but there were no differences among the groups (see figure 7.10). Thus, exercise was found to be as effective as traditional psychotherapy, but there was no additional benefit when exercise was added to psychotherapy.

Aerobic exercise was compared to standard medication in a training study of 156 older men and women who were clinically diagnosed with major depressive disorder (Blumenthal et al. 1999). Participants were randomly assigned to aerobic exercise, antidepressants, or combined exercise and medication. After the 16-week program, all three groups demonstrated similar decreases in depression that were statistically and clinically significant. The medication-only group exhibited the fastest initial response; but

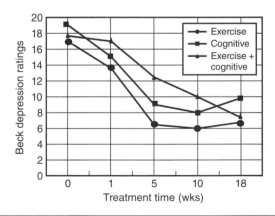

Figure 7.10 Changes in self-reported symptoms of depression for men and women randomly assigned to supervised running, individual cognitive psychotherapy, or running plus psychotherapy.

Data from Fremont and Craighead 1987.

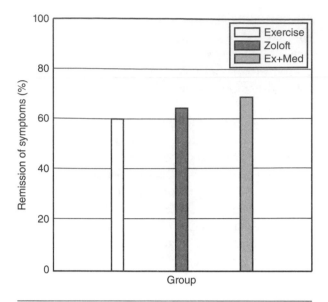

Figure 7.11 Remission rates after 16 weeks for groups of older men and women clinically diagnosed with major depressive disorder randomly assigned to groups receiving antidepressant medication, aerobic exercise, or aerobic exercise plus medication.

Data from Blumenthal et al. 1999.

by the end of the program, the exercise treatment was equally effective in reducing depression in this older sample (see figure 7.11). A follow-up study of these older men and women reported that patients in the exercise group were more likely to be fully recovered and less likely to have relapsed into depression 6 months after treatment than the drug treatment patients were (Babyak et al. 2000).

How Much Is Enough?

It is important to learn how much physical activity is minimally or optimally needed to help protect against or treat depression. At present, there does not seem to be a clear dose–response relationship between the intensity or total amount of daily physical activity and depression. On balance, though, it appears that being sedentary increases the risk for depression but that high levels of exercise may not be more protective against depression than lower levels.

In the Canada Fitness Survey (Stephens 1988), people were seemingly protected from symptoms of depression when their daily leisure energy expenditure was at least 1 kilocalorie per kilogram of body weight per day, which is a low

level of activity (e.g., about 20 min of walking). The risk of depression was not further reduced when the energy expenditure was raised to 2 to 5 kilocalories per kilogram of body weight per day.

Data from the Harvard alumni study (Paffenbarger, Lee, and Leung 1994) did suggest a dose-dependent reduction in depression with increased exercise; this occurred after more than 3 hours of vigorous sports or 2,500 kilocalories of expenditure per week (see figure 7.12). However, the significance of those findings is limited, because fewer than 1 in 10 adults in the United States expend this much energy in leisure-time physical activity.

The effects of setting and exercise intensity on depressive mood were examined in a study of 357 healthy older adults without clinical depression (King, Taylor, and Haskell 1993). Sedentary men and women ages 50 to 65 were randomly assigned to one of three exercise training programs (i.e., high-intensity group exercise, high-intensity home exercise, and low-intensity home exercise). After 12 months, no

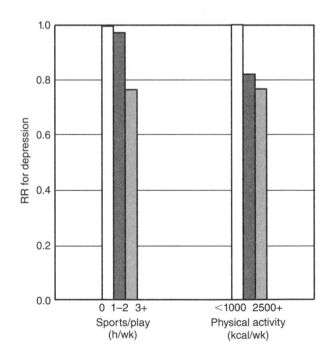

Figure 7.12 The analysis of activity habits from 1962 through 1966 and the incidence of depression during 23- to 27-year follow-ups among Harvard alumni (*n* = 10,201 males) shows that relative risk (RR) for depression was improved with some regular activity.

Data from Puffenbarger, Lee, and Leung 1994.

Exercise Can Benefit Depression During Recovery From Physical Illness

About a dozen experiments have shown that patients recovering from a heart attack report a moderate reduction in self-rated depression (about 1/2 SD) when they participate in a cardiac rehabilitation exercise program (Kugler, Seelbach, and Kruskemper 1994). Improvements in symptoms of depression have also been reported among breast cancer survivors who exercised (Segar et al. 1998).

significant differences among the groups were observed. However, subsequent data analysis revealed an inverse relationship between the level of exercise participation and depression scores independent of exercise format and intensity.

About three-fourths of the randomized controlled trials of healthy adults and nonpsychiatric medical patients used a moderate-to-vigorous exercise intensity of 60% to 80% of people's aerobic capacity or maximal strength that occurred 3 days per week. Intensity was lower or the frequency was 2 days per week in the other studies. The average duration of each session was about 35 minutes, but it was less than 30 minutes in a fourth of the studies and more than 1 hour in another fourth of the studies. However, fewer than half the studies were clear about how the time was partitioned into warm-up, exercise, and cool-down. Nonetheless, reductions in depression symptoms have not consistently differed across these varying features of exercise. However, those studies did not experimentally examine whether the apparently antidepressant effects of physical activity depend on the type or amount of physical activity. Two of three well-executed studies of depressed patients have shown a dose–response effect on symptom reduction.

Aerobic Exercise DOSE Study

The DOSE study was the first randomized controlled trial designed to test the dose–response relationship between aerobic exercise and reduction in depressions symptoms in patients (Dunn et al. 2005). Eighty adults diagnosed with mild-to-moderate major depressive disorder were assigned to either a placebo control (3 days per week of flexibility exercise) or to one of four solitary aerobic exercise treatments conducted in a supervised laboratory, which varied by energy expenditure each session and weekly as follows: low dose (7.0 kcal/kg/week, or about 100 to 150 calories each session) or high dose (17.5 kcal/kg/week, or about 250 to 400 calories each session) and a weekly frequency of either 3 days or 5 days. The primary outcome was the score on a physician diagnostic rating scale of depression symptoms. Depression scores at 12 weeks were reduced by 47% from baseline in the high-dose group, compared with 30% and 29% for the low-dose and control groups, respectively. There was no main effect of exercise frequency at 12 weeks, but figure 7.13 shows that people in the high-dose group who exercised 5 days a week were about twice as likely to have a favorable response (i.e., a 50% or more reduction in their symptoms) and a remission in symptoms (i.e., no longer have enough symptoms to be judged as depressed).

Resistance Exercise Dose Study

Sixty community-dwelling adults aged 60 or older who had major or minor depression were randomized to usual care by a physician or to supervised progressive resistance exercise of high intensity (80% maximal load) or low intensity (20% maximal load) 3 days per week for 8 weeks (Singh et al. 2005). The rate of favorable response (i.e., a 50% reduction in physician-rated symptoms) in the high-intensity group (61% of those patients) was twice that of the low-intensity group (29%) and of the standard care group (21%).

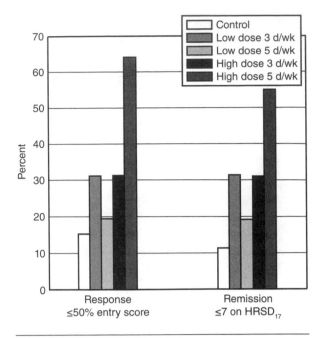

Figure 7.13 Changes in depression response and remission rates across two doses of exercise treatment.

Adapted from *American Journal of Preventive Medicine,* Vol. 28(1), A.L. Dunn et al., 2005, "Exercise treatment for depression: Efficacy and dose response," pgs. 1-8, copyright 2005, with permission from Elsevier.

DEMO Trial

The DEMO trial was a randomized pragmatic trial for patients with unipolar depression conducted from January 2005 through July 2007. Patients were referred from general practitioners or psychiatrists and were eligible if they fulfilled ICD-10 criteria for unipolar depression and were between 18 and 55 years old. Patients (*N* = 165) were allocated to two weekly sessions of supervised strength, aerobic, or relaxation training during a 4-month period (Krogh et al. 2009). The primary outcome measure was the

> **E**xcessive exercise training in athletics (i.e., overtraining) can induce depressive states in some athletes (Morgan 1994b). A majority of youth and adults are sedentary, though, so depression resulting from overtraining is not a concern for the general population.

> **B**eing sedentary increases the risk for depression, but high levels of physical activity may not be any more protective than moderate amounts of physical activity.

17-item Hamilton Rating Scale for Depression (HAM-D[17]), the secondary outcome measure was the percentage of days absent from work during the last 10 working days, and the tertiary outcome measure was cognitive abilities. Despite an increase in strength in the resistance group and maximal oxygen uptake in the aerobic group, changes in depression symptoms, or cognitive abilities, after 4 months were not different from those in the relaxation group. However, 40% of the participants left the study, and those who remained averaged just 1 day of supervised exercise each week, so the exposure to exercise may have been insufficient to affect symptoms. Exercise outside the program wasn't verified, so the fitness scores that were based on performance, not objective physiological criteria, might have improved because of a motivation to perform better the second time they were tested.

Although a few studies have tested the effects of resistance or flexibility exercise on depression, most have used jogging as the mode of activity; a few used cycling. Exercise training usually was prescribed based on the guidelines of the American College of Sports Medicine for the types and amounts of exercise recommended for cardiorespiratory fitness in otherwise healthy people (see table 15.4). Because no adverse effects were reported in these studies, the following exercise guidelines should be appropriate for people with depression who are otherwise healthy:

- 3 to 5 days a week
- 20 to 60 min each session
- 55% to 90% of maximal heart rate

People beginning an exercise program should always increase the intensity and length of their workouts gradually, but gradual progress is espe-

Weaknesses in research on exercise and depression include using subjects who were not depressed, measuring depression only with self-report, not including a placebo control group, and inadequately documenting the exercise stimulus used in the training protocol.

cially important for someone who is depressed. Gradual progress helps to maximize feelings of success, as well as to control and minimize potential feelings of failure that can arise if the person can't sustain the program because it calls for too quick a progression. It is important to remember that continued participation is more important for reducing depression than increasing fitness is.

PHARMACOTHERAPY

More than 30 drugs are being used worldwide to treat depression (see Common Antidepressant Drugs). In 2005, an estimated 27 million Americans used antidepressant medication, including 2.5% of children ages 6 to 17 (Olfson and Marcus 2009). Half the patients used the drugs for back or nerve pain, fatigue, sleep difficulties, or other problems aside from depression. Among American users of antidepressants, the percentage receiving psychotherapy fell from 31.5% in 1996 to less than 20% in 2005. About 80% of patients were treated by doctors other than psychiatrists.

The most common drugs used to treat depression are tricyclics, introduced in the 1940s, which block the reuptake of monoamines released by brain neurons; monoamine oxidase inhibitors (MAOIs), introduced in the 1950s, which block the deamination (i.e., metabolism) of monoamines after neuronal release; and selective serotonin reuptake inhibitors (SSRIs), introduced in the late 1980s, which block the reentry of serotonin into the neuron after release. The SSRIs are currently the most popular, not so much because they are more effective than the others but because they have fewer side effects (e.g., less sedation, dry mouth, dizziness, faintness, stomach upsets, and weight gain) than do the tricyclics and MAOIs.

During the 1990s, selective norepinephrine reuptake inhibitors (SNRIs; e.g., reboxetine), which selectively block the reuptake of norepinephrine, and drugs that simultaneously block the reuptake of both norepinephrine and serotonin (e.g., venlafaxine) or that block the reuptake of dopamine (e.g., amineptine and bupropion) more than norepinephrine and serotonin became popular. Some other tetracyclic antidepressants (also known as noradrenergic and specific serotonin antidepressants [NaSSAs]), first introduced in the 1970s, have a different chemical structure from tricyclics and MAOIs. They do not affect the reuptake or metabolism of monoamines; rather, they block receptors (e.g., mianserin blocks 5-HT2 [serotonin] receptors, and mirtazapine blocks α-2 [norepinephrine] autoreceptors). By blocking α-2 adrenergic autoreceptors, as well as α-1 and 5-HT3 receptors, NaSSAs enhance adrenergic and serotonergic neurotransmission, especially 5-HT1A-mediated transmission.

MECHANISMS

There is ample evidence that exercise is associated with decreases in depression, but we are still discovering the underlying reasons for these antidepressant effects. Explanations for this association are based on social, cognitive, and biological mechanisms. Possible social cognitive explanations for antidepressant effects associated with exercise programs include subjective

Tetracyclic Noradrenergic and Specific Serotonin Antidepressants

Mianserin (Bolvidon, Norval, Tolvon)

Mirtazapine (Remeron, Avanza, Zispin)

Setiptiline (Tecipul)

Recommendations for Supervising Exercise Training of Persons With Depression

- *Be familiar with the symptoms and basic treatment of mental disorders and have referral sources on hand.* If someone expresses emotional or psychological problems that seem to be beyond normal adjustment issues, you may want to express concern and have available some names and numbers of local resources to let the person know that professional help is available. Be tactful! It is important for all health care providers to be knowledgeable about how to recognize and respond to suicidal ideation. Familiarize yourself with commonly prescribed medications for depression. People may feel more comfortable reporting information about medications rather than providing a psychiatric diagnosis on the intake. Also, some medications may have side effects, such as weight gain or fatigue, that may influence a person's motivation to exercise.

- *Avoid minimizing the person's feelings or concerns.* Most people prefer someone who simply listens and exhibits compassion rather than someone who attempts to soothe or give advice. For person-centered psychotherapy, the core conditions for change are genuineness, empathy, and warmth. Avoid making your regard for the patient dependent upon the person's meeting your standards for exercise participation.

- *Establish boundaries in your relationships with your patients.* As you develop a rapport with your patients, it is likely that you will encounter someone who begins to think of you as a counselor. Be supportive and encouraging while avoiding fostering dependence. For most people you work with, this will not be a problem. However, a person with a mental disorder may latch onto the first individual who seems to take a sincere interest in his or her life, and boundaries may be difficult to establish. It is your responsibility to set the limits of your relationship with patients according to professional ethics and what is comfortable for you.

- *Assess current physical activity habits and fitness.* Because individuals with depression have difficulty managing time and accomplishing daily tasks, they may overestimate the amount and intensity of physical activity. Any activity may seem like a tremendous burden. For individuals who exhibit motor retardation and hypersomnia, daily activity may be reduced beyond that of a typical sedentary person and consequently their fitness may be low. People in this situation may question their ability to perform *any* exercise and should be reassured that the program will be designed specifically for them.

- *Determine the person's motivation for exercise.* What by-product of exercise has meaning for this person? Is the motivation internal or external? Are there specific goals the person wants to accomplish? Are these goals realistic? It is important to consider the individual's motivation in the context of his or her mental state in order to establish goals, prescribe the appropriate exercise, promote adherence, and help the person develop a positive perception of exercise and self.

- *Make the exercise enjoyable and non-threatening.* Since low motivation, fatigue, and reduced pleasure are core symptoms of depression, it is important to make the activity as pleasurable as possible. One way to do this is to find out what activities the individual has enjoyed in the past and create an environment that reflects his or her interests. Identify and minimize the features of exercise that the person finds intimidating. One individual may enjoy the social aspect of group aerobics while another finds a group atmosphere threatening. And although you want to avoid making the exercise too hard, it is also important to avoid making the exercise so easy that it seems like a waste of time or a "non-accomplishment."

(continued)

Recommendations . . . (continued)

• *Make the exercise accessible.* Getting the person to the exercise session may be the biggest hurdle. Discuss and develop plans for overcoming the barriers that could prevent the individual from attending an exercise session (time, transportation, work and family conflicts, etc). This step may require you to help the individual problem solve at the most basic level. For example, you may have to help work out an alternative plan if the person's spouse has to use the car at the scheduled exercise time.

• *Encourage personal responsibility by including the person in the planning of the exercise program.* The degree of control that the patient is willing or able to handle will vary with the individual. Avoid overwhelming people by giving them too much responsibility, but at the same time try to promote a sense of independence and accomplishment. Watch for cues that will let you know what is right for each person, and be ready to give or take more control as needed. Don't let the individual give you the credit for his or her success. Encourage the person to take pride in his or her accomplishments, no matter how small.

• *Be prepared for nonadherence and excuses.* It is important to be nonjudgmental. Avoid blaming, and try to minimize the opportunity for guilt and self-blame. Don't allow the individual to magnify a lapse into a total sense of failure. Plan for lapses and trouble situations, and problem solve in advance with the patient's input. Don't accept vague excuses; instead, identify a concrete, modifiable cause for the lapse and develop strategies to overcome the barrier. View lapses as a learning process, and establish an opportunity for success as soon as possible after a lapse.

• *Encourage the person to increase physical activity outside the established exercise sessions.* Set small, readily attainable activity goals (established by joint agreement) that the person can accomplish between sessions. Have the person keep a record of his or her activity habits, barriers/setbacks, exercise accomplishments, and so on to use as a tool for future problem-solving sessions. For example, use of step counters is a simple and inexpensive way to encourage self-monitoring and goal setting.

• *Watch for sabotage.* Habits, whether psychological or exercise-related, become comfortable, and any departure from that "comfort zone" may be resisted by the patient or by significant others who depend on that person to behave in a certain way. Thus, there may be subtle attempts by the patient or others to discourage change, and these potential deterrents of change should be identified and addressed directly.

• *Be aware of what behavior is being reinforced.* For many people, negative attention is better than no attention. If you always express concern for missed sessions or are more attentive when people appear anxious/depressed, then that behavior may increase. Positively reinforce the desired behavior in a way that is meaningful for the individual. Remember that what is reinforcing for one person may not be reinforcing for another.

Reprinted, by permission, from H.A. O'Neal, A.L. Dunn, and E.W. Martinsen, 2000, "Depression and exercise," *International Journal of Sport Psychology* 31(2): 133-135.

expectations, diversion from stressful stimuli, attention, improved self-image, feelings of control, social interaction, and social support (Ernst, Rand, and Stevinson 1998). Although plausible, these explanations have not been empirically tested in well-designed studies (O'Neal, Dunn, and Martinsen 2000). Also, even if shown to be true, they would not provide an explanation of a direct effect of physical activity independent of the setting in which the physical activity occurred. For example, in one study, 30 mildly depressed elderly men and women were randomly assigned to either 20 min of outdoor walking with a student or 20 min of social

Common Antidepressant Drugs

Tricyclics
Anafranil (clomipramine)
Asendin (amoxapine)
Aventyl (nortriptyline)
Elavil (amitriptyline)
Norpramin (desipramine)
Pamelor (nortriptyline)
Sinequan (doxepin)
Surmontil (trimipramine)
Tofranil (imipramine)
Vivactil (protriptyline)

Monoamine Oxidase Inhibitors
Marplan (isocarboxazid)
Nardil (phenelzine sulfate)
Parnate (tranylcypromine sulfate)

Selective Serotonin Reuptake Inhibitors
Celexa (citalopram)
Desyrel (trazodone); now available as generic
Lexapro (escitalopram)
Ludiomil (maprotiline)
Paxil (paroxetine)

Prozac (fluoxetine)
Selfemra (fluoxetine)
Zoloft (sertraline)

Selective Serotonin and Noradrenaline Reuptake Inhibitors
Cymbalta (duloxetine); for generalized anxiety disorder
Effexor (venlafaxine); for generalized anxiety disorder
Luvox (fluvoxamine)
Prixtiq (sustained-release desvenlafaxine)
Serzone (nefazodone)

Dopamine Agonists
Wellbutrin (bupropion); for panic disorder
Zyban (sustained-release bupropion)

The generic name of each drug appears in parentheses. Side effects include low blood pressure, blurred vision, irregular heartbeat, stomach and gastrointestinal upsets, male sexual dysfunction, and toxicity after extended use.

---

contact with a student twice weekly for 6 weeks, or to a wait-list control group (McNeil, LeBlanc, and Joyner 1991). As figure 7.14 shows, the reductions in depression after walking were the same as after merely meeting weekly with a student. Hence, it is possible that the social contact with the student was responsible for the depression reduction in both conditions. Walking might have been superfluous to the antidepressant effect.

Biological mechanisms offer more potential for establishing a direct, causal relationship. However, even biological explanations might not directly support an independent effect of exercise on reducing depression. For example, bright light treatment is effective for some depression; thus, exercising in bright sunlight might reduce depression more because of the light exposure than because of the exercise. Nonetheless, to support biological plausibility, explanations for reductions in depression with increased physical activity should be consistent with what is known about the etiology of depression and the biological adaptations that occur with physical activity.

Exercise may decrease depression because of psychosocial benefits, such as enhanced self-esteem or increased social support.

Proposed Psychosocial Mechanisms for Effects of Exercise on Depression

Subjective expectations: Prevailing folk wisdom is that exercise makes you feel better, so people might begin exercise with the expectation that their moods will improve (placebo effect).

- *Diversion from stressful stimuli*: Decreases in anxiety and depression may be explained by a "time-out," or distraction, from worries and concerns during an exercise session. The psychological respite from stress emotions may have residual effects that are strengthened with each exercise session, and the mood improvement can reinforce repeated bouts of activity.

- *Attention*: People involved in exercise programs typically have one-on-one contact with fitness professionals and other participants. The positive attention from others may foster a sense of value and self-worth because the person feels important to others.

- *Improved self-image*: Physical adaptations to regular exercise include some cosmetic benefits, such as increased muscle tone, in addition to improved exercise tolerance.

Physical self-concept can be enhanced, and along with it self-esteem, which is a critical psychological variable in mental health.

- *Feelings of control*: Feelings of helplessness and hopelessness are core in depression. Participation in exercise enables depressed people to exert control over one aspect of their lives. Reestablishing a sense of power in one area may transfer to perceptions of control in other areas of life and increase a sense of hope.

- *Social interaction*: Social isolation can be a contributing and sustaining factor in depression, and participating in exercise programs in a hospital, community center, or commercial fitness center can provide personal contact that may decrease a sense of isolation.

- *Social support*: Exercising with others can offer depressed people opportunities for tangible and intangible validation that they are important to others, as well as instilling a sense of being part of a community.

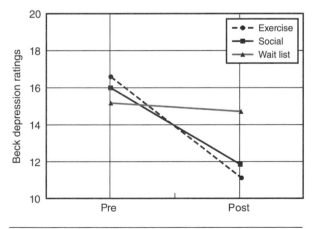

Figure 7.14 Reduction of depression after an exercise program (walking) versus regularly scheduled social contact with another person.

Reprinted, by permission, J.K. McNeil, E.M. LeBlanc, and M. Joyner, 1991, "The effect of exercise on depressive symptoms in the moderately depressed elderly," *Psychology and Aging* 6(3): 487-488.

Neurobiology of Depression

Some background on the etiology of depression can help in making the link between changes in symptoms of depression and exercise adaptations. The two most prominent neurobiological models of depression are the monoamine depletion hypothesis and the hypothalamic-pituitary-adrenal (HPA) axis model.

> The biological basis of depression is centered in dysregulation of the monoamine system and the HPA axis.

Monoamine Depletion Hypothesis

Critical insight into the neurobiology of depression began to develop in the 1950s when unexpected psychological side effects were noted from medications prescribed for physical illnesses. Depressive symptoms were found in 15% of hypertensive patients treated with reserpine. Reserpine controls blood pressure by inactivating storage granules containing norepinephrine (NE) and serotonin (5-HT) in peripheral nerves, thus depleting NE and serotonin intracellularly. Because it is an alkaloid, reserpine can cross the blood–brain barrier. Hence, a side effect appeared to be the depletion of NE and serotonin in the brain, contributing to depressed mood in some people. About the same time, improved mood was observed as a side effect of treating tuberculosis with iproniazid, which inhibits monoamine oxidase (MAO), an enzyme that degrades NE and 5-HT. Studies conducted in the 1960s and 1970s showed reduced levels of metabolites of NE (i.e., MHPG, see chapter 3) and metabolites of serotonin (i.e., 5-HIAA) in some depressed populations compared to people without clinical disorders. In addition, patients who had bipolar depression secreted low levels of MHPG (NE metabolite) when depressed and above-normal levels when manic. The evidence for a relationship between the levels of NE, serotonin, or both, and depression led to the **monoamine depletion hypothesis** of depression.

According to the monoamine depletion hypothesis, depression is caused by a deficiency of NE at central **adrenergic** receptors, or a deficiency of serotonin, or both, and mania results from excessive NE. Norepinephrine and serotonin, as discussed previously, are major neurotransmitters whose functions in modulating most brain areas involved in stress and mood make them prime candidates in the etiology of depression (see table 7.2 and Biogenic Amines in chapter 3). In addition, a structural and functional relationship exists between **noradrenergic** and serotonergic systems. For example, there are projections from the locus coeruleus (LC), the main NE-producing cell in the brain stem, to the raphe nuclei that synthesize brain serotonin, as well as to serotonin-producing cells surrounding the LC.

In support of the depletion hypothesis, the primary action of several antidepressant medications is to increase levels of NE, serotonin, or both. Most common antidepressant drugs upregulate central nervous system α-adrenergic and serotonergic receptors, down-regulate β-adrenergic receptors, and/or desensitize the postsynaptic second messenger (adenylate cyclase), or prevent the metabolism of neurotransmitters after they are released (see table 7.3). Antidepressants are significantly more

Table 7.2 Functions of Norepinephrine and Serotonin in the Central Nervous System

Norepinephrine	Serotonin
Hormonal release	Sensory perception
Cardiovascular functioning	Regulation of pain
Rapid eye movement sleep	Fatigue
Analgesic responses	Appetitive behavior
Arousal	Periodicity of sleep
Reward	Temperature regulation
Sexual behavior	Corticosteroid activity
Vigilance	Dreams
Regulation of mood	

Table 7.3 Classes of Antidepressant Drugs

Drug class	Actions
Tricyclics (TCAs)	Alter the brain's responses to the neurotransmitters norepinephrine (NE) and serotonin (i.e., prevent reuptake of NE and serotonin by blocking presynaptic receptors). Keep neurotransmitters in contact with postsynaptic receptors, which prolongs the effects.
Monoamine oxidase inhibitors (MAOIs)	Block the action of an enzyme (MAO) that breaks down the transmitters NE, dopamine, and serotonin within the neuron.
Selective serotonin reuptake inhibitors (SSRIs)	Target the serotonergic system and enhance the activity of serotonin by preventing its reuptake by the neuron after release into the synapse.

effective than placebo for treating depressive disorders (Williams et al. 2000). Drug treatment alters the levels of NE and serotonin within hours—but changes in symptoms do not occur for about 2 to 3 weeks.

The delay in symptom reduction when levels of neurotransmitters were increased challenged the monamine depletion hypothesis. The etiology and maintenance of depression are not as simple as a deficiency of NE or serotonin, and ensuing studies have not supported the depletion of neurotransmitters as a cause of depression. For example, some depressed patients have high or normal levels of MHPG, and lower levels of MHPG in the cerebral spinal fluid (CSF) have not been verified. Two effective treatments for depression, electroconvulsive shock treatment and the drug iprindole, do not affect monoamine levels (Maas 1979).

The monoamine model was modified to describe depression as a function of **dysregulation** of the noradrenergic and serotonergic systems rather than only a matter of decreased transmitter levels. Depression is thought to result from a disruption in these neurotransmitter systems' self-regulating abilities and from the overstimulation of neural centers such as the prefrontal cortex, amygdala, hippocampus, and periventricular gray. A major proposed site of dysregulation is the LC.

A key response to low levels of NE is up-regulation (i.e., an increase in the number or sensitivity) of postsynaptic β-1 receptors for NE. That response can then lead to a hyper-responsiveness of neurons to NE when it is released into the synapse. A hallmark feature of a therapeutic response to antidepressant drugs is the down-regulation of β-1 receptors and a return to normal sensitivity to NE. An intact brain serotonergic system is needed for that response.

In addition, presynaptic α-2 autoreceptors are normally involved in negative feedback to control the release of NE. With decreased levels of NE, there is decreased self-inhibition of the LC by its α-2 autoreceptors. Negative feedback is removed, leading to the excessive release of NE from LC neurons. That response can lead to a temporary depletion of NE in the brain because of the excessive firing of NE cells during stress. Because the main action of NE is to modulate the firing rates of other cells in the brain by inhibition, the result can be a hyperactivity of the neural centers that regulate negative moods such as depression.

Much of the physiological research on depression has focused on the brain monoaminergic systems, particularly noradrenergic and serotonergic systems. However, the monoamine dopamine (DA) should also be considered in the etiology of depression (O'Neal, Dunn, and Martinsen 2000). A main area of DA-producing cells in the brain is the ventral tegmental area (VTA). Electrical stimulation of the VTA and the surrounding portions of the hypothalmus produces pleasure. Although NE is not a major neurotransmitter in the VTA, the depletion of brain NE appears to indirectly suppress the normal activity of DA in the VTA. The DA system plays a critical role in reward, motivation, and motor functions. For example, natural rewards and reinforcement involve the release of DA in the nucleus accumbens, where some DA receptors contain encephalin and dynorphin opioids that help regulate motivation and pleasure (see chapter 3).

Thus, dysregulation of this system may contribute to the anhedonia (i.e., loss of pleasure) and psychomotor disturbances that are observed in depression. For example, disturbances in dopaminergic projections to limbic structures have been shown in response to prolonged elevations in corticotropin-releasing hormone (CRH) and cortisol with chronic stress (Chrousos 1998), and certain antidepressant drugs influence dopaminergic activity by targeting DA receptors or altering DA metabolism (Willner 1995).

Hypothalamic-Pituitary-Adrenal (HPA) Axis Model

The integration of neurobiological systems (i.e., HPA axis and monoamine) in depression is illustrated by the need for adequate concentrations of **glucocorticoids** for normal NE function (Gold and Chrousos 1999). There is considerable evidence that the HPA axis plays an integral role in the etiology of depression. For example, symptoms of depression, such as weight loss and sleep disturbances, can be directly linked to disruptions in the HPA axis.

The HPA axis plays a major role in the stress response (see chapter 4), and a dysregulation in the stress response has been implicated in the etiology of depression. When a real or imagined threat is perceived, the paraventricular nucleus (PVN) of the hypothalamus releases CRH into the median eminence of the anterior pituitary. Corticotropin-releasing hormone acts on the pituitary to signal the release of adrenocorticotropic hormone (ACTH) and β-endorphin from the precursor molecule, proopiomelanocorticotropin. Adrenocorticotropic hormone then exerts its effect on the adrenal gland to stimulate the increased synthesis and release of cortisol from the adrenal cortex. The integrated function of this system is to prepare the body for fight or flight. (Please refer to chapter 3 and see chapter 4 for a more detailed description of the physiological response to stress.)

Although the activation of this system is critical for an appropriate stress response, excess activation of the HPA axis may play a role in the development of depression. In fact, symptoms of melancholia resemble a state of profound stress and can be precipitated by stress (Gold

> ### Functions of the Hypothalamic-Pituitary-Adrenal (HPA) Axis
>
> - Regulation of hunger and satiety
> - Sexual behavior
> - Sleep
> - Growth
> - Hormonal secretions
> - Regulation of the physiological response to stress

and Chrousos 1999). Hippocampal cells contain glucocorticoid receptors that mediate the suppression of the CRH neuron in the hypothalamus (see figure 7.15). Normally, when high levels of cortisol feed back to glucocorticoid receptors at the level of the hippocampus and hypothalamus, there is a subsequent *reduction* in the production of CRH and corticosteroid secretions (i.e., negative feedback—output inhibits the activity of the initial input). However, hypercortisolism can damage the hippocampal glucocorticoid receptors that inhibit feedback from the HPA axis, down-regulating the hippocampal receptors and leading to the overactivation of the HPA axis. Hypercortisolism may also result in abnormally high levels of cortisol and ACTH by altering the brain stem monoaminergic system or other neural systems that regulate HPA function, such as the amygdala and prefrontal cortex (Gold and Chrousos 1999). Indeed, hypercortisolism is found in about 50% of depressed patients. With depression, there is also an overall increase in ACTH, a loss of sensitivity in steroid-negative feedback, and an increased sensitivity to all doses of CRH. Because CRH and glucocorticoids influence the limbic structures important in emotional responding, including the nucleus accumbens, amygdala, and hippocampus, elevated levels of CRH and cortisol under conditions of chronic stress may disrupt functioning in the brain regions that regulate emotion (Gold and Chrousos 1999).

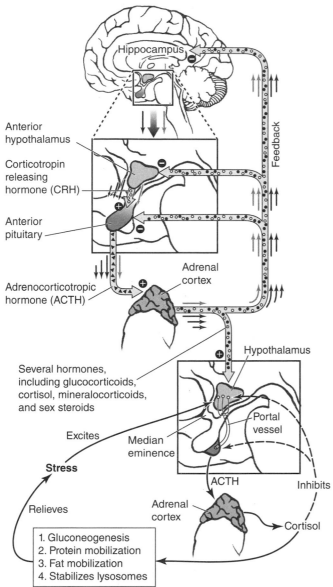

Anterior hypothalamus releases CRH (circadian rhythms and in response to physical and mental stress) into the hypothalamic-hypophyseal portal vessels to travel to the *anterior pituitary*. Receptors for cortisol provide feedback inhibition of CRH release. ⊖

Anterior pituitary responds to CRH by the co-secretion of *ACTH* and ß-*endorphin* into the circulation. ⊕Receptors for cortisol provide feedback inhibition of ACTH release.⊕

Adrenal cortex is activated by *ACTH*⊕to secrete *cortisol*.

Cortisol affects metabolism of carbohydrate, protein, and fat and is also involved in stress response and depression.

Elevated levels of cortisol feed back to receptors on the hippocampus and signals from the hippocampus inhibit the secretion of CRH by the anterior hypothalamus. There are also cortisol receptors on the anterior hypothalamus and anterior pituitary that are involved in feedback inhibition of CRH and ACTH, respectively, with high levels of cortisol. Thus, the outcome of elevated cortisol levels is an eventual reduction in secretion to return levels to normal.

Abnormal pattern. High levels of cortisol damage hippocampus receptors, removing feedback inhibition of the HPA axis. Continued release of CRH results in high levels of ACTH and sustained oversecretion of cortisol.

Figure 7.15 Actions and effects of corticotropin-releasing hormone on the hypothalamic-pituitary-adrenal (HPA) axis (normal and abnormal patterns).

Redrawn, by permission, from M.R. Rosenzweig, A.L. Leiman, and S.M. Breedlove, 1999, *Biological psychology: An introduction to behaviorial, cognitive, and clinical neuroscience,* 2nd ed. (Sunderland, MA: Sinauer Associates), 125.

Evidence for the Biological Plausibility of Exercise Affecting Depression

There are virtually no studies examining the biological mechanisms that could explain the antidepressant effects of physical activity and exercise among humans. However, several encouraging lines of research using the methods of neuroscience and animal models of stress and depression have emerged in exercise psychology during the past decade.

Monoamine Dysregulation Hypothesis

According to the **monoamine dysregulation hypothesis**, depression is the result of a dysregulation in the biogenic monoamine system. Thus, exercise may decrease depression by exerting

> **E**xercise may decrease depression through adaptations such as the increased synthesis of NE and serotonin in the central nervous system.

a regulatory influence on this neurotransmitter system. For example, there is some evidence that chronic exercise affects NE and 5-HT receptors on the brain stem, and brain stem NE neurons project to the ventral tegmentum area, a major reward center. Exercise adaptations, such as the increased synthesis of monoamines, could affect limbic structures through a connection with motor neurons; and sensory afferents from muscles could stimulate higher brain centers by way of the thalamus.

The aim of a number of human and animal studies has been to describe the effects of exercise on NE and its synthesis and metabolism. In humans, changes in brain NE activity after acute physical activity have been estimated by measuring levels of MHPG (the primary NE metabolite) in urine, plasma, or (rarely) cerebral spinal fluid. Studies with depressed and nondepressed subjects have found either an increase or no change in levels of urinary MHPG after acute exercise. The meaning of these studies for understanding exercise and depression is unclear, though. For example, at rest only about one-third of the MHPG in peripheral blood or urine comes from the metabolism of brain NE. In acute exercise that is of light to moderate intensity, NE levels have been shown to increase two- to sixfold, but most of this increase comes not from the brain but from sympathetic postganglionic nerve endings innervating the heart, with some coming from the exercising skeletal muscles. This increase in NE is related to biological adjustments to meet the strain of exercise. Levels and changes in NE or serotonin in specific brain regions must be assessed to determine the central effects of exercise training. But this is understandably difficult in human research, and the use of brain imaging methods to study the effects of exercise on depression has not yet been reported.

Animal research has provided better evidence for a mediating effect of exercise on monoaminergic systems implicated in depression. Studies have shown transient increases in brain 5-HT and NE levels during acute exercise (see figure 7.16) and adaptations in brain monoamine systems after chronic exercise in rats (Dishman, Renner, et al. 2000; Dunn and Dishman 1991; Dunn, Reigle, et al. 1996). Also, chronic exercise of moderate intensity has been accompanied by the down-regulation of β-adrenergic receptors in the brain cortex (Yoo et al. 2000; Yoo et al. 1999), comparable to the effects of antidepressant drug treatment. A key action of antidepressant drugs known as selective serotonin reuptake inhibitors (SSRIs) is the inhibition of the serotonin transporter (SERT), a protein that transports serotonin molecules back into the serotonin cell after release. This blocks reuptake, leaving serotonin in the synapse longer and presumably providing more molecules for binding with 5-HT receptors postsynaptically (see figure 7.17).

Researchers treated neonatal male rats with clomipramine, a serotonin reuptake inhibitor that causes long-term depletion of brain NE and adult-onset depression in the rat. After reaching maturity, the rats that had exercised for 12 weeks by running either in activity wheels or on a treadmill had increased levels of NE in the brain frontal cortex compared to the sedentary controls (Yoo et al. 2000). Both exercise groups had increased levels of NE, although the activity-wheel runners had a therapeutic decrease in β-adrenergic receptors that was equal to the effect of an antidepressant drug and had improved sexual performance, a behavioral sign of an antidepressant effect.

A common model of human depression in animal studies is repeated exposure to uncontrollable, inescapable stress that results in the depletion of brain NE or 5-HT and subsequent deficits in the animals' behavior to escape the stress when escape becomes possible. The first study to use that model after chronic exercise showed that sedentary rats had lower NE and 5-HIAA levels in the LC, hippocampus, and amygdala after exposure to uncontrollable, inescapable foot shock when compared to rats that had been permitted to run on activity wheels for 6 weeks (Dishman et al. 1997). The sedentary animals also exhib-

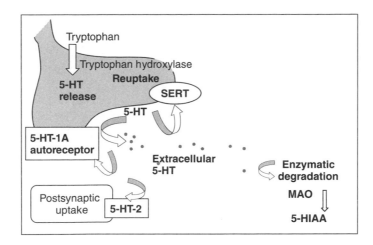

Figure 7.16 Diagram of a serotonin synapse that shows the possible fates of serotonin after it is released by the presynaptic neuron: postsynaptic uptake, binding with presynaptic autoreceptors, and reuptake into presynaptic neuron via actions of SERT (serotonin transporter).

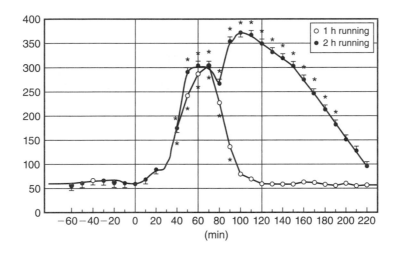

Figure 7.17 Changes in norepinephrine levels during treadmill running after treadmill exercise training.
Data from Pagliari and Peyrin 1995.

ited 28% higher 5-HT in the amygdala after foot shock. The activity-wheel runners subsequently exhibited a quicker escape from controllable foot shock than the sedentary animals did, indicating an antidepressant effect of the wheel running. Later research found similar benefits of wheel running for reducing this so-called learned helplessness (Greenwood et al. 2003).

There is evidence that treadmill running acutely increases dopamine release and turnover and chronically up-regulates DA D2 receptors in the striatum of rats, but the effects of exercise on striatal dopamine activity have not yet been shown in humans (see Dishman, Berthoud, et al. 2006 and Knab and Lightfoot 2010

for reviews). Those changes were reported to occur in parts of the striatum, which regulates locomotion, rather than the VTA or nucleus accumbens, which regulate motivational drive. In contrast to the effects of treadmill running, which is mainly forced, striatal DA activity has been reduced after chronic exposure to wheel running in highly fit rats (Waters et al. 2008), whereas gene expression for D2 receptors was unchanged in the nucleus of mice (Knab et al. 2009) but decreased in the nucleus accumbens of rats (Greenwood et al. 2011). So, on balance, it is not known whether exercise affects DA in the brain regions most involved with regulating moods such as depression.

Some new evidence suggests that genetic variation (i.e., combinations of different alleles, or forms, of a gene inherited from each parent) in the serotonin system may interact with physical activity levels to influence depression symptoms. For example, the short allele of the serotonin transporter gene is associated with the lower metabolism of serotonin and may increase the risk of elevated depressive symptoms. In a recent cross-sectional study (Rethorst et al. 2011), college students who had the short allele from at least one parent and relatively low physical activity also reported more depressive symptoms on the Beck Depression Inventory than those who also reported similarly low physical activity and had the long allele from both parents. However, contrary to expectations, among students who reported high physical activity, those with at least one short allele had lower depressive symptoms than those with both long alleles. Nonetheless, after 5 weeks of aerobic exercise training, students with at least one long allele had larger reductions in depression symptoms than those who were homozygous for the short allele (Rethorst et al. 2010).

Hypothalamic-Pituitary-Adrenal Cortical (HPA) Axis Hypothesis

Chronic exercise training results in a diminished endocrine response during standard exercise (Richter and Sutton 1994). Thus, the effects of physical activity on the regulation of the HPA axis may be another means by which exercise affects depression. Animal studies provide some support for exercise-induced effects on the HPA axis that could be related to antidepressant effects. For example, treadmill-trained female rats had attenuated ACTH and corticosterone responses to treadmill running but a hyperresponsiveness of ACTH to immobilization stress (White-Welkley et al. 1995) and foot shock (White-Welkley et al. 1996). Whether this hyperresponsiveness of ACTH is a healthful adaptation and whether it is attributable to increased CRH or other factors that affect CRH release are not known. Altered CRH activity with exercise would be particularly relevant for depression, because CRH increases the activity of the brain stem LC. Recall that the LC plays a key regulatory role in modulating brain and peripheral sympathetic nervous system

> **A**daptations in the HPA axis from exercise training may help to reregulate disruptions that have fostered biological contributions to depression, but research on this issue is limited.

responses to appetitive and aversive behaviors that are central to depression.

Other Biologically Based Hypotheses

Aside from the hypotheses presented in chapter 5 on affect, mood, and emotion (i.e., that increased brain blood flow, body temperature, and endorphins during acute exercise might explain changes in mood), new areas of research implicate other potential biological mechanisms for the positive effects of exercise on depression. For example, neurotrophic peptides such as brain-derived neurotrophic factor (BDNF) and VGF enhance the growth and maintenance of several neuronal systems, and might have an important role in the neuropathology and treatment of depression (Hunsberger et al. 2007; Russo-Neustadt 2003). Animal studies of chronic exercise have demonstrated increased gene expression for VGF and BDNF in the hippocampus, which is involved with contextual memories (e.g., Adlard and Cotman 2004), and the ventral tegmental area of the mesolimbic system, which helps modulate motivation (Van Hoomissen, Chambliss, Holmes, and Dishman 2003).

SUMMARY

Major depression is a common mental health disorder that can have serious effects; it is characterized by significant distress or impairment in social or occupational functioning, or both. Traditional treatments for depression are time-consuming, costly, and often ineffective. Side effects of pharmacological interventions may include fatigue, cardiovascular complications, and possible addiction. Thus, exercise may be a desirable alternative or adjunct treatment. Overall, the literature supports some effect of exercise on reducing the primary risk of depression and alleviating symptoms in people diagnosed as having mild-to-moderate depression. In some studies, reductions in depression after exercise training have been as great as those seen after psychotherapy or drug therapy.

However, the specific parameters of exercise type, frequency, and intensity necessary for optimizing positive effects are not yet established. Well-controlled studies that encompass a range of demographic groups and fully consider subject characteristics still are needed for determining whether the apparently protective effect of exercise against the risk of developing depression is an independent one and is consistent across sex, age, race and ethnicity, education, socioeconomic level, and mental status. People with depression typically have reduced levels of muscular endurance (Morgan 1968), physical working capacity (Morgan 1969), and cardiorespiratory fitness (O'Neal, Dunn, and Martinsen 2000; Martinsen, Strand, et al. 1989) compared to mentally healthy people. But it is possible to implement a carefully graduated exercise program successfully with proper attention to unique problems of treatment adherence. Also, people who maintain their cardiorespiratory fitness during middle age reduce their odds of developing depressive symptoms.

Although recent randomized controlled trials have added credence to the view that moderately intense exercise is an effective approach to reducing symptoms of mild-to-moderate depression, exercise is not yet medically recognized as a treatment for depression (American Psychiatric Association 2000). Understanding the mechanisms, especially the neurobiological mechanisms, whereby exercise directly and independently reduces depression is one of the next frontiers of exercise psychology.

WEBSITES

www.ndmda.org

www.psychologyinfo.com/depression

www.nimh.nih.gov/health/topics/depression/index.
   shtml

Exercise and Cognitive Function

Deciding to adopt and maintain regular exercise or an active lifestyle is a smart thing to do, but what about the effects of exercise on intellectual function? Can exercise make you smarter? The relationship between exercise and cognition is a relatively new area of research and practice, but academic interest in human cognition can be traced historically to the second century BC and Aristotle's *On Memory and Reminiscence* (Sorabji 2004). In this treatise, Aristotle conceptualized mental processes as operations that could be studied empirically. Since then, scientists have examined the process and manifestations of cognitive processes from perceptual assessments to changes in the structure and function of the brain and the consequent effects on behavior.

Cognitive processes are affected by genetics, developmental factors, and environmental experiences. This chapter focuses on environmental influences in the context of exercise behavior and provides the foundation for understanding the relationship between exercise and our ability to reason, remember, and respond. Evidence for effects on various healthy and clinical populations and age groups are presented and discussed. Possible mechanisms, mediators, and moderators are presented, and issues in addressing the relationship between exercise and cognitive function are summarized.

DEFINITION

Aristotle's views on the study of cognition influenced philosophers in 15th- and 16th-century Europe who were instrumental in the emergence of the scientific method. For example, one of René Descartes' contributions to psychology was his view that cognition could be understood via direct observation and measurement, and that the brain was the mediator of behavior (Hergenhahn 1992). Contemporary researchers use *cognition* as a general term

> *Cognition* is from the Latin *cognoscere*, which means, "to know," "to conceptualize," or "to recognize." It is the process of thought.

for any process that reflects a person's knowledge or awareness, and it includes perceiving, remembering, judging, and reasoning (Wilson, Caldwell, and Russell 2007). Cognition reflects the integration of numerous mental processes that are hypothesized to interact in a hierarchical fashion. Processes high in the hierarchy include those that are associated with consciousness, such as planning to run a marathon, and goal-directed actions, such as choosing to run instead of playing a video game. Lower-level processes govern automatic and reflexive behaviors.

> The ancient Greeks asserted that a healthy body contributes to a healthy mind: *Mens sana in corpora sano*. However, only recently have we begun to evaluate systematically the association between exercise and cognition in empirical studies.

MEASUREMENT

Several hundred tests have been developed over the past 150 years to measure mental processes. Some evaluate cognition at a global level (e.g., general intelligence); others isolate and explore the operations of specific processes (e.g., attention). Tests most often used by exercise scientists are drawn from four overlapping research domains: educational psychology, experimental psychology, clinical neuropsychology, and neurophysiology.

> **T**he first test to measure intellectual functioning was the Binet-Simon test, published in 1905.

Educational Psychology and Psychometrics

In the very early years of the 20th century, the French government led an initiative to evaluate how the children who lived in Paris benefited from universal education. The first test designed to measure individual differences in intellectual function is credited to Alfred Binet, a French psychologist. The Binet-Simon (1905) test consisted of 30 items believed to assess higher-level mental processes, such as reasoning and problem solving, that were ranked in order of difficulty and scored on a pass/fail basis. The derivation of age-graded norms permitted a child's mental age to be determined. Binet's pioneering conceptualization of intelligence and his insightful selection and organization of test items contributed substantially to the evolution of the field of psychometrics, which was discussed in chapter 2. Psychometrists have, over the past century, explored the structure of human intelligence using increasingly sophisticated quantitative methods of measuring human performance (Wasserman and Tulsky 2005). An example of the factor structure of an intelligence test is seen in figure 8.1. The rise of psychometrics led to the development of numerous intelligence tests (e.g., Stanford-Binet Scales, Wechsler Intelligence Scales, Kaufman Assessment Battery for Children) that have been used worldwide to measure and characterize the abilities of millions of people.

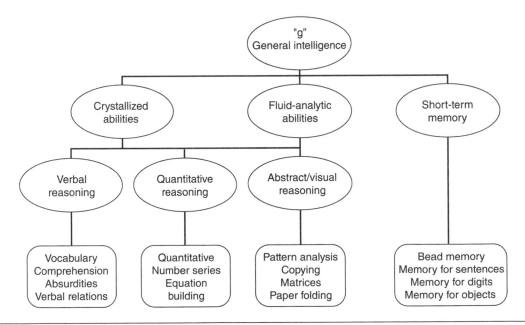

Figure 8.1 The factor structure of the Stanford-Binet IQ test. General intelligence (g) is a single score derived from measuring performance on individual test items (e.g., vocabulary, number series, memory for objects). Correlations among item scores provide the basis for inferring mental constructs hypothesized to underlie individuals' adaptive thought and behavior (e.g., reasoning, abilities, and memory).

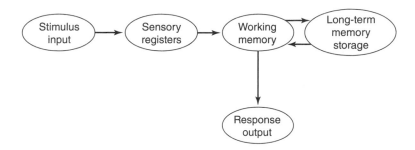

Figure 8.2 Information-processing model. Environmental information affects sensory receptors and flows into short-term, working memory where it is manipulated via control processes (e.g., rehearsal) using memories drawn from long-term memory stores. Executive processes involved in goal-directed action then configure behavioral actions

Experimental Psychology

The academic discipline of psychology initiated in Germany in 1872 by Wilhelm Wundt focused on understanding the complexities of the mind by studying its components. Tests of memory and **mental chronometry**, which used measures of reaction time to fractionate mental processes, provided Wundt and his students with methods to study the structure of cognition. Mental processes and corresponding subjective experiences were examined under highly controlled laboratory conditions. Research conducted by many contemporary experimental psychologists continues this tradition of component analysis (Detterman 1986).

Modern cognitive psychology emerged in the 1960s as a method that focused on how information is encoded, stored, processed, and manipulated, and how it leads to behavior. Researchers interested in encoding processes typically employ perceptual tests that measure how sensory systems change raw physical energy into perceptions that have meaning. Visual and auditory organs, for example, scan and inspect the outside world. Inspection-time methods (Nettelbeck and Wilson 1997) and scanning protocols (Sternberg 1969) have been developed that isolate perceptual processes. Information storage and processing are typically studied using classical tests of short- and long-term memory that can be traced to methods developed by Hermann Ebbinghaus in the mid-19th century (e.g., Brown-Peterson tests).

The construct of **working memory** evolved in the 1980s from theorizing about the functions of short-term memory (Baddeley 1986). Work-ing memory refers to the temporary storage and manipulation of information necessary for complex tasks such as learning, language comprehension, and reasoning. Tests of attention provide researchers with methods to explore and assess how information is manipulated. These tests examine mental processes that influence encoding and the operations of memory systems.

Other methods are used to assess how information leads to behavior. Tests of **executive function** assess the mental processes that are central to decision making, goal planning, and choosing behavior (Miyake et al. 2000; Naglieri and Johnson 2000; Posner and Dahaene 1994). These processes have also been classified as **metacognition**, which refers to the higher-order thinking that controls the thought processes required for problem solving (Borkowski, Carr, and Pressely 1987; Flavell 1979). Figure 8.2 provides an example of a generic information-processing model that highlights the processes involved in stimulus extraction, manipulation, and response preparation. The operations of these lower-level mental processes can be modified by attentional processing and motivation.

Clinical Neuropsychology

The way disease and injury affect cognition and behavior has long been a focus of interest by physicians. In the third century BC, Hippocrates explained disorders of thought and reasoning as imbalances in the four bodily humors: blood, black bile, yellow bile, and phlegm. He believed that imbalances in these humors altered the brain and affected emotion and perception. Galen, a second-century AD Roman physician, extended Hippocrates' naturalistic explanation of mental function by linking personality attributes to body humors. As described in chapter 5, contemporary biologically based personality theories reflect these early conceptualizations of humoral balance (e.g., Eysenck 1990).

A wide variety of tests have been developed to assess cognitive function in clinical populations, such as people who have Alzheimer's disease or have suffered a concussion. A comprehensive review of the neurocognitive literature by Lezak and her colleagues documents over 400 behavioral tests designed to assess a variety of cognitive functions, such as mental flexibility and processing speed (Lezak, Howieson, and Loring 2004).

NEUROPHYSIOLOGICAL MEASURES

In contrast to the measurement methods described earlier, which infer cognitive processes from the observation of behavior, there has been a longstanding interest in direct measures of brain activity. Researchers have used methods to measure cortical brain activity (e.g., electroencephalography [EEG]) for many decades. Considerable technological advances have been made during the past two decades that provide increasingly precise measures of brain structures and function.

Structures of the Brain Implicated in Executive Function and Memory

The **frontal lobe** receives multiple inputs from cortical and subcortical areas and integrates information in ways that lead to unified, goal-directed behavior.

The **dorsolateral prefrontal cortex** receives input from the parietal cortex, the premotor cortex, and the basal ganglia. This region of the frontal lobe has been linked to goal selection, planning, sequencing, verbal and spatial working memory, self-monitoring, and self-awareness.

The **ventrolateral prefrontal cortex** receives input from the temporal cortex. This region plays a role in analyzing features and attributes of environmental information in ways that conform to the execution of goal-directed actions. The left ventrolateral prefrontal region has been associated with working memory processes, which involve the maintenance of information while blocking distractions. The right ventrolateral prefrontal region has been linked to vigilance and the detection of conditions that pose a potential threat.

The **orbitofrontal cortex** is closely connected to the limbic system, especially the amygdala. This region plays a role in the inhibition of inappropriate responses and is implicated in judging the likelihood of reward and risk. Processes in this region are believed to underpin emotional and social behavior.

The **anterior cingulate cortex** is involved in monitoring and detecting behavioral errors and is involved in conflict detection processes. This region is part of a network that is involved in stimulus processing and memory updating.

The limbic system is a complex structure that is linked to emotion, learning, and memory.

The amygdala is a cluster of nuclei in the limbic system that influence emotional behaviors and memories associated with emotional situations. Emotional experiences are learned rapidly, and memories elicit fear and anxiety responses (tachycardia, increased respiration, stress-hormone release).

The hippocampus is a structure in the limbic system involved in the formation of long-term memories. The activation of neurons in the hippocampus can result in long-term potentiation and the consolidation and storage of memories of the context of experiences and associated information.

As described in chapters 2 and 3, exercise researchers employ a wide variety of techniques to assess the role of physical activity, level of physical fitness, and training interventions on brain function in both healthy and clinical populations. Each method captures slightly different perspectives of the brain, and together they enable the mapping of neural networks that operate during information processing, memory, and attentional processing (O'Reilly 2010; Posner and Raichle 1997). The capacity to measure changes in brain activity while people are performing specific cognitive tests provides researchers with converging evidence for the impact of exercise on cognitive function. Further, assays of animal brains (typically rodents) provide information concerning the effects of physical activity on metabolic changes that occur between and within brain cells that may underlie animal learning and performance (Dishman, Berthoud, et al. 2006; Meeusen and De Meirleir 1995).

> The multidimensionality of cognitive function and the diversity of assessment methods present a special challenge when interpreting evidence regarding the effect of physical activity and exercise on cognitive function.

RESEARCH

Numerous narrative and meta-analytic reviews indicate that both acute bouts of exercise and chronic exercise training influence cognitive function. The first comprehensive meta-analytic review of studies on exercise and cognition was conducted in 1997 (Etnier et al. 1997). An analysis of 134 cross-sectional, correlational, and experimental studies revealed an overall mean effect size (ES) of 0.25, suggesting that exercise exerts a small but significant effect on mental function. Moderator analyses revealed that the strength of the association depended on a number of factors. Significantly smaller effect sizes were found in studies that employed acute exercise bouts (ES = 0.16) than in those that

employed chronic exercise training programs (ES = 0.33). As seen in the following list, several narrative and quantitative reviews have focused on acute and chronic exercise training protocols.

Acute Exercise and Cognition: Narrative Reviews

Tomporowski and Ellis (1986): Examined 27 published experiments.

Method: Studies grouped into four categories:
- Very brief, high-intensity (isometric) exercise
- Short-duration, high-intensity, anaerobic exercise
- Short-duration, moderate-intensity, aerobic exercise
- Long-duration, aerobic exercise

Conclusions:
- Many studies lacked adequate methodological controls.
- There was insufficient support for an exercise–cognition relation.

McMorris and Graydon (2000): Evaluated 23 published experiments.

Method: Studies grouped into three categories:
- Rest vs. submaximal exercise
- Rest vs. maximal exercise
- Submaximal vs. maximal exercise

Conclusions:
- Increased response speed was associated with exercise performed up to anaerobic threshold.
- There was no effect of exercise intensity on response accuracy.
- There was no support for the unidimensional inverted-U hypothesis.

Brisswalter, Collardeau, and Arcelin (2002): Evaluated 7 published studies.

Method: Studies grouped into three categories:
- Exercise intensity
- Exercise duration
- Level of participants' physical fitness

Conclusions:

- Cognitive performance improved on simple and complex mental tasks during moderately intense exercise (~40%-80% $\dot{V}O_2$max) performed for less than 20 min.

- There was no relation between the level of aerobic fitness and cognitive performance during exercise.

Tomporowski (2003a): Evaluated 43 published experiments.

Method: Studies grouped into three categories:

- Intense anaerobic exercise
- Short-duration aerobic and anaerobic exercise
- Steady-state aerobic exercise

Conclusions:

- Cognitive function was resistant to change during putative exercise-induced fatigue conditions.

- Response speed, response accuracy, and executive processing were facilitated during and after steady-state, moderate levels of exercise.

- There were no exercise-related changes in memory storage.

- There was no support for the unidimensional inverted-U hypothesis.

Acute Exercise and Cognition: Meta-Analytic Reviews

Etnier et al. (1997): Examined 134 published and unpublished studies.

Method: Identified 371 effects from acute-exercise studies.

Conclusions:

- Acute exercise led to small but significant improvements in cognitive performance (ES = 0.16).

- The effect size depended on the cognitive test employed.

- There was no support for the unidimensional inverted-U hypothesis.

- Cognitive function was not affected by putative exercise-induced fatigue conditions.

- Exercise reduced simple reaction time and lengthened choice reaction time.

Lambourne and Tomporowski (2010): Examined 40 published within-subject experiments.

Method: Separate analyses were conducted for studies that assessed cognition during and after exercise.

- A total of 126 effects from 21 studies were used to assess cognitive performance during exercise.

- A total of 109 effects from 29 studies assessed cognitive performance following exercise.

Conclusions:

- During exercise there was an impairment in cognitive performance ($d = -0.14$; 95% CI = -0.26 to -0.01); mediator analyses revealed that performance was biphasic with performance declines during the first 20 min of exercise and performance improvements after that point.

- Performance on simple, choice, and discriminant response time improved during steady-state aerobic exercise but declined during anaerobic exercise.

- Effect size depended on the cognitive test employed, with the greatest impact on automatic processing and minimal effects on executive processes.

- After exercise, there was an improvement in cognitive performance ($d = 0.20$; 95% CI = 0.14-0.25); mediator analyses revealed that effect sizes were greater for cycling than for running protocols.

McMorris et al. (2011): Examined 38 effects from 24 experiments that assessed working memory during moderate levels of aerobic exercise (~50%-75% $\dot{V}O_2$max).

Methods: Separate analyses were conducted to assess changes in response time and response accuracy during exercise.

Conclusions:

- Exercise led to large increases in response speed ($g = -1.41$; 95% CI = -1.74 to -1.08).
- Exercise led to low-to-moderate decreases in response accuracy ($g = 0.40$; 95% CI = 0.08-0.72).

Chronic Exercise and Cognition: Narrative Reviews

Folkins and Sims (1981): Examined 12 studies.

Method: Examined studies conducted with children, young adults, and older adults.

Conclusions:

- There was little evidence that physical fitness training influenced children's and young adults' performance on general tests of intelligence and academic performance.
- Two studies demonstrated improvements in geriatric mental patients.

Chodzko-Zajko and Moore (1994): Examined 35 studies.

Method: Examined 23 cross-sectional and 12 chronic exercise studies conducted with older adults.

Conclusions:

- Physical fitness was associated with enhancements in cognitive processing speed.
- There was insufficient evidence that physical fitness training influenced older adults' cognitive performance.

Chronic Exercise and Cognition: Meta-Analytic Reviews

Etnier et al. (1997): Examined 134 cross-sectional, quasi-experimental, and experimental published and unpublished studies.

Method: Identified 358 effects from chronic exercise studies.

Conclusions:

- Exercise training was associated with moderate improvements in cognition (ES = 0.53).
- Randomized experiments ($n = 17$) evidenced a smaller, but significant effect (ES = 0.18).
- Effects were not related to physical fitness.
- The effects were moderated by age.

Etnier et al. (2006): Examined 37 cross-sectional, within-subject, and between-group studies.

Method: Identified 571 effects from chronic exercise studies.

Conclusions:

- Exercise training was associated with small improvements in cognition (ES = 0.34; SD = 0.34).
- Eight cross-sectional studies yielded 27 effects and an average ES of 0.40 (SD = 0.67).
- Thirty within-subject experiments yielded 106 effects and an average ES of 0.25 (SD = 0.35).
- Twenty-four between-group experiments yielded 78 effects and an average ES of 0.27 (SD = 0.50).
- Regression analysis suggested that aerobic fitness was not a predictor of change in cognitive performance.

Colcombe and Kramer (2003): Examined 18 intervention experiments conducted with nonclinical and clinical older adults (55 years and older).

Method: Identified 197 effects studies and coded them into four categories: speed, visuospatial, controlled processing, and executive processing.

Conclusions:

- Exercise training was associated with moderate improvements in cognition (g = 0.48; SE = 0.028).

- Training significantly influenced speed (g = 0.27; SE = 0.50), visuospatial (g = 0.43; SE = 0.062), controlled processing (ES = 0.46; SE = 0.035), and executive processing (g = 0.68; SE = 0.052).

- Clinical and nonclinical samples showed similar improvements.

Angevaren et al. (2008): Examined 11 randomized controlled trials with nonclinical adults 55 years and older.

Method: Effects were coded into 11 categories.

Conclusions:

- Two of 11 comparisons yielded significant results.

- Large effects were found on motor function (ES = 1.17; 95% CI = 0.19-2.15). Moderate effects were observed for cognitive speed (ES = 0.26; 95% CI = 0.04-0.48), auditory attention (ES = 0.50; 95% CI = 0.13 to 0.91), and visual attention (ES = 0.26; 95% CI = 0.02-0.49).

- Cognitive function was not associated with aerobic fitness improvement.

Acute Exercise and Cognition

Sport psychologists have addressed the effects of arousal on attention and performance, and likewise, the effects of arousal on mental function have long been of interest to psychologists (see van der Molen 1996 for an excellent historical review of arousal theories). In 1908, Robert Yerkes and John Dodson introduced the inverted-U hypothesis to describe the relationship between arousal and performance. In its most basic form, arousal theories predict that individual performance will improve to an optimal level as arousal increases and deteriorate with additional increases in arousal. More elaborate contemporary theories (Hockey 1997; Kahneman 1973; and Sanders 1998) consider levels of processing and the allocation of resources (i.e., mental and physiological) and how these resources are used to explain how arousal affects cognition and subsequent behavior. Neuropsychological extensions of classical arousal theory have also been recently presented (Pfaff 2006).

The narrative and quantitative reviews described earlier suggest that although there is little support for the inverted-U hypothesis, exercise-induced arousal does influence cognitive function. In general, cognitive functions are facilitated after acute exercise bouts, but the influence on behavioral tests appears to be quite brief (Lambourne and Tomporowski 2010). After approximately 20 minutes of moderately intense, continuous aerobic exercise, sensory processing improves and the speed of executing well-learned, automated behaviors (e.g., simple, choice, discriminant response time [RT]) increases (Lambourne and Tomporowski 2010). Response speed also increases during the performance of executive function tests; however, response accuracy decreases (McMorris et al. 2011). Relatively brief, intense anaerobic exercise that produces subjective reports of fatigue have little impact on cognitive performance (Brisswalter, Collardeau, and Arcelin 2002; McMorris and Graydon 2000; Tomporowski 2003); however, long-duration exercise that leads to carbohydrate depletion and dehydration impairs memory and multiple components of cognition (Brisswalter, Collardeau, and Arcelin 2002; Tomporowski 2003).

Neurophysiological studies provide more information about the mechanisms for effects of exercise on cognitive function. Researchers have measured brain activation both during and immediately after individual exercise bouts. Measuring brain activation during exercise is made difficult by the large changes in electrical potential that accompany muscle contraction and head and eye movements, which make the small changes in cortical activation that are measured in microvolts difficult to detect and monitor (Luck 2005). The results of the few studies that have examined neural activity during exercise using event-related potentials (ERP) methodologies (Grego et al. 2004; Pontifex and Hillman 2007; Yagi et al. 1999) have been consistent, showing a slowing of processing speed and decreased response accuracy on behavioral tests (Pontifex and Hillman 2007). These changes are thought to be due to the allocation of attentional resources to the control of movement and away from cognitive task performance.

In contrast, numerous studies in which cortical activation was measured after exercise have uniformly shown changes in brain activation patterns in children and young adults that reflect improved cognitive processing and executive control (Kamijo 2009). In particular, postexercise increases in P3 amplitude, which reflect accessing and updating working memory, and shortening of P3 latency, which is viewed as stimulus evaluation speed, are typically observed during discrimination tasks. The modulation of the event-related negativity (ERN) wave pattern of an ERP is seen during response-inhibition tasks and is interpreted as an index of executive control (Hillman, Erickson, and Kramer 2008).

> **I**nformation processing speeds up during acute exercise, but errors increase for tasks that involve working memory and executive control.

In summary, results obtained from both behavioral and neurophysiological studies provide convergent evidence for the impact of acute exercise on cognitive function. During exercise, information processing speeds are accelerated, but at a cost of increased errors on tasks that involve working memory and executive control. Immediately after exercise, cognitive performance measured in terms of speed and accuracy shows transient facilitation; however, measures of cortical activity suggest that the effects may last for longer periods. Cortical activity alterations have been reported after delays of 24 minutes in children (Hillman, Pontifex, et al. 2009) and up to 60 minutes in young adults (Hillman, Snook, and Jerome 2003).

Evidence From Cross-Sectional Studies

Considerable research has examined the relation between physical fitness or physical activity and mental abilities. Historically, the bulk of research has focused on age-related changes in mental function. In the United States, several large-scale reviews of studies have focused on older adults' cognitive abilities, and evidence suggests that physical activity and level of physical fitness modify age-related loss of cognitive function and delay the onset of dementia and other diseases of aging (Hamer and Chida 2009; Lindwall, Rennemark, and Berggren 2008; Paterson and Warburton 2010; Sturman et al. 2005). More recently, cross-sectional research has addressed the physical fitness–cognition relation in children, and several large-scale studies have reported associations between children's physical activity and academic achievement (California Department of Education 2005; Carlson et al. 2008; Chomitz et al. 2009; Roberts, Freed, and McCarthy 2010).

Studies conducted with smaller groups under more controlled conditions than national studies have consistently shown benefits of physical activity or physical fitness in children, young adults, and older adults based on a wide range of cognitive tests. Further, physical fitness levels have been linked to neuropsychological functions and brain structure. In older adults, higher cardiorespiratory fitness is associated with measures of cortical activation in brain areas involved in executive control, response inhibition, and movement control (Hillman, Erickson, and Kramer 2008). Neuroimaging studies report that physical activity and physical fitness are positively associated with recruitment in prefrontal and parietal cortices (Prakash et al. 2011), prefrontal and temporal cortical gray matter volume (Colcombe et al. 2006), hippocampal volume (Colcombe et al. 2004), and cerebral blood volume (Pereira et al. 2007), all of which are implicated in brain health and cognitive function.

In children, Hillman, Buck, and colleagues (2009) observed fitness-related differences in several indexes of cortical activity thought to affect executive control and information processing.

A recent review of neuroimaging studies conducted with children suggests that physical fitness is associated with the volume of specific brain regions, in particular the dorsal striatum, which is part of the basal ganglia and involved with executive control and response resolution, and the hippocampus, which is critical for long-term memory (Chaddock et al. 2011). In addition, functional magnetic resonance imaging (fMRI) recordings show that more physically fit children have greater prefrontal activation in areas associated with executive control compared to less fit children. In summary, cross-sectional studies provide clear evidence for a positive relation between physical fitness and cognitive test performance and suggest that several brain systems may underlie the association.

Evidence From Chronic Training Studies

The vast majority of published studies on cognition and exercise have employed aerobic training as the exercise intervention. The assumption has been that routine exercise improves cardiorespiratory function that, in turn, facilitates the brain functions that underlie mental processes. In many studies, measures of cardiorespiratory function have been presented as the gold standard to quantify the impact of exercise training. However, because changes in aerobic fitness are not necessary to realize reductions in the symptoms of depression (see chapter 7), changes in aerobic fitness have not been consistently associated with improvements in cognitive function (Etnier et al. 1997; Etnier et al. 2006). Meta-analyses have consistently reported small but significant overall effect sizes for chronic exercise, but a meta-regression analysis designed to address directly the cardiorespiratory hypothesis found little support for the relation (Etnier et al. 2006). As described later in this chapter, contemporary researchers are beginning to consider other physiological, psychosocial, and psychological factors that may mediate exercise-induced changes in cognitive function. A recent review of the effects of resistance training, for example, concluded that strength training interventions may facilitate older adults' cognition

and especially memory functions (O'Connor, Herring, and Caravalho 2010).

Exercise training effects have been hypothesized to be robust at the two ends of the life span continuum (Dustman, Emmerson, and Shearer 1994; Hertzog et al. 2009). The aging brain is marked by deterioration of gray and white matter tissue, with the greatest deterioration occurring in the prefrontal cortical areas that underlie executive processing and planning (Erickson and Kramer 2009; West 1996). Exercise has long been thought to ameliorate age-related cognitive decline, and a number of studies have assessed its impact on nonclinical and clinical populations. Several meta-analyses support the benefits of exercise training on older adults' mental function; however, the patterns of effects are not consistent across studies. Reviews by Etnier and her colleagues (1997, 2006) found that specific age ranges mediated the effects of exercise, but the relations are difficult to interpret. Colcombe and Kramer's (2003) review of 18 studies conducted with healthy and clinically impaired older adults suggests that exercise training enhances multiple cognitive processes, with the greatest benefit for executive functioning. However, Angevaren and colleagues' (2008) evaluation of 11 randomized controlled trials with nonclinically impaired older adults revealed that exercise affected only a few basic cognitive processes and exerted minimal influence on higher-level attentional or executive processes. Heyn, Abreu, and Ottenbacher (2004) reviewed studies conducted with clinically impaired, frail older adults (mean age 80) and suggested that this population may gain both physical and mental benefits from exercise training. The benefit of exercise on people with Alzheimer's disease was reported in a narrative review by Eggermont and colleagues (2006); however, the effect may differ for people who have cardiovascular risk factors.

The lack of agreement among these reviews and meta-analyses may be explained in terms of differences in study selection, coding methods, and the delivery of exercise interventions. Although there are inconsistencies among the reviews, there is sufficient evidence to conclude that exercise training benefits healthy older adults' mental processes.

Evidence From Neuropsychological Studies

Training studies provide evidence for a causal relation between exercise and changes in brain systems that underlie cognitive function. Kramer and colleagues (2002) observed that aerobic exercise training was associated with older adults' (60-75 years) improved executive control processing (e.g., scheduling, planning, inhibition, and working memory). A replication of the study using fMRI brain imaging methods revealed that 6 months of aerobic training enhanced inhibition processes during a behavioral test and altered brain activation in areas predicted to be influenced based on the task's cognitive requirements (i.e., anterior cingulate cortex, middle frontal gyrus, superior frontal gyrus, and superior and inferior parietal lobules) (Colcombe et al. 2004).

Less studied are the effects of exercise training on children's mental development. Evidence from several areas of research indicates that the emergence of children's neural organization can be influenced by environmental experiences and physical activity (van Praag 2009), and developmental psychologists provide compelling evidence for the role of motor activity on cognition (Thelen 2004). Narrative reviews link exercise training to improvements in information processing, attention, and executive function (Chaddock et al. 2011; Tomporowski et al. 2008). A meta-analytic review of acute and chronic interventions reported in 44 studies yielded an overall effect size of 0.32, suggesting a significant positive relation between physical activity and cognitive functioning in children (Sibley and Etnier 2003).

An experiment that addressed the hypothesis that chronic exercise training exerts its greatest improvements on executive function was conducted with sedentary and overweight children (N = 171; mean age 9.3) assigned randomly to a low-dose (20 min/day) or high-dose (40 min/day) 13-week after-school program, or to a non-intervention control group (Davis et al. 2011). A standardized cognitive test, which provided separate indexes of executive function, attention, memory, and perceptual organization, and a standardized test of academic achievement were

administered at baseline and posttest. A dose-related exercise effect on children's performance of executive processing tests (ES = 0.30) and significant improvements in academic achievement (mathematics) were observed (see figure 8.3). Neuroimaging (fMRI) was conducted before and after training on a subgroup of children (control n = 9; exercise n = 10). During the performance of a response-inhibition task, children who exercised showed increased bilateral prefrontal cortex activity and decreased activity in the bilateral posterior parietal cortex, compared to controls. The findings are consistent with those conducted with older adults and add evidence of a dose–response effect.

The relation between exercise training and children's academic performance has been of interest to educators for many years. An early experiment conducted in an elementary school setting revealed that an 8-month intensive physical education program improved children's performance on a standardized test of academic

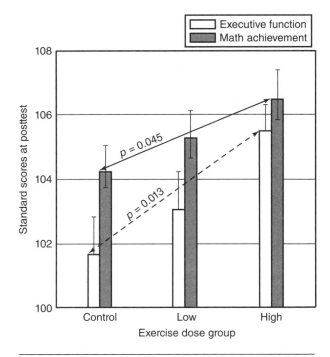

Figure 8.3 Overweight children's executive function and math academic achievement (SE) test performance at posttest showing dose–response effects of 20 min and 40 min aerobic exercise sessions compared to control.

Reprinted, by permission, C.L. Davis et al., 2011, "Exercise improves executive function and academic achievement and alters brain activation in overweight children: A randomized, controlled trial," *Health Psychology* 30: 96.

achievement compared to tradition physical education classes (Ismail 1967). Similar findings have been reported recently (Donnelly and Lambourne 2011), and these results have been highlighted by proponents of increased physical activity in school and after-school settings (Morabia and Costanza 2011).

The majority of experiments conducted to assess the exercise–cognition relation have focused on either older adults or children under the supposition that these populations, because of declining or underdeveloped resources, would evidence the most robust gains from exercise interventions. There is reason to believe, however, that exercise training may improve cognitive function across the life span. Pereira and colleagues (2007) found that 3 months of aerobic training improved 10 young adults' (mean age 33) free recall memory, and the changes were related to increased cerebral blood volume in the hippocampal dentate gyrus. Similarly, Stroth and colleagues (2009) observed that spatial, but not verbal, memory improved in young adults (mean age 19.6) after 6 weeks of aerobic exercise training compared to controls. Likewise, Masley, Roetzheim, and Gualtieri (2009) reported that a 10-week aerobic exercise program led to dose-related improvements in the executive processes

of 71 middle-aged adults (mean age 47.8). These findings replicate studies conducted with animals and provide evidence of the benefits of exercise on spatial memory and learning. They also suggest that exercise training may benefit cognitive performance across the life span.

MECHANISMS

Early research conducted to assess the exercise–cognition relation was descriptive and atheoretical (Tomporowski and Ellis 1986). As evidence has accumulated, researchers have begun to propose various explanations for the relation. Spirduso, Poon, and Chodzko-Kajko (2008) introduced a conceptual model that identifies factors that mediate and moderate the relation between physical activity and cognition in older adult populations. The model has been extended to children (Tomporowski, Lambourne, and Okumura 2011) (see figure 8.4), and it is useful for highlighting the complexities faced by contemporary researchers. Changes in cognition brought about by exercise have been explained in terms of their direct biological effects on the body and their indirect effects via physical resources and mental resources. *Resources* and ***brain plasticity*** are terms often used

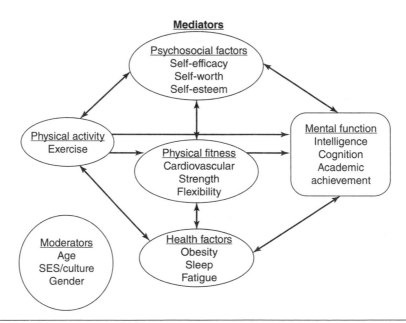

Figure 8.4 Mediators and moderators that may play a role in physical activity effects on cognitive function (SES = socioeconomic status).

Reprinted, by permission, from P.D. Tomporowski, K. Lambourne, and M.S. Okamura, 2011, "Physical activity interventions and children's mental function: An introduction and overview," *Preventive Medicine* 52: S7.

interchangeably to describe how people learn to adapt to environmental conditions and challenges (Hertzog et al. 2009; Hillman, Erickson, and Kramer 2008; Noack et al. 2009).

The notion of resource allocation is central to a number of influential cognitive theories (Baltes, Staudinger, and Lindenberger 1999; Kahneman 1973). Resources reflect the capacity to perform a given task, and resource allocation is determined by individual differences, environmental factors, and motivation. People with fewer resources are predicted to benefit more from exercise than healthy people who have sufficient resources to engage and adapt cognitively in an ever-changing, challenging environment. This assumption has led many researchers to evaluate exercise's ameliorative effects on symptoms associated with disease, injury, and stress (e.g., fatigue, mental confusion, and reductions in energy).

Biological Explanations

Early gerontology researchers commonly thought that exercise improves cognition because it leads to greater brain oxygenation and the regulation of neurotransmitter production (Spirduso 1980; Stones and Kozma 1988). Dustman and colleagues (1994) provided the first systematic review of studies that examined neuropsychological function in older adults. Of particular interest in these studies was cerebral metabolism (i.e., blood flow, oxygen consumption, and glucose utilization) and how it was altered by physical activity. Dustman and colleagues concluded that cross-sectional studies associated physical fitness with faster information processing, as measured by EEG and ERP methods; however, the results of training studies were inconclusive.

Changes in brain structure may be how cognition is affected as a consequence of exercise, and several mechanisms to drive these changes have been hypothesized. Drawing on a large animal literature and available research conducted with humans, researchers linked four mechanisms to changes in older adults' cognitive function: (1) vascular plasticity and angiogenesis (i.e., the growth of new capillaries), which may improve cerebral blood flow, oxygen extraction, and glucose utilization; (2) synaptogenesis, which involves modification of dendritic spines in ways

that enhance the efficiency of neural networks; (3) neurogenesis, or the creation and proliferation of neurons, particularly in the hippocampus; and (4) glial cell plasticity and the enhancement of other brain cells that support neuronal activities (Churchill et al. 2002). Additional biological mechanisms include the roles of neurotrophic factors, such as brain-derived neurotrophic factor (BDNF), nerve growth factor, and galanin (Dishman, Berthoud et al. 2006). Brain structures, including those involved in the initiation and control of movement, may also be altered by exercise (Anderson et al. 2003). Recent studies that have examined neuron function at molecular levels have revealed how exercise may regulate the operations of intracellular signaling systems and affect neuron function (van Praag 2009; Vaynman and Gomez-Pinilla 2006).

Substantial advances have been made in understanding brain structure and function, and contemporary researchers have made many attempts to link the alteration of brain systems to altered behavior and cognitive function. The extent to which brain activity can be mapped onto cognition and behavior has been a topic of discussion for some time, however (Diamond 1991). Concerns have been raised about interpretations of the results of imaging methods, and scientists have argued about the conclusions drawn from biological data. Nevertheless, the bulk of the evidence supports the view that exercise leads to biological changes that have a positive influence on cognitive function.

Resource Explanations

Exercise can also influence mental functioning indirectly, and potential mediators have been identified, such as changes in physical and mental resources. Physical resources are homeostatic, and their allocation is reflected in changes in energy and fatigue. Historically, exercise has been prescribed to rejuvenate energy levels, regulate sleep patterns, and improve the functional capacity of the body—all of which presumably result in improved clarity of thought and reasoning. Agents that reverse reductions in physical resources are of interest to those interested in athletic performance, work behavior, industrial accidents, and transportation. A number of studies have examined how sleep deprivation leads to fatigue and influences cognitive function. A meta-analysis of 70 studies that examined sleep deprivation ranging from 24 to 48 hours revealed that the effects were task dependent, with large effects on simple detection tasks ($g = -0.78$; 95% CI = -0.96 to -0.60), moderate effects on working memory tasks ($g = -0.55$; 95% CI = -0.74 to -0.37), and small, nonsignificant effects on high-level reasoning tasks (Lim and Dinges 2010). Compared to the large number of studies that have examined the effects of psychopharmacological agents on physical fatigue and cognitive performance, very few studies have assessed exercise as a countermeasure. Further, the results of those studies are inconsistent; some show positive effects (Englund et al. 1985), and others show null effects (LeDuc, Caldwell, and Ruyak 2000). There is evidence that chronic exercise alters sleep patterns in people with sleep complaints (King et al. 2008; Li et al. 2004), discussed in chapter 10, and it is plausible that sleep regulation benefits cognitive function (Vitiello 2008); however, empirical support for the relation is lacking.

Environmental events and stressors affect mental resources, which determine one's capacity to initiate and sustain mental processing. Biological responses to stressors have been studied extensively, and the impact of exercise on stress is described in chapter 4. Cognitive responses to stress can also be evaluated, and there is clear evidence for declines in many aspects of cognitive function in people with nonclinical levels of depression and anxiety. A meta-analysis of 14 studies by McDermott and Ebmeir (2009) revealed that the severity of depression was related to executive function, episodic memory, and processing speed. Interpreting the effects of exercise interventions on depressed people's cognitive function is not straightforward because there are differences between prodromal and mild transitory episodes of depressive symptoms and major depressive disorder, which is associated with the degradation of cognition-related brain structures (described later). Further, the outcome measures employed in most exercise training studies have been limited to measures of depression symptoms and have not included assessments of cognition (Deslandes et al.

Exercise training may indirectly influence cognition through the allocation of physical or mental resources. However, the strength of the relation between exercise and specific resources remains to be determined. Statistical methods, such as structural equation modeling (see chapter 2), may be useful for exploring exercise effects.

2009). The results of intervention studies that do include measures of cognition are mixed; some show positive gains (Khatri et al. 2001), and others, null effects (Hoffman et al. 2008). Likewise, exercise treatment studies that have focused on anxiety symptoms do not include outcome measures that isolate the effects on cognitive functions.

DISEASE STATES, EXERCISE, AND COGNITION

Many diseases, infections, and environmental conditions produce brain damage and negatively affect cognitive function, presumably via reductions in physical and mental resources. Exercise has been employed as a therapy for a limited number of these conditions. Emphasis has focused on diseases that are progressive and show only limited response to pharmacological therapies, such as Alzheimer's disease, multiple sclerosis, and Parkinson's disease. Researchers have also focused on cardiovascular disease and disorders that affect cerebral blood flow. Further, limited research has addressed the impact of exercise therapies on biologically based psychological disorders, such as depression.

Exercise and Cognition in Clinical Populations: Reviews

Eggermont et al. (2006): Evaluated eight clinical studies of individuals with Alzheimer's disease.

Method: Examined the effects of exercise training on cognition, particularly attention, memory, communication, executive function, and global mental functioning.

Conclusions:

- Seven of eight studies showed positive effects.
- Suggested that beneficial effects of exercise may depend on cardiovascular risk factors.

Hamer and Chida (2009): Evaluated 16 prospective studies in terms of dementia, Alzheimer's disease, and Parkinson's disease.

Method: Tracked 163,797 nondemented men and women at baseline with 3,219 cases at follow-up.

Conclusions:

- Physical activity reduces the risk of dementia by 28% and that of Alzheimer's by 45%.
- Physical activity was not associated with an increased risk of Parkinson's disease.

Exercise and Cognition in Clinical Populations: Meta-Analysis

Heyn, Abreu, and Ottenbacher (2004): Evaluated 30 randomized controlled trials with clinically impaired people 65 years old and older.

Method: Isolated 12 effects.

Conclusions:

- Exercise training improved cognitive performance by a moderate amount (ES = 0.57; 95% CI = 0.38-0.75).
- Frail sedentary adults exhibit good short-term responses to exercise.

Alzheimer's Disease

Alzheimer's disease (AD) is the most common form of dementia; it is an incurable, degenerative, and terminal disease that is characterized by memory loss and mental confusion. Alzheimer's disease is distinguished from other types of dementia (e.g., vascular dementia, multi-infarct dementia, Lewy body dementia, and frontal–temporal lobe dementia) by the presence of β-amyloid plaques outside neurons and neurofibril tangles within neurons. Brain shrinkage is typically observed first in the hippocampal regions, which helps explain the memory-encoding difficulties that are the trademark of Alzheimer's disease.

Research demonstrating the modification of brain structures and improved cognitive performance in healthy older adults after chronic exercise training has provided the impetus for experiments to assess how cognitive decline associated with AD might be delayed or mitigated. Although the evidence is convincing that exercise has a beneficial effect on brain structure and cognitive function in healthy older adults, the benefits of physical activity on people who evidence symptoms of dementia have been questioned (Briones 2006). The progression of dementia from prodromal, to mild, to severe involvement may take a decade, and the onset and rate of progression are affected by a variety of factors (Polidori, Nelles, and Pientka 2010). Results of recent randomized trials do, however, lend credence to the exercise–cognition relation in adults who may be at risk for Alzheimer's disease or who have mild dementia.

Lautenschlager and colleagues (2008) assigned older adults at risk for Alzheimer's disease to either a 6-month, home-based exercise or an educational control intervention. The Alzheimer Disease Assessment Scale (ADAS), consisting of 11 cognitive tests, and the Cognitive Battery to Establish a Registry for Alzheimer's Disease were administered at baseline, immediately following the interventions, and at 12 and 18 months after the interventions. Exercisers' overall ADAS scores and delayed-recall memory were better than those of controls immediately after the intervention. The effect size was small but remained, though attenuated, on follow-up assessments.

A comparison between 75 control adults and 77 older adults with mild dementia (mean age ~75) after 6 and 12 months of a structured walking program did not show any change in cognitive function (van Uffelen et al. 2011). However, adherence to the physical activity program was positively related to improved memory in men and improved attention in women. Baker and colleagues (2010) evaluated the impact of 6-month aerobic exercise and stretching control interventions on 33 sedentary older adults (mean age 70) with mild cognitive impairment. There were no group differences when measured after 3 months of intervention; however, postintervention measures revealed improvements in the measures of executive function, but not memory. There was evidence that women's gains (ES = 0.72) were greater than those of men (ES = 0.33).

It is plausible that exercise may influence vascular functions and alter symptoms of Alzheimer's disease. Regional hypoperfusion is linked to reduced brain metabolism and dementia, and exercise has been associated with increased cerebral blood flow. However, the effects of exercise on brain physiology may be moderated by a number of factors. There is evidence that cardiovascular risk factors may modify the effects of exercise on cognitive function (Eggermont et al. 2006). Genetic factors may differentiate exercise effects, as well. For example, the protein apolipoprotein E4 (ApoE4) plays a role in cerebral metabolism and has been linked to the onset of dementia. A recent cross-sectional imaging study suggests that aerobic fitness may be particularly beneficial for memory functions in older adults with ApoE4 alleles (Smith, Nielson, et al. 2010). Additional research in this area is warranted. Even if exercise can just delay the onset of dementia, the societal impact would be significant; it has been estimated that offsetting dementia by 12 months would result in 9.2 million fewer cases of AD worldwide (Lautenschlager et al. 2008).

Multiple Sclerosis

Multiple sclerosis is a chronic, inflammatory, demyelinating disease of the central nervous system. All cognitive domains can be impaired, but impairment of mental speed, cognitive flexibility, sustained attention, and memory retrieval is quite common in multiple sclerosis (Bol et al. 2009). Historically, people with multiple sclerosis have been advised to avoid exercise, because the belief was that it would increase fatigue and exacerbate symptoms. More recently, exercise has been found to reduce the symptoms of

In April 2010, an independent panel of experts convened by the U.S. National Institutes of Health issued an extensive report of factors thought to prevent the onset or reduce the impact of Alzheimer's disease. The panel examined 25 systematic reviews and 250 primary studies and grouped them into five categories: (1) nutritional factors; (2) medical factors (including prescription and nonprescription medications); (3) social, economic, and behavior factors (including physical activity); (4) toxic environmental factors; and (5) genetics. Only a few of the many factors evaluated were found to be associated with positive outcomes. Cognitive engagement and physical activity showed a fairly consistent association with a decreased risk of Alzheimer's disease and cognitive decline. The associations, however, were small to moderate, and the quality of studies reviewed was typically low (Williams et al. 2010).

depression and fatigue; however, the effects of exercise on cognition have not been sufficiently explored. A randomized controlled trial that compared individuals on a wait list (*n* = 20), a 6-month aerobic exercise program (*n* = 15), and a 6-month yoga program (*n* = 22) found that both activity conditions reduced fatigue symptoms but did not influence performance on tests that comprised a battery of attentional and executive function tasks (Oken et al. 2004). A study conducted with a small group of 20 patients who completed either yoga training or rock climbing found that yoga favorably influenced selective attention but had no effects on tests of executive function. Exercise did not influence performance on any test (Velikonja et al. 2010).

Parkinson's Disease

Parkinson's disease is a progressive disorder of the nervous system that is most characterized by movement problems. Most representative is bradykinesia, or a slowing of movement, which reflects the loss of the ability to plan, initiate, and execute motion. Additional symptoms include tremor, muscle rigidity, and speech changes. Paralleling these gradually debilitating symptoms are declines in cognitive function. The disorder is linked to the degeneration of the substantia nigra and a decline in dopamine production that is critical for basal ganglia structures and their connections to prefrontal regions, in particular the nigrostriatal, thalamus-cortical circuit (Tanaka et al. 2009). nigrostriatal Recent fMRI imaging studies reveal that Parkinson's disease leads to reductions in the activation of the mid-dorsal frontal cortex, which is central to working memory processes (Lewis et al. 2003; Owen 2004).

Physical activity is one of many interventions that have been thought to ameliorate Parkinson's disease symptoms. The empirical research on exercise effects is limited; only one study has addressed this relationship. Tanaka and colleagues (2009) assigned 10 adults with mild Parkinson's disease to a 6-month exercise program that consisted of multiple types of activities designed to maintain heart rate between 60% and 80% of age-related maximum. Participants exercised 60 min, three times per week. The 10 adults assigned to the control condition maintained their normal routines and did not participate in exercise activities. Measures obtained from the Wisconsin Card Sort Test and a subscale of the WAIS that measured attention, administered before and after the intervention, showed exercise-related improvements. The pattern of test performance suggested that exercise enhances the mental flexibility and response inhibition in people with Parkinson's disease. The mechanisms by which chronic physical activity may influence brain structure and neuromodulators would be expected to have similar effects on people with Parkinson's disease. The long-term effectiveness of exercise on the course of the disorder is unknown.

Cardiovascular Diseases

Cardiovascular diseases (atherosclerosis) influence the heart's capacity to deliver blood and nutrients throughout the body. Reduced or irregular blood flow to the brain has been implicated in changes in cognitive function. The activation of neurons requires a constant supply of glucose, which makes them vulnerable to disruptions in metabolic resources. Hypertension is associated with subtle deficits in cognitive function (Elias and Goodell 2010), which may be made worse by obesity (Gunstad et al. 2009).

A randomized controlled experiment assessed the impact of a combination of 4 months of aerobic exercise and diet, and diet alone, on the cognitive function of overweight adults who were pre- or moderately hypertensive (Smith, Blumenthal, et al. 2010). Improvements in executive function, memory, and learning were found for those assigned to the combined diet and exercise group ($n = 43$) when compared to controls ($d = 0.56$); no improvements on these tests were observed for those who only dieted. The lack of an exercise control condition limits the interpretation of this experiment, however. A previous experiment designed to assess the effects of aerobic exercise treatment on memory functions in people with mild hypertension failed to observe any change (Pierce et al. 1993). Several researchers have suggested that diets high in fat that lead to overweight may negatively affect cognitive function (Molteni et al. 2002; Wolf et al. 2007); exercise in conjunction with reduced caloric intake may ameliorate the condition.

Chronic Obstructive Pulmonary Disorder

Chronic obstructive pulmonary disorder (COPD) is a disease caused by damage to lung airways that interferes with the exchange of oxygen and carbon dioxide. Most COPD is caused by long-term smoking. The symptoms of COPD are similar to those of asthma; however, asthma is intermittent and reversed with medication, whereas the effects of COPD are largely irreversible. People with mild COPD experience dyspnea, or labored breathing, during heavy exertion; those with moderate to severe involvement report leg fatigue and discomfort when physically active (Rochester 2003). Also associated with COPD are declines in memory, abstract reasoning, reaction time, and complex visual–motor processes

(Emery 2008). A decline in arterial desaturation and reduced transportation of oxygen to the brain and the resulting hypoxemia have been hypothesized to cause reduced cognitive function.

Cross-sectional studies indicate that the aerobic fitness of people with COPD is positively related to cognitive function (Emery et al. 1991; Emery et al. 1998; Etnier et al. 1999), and longitudinal studies have found that COPD patients who adhere to routine exercise programs over a 12-month period maintain executive functions, whereas those who stop exercising evidence decline (Emery et al. 2003). Exercise interventions have been found to affect aspects of executive function, particularly verbal fluency, in older adults with COPD (Emery 1994; Etnier and Berry 2001); however, the lack of adequate control conditions limits the interpretation of these findings.

A randomized controlled experiment conducted with older adults (mean age 66.6) assessed the effects of 10 weeks of exercise activities performed in conjunction with educational and stress management programs ($n = 29$), educational and stress management alone ($n = 25$), and wait-list control ($n = 25$) on respiratory function, aerobic fitness, and cognitive function (Emery et al. 1998). Postintervention verbal fluency performance improved for those assigned to the exercise condition compared to control conditions. There were no exercise-related changes in attention, motor speed, or executive function measured by a switching task. In sum, the effects of chronic exercise training provide preliminary, but limited, evidence of an exercise–cognition relation, particularly related to executive functions (Emery 2008).

Similarly, acute bouts of exercise may have selective effects on older adults' cognitive function. Emery and colleagues (2001) assessed the short-term aftereffects of an acute bout of aerobic exercise on the cognitive function of 29 older adults (mean age 67) with COPD matched with those without COPD. Twenty minutes of cycling enhanced the verbal fluency of those with COPD but had no effect on healthy people. Given the hypoxia that characterizes COPD, these people might be especially sensitive to the benefits derived from both acute and chronic exercise.

Major Depressive Disorder

Considerable research has been conducted to identify the causes of major depressive disorder and how it can be prevented and treated, and research has confirmed established benefits of exercise for reducing risk and ameliorating symptoms (see chapter 7). Although major depression is expressed most clearly in affect and withdrawal behaviors, it also results in disturbances in memory and concentration. Depression can present itself at any point across the life span; however, onset is most common in the third decade and increases again in later life.

A meta-analysis of neuropsychological studies suggests that early-onset depression is characterized by hippocampal loss and deficits in memory consolidation, whereas late-onset depression, defined as onset after 65 years, is linked to the disruption of the frontostriatal structures critical for executive function and processing speed (Herrmann, Goodwin, and Ebmeier 2007). The impoverished activity in prefrontal circuitry suggests that people with late-onset depression would be particularly sensitive to the beneficial effects of exercise training. Initial research provided support for this prediction.

A randomized controlled experiment conducted by Khatri and colleagues (2001) compared the cognitive test performance of clinically depressed men and women (mean age 57) after 4 months of participation in a supervised aerobic exercise program that consisted of 45 min of aerobics, three times per week, or drug treatment (sertraline, a selective serotonin reuptake inhibitor). Symptoms of depression were reduced in both groups; however, those who exercised showed improved performance on memory and executive function tests, suggesting that exercise benefits selective cognitive functions. The researchers recognized the lack of a nondrug comparison group in this study as a limitation, and noted that differences in cognitive performance could have been due to drug-related declines in cognitive function. This alternative explanation was supported in a systematic replication of the experiment by Hoffman and colleagues (2008), which compared the cognitive performance of 202 clinically depressed middle-aged men and

> **M**ajor depression is a significant health burden, and most studies conducted to assess the effects of physical activity interventions on its symptoms report general assessments of participants' well-being and mental status; however, only a few have included tests that are sensitive to neurocognitive processing and designed to test the exercise–cognition relation.

women (mean age 51.7) assigned to either exercise, drug therapy (sertraline), or drug placebo conditions. As in the prior study, improvements in executive function tests were detected when comparisons were made between exercise and drug conditions; however, comparisons between exercise and placebo conditions failed to yield differences, suggesting that the results of the prior research may have resulted from drug-induced neurocognitive declines rather than exercise-related improvements.

In summary, exercise has been prescribed as a treatment for a wide number of diseases and disorders, and a comprehensive review is beyond the scope of this chapter. General conclusions, however, can be drawn from the studies evaluated so far. The structures of the central nervous system are affected differently by various diseases and environmental insults, although there is also evidence that exercise can affect brain structure and function. Thus, it is possible that systematic exercise can exert global effects on brain integrity and function, particularly on the developing nervous systems of the young; however, the available data suggest that, in adults, exercise training affects select cognitive functions. Exercise treatments may benefit people with conditions that alter prefrontal brain networks that underlie executive processes; however, as discussed in the next section, a number of factors may alter the magnitude of the effect. Information concerning exercise-related changes in human memory among diseased patients is limited, and additional research is needed to verify that changes in hippocampal

stuctures significantly affect memory in those with Alzheimer's disease or other dementias.

FACTORS THAT MODERATE THE EFFECTS OF EXERCISE

A moderator, as defined in chapter 2, is a variable outside the causal pathway between an independent and dependent variable that influences how an intervention affects the outcome. The influence of exercise on cognition is not an all-or-nothing relation. The degree or amount that cognition is affected by exercise may be influenced, or moderated, by many factors. Factors that have been hypothesized to moderate the exercise–cognition relation include age, sex, and level of intelligence.

Age

At maturity, the human brain has approximately 100 billion cells, the vast majority of which emerge and organize in an orderly fashion over the first two decades of life (Casey, Galvan, and Hare 2005). Traditionally, children's physical and mental progression has been thought to follow a structured set of milestones, or stages. Recent neurocognitive studies reveal, however, that people's mental processes emerge at different points in time, and all of us have our own developmental trajectories (Best, Miller, and Jones 2009; Diamond 2006, Diamond and Lee 2011). Further, these trajectories can be influenced by environmental experiences.

A recent developmental view (Best 2010) highlights the emergence of motor movement control and skills, memory, language acquisition, and executive processes and how they may influence the way exercise affects cognitive development. Through play and games, children learn predictive relations between action and outcomes, because controlled movements require the selection, ordering, and temporal sequencing of muscle contractions. The structure of exercise activities and their ensuing mental representations may modify and shape the way children and adolescents process information and plan behaviors. Mental processing speed reaches its apex during young adulthood, but mental slowing begins during the third decade of life and continues gradually over the remainder of life (Salthouse 1988). With increasing age, reduced processing speeds are often compensated for by changes in metacognitive, or higher-level, response strategies (Baltes, Staudinger, and Lindenberger 1999). The magnitude of the effects of exercise training on cognition would be expected to reflect the widespread changes in neurological integrity and the availability of metacognitive processes during adulthood. Recent advances in developmental psychology implicate the importance of physical activity in growth and mental function; however, until very recently, relatively few studies addressed the relation (see the following list).

Exercise and Cognitive Development: Reviews

Tomporowski (2003): Evaluated 20 published studies conducted with children and adolescents.

Method: Isolated 17 studies with children with clinical disorders (attention-deficit/ hyperactivity disorder, autism and learning disorders, behavioral disorders, and developmental delay) and 4 studies with children without clinical disorders.

Conclusions:

- School-based physical activity programs do not interfere with academic performance.
- Cognitive performance may improve after vigorous physical activity.
- Exercise may exert some benefit for disorders characterized by impulse control.

Tomporowski et al. (2008): Evaluated 16 correlational and experimental studies with children and adolescents.

Method: Grouped studies into three categories: intelligence, cognition, and academic achievement.

Conclusions:

- Global measures of intellectual function and academic achievement fail to detect effects of exercise training.

- Process-specific tests often report positive effects of exercise training.
- The roles of contextual and psychosocial factors have not been identified.

Exercise and Cognitive Development: Meta-Analysis

Sibley and Etnier (2003): Examined 44 published and unpublished studies with children and adolescents.

Method: Isolated 125 effects and coded for research design, age group, exercise type, and cognitive test.

Conclusions:

- The overall effect of exercise on cognition was $g = 0.32$ (SD = 0.27).
- Age-moderated exercise effects (ES = 0.40-0.48) with middle-school children were the largest effects.
- Significant change occurred in all cognitive tests (ES = 0.17-0.49) except memory (ES = 0.03).

Sex

A meta-analysis of exercise experiments conducted with older adults (Colcombe and Kramer 2003) reported that greater cognitive gains were derived by women than by men. Sex-related differences in hormone production, particularly in older adult women, have been thought to influence brain structure and cognitive function (Erickson et al. 2007). However, a national study of 839 older Swedish adults found that cognitive performance in men, but not women, was positively related to light, but not heavy, physical activity routines (Lindwall, Rennemark, and Berggren 2008). The information currently available is insufficient to predict whether sex may affect exercise intervention outcomes.

Intelligence

People with developmental delays are characterized by slow information-processing speed and less effective memory-encoding abilities than people with average intelligence. Following the notion of resource capacity and allocation, researchers have suggested that people with developmental disabilities might be particularly sensitive to the beneficial effects of exercise training. Although this theory is plausible, recent reviews (Tomporowski, Naglieri, and Lambourne 2010; Zagrodnik and Horvat 2009) of controlled experiments failed to find empirical support for the exercise–cognition relation. However, the majority of studies that have been conducted have used global measures of cognitive function (e.g., general intelligence tests), which may lack sensitivity. The area is understudied, particularly with regard to specific mental processes such as executive function and memory.

In summary, useful psychological theories serve two purposes: they summarize the results of observations made by researchers, and they provide a basis for making predictions about causal relations. Great strides have been made in theory development over the past three decades. Competing neuropsychological, cognitive, social, and behavioral theories are currently guiding research conducted by exercise psychologists. As the size of the database increases, it will be vital for exercise scientists who are interested in the relation between exercise and cognition to address how individual differences play a role in predicting behavioral change.

ISSUES IN RESEARCH

The number of studies conducted to evaluate whether exercise can enhance mental functioning has increased dramatically over the past decade. The results of some studies have been summarized in the media and popular magazines and have drawn considerable attention from the general public, educators, and policy makers. Exercise-based interventions have been promoted for a wide range of target groups: children, older adults, people with physical and mental disorders, and others. Scientists by nature tend to be conservative when making predictions about the application of research findings obtained under controlled laboratory conditions to real-world conditions. Before promoting the benefits of exercise in mental functioning, it is important to gather proof that interventions produce meaningful changes in cognition and that the changes are enduring.

Proof of Claim

The interest in interventions that improve mental functions has been longstanding. Over the centuries, many miracle drugs, diets, and lifestyle behaviors have been proposed to augment or restore the human body and mind. Indeed, at one point in the early 20th century, daily doses of radium were believed to promote health and prevent the effects of aging; many people ingested toxic levels on a daily basis. Today, as in the past, people are drawn to activities proposed to promote physical and mental health; routine exercise is only one of many considered to have salutary benefits.

Two recent comprehensive reviews of treatments designed to improve cognition addressed issues regarding "proof of claim." A monograph published by Hertzog and his colleagues in *Psychological Science in the Public Interest* (Hertzog et al. 2009) described a life span approach to examining the effectiveness of cognitive enrichment (i.e., intellectual, physical, and social activities) and mental training interventions in producing meaningful positive mental health outcomes. Noack and colleagues' 2009 review focused on rehabilitation issues for older adults. Treatment effectiveness was evaluated in light of four criteria shown in the sidebar Intervention Effectiveness. The examination of longitudinal studies led reviewers to conclude that enriched lifestyles that included mentally engaging activities and physical activity contribute to cognitive functioning. Successful intervention programs are characterized by training that requires participants to exert cognitive effort and metacognitive, or higher-order, processing. The notion that challenging experiences, both mental and physical, benefit cognitive function has been voiced previously (Tomporowski 1997).

Studies that compare the independent effects of exercise interventions and mental enrichment interventions on cognitive function will be important contributions to the literature. Few randomized controlled experiments have included nonexercise conditions that systematically control for mentally engaging activities. Interventions that combine physical activity and mental engagement have been hypothesized to have synergetic effects on cognitive function

Intervention Effectiveness

Criteria used to judge "proof of claim" (Hertzog et al. 2009, 17):

1. *Positive transfer.* Will learning acquired in one context influence the acquisition of a new skill, the execution of a novel task, or task performance in a different context?

   Transfer reflects the degree to which knowledge gained in one situation (e.g., the school classroom) is employed in other settings (e.g., work). Cognitive training programs directed at learning new cognitive skills often show large improvements in performance in the task being trained (e.g., crossword puzzles) but very low transfer to other tasks (e.g., Sudoku puzzles). Programs designed to impact general abilities provide the best evidence of transfer.

2. *Maintenance of intervention effects over time.* How long will the effects of the intervention last?

   Interventions may alter performance during training; however, it is important to determine whether the effects of training continue once the intervention has been terminated. A variety of noncognitive factors can modify people's behaviors when they are participating in training programs. At issue is whether the learning gained from training continues to be utilized.

3. *Application of intervention gains to everyday life.* Do individuals alter decision making and strategy use when faced with routine daily challenges?

   Cognitive training programs that teach memory strategies (e.g., mnemonic training) have shown marked and impressive gains in individuals' laboratory performance. The significance of training effects, however, is reflected by the extent to which newly acquired cognitive strategies are selected and used effectively to solve routine daily challenges.

4. *Generalization to the larger population.* Will the training program produce similar outcomes for all individuals?

   Participants in laboratory studies of cognitive training are seldom randomly selected from the general population. As sampling bias may influence the impact of training programs, the degree to which programs translate widely needs to be determined.

(Schaefer, Huxhold, and Lindenberger 2006; Tomporowski, McCullick, and Horvat 2010); however, empirical support is limited.

What Makes Exercise Special?

Noack and colleagues (2009) contrasted the effectiveness of cognitive and physical activity treatments and noted that exercise programs consistently produced greater transfer of cognitive performance. The reviewers drew on the **neurogenic reserve hypothesis** (Kempermann 2008), developed on the basis of animal studies, to explain why exercise training may be unique. Exercise leads to a cascade of neurological changes in the brain and an increase in the number of neurons in the dentate gyrus of the hippocampus. The increased numbers of hippocampal neurons establish a resource pool that enables people to respond adaptively to environmental challenges. However, the increase in hippocampal cells is not the only important result; people's experiences, in turn, alter hippocampal cell functions and alter the neurological pathways that underlie learning. Thus, conditions under which cognitive challenge is combined with physical activity are predicted to maintain the neurogenic reserve and plasticity. The neurogenic reserve hypothesis predicts that combinations of physical activity and cognitive engagement are particularly important early in the life span because the reserve developed provides resources in later life. "Broad ranges of physical activity early in life would not only help to build a highly optimized hippocampal network adapted to a complex life . . . [but] would also contribute to a neurogenic reserve by keeping precursor cells in cycle" (Kempermann 2008, 167).

Very few chronic exercise studies provide detailed descriptions of the interventions employed. Most simply describe interventions as aerobic or nonaerobic exercises. Participants' cognitive engagement during solitary treadmill walking would be expected to differ from dance-based activities performed in a group context. A fine-grain examination of the cognitive demand elicited during exercise training may help resolve, at least in part, the discrepancies that exist among study outcomes.

Does Exercise Training Influence Performance or Learning?

Exercise interventions often change participants' behaviors. Psychologists make clear distinctions between changes in behavior due to learning, which are relatively permanent changes in response potential that are acquired from experience, and changes in behavior due to performance, which are transitory because they result from noncognitive factors. Three sources of behavioral change have been identified: (1) daily variation of fatigue, mood, or motivation; (2) the use of existing strategies or mnemonic skills; and (3) the alteration of basic abilities (Noack et al. 2009). Participants who volunteer for exercise studies are aware of treatment conditions, and their expectancies may alter their cognitive test performances. Likewise, the energizing effects of acute bouts of exercise or the physical adaptations that occur with chronic exercise may affect neural speed, selection, and the use of decision-making strategies that are central to many tests of executive function. The enhancement of cognitive test performance, however, lasts only as long as the physiological perturbations. Repeated bouts of acute exercise

may also alter neural integrity in ways that lead to learning via relatively permanent alterations in cortical and subcortical networks. These three sources of change do not operate in isolation, which makes conclusions concerning performance or learning difficult to determine.

The distinction between performance (skills) and learning (abilities) is important because it reflects both transfer and generalization. Improvements in physical and mental skills are clearly important in everyday life, and humans strive to achieve and maintain expertise through practice. Skills, however, are domain specific and useful only within specific contexts. Abilities are individual traits that underlie adaptive problem solving, which crosses multiple knowledge domains (Carroll 1993). Currently, the bulk of the evidence that supports the exercise–cognition relation in humans comes from behavioral tests of executive processing that emphasize response selection, speed, and accuracy. Only a few studies have reported changes in memory functions. Evidence from recent neurological studies is beginning to shed light on the performance–learning issue. Experiments designed to assess learning effects via transfer and retention manipulations would advance the field.

Dose—Response Studies?

Research evidence shows that changes in brain integrity (e.g., neurotransmitters, neuromodulators, vascularization, neurogenesis) follow exercise training. At this time, however, the effect of multiple acute exercise bouts on cognitive function is not well understood. Historically, researchers have employed guidelines developed by exercise physiologists to improve adults' cardiorespiratory function. The majority of studies have employed aerobic programs in which participants' cognitive functions are measured before and after several months of exercise performed at intensities, durations, and frequencies required for a training effect. Evidence supporting the cardiorespiratory hypothesis is lacking (Etnier et al. 2006), however, and alternative explanations have yet to emerge.

Experimental evidence of the effect of exercise training duration on cognitive function is also lacking. These data are particularly important for program development in educational, rehabilitative, health, and human performance settings. Davis and colleagues (2011) observed a linear relation between the length of exercise bouts (20 min vs. 40 min) and improved executive function and academic achievement in overweight children. Similarly, Masley and colleagues (2009) assessed healthy middle-aged adults' (mean age ~47) cognitive function before and after 10 weeks of aerobic exercise participation and found the greatest gains in executive function in those who exercised 5 to 7 times weekly compared to those who exercised 3 or 4 times and fewer than 2 times weekly. Researchers need to determine whether a threshold of physical activity must be met to accrue cognitive benefits.

SUMMARY

Exercise appears to benefit human cognition. Although advances in understanding the underlying mechanisms have been made, unambiguous explanations for the relation are lacking. Physical activity may benefit cognition directly via effects on a wide number of physiological structures that operate at multiple levels of functioning (e.g., molecular, cellular, organ, or systems). Recent advances in neuropsychology have highlighted the importance of brain networks that are influenced by exercise training. However, the exercise–cognition relation is very complex, and the roles of multiple environmental factors as well as individuals' past learning experiences are clearly influential. Exercise interventions appear to influence specific cognitive functions, and the size of the effect may depend on a variety of moderating factors. It is also important to realize that when the benefits of exercise interventions have been documented, the magnitudes of the effects consistently range between small and moderate.

Taken together, the available data suggest that exercise, although beneficial for mental function, is not the panacea described in articles published in the popular press. Many issues must yet be addressed to further our understanding of the pathways by which physical activity modifies biological systems, and of how those adaptations alter mental activity and, ultimately, behavior.

WEBSITES

www.fi.edu/learn/brain/exercise.html

www.johnratey.com/newsite/index.html

www.apa.org/topics/children/healthy-eating.aspx

http://consensus.nih.gov/2010/alzstatement.htm

chapter
9

Energy and Fatigue

A working mother of two young children often feels too tired to exercise, but when she does, even if it is a low-intensity walk around the neighborhood or some digging in the garden, afterward she feels a short-term energy boost. Medical patients, such as those with cancer, depression, or heart disease, often are sedentary and feel persistent fatigue. People with these conditions usually realize long-lasting improvements in energy within a few weeks of starting to exercise regularly. A highly energetic college athlete, able to perform two vigorous swimming bouts each day for months, may increase her exercise training to an even higher level for several weeks and induce feelings of intense, relatively persistent **fatigue**. These examples illustrate some of the potential complexities in the relationship between physical activity and feelings of energy and fatigue.

This chapter focuses on the influence of acute and chronic physical activity on feelings of energy and fatigue. The chapter begins by defining these feelings, describing how they have been conceptualized, commenting on their measurement, and discussing their importance. This background information is followed by a summary of what is known about how physical activity relates to feelings of energy and fatigue.

DEFINITIONS

The term *energy* can be defined as subjective feelings of having the capacity to complete mental or physical activities. The term *fatigue* can be defined as subjective feelings of having a reduced capacity to complete mental or physical activities. Feelings of energy are often described as feeling energetic and vigorous. Feelings of

> The word *energy* stems from the Latin and Greek words *energia* and *energos,* which come from the roots *en* (meaning "more") and *erg* (mean "work").
>
> The word *fatigue* stems from the Latin word *fatigare,* which comes from the root *fati* (meaning "enough") and from the French *fatiguer,* meaning "to tire or exhaust with labor."

fatigue are often described in terms of exhaustion and tiredness. Because feelings are subjective, they are properly described as symptoms of energy or symptoms of fatigue, although some authors use the phrases *mental energy* and *mental fatigue* to clarify that they are not referring to exercise-related fatigue.

A BRIEF HISTORY

Recorded historical ideas about the mental aspects of energy and fatigue date back at least to Aristotle's conception of *actus et potential* during the fourth century BC. He argued that mental energy is the power source for activating all the operations of the mind. Modern English words describing energy and fatigue can be traced to the 17th century. The word *energy* stems from the Latin and Greek words *energia* and *energos*. These come from the roots *en* (meaning "more") and *erg* (meaning "work"). The word *fatigue* stems from the Latin and French words *fatigare* and *fatiguer*, and comes from the root *fati* (meaning, in Latin, "enough," and in French, "to tire or exhaust with labor").

The concept of psychic energy played a central role in Sigmund Freud's influential psychoanalytic theory of personality, which was formalized in the 1920s. In 1921 psychologist Bernard Muscio struggled with the challenges of defining and measuring fatigue and concluded that "the term mental fatigue should be absolutely banished from scientific discussion, and attempts to develop a test of mental fatigue should be abandoned" (Muscio 1921). Despite that extreme position, psychologists in the mid-20th century, such as Elizabeth Duffy, generated theories of arousal, a concept similar to that of mental energy, that argued that arousal played a central role in broadly influencing most if not all affect, behaviors, and emotions.

In recent years researchers have attempted to explain mental fatigue more narrowly and from cognitive, illness (e.g., cancer-related fatigue), and biological perspectives (Dawson et al. 2011; Deluca 2005; Stahl 2002; van der Linden 2011; Watanabe et al. 2010). Today the interest in feelings of energy and fatigue appears to be at an all-time high in part because so many people feel too tired to function optimally. Contributing to the high prevalence of fatigue has been the revolution in technology. Internet access has motivated many to expand their engagement in social, occupational, and other cognitive activities, often taking time away from mental energy–promoting activities such as sleep and physical activity.

CONCEPTUAL FRAMEWORK

The layperson often makes a distinction between physical fatigue (associated with high-intensity skeletal muscle activity) and mental fatigue. Here our focus is on the mental aspects of fatigue. The distinction between physical and mental fatigue can be useful for discussion purposes, but it is important to recognize that such a dichotomy is philosophically and technically inappropriate. Feelings of energy and fatigue that we define as either mental or physical are both caused in part by electrochemical events within brain neural circuits. These events are modifiable by signals originating outside of the brain, such as information received from the activation of sensory receptors located in skeletal muscles.

There are two broad types of energy and fatigue: acute (states) and chronic (traits or trait-like). Energy and fatigue states fluctuate over the day and are influenced by daily acute events such as a single night's sleep length, an afternoon of difficult work requiring high concentration, or a single bout of exercise. Chronic energy or fatigue refers to longer-lasting experiences, including relatively permanent aspects of a person's personality. Perhaps you know someone whom you think of as always having a high degree of energy. Chronic energy and fatigue levels are changeable, but doing so requires usually a more substantial stimulus, such as a medical illness or a persistent change in behavior (e.g., a long-term change in sleep, diet, or physical activity patterns).

If the dominant feeling a person experiences is fatigue, then that person typically lacks feelings of energy, and vice versa. Energy and fatigue feelings are not always this simple, however. A woman might feel both fatigued and energized when her child is born after a long labor. This occasional presence of mixed feelings is of potential interest to scientists because it implies that the brain neural circuits underlying feelings of energy are separate from those underlying feelings of fatigue. If this is true, the effects of exercise on feelings of energy may be independent of its effects on feelings of fatigue.

> **A** reciprocal relationship between energy and fatigue is reasonable, but mixed feelings (e.g., feeling fatigued and energized at the same time) suggest the possibility of separate neural circuits for energy and fatigue.

MEASUREMENT

There is no objective measure of energy or fatigue feelings that is widely recognized as valid. The consensus criterion is a measure of self-reported energy or fatigue feelings obtained from an interview or, more commonly, a questionnaire. Questionnaires using one of three types of scales are often used. Researchers and psychologists use **unipolar scales** that conceptualize energy and fatigue as separate constructs scaled in categories ranging from *the absence of the feeling* to *an extremely intense feeling*. This type of measure allows for the assessment of mixed feelings of energy and fatigue. The vigor and fatigue subscales of the Profile of Mood States questionnaire are examples of widely used unipolar scales designed to measure the intensity of energy and fatigue feelings. These scales could measure mixed feelings of fatigue and energy that you might experience immediately after completing your first 26.2-mile marathon run.

> **R**unners at the finish line of the Boston Marathon may experience both intense fatigue and energy.

The vitality subscale of the popular SF-36 Health Survey, which conceptualizes energy and fatigue on opposite ends of a single continuum, is a **bipolar scale**. For example, with this bipolar scale, to earn the highest vitality score, a person must report feeling energetic all of the time and feeling fatigued none of the time. If fatigue is present some of the time, then the overall vitality score is reduced. This vitality scale is commonly used in studies of exercise training that seek to quantify changes in the recalled frequency of energy and fatigue feelings.

A third approach uses **multidimensional scales** that simultaneously measure fatigue and other related constructs. Multidimensional scales are frequently used in studies of exercise training with medical patients. The Fatigue Symptom Inventory, for example, was designed to measure fatigue among cancer patients. It obtains information not only about fatigue but also about how much a patient perceives that fatigue is interfering with his or her daily life, including the ability to work, concentrate, enjoy life, and maintain good relationships with other people.

Although multidimensional measures often provide a good assessment of fatigue-related functioning, the failure to focus questions solely on energy and fatigue can introduce substantial error in the measurement of energy and fatigue feelings per se.

The measurement of fatigue, and other medically important symptoms such as pain, in medical patients is sometimes called a patient-reported outcome (PRO). Because of the medical importance of PROs, the U.S. National Institutes of Health (NIH) has devoted funding to an initiative aimed at improving the way PROs are measured in patients by using a rigorously tested web-based computer adaptive testing system. The advantage of computer adaptive testing over paper-and-pencil questionnaires is that it can obtain greater measurement precision with fewer questions by tailoring each new question based on previous answers. The NIH initiative is called Patient Reported Outcomes Measurement Information System (PROMIS), and a website with more information is provided at the end of this chapter.

Ideally, mental energy and fatigue should be measured objectively. Among the best currently available objective measures related to energy and fatigue are performances on vigilance tasks. These are cognitive tests of a specific type of attention. An example of a vigilance task is pressing a computer key every time the letter Q appears on a screen immediately after the letter M when a series of letters are presented every second. A unique feature of vigilance tests is that they involve extended concentration for relatively long periods; for instance, from 20 minutes to several hours. Over time, vigilance performance decreases: a key press is missed, or it takes a longer time to press the key in response to a letter Q.

> **A** patient-reported outcome (PRO) can be fatigue, pain, or other aspects of a patient's health based on information gathered directly from the patient without interpretation by anyone else.

Studies have shown that fatigue-causing events, such as a night without sleep, reduce vigilance performance and that a moderate correlation exists between decrements in objective vigilance performance and both increases in feelings of fatigue and decreases in feelings of energy. For example, 143 U.S. Army rangers completed a 12-mile (19.3 km) walk with 38-pound (17.2 kg) backpacks followed 30 minutes later by an unloaded 3-mile (4.8 km) run and four hours later by another unloaded 3-mile (4.8 km) run (Lieberman, Falco, and Slade 2002). Before, during, and after these activities, the soldiers completed the Profile of Mood States (POMS) and responded with a button press to sounds presented by a wristwatch monitor. The accuracy and speed with which they responded to the sounds were used as measures of vigilance. These men also were randomly assigned to receive either a placebo beverage or a beverage containing either 6% or 12% carbohydrate. Vigilance was improved in a dose–response manner with the administration of carbohydrate, and the subjective vigor scores corroborated the objective results obtained from the monitor.

Causes and Correlates of Fatigue Symptoms

The fact that a large number of environmental, social, behavioral, individual, and physiological variables have been linked to feelings of energy and fatigue complicates our ability to fully understand the influence of physical activity on these feelings. The complexity of fatigue becomes obvious after reviewing the next paragraph, which enumerates these diverse but key variables thought to affect energy and fatigue symptoms.

Each day sustained wakefulness contributes to gradually increasing feelings of fatigue from the time we wake up to bedtime. Chronic sleep loss contributes to increased feelings of fatigue that can accumulate over multiple days. Active engagement in a cognitive task that requires sustained attention increases feelings of fatigue over time. Even more fatigue provoking is sustaining attention over many hours either while engaging in a single complex task or switching among several complex tasks, as is required in

many jobs. Physical or social situations perceived as interesting or threatening result in a reduction of fatigue symptoms. People with neurotic personality types are characterized by elevated fatigue symptoms. Some environmental conditions, such as those involving exposure to bright or varying light, are energizing, whereas other environments, such as those with constant dim lighting or total darkness, promote fatigue. Some sounds, such as your favorite upbeat music, help you feel more energetic, but other sounds, such as sustained exposure to loud industrial noise, can be fatiguing. Symptoms of fatigue are negatively associated with motivation to perform both cognitive and physical work. Decreased feelings of fatigue result from the ingestion of stimulants, such as caffeine, nicotine, and amphetamines (e.g., Adderall). Other drugs, such as antihypertensives, can produce fatigue. Still others, such as alcohol, can both increase and then later decrease feelings of energy. Acute and chronic food restriction produces increased feelings of fatigue. Eating, depending on what is consumed and when, can generate feelings of either energy or fatigue. At some point, pregnancy increases feelings of fatigue for most women; it is minor and transient for some and severe and debilitating for others. Fatigue is also common after a traumatic head injury. Fatigue symptoms frequently are elevated as a result of psychological or physiological pathologies that cause medical illnesses (See Examples of Illnesses Characterized by Increased Symptoms of Fatigue). Also, studies of mono- and dizygotic twin pairs show that about half of the variation in chronic fatigue states can be attributed to genetic factors. In short, brain circuits that generate feelings of energy and fatigue do so by integrating information from a wide variety of sources, including psychobiological responses and adaptations to acute and chronic physical activity.

Prevalence of Severe Fatigue

Prolonged, elevated symptoms of fatigue are a widespread problem in the United States and across the world. Symptoms of fatigue are normally distributed in the population, but the prevalence of fatigue as a public health problem

Examples of Illnesses Characterized by Increased Symptoms of Fatigue

- Allergies (e.g., hay fever)
- Anemia
- Anorexia
- Anxiety disorders
- Asthma
- Cancers
- Coronary heart disease
- Chronic fatigue syndrome
- Chronic obstructive pulmonary disease
- Chronic pain
- Diabetes
- Depressive disorders

- Fibromyalgia
- Heart failure
- Acute (e.g., influenza, mononucleosis) and chronic (e.g., giardiasis, HIV) infections
- Multiple sclerosis
- Obesity
- Parkinson's disease
- Sleep disorders
- Stroke
- Substance abuse
- Thyroid disease

depends on how it is defined. For example, a study of 4,591 middle-aged American men and women showed that 37% reported at least one bout of prolonged fatigue during their lifetimes. The prevalence of fatigue was lower when stricter definitions were used. The prevalence of fatigue was 23% and 16% when symptoms were required to be elevated for greater than 1 and 6 months, respectively. About 20% of primary care patients complain of a recent history of prolonged fatigue. Women are two to three times more likely to experience fatigue problems than men are, regardless of how it is defined.

Only ~1% of the U.S. population, a small percentage but equating to ~3.1 million Americans, suffer from **chronic fatigue syndrome**, a disorder characterized by severe and disabling fatigue lasting at least 6 months and accompanied by widespread infectious and rheumatological pain and psychological symptoms. Anxious or depressed people are six to seven times more likely to suffer from severe fatigue, yet when fatigue is present, it is more difficult for physicians to diagnose a major depressive disorder. Elevated fatigue is the most common symptom among cancer patients, and these feelings persist for months and even years after treatment in about one-third of cancer patients.

The prevalence of persistent fatigue is not uniform across the globe. For example, the results of one study of people residing in 14 countries showed that among people from less economically developed countries such as Nigeria, the prevalence of fatigue was lower than average (Skapinakis, Lewis, and Mavreas 2003). However, the percentage of those with unexplained fatigue who complain about it to a physician was higher in economically poorer countries compared to people living in economically well-developed countries. In sum, feelings of fatigue and low energy affect a large number of people, especially women, anxious and depressed people, and those coping with medical illnesses or living in industrialized countries.

Feelings of low energy and fatigue are clearly significant for both individuals and society. For individuals they can have a negative impact on a wide range of concerns including learning, interpersonal relationships, health, quality of life, and work productivity. Because of the effects on work productivity, low energy and fatigue negatively affect the health of the economy.

Feeling energetic may be part of our evolutionary heritage; it is logical to assume that highly energetic people would have had greater success in acquiring food, shelter, and mates than those with little energy. Fatigue may have contributed to the success of our species independently of feelings of energy. Assuming that feelings of fatigue represent either the presence of an illness or a state of suboptimal mental or physical capability, fatigue symptoms could signal the need for greater than normal rest. Attention to fatigue symptoms may have allowed our ancestors to more successfully pass on their genes by delaying the competition for resources until they were enjoying more effective mental and physical states.

Beyond the speculation about the role of feelings of energy and fatigue in our evolution, these symptoms are important in other ways. Children with low energy and fatigue do poorly in school compared to energetic youngsters. People dealing with fatigue problems have a lower quality of life characterized by reduced physical and mental functioning compared to those without fatigue.

Elevated symptoms of low energy and fatigue are viewed as particularly important by patients and represent one of the top reasons people seek medical help. This concern is logical for many people including older adults for whom fatigue symptoms are independently associated with an increased risk of mortality. Yet, many physicians consider elevated fatigue symptoms relatively unimportant, perhaps because they are so common and the symptoms do not easily contribute to a specific diagnosis. Physicians, however, often do not have the healthiest attitude toward fatigue. Their jobs often require them to work long hours with inadequate sleep, and many are proud of their toughness in dealing with fatigue. Yet a survey of nearly 3,000 physicians in training (i.e., medical residents) found that one in five admitted fatigue-related poor performance that injured a patient. Accidents of all types, including those resulting in loss of life or catastrophic environmental and economic losses (e.g., the Chernobyl nuclear accident), have often been precipitated in part by attempts to ignore symptoms of fatigue.

Epidemiological Evidence

More than a dozen population-based studies testing over 150,000 participants have measured feelings of fatigue and compared adults who were physically active in their leisure time to those who were not. The results are highly consistent. All studies examined, regardless of the age or health status of participants or the country in which the study was conducted, showed that inactive people reported feeling less energetic or more fatigued than more active people did. Figure 9.1 shows the consistency of results across age from adolescents to older adult men living in European nations.

Overall, physically active people had a 40% reduced risk of experiencing fatigue compared to inactive people (Puetz 2006). The effect was robust in that it remained meaningful in cross-sectional studies after making statistical adjustments for potential confounding factors such as smoking and alcohol use. The effect also was consistently observed in prospective studies. For example, one investigation of 128 older adults, including 54 centenarians, found that physical inactivity was a strong predictor of increases in fatigue over 1.5 to 5 years (Martin et al. 2006).

Walking is the most common form of physical activity. Among U.S. adults, those who never walk are more than four times more likely to report a perceived lack of energy to exercise than those who do walk (Eyler et al. 2003). The epidemiological evidence suggests a negatively accelerating dose–response relationship between typical leisure-time physical activity and **energy symptoms**, as illustrated in figure 9.2.

One limitation of epidemiological evidence is the potential for substantial error in measuring physical activity from short self-reports. Given that one consequence of increased vigorous exercise is an increase in physical fitness ($\dot{V}O_2max$), which can be measured objectively and with less error than self-reported physical activity, it is notable that a study of 427 older workers showed a statistically meaningful tendency for the more fit people to report a higher frequency of feeling energetic (Strijk et al. 2010).

To complicate matters, an inverted-U relationship between physical activity and feelings of energy is found when the data include people engaged in exercise training at a very high level, such as those training for endurance sports. For instance, a study of 1,880 boys and girls aged 11 to 14 who were followed for more than two years found that being sedentary for more than

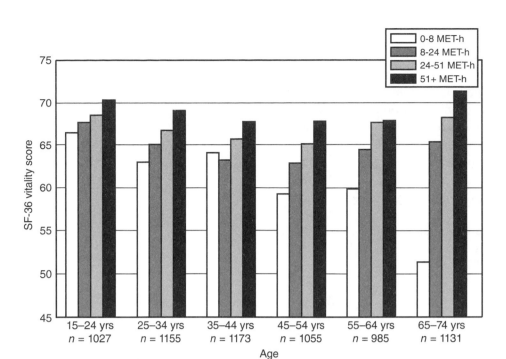

Figure 9.1 Association between the self-reported prior week's physical activity (MET-hours/week) and feelings of energy (measured by the SF-36) among 6,526 men aged 15 and older living in 1 of 16 European Union member nations.

Adapted from Abu-Omar, Rutten, and Lehtinen 2004.

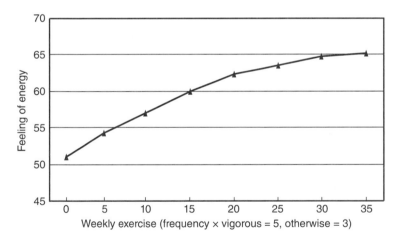

Figure 9.2 Association between weekly exercise and feelings of energy (assessed from SF-36 vitality scores) among 39,325 adult Australian women. For comparison, on the same measure from a representative sample of 1,412 adult U.S. women, the mean and standard deviation scores are 58 and 21, respectively.

Adapted from Brown et al. 2000.

four hours per day or being highly physically active were both associated with an increased likelihood of reporting persistent fatigue (Viner et al. 2008).

Some epidemiological evidence suggests that fatigue is a barrier to participating in physical activity. A random sample of 1,818 U.S. adults revealed that ~20% reported they were too tired

to exercise regularly (Brownson et al. 2001). Another study found that increases in symptoms of fatigue over 6 months among 263 people with relapsing-remitting multiple sclerosis were significantly associated with reductions in physical activity (Motl et al. 2011). A separate investigation learned that people reporting frequent fatigue usually were only contemplating being physically active rather than actually engaging in the behavior.

In sum, a substantial body of epidemiological evidence supports a link between physical inactivity and feelings of fatigue and low energy. However, experimental evidence is needed to determine conclusively whether physical inactivity causes people to lack energy.

Experimental Evidence

Experiments can provide evidence of whether physical activity can cause changes in feelings of energy and fatigue. The most common type of experiment involves increased physical activity, either exercise training or a single bout of exercise. As important as determining whether exercise causes changes in energy and fatigue is discovering what happens when people stop exercising.

Reductions in Physical Activity

Periods of reduced physical activity are common among regularly active people. Some decide to spend more time on other things and become couch potatoes. Others are injured or undergo surgery, and their recovery requires some time off from their usual physical activities. Many women reduce their level of physical activity during pregnancy. Those who are able to maintain their prepregnancy levels of physical activity appear to enjoy more mood stability, including greater feelings of energy and fatigue (Poudevigne and O'Connor 1995). Annually, about 1 million U.S. women undergo extended bed rest in the hopes it will contribute to a positive outcome associated with a multiple-birth pregnancy or a pregnancy with complications. Unfortunately, current evidence shows no clear benefit of bed rest, but multiple adverse side effects, including loss of muscle function and mass and increased insulin resistance and risk for thromboembolic disease.

If physical activity causes people to feel more energetic, then when physically active people stop being active, this should cause them to feel more fatigued. A small number of studies involving 3 to 20 days of bed rest or exercise abstinence have found increased symptoms of fatigue and low energy compared to control

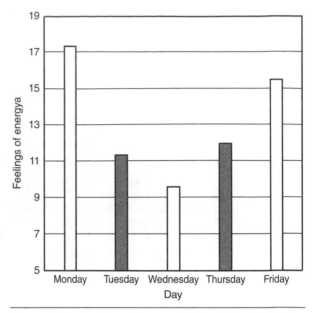

Figure 9.3 Feelings of energy before (Monday), after (Friday), and during 3 days (Tuesday through Thursday) of exercise abstinence among highly active adults (45 minutes per day, 6 or 7 days per week).

Based on Mondin et al. 1996.

conditions involving usual levels of physical activity. As an example, one study's results are summarized in figure 9.3.

Increases in Physical Activity

Dozens of studies have examined the effects of acute exercise on mood including feelings of energy and fatigue, primarily among college students (Yeung 1996). After typical short-duration (~20-40 min) low- to moderate-intensity exercise, feelings of energy are increased but feelings of fatigue remain unchanged. The increase in energy has been observed with most modes of exercise, including walking, cycling, swimming, resistance exercise, yoga, and martial arts (Herring and O'Connor 2009). This improvement has been found with exercise bouts as short as 10 minutes (Osei-Tutu and Campagna 2005), although some evidence indicates that 30 minutes is a more effective stimulus for enhancing feelings of vigor (Hansen, Stevens, and Coast 2001).

Immediately after short-duration exercise at very high intensities, feelings of fatigue may increase. The magnitude of this change is intensity dependent; the greatest increases in feelings of fatigue are observed with the highest-intensity exercise. This effect is transient; as recovery time continues, feelings of fatigue gradually return to preexercise levels. With longer acute exercise durations (>2 hours), increased feelings of fatigue and reduced feelings of energy can be experienced even with low-intensity exercise. This effect is moderated by fitness level; highly fit people can exercise at a low intensity for several hours without feeling much fatigue.

The improvements in energy and fatigue symptoms with acute exercise are realized by men and women of all ages, although some evidence suggests that regular exercisers exhibit these improvements most reliably (Hoffman and Hoffman 2008). Improvements in feelings of energy and fatigue after a single bout of exercise also have been documented among those with a variety of medical illnesses including patients with depression, multiple sclerosis, and obesity (Bartholomew, Morrison, and Ciccolo 2005). A few studies have examined the influence of a single bout of exercise on fatigue operationalized by changes in objective vigilance performance. The results have not consistently produced the expected improvement in vigilance after low- to moderate-intensity exercise or reductions in vigilance after high-intensity exercise (Lambourne and Tomporowski 2010).

Few studies have compared the effects of an acute bout of exercise on feelings of energy and fatigue to other experiences that might also affect these symptoms. One study reported that a 10-minute afternoon walk improved feelings of energy to a greater extent than did eating a candy bar (Thayer 1987).

At least 70 randomized controlled trial experiments have examined the influence of exercise

To get a quick energy boost, you could take a walk, listen to music, have an energy drink, socialize, or take a nap. Although any of these might help, more research is needed to learn how these methods of managing fatigue compare in both the short term and the long term.

training performed by sedentary people on symptoms of energy and fatigue. Analyses of these experiments have found that compared to inactive control participants, those who participated in 6 to 20 weeks of exercise training 2 to 5 days per week experienced decreased feelings of fatigue. Improvements in exercise and fatigue symptoms favored the exercise group in 94% of 70 trials. The overall average effect of 0.37 standard deviation is a meaningful magnitude of improvement (Puetz, O'Connor, and Dishman 2006). Improvements in feelings of energy and fatigue have been reported in supervised exercise programs held in medical clinics and in worksite and home-based exercise programs.

The ideal exercise dose needed to produce improvements in feelings of energy and fatigue is uncertain. Among the best evidence addressing this issue comes from a 6-month randomized controlled trial including 430 sedentary, overweight, and obese postmenopausal women (Martin et al. 2009). It was found that feelings of energy improved after aerobic exercise training (treadmill or semirecumbent cycling at a low intensity [50% aerobic capacity] three or four times each week) that expended 4, 8, or 12 kilocalories per kilogram of body weight each week. Those amounts of physical activity approximated 50%, 100%, and 150% of the levels recommended by the U.S. National Institutes of Health. These results show that both high and low exercise doses at a low intensity can produce improved feelings of energy. A summary of these findings is presented in figure 9.4.

More than three-quarters of the experiments investigating the influence of regular exercise on symptoms of energy and fatigue involved walking, cycling, and running modes, but the largest improvements occurred in the strength training studies. Results from at least 10 trials now support the conclusion that strength training alone is associated with improvements in symptoms of energy and fatigue (O'Connor, Herring, and Caravalho 2010).

Most of these randomized controlled trial experiments involved medical patients. Exercise training improved fatigue to some degree for all patient groups studied. Psychiatric and cardiac patients showed the largest improvements. In recent years researchers have paid increased

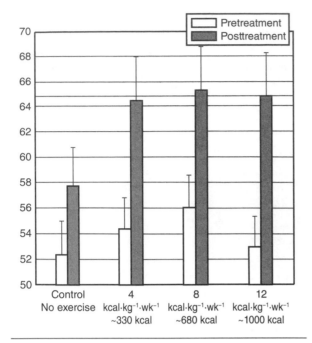

Figure 9.4 Results of a randomized controlled trial examining the influence of three or four training sessions per week for 6 months at one of three doses of physical activity on feelings of energy (SF-36 vitality scores) among 464 sedentary, overweight, postmenopausal women with an average age of 57. The solid horizontal line indicates national norms for American women aged 55 to 64 for SF-36 vitality scores.

Adapted from Martin et al. 2009.

Years ago, cancer patients were told to rest to optimize their well-being. Accumulated evidence in this "hot" research area now suggests that low- to moderate-intensity exercise, performed before, during, and after treatment, can improve the quality of life of breast and prostate cancer patients and survivors, including enhancing their feelings of energy.

attention to learning the extent to which regular exercise might help improve the quality of life of cancer patients, especially those with prostate or breast cancer. The results of one of these investigations with breast cancer patients are illustrated in figure 9.5. These studies typically involve moderate-intensity, supervised aerobic

exercise of ~45 minutes per session, 3 days per week, for 12 weeks. A review of 43 studies of cancer patients undergoing treatment and 27 studies of cancer survivors found that exercise training reduced cancer-related fatigue among patients within these two categories by 0.32 and 0.38 standard deviations, respectively (Puetz and Herring, 2012). The magnitude of these improvements was similar to the magnitude of improvements realized with either drug or psychotherapy aimed at treating fatigue in cancer patients.

It is logical to think that if regular exercise improves feelings of energy, then people suffering from fatigue would benefit the most from getting off the couch. Feelings of energy were improved by ~20% after 6 weeks of low and moderate exercise training in one experiment of sedentary adults who initially reported persistent feelings of fatigue without a well-defined medical condition. In that study (Puetz, Flowers, and O'Connor 2008), improvements in fatigue symptoms were larger than those for energy symptoms, and the improvements in fatigue were realized sooner (within 3 weeks)

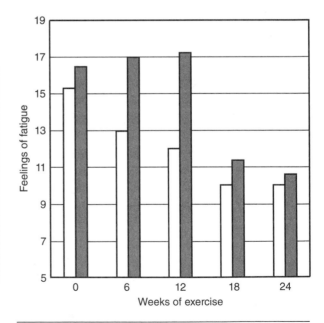

Figure 9.5 Feelings of fatigue in breast cancer survivors randomly assigned to start a 12-week exercise program immediately after baseline testing (weeks 0 to 12, open bars, $n = 29$) or after waiting for 12 weeks and then exercising from weeks 12 to 24 (shaded bars, $n = 29$).

Adapted from Milne et al. 2008.

than those for energy (which occurred primarily at week 6).

Patients with chronic fatigue syndrome (CFS) and related comorbid conditions such as fibromyalgia are physically inactive compared to healthy adults, which can lead to a reduced level of physical fitness. Many CFS patients avoid exercise because they believe it exacerbates their disease symptoms. Some experts have hypothesized that chronic fatigue is promulgated in part by psychobiological consequences resulting from physical inactivity. Randomized controlled trials show that 12 weeks of low- to moderate-intensity graded exercise training improves fatigue symptoms among those with CFS. In the largest trial to date, the rate of adverse reactions to exercise was low and similar to that found with usual medical care (White et al. 2011). Approximately 30% had recovered from CFS after participating in graded exercise training for one year. Exercise can be especially difficult for people who suffer from the combination of CFS and fibromyalgia, and studies show that exercise is more effortful and painful for this group than for those with CFS only (Cook et al. 2006).

Exercise compares favorably to other treatments for chronic fatigue. Nonpharmacological approaches to treating fatigue, such as cognitive behavioral therapy and exercise, are preferred as a first-line therapy over drug treatments in part because of the greater potential for adverse side effects with psychostimulants (e.g., amphetamine, methylphenidate and modafinil). As the name suggests, cognitive behavioral therapy focuses both on (1) teaching patients to cognitively appraise situations appropriately and thereby cope better with fatigue and (2) having patients avoid maladaptive behaviors that might contribute to fatigue (e.g., chronically drinking coffee in the evening and consequently experiencing poor sleep). Although exercise therapy has not been compared to cognitive behavioral therapy frequently, in one large study (Donta et al. 2003) that compared the two treatments, exercise training improved fatigue symptoms to a larger degree than did cognitive behavioral therapy, and there was no advantage to combining exercise and cognitive behavioral therapy. The results of this study are illustrated in figure 9.6.

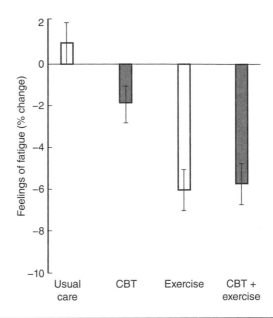

Figure 9.6 Influence on fatigue symptoms of 12 weeks of aerobic exercise training (n = 265; 60 min, 3 times/week) compared to a usual care control condition (n = 270), cognitive behavioral therapy (CBT; n = 286), and exercise plus CBT (n = 266). Participants were U.S. veterans with Gulf War illness.

Data from Donta et al. 2003.

MECHANISMS

Our current understanding of the biological mechanisms by which exercise influences feelings of energy and fatigue is poor in part because few studies have been specifically designed for that purpose. Changes in feelings of energy and fatigue after decreases in physical activity or after exercise training appear to be unrelated to peripheral physiological changes such as reductions in body fat or increases in aerobic fitness. This is logical because fatigue symptoms are generated by brain neural circuits that are unlikely to be influenced by, for instance, the cardiovascular (e.g., increased blood volume) and metabolic (e.g., increased skeletal muscle mitochondria) adaptations that contribute to aerobic fitness. A more logical approach is to consider, as plausible biological mechanisms, changes in the brain that occur concurrently with changes in symptoms of energy and fatigue.

The effects of exercise on brain activity measured using electroencephalography (EEG) have been a dominant approach to date. In a study conducted in France (Grego et al. 2004), well-trained cyclists cycled at a moderate intensity for three hours. Before and after, EEG in response to two different sounds was measured 300 milliseconds after the tones. The amplitude of the P300 wave was increased during exercise compared to at rest before exercise. Because prior research has shown that the amplitude of the P300 wave is related to the amount of attentional resources, one interpretation of the results is that biological circuits underlying attention and energy were affected by the exercise.

Other investigations (Petruzzello, Hall, and Ekkekakis 2001; Woo et al. 2009) have linked energy and fatigue symptom reports to EEG. One of these studies examined whether transient changes in feelings of energy and fatigue after 20 minutes of low- and moderate-intensity cycling performed at weeks 1, 3, and 6 of a 6-week exercise training program were related to EEG among adults who started the program with elevated fatigue (Dishman, Thom et al. 2010). Fatigue symptoms were improved after an acute bout of low-intensity exercise during both week 3 and week 6. Feelings of energy were improved at every testing week after acute exercise of both intensities. Half of the effect of acute exercise on improved energy feelings was mediated by EEG changes in the theta frequency range (i.e., the component of the EEG oscillating from four to seven times per second) measured in the posterior part of the brain.

These results support the idea that exercise-induced improvements in energy symptoms have a biological basis. Research of this type is a priority for better understanding the brain basis of exercise-induced changes in energy and fatigue and ruling out, or ruling in, alternative hypotheses such as the idea that improvements in these symptoms are placebo effects driven by biased symptom reports from people who have strong expectations of psychological improvements after exercise.

Several approaches, rarely used in exercise studies to date, including functional neuroimaging and psychopharmacological studies, suggest plausible biological mechanisms by which exercise could influence fatigue symptoms. Several functional neuroimaging studies have examined the association between blood flow and measures of fatigue among fatigued and nonfatigued

people while they performed mentally fatiguing (vigilance) and nonfatiguing (finger tapping) tasks at rest (Cook et al. 2007). The best neuroimaging evidence to date suggests that energy and fatigue symptoms are most strongly related to blood flow in the cingulate, cerebellum, basal ganglia, and parietal brain areas (Genova, Wylie, and DeLuca 2011). Even though overall brain blood flow is not changed with low- to moderate-intensity exercise, regional increases in blood flow with exercise at these intensities have been reported for the cingulate and cerebellum (in exercising pigs) as well as the insular cortex and prefrontal cortex (Rooks et al. 2010).

Research psychiatrists take a different approach to understanding fatigue. They give psychoactive drugs to patients and examine the effects on various moods and symptoms, including energy and fatigue. Studies using a psychopharmacological approach with human test subjects have implicated several brain neurotransmitter systems as important biological contributors to energy and fatigue symptoms (Stahl 2002). Methylphenidate (Ritalin), which increases brain dopamine (DA) levels, is associated with enhanced feelings of energy. Other medications that increase brain norepinephrine (NE) or increase both DA and NE, such as fluoxetine (Prozac), sertraline (Zoloft) and bupropion (Wellbutrin), can reduce fatigue and increase energy symptoms (Demyttenaere, De Fruyt, and Stahl 2005). Medications that increase brain histamine levels, such as modafinil (Provigil), increase feelings of energy, whereas medications that prevent the action of histamines, such as first-generation antihistamines (e.g., Mepyramine, a drug that can cross the blood–brain barrier), produce symptoms of fatigue.

The psychopharmacological approach has implicated a great number of brain areas and circuits as potentially involved in symptoms of energy and fatigue because the DA, NE, and histamine systems have axons that project widely throughout the brain. Projections from the DA, NE, and histamine cell bodies to higher brain areas, such as the dorsolateral prefrontal cortex, are thought to contribute to the reduced cognitive performance (on executive function and vigilance tasks) that occurs with fatigue. Projections involving the nucleus accumbens can influence general motivation and the specific motivation to engage in exercise (Salamone et al. 2007). Projections to the hypothalamus can influence a host of releasing factors that ultimately affect hormones, such as cortisol, which can influence brain neural circuits either directly, because of the presence of cortisol receptors on brain neural tissue, or indirectly by affecting aspects of the immune system. For example, cortisol influences proinflammatory cytokines (e.g., tumor necrosis factor-alpha [TNF-α] and several interleukins [IL-1, IL-6, IL-8]), which have been suggested as potential contributors to fatigue. **Cytokines** are a family of cell-signaling molecules that are present in most cells in the body and can act on brain neural tissue and cause neurochemical and neuroendocrine changes. Although it is plausible that regular exercise could reduce brain levels of proinflammatory cytokines and thereby reduce symptoms of fatigue, the currently available evidence reveals uncertainty about whether that occurs (Cotman, Berchtold, and Christie 2007).

SUMMARY

Energy and fatigue symptoms are important because of their influence on accidents, learning, quality of life, and work productivity. Even though these symptoms are influenced by a myriad of factors, the overall weight of the available epidemiological and experimental evidence clearly shows a consistent link between physical activity and feelings of energy and fatigue.

Physically inactive people tend to report more severe fatigue and low energy symptoms than do those who are regularly active. An acute bout of low- to moderate-intensity exercise improves feelings of energy. Low- to moderate-intensity exercise training improves feelings of energy and fatigue among normal adults as well as those with persistent fatigue and those with a variety of medical illnesses, including chronic fatigue syndrome. Exercise training doses from 50% to 150% of what is recommended for health are associated with improvements in feelings of energy and fatigue if the exercise intensity is maintained at a low level. Very high training intensities or durations (or both), such as those engaged in by endurance athletes, can produce intense and prolonged feelings of fatigue and low energy. The biological mechanisms by which physical activity alters feelings of energy and fatigue are poorly understood but likely involve complex interactions among multiple neurotransmitter systems, brain circuits, and cell-signaling molecules.

WEBSITES

www.cancer.gov/cancertopics/pdq/supportivecare/
   fatigue/patient

www.nlm.nih.gov/medlineplus/fatigue.html

www.ncfsfa.org

www.cdc.gov/cfs

chapter 10

Sleep

One-third of humans' lives is spent asleep, so understanding ways to improve the quality of sleep is an important area of research. Most people assume that they will sleep well after spending a day doing hard manual labor. That assumption seems to have led to the belief that exercise will also foster a good night's sleep. Although exercise is a habit that can promote sleep, and it is recommended by the U.S. National Sleep Foundation (see Recommendations for Promoting Sleep), there is surprisingly little **empirical research** on exercise in relation to disturbed sleep. This chapter provides information about what sleep is, how it is measured, and what factors influence it. We review research on sleep and exercise and address possible mechanisms for the influence of exercise on sleep.

SLEEP DISTURBANCES

Poor sleep can impair health, and many medical conditions and chronic diseases (e.g., heart disease and diabetes) are associated with poor sleep. The most studied of the 70 or so sleep disorders are insomnia and obstructive sleep apnea (interrupted breathing). Insomnia is the perception that sleep is inadequate (poor quantity or quality). It can result from and contribute to emotional distress and can impair daytime function (National Institutes of Health 2010). There are several types of insomnia, which can co-occur.

The types of insomnia include sleep-onset insomnia (trouble falling asleep) and two forms of sleep-maintenance insomnia (awaking frequently or staying awake during the night and waking up early without being able to go back to sleep). Acute insomnia lasts 1 to 3 nights, short-term insomnia lasts 3 nights to 1 month, and chronic insomnia lasts longer than 1 month. Acute insomnia is often caused by emotional or physical discomfort and can become chronic if not successfully treated. Insomnia can be the primary disorder (the least prevalent form), or it can be secondary (i.e., be comorbid) to other health conditions (the most prevalent form). Typically, people with insomnia underestimate

Recommendations for Promoting Sleep

- The most important recommendation is to maintain regular bed and wake times, including on weekends.
- Avoid stimulants such as caffeine and nicotine within 3 to 4 hours of bedtime.
- Avoid alcohol close to bedtime. Although it speeds onset of sleep, it disrupts the second half of the sleep cycle.
- Make sure your bedroom is dark, quiet, and neither too hot nor too cold.
- Avoid heavy meals and lots of fluids close to bedtime.
- Establish a regular, relaxing bedtime routine.
- Associate your bed with sleep; don't use it for watching TV.
- Avoid daytime napping.
- Participate in regular exercise.

Adapted from the National Sleep Foundation, www.sleepfoundation.org.

their ability to sleep when sleep patterns are measured objectively by polysomnography (National Institutes of Health 2010).

PREVALENCE AND IMPACT OF SLEEP DISTURBANCES

About one-third of the people in the United States report having sleep problems, even though only about 15% are diagnosed with insomnia. Sleep-maintenance insomnia is more common than sleep-onset insomnia. In the 2009 Sleep in America Poll conducted by the National Sleep Foundation, nighttime awakenings and poor sleep quality (i.e., not feeling restored after sleep) were the most common complaints.

In the National Comorbidity Survey Replication, 12-month prevalence rates of sleep problems ranged from 16.4% to 25% for difficulty initiating or maintaining sleep, early morning awakening, and nonrestorative sleep. About 36% of people reported at least one of those problems (Roth et al. 2006). They were about three to four times more likely to also be diagnosed with anxiety, mood, or substance disorders that were associated with social role impairments, especially in people who reported nonrestorative sleep. Worldwide, nearly 75% of insomnia patients report problems staying asleep or waking up too early, whereas about 60% say they have problems falling asleep. About half say their quality of sleep is poor (e.g., not restful).

Patients who have insomnia have more emergency department and physician visits, laboratory tests, and prescription drugs filled than people who do not have insomnia. Thus, insomnia contributes to both direct and indirect

Risk factors for insomnia include female sex (especially during the menopause transition); increasing age, especially ages 45 to 54 and after age 85; and shift work, which can disrupt circadian sleep–wake cycles.
Adapted from Rosekind and Gregory 2010.

health care costs. Insomnia also has been shown to negatively affect daytime functioning, including workplace productivity, as well as workplace and public safety (Rosekind and Gregory 2010). The annual direct cost of insomnia treatment in the United States was estimated at $13.9 billion in 1995 (Chilcott and Shapiro 1996).

A more recent retrospective observational study of medical claims for inpatient, outpatient, pharmacy, and emergency department services found the direct costs (in 2003 U.S. dollars) of 6 months of treatment for insomnia to be $924 per patient for ages 18 to 64 and $1,143 per patient for ages 65 and older (Ozminkowski, Wang, and Walsh 2007).

In the United States, direct and indirect medical costs are about $1,200 greater for insomnia patients than for other patients during the 6 months before diagnosis.

Only about 5% to 20% of people who experience sleep disturbances seek help from a primary care physician; about half of those who seek treatment receive a drug prescription, usually a hypnotic or anxiolytic benzodiazepine. Many who do not seek treatment purchase over-the-counter sleep aids or use caffeine to overcome daytime sleepiness resulting from poor sleep or alcohol to get to sleep at night, which can worsen the sleep problem in the long term (Kripke et al. 1998).

So-called natural sleep-promoting agents have unestablished efficacy and may carry health risks. For example, melatonin has been promoted as a miracle sleep drug, but evidence that it promotes sleep is limited. For older adults whose sleep problems can be attributed to advanced circadian phase (i.e., early sleep and early awakening), taking melatonin at night could worsen sleep problems by further advancing the circadian phase. Negative side effects of melatonin, including nausea, nightmares, and headaches, may offset its potential benefits (Guardiola-Lemaitre 1997). Natural melatonin has several limitations as a sleep aid, including that it is quickly metabolized. Melatonin analogs, such as ramelteon, may prove more effective as sleep aids than natural melatonin.

Pharmacological treatments for insomnia include self-prescribed treatments, such as over-the-counter sleep aids, alcohol, and "natural" treatments (e.g., valerian, chamomile, and St. John's wort). Although widely used, over-the-counter sleep aids such as those containing antihistamines (diphenhydramine or hydroxyzine) have adverse side effects, including cognitive impairment and residual day-after effects. The most common prescription drugs for insomnia include benzodiazepines, nonbenzodiazepine hypnotics, and ramelteon, as well as some antidepressants, particularly serotonergic drugs (Rosekind and Gregory 2010).

Understanding the actions of effective insomnia drugs can help guide the study of mechanisms by which exercise aids sleep in people with insomnia. Benzodiazepines (BZDs) are agonists of γ-aminobutyric acid A (GABA$_A$) receptors and are the first-line drug choice for the short-term management of insomnia, especially for reducing the time to sleep onset (sleep latency) and the number of nighttime awakenings. However, long-term use is discouraged because they can impair memory and lead to rebound sleepiness. Non-BZD hypnotics produce similar hypnotic effects as benzodiazepines with fewer side effects. Both BZD and non-BZD hypnotics can be addictive. Ramelteon, a melatonin receptor agonist, is used for sleep-onset insomnia, especially in the treatment of circadian disruptions induced by shift work and jet lag. Some antidepressants are prescribed for the treatment of insomnia because they have sedative effects. Trazodone and mirtazapine are sedating by acting as serotonin receptor agonists or as antihistamines (Rosekind and Gregory 2010). Antagonists of 5-HT2 serotonin receptors have improved deep sleep and sleep quality (e.g., ritanserin) in people with insomnia (Monti 2010).

Common Drugs Used to Treat Insomnia

Benzodiazepines

Dalman (flurazepam)

Doral, Dormalin (quazepam)

Halcion (triazolam)

ProSom, Eurodin (estazolam)

Restoril (temazepam)

Nonbenzodiazepine Hypnotics

Ambien, Edluar (zolpidem)

Sepracor (eszopiclone)

Sonata (zeloplon)

Tricyclics

Elavil (amitriptyline)

Sinequan (doxepin)

Monoamine Oxidase Inhibitors

Desyrel (trazodone)

Tetracyclics

Remeron, Avanza, Zispin (mirtazapine)

Melatonin Receptor Agonist

Rozerem (ramelteon)

A BRIEF HISTORY

In 1913, French scientist Henri Pieron wrote a book titled *Le Probleme Physiologique du Sommeil* (which translates to *The Physiological Problem of Sleep*), the first text to use a physiological approach to describe sleep. Dr. Nathaniel Kleitman, generally acknowledged as the father of American sleep research, began research on the regulation of sleep, wakefulness, and circadian rhythms at the University of Chicago in the 1920s. Kleitman's seminal studies included research on the effects of sleep deprivation. In 1953 he and one of his students, Dr. Eugene

Research on sleep began in the 1920s, and REM sleep was identified in the early 1950s, but sleep research is still developing.

Aserinsky, discovered rapid eye movement (REM) during sleep.

Another of Kleitman's students, Dr. William C. Dement, described the "cyclical" nature of nocturnal sleep in 1955, and in 1957 and 1958 established the relationship between REM sleep and dreaming. Today, over 1,800 accredited sleep disorder centers and laboratories in the United States alone recognize and treat sleep disorders (Epstein and Valentine 2010). Against this historical background, scientific research into the effects of exercise on sleep is in its infancy (Youngstedt 1997, 2000).

DEFINITIONS

Sleep is a state of reversible unconsciousness characterized by little movement and reduced responses to external stimuli. All mammals sleep, and it is believed that lowered brain metabolism during slow-wave sleep provides a rest period for the brain. Dreaming is thought to occur primarily during **rapid eye movement (REM) sleep**; and although there is debate over the purpose of dreams, REM sleep appears critical. The critical nature of REM sleep is based on a rebound phenomenon that occurs after REM deprivation in which more time than normal is spent in REM sleep. One night of sleep deprivation has a significant effect on cognitive function and mood, but little impact on the ability to perform physical exercise. Multiple nights of sleep deprivation can provoke perceptual distortions and hallucinations.

Being asleep is not analogous to putting your body and brain on hold. Sleep consists of a variety of stages with corresponding neural, physiological, and behavioral patterns. On the basis of polysomnographic studies, sleep has been divided into periods of REM sleep and

> **S**tages of sleep are identified by corresponding neural, physiological, and behavioral patterns, although the most familiar to the general public is REM sleep, during which most dreaming occurs.

four stages of non-REM (NREM) sleep during which sleep progressively deepens. Stages 3 and 4 combined constitute **slow-wave sleep (SWS)**, when people are hardest to awaken. About 75% of the night's sleep is NREM (~5% stage 1, ~50% stage 2, and ~20% SWS). During sleep, the activity of the brain cortex fluctuates along a continuum from synchronous, low-frequency, high-amplitude activity to asynchronous, high-frequency, low-amplitude activity (see figure 10.1). This continuum can be delineated by corresponding periods of δ (0.5-3 Hz), θ (3.5-7.5 Hz), α (8-12 Hz), and β (13-30 Hz) activity (one wave per second is 1 Hz). **Alpha wave** activity is commonly described as relaxed wakefulness.

Sleep progresses from drowsiness to stage 1, marked by θ activity, which usually lasts 1 to 7 min. Stage 2 occurs later, denoted by θ activity, sleep spindles (short bursts of 12-14 Hz), and K complexes (sudden sharp spikes).

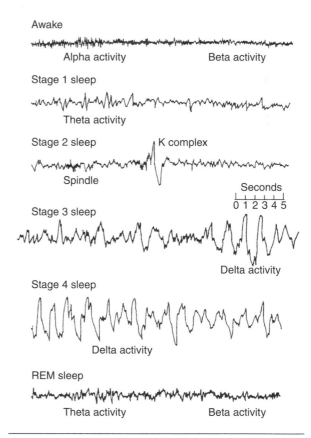

Figure 10.1 Fluctuations in brain activity during various stages of sleep.

Reprinted, by permission of Oxford University Press, from J.A. Horne, 1988, *Why we sleep: The functions of sleep in humans and other mammals* (Oxford, UK: Oxford University Press), ©1988 by James Horne.

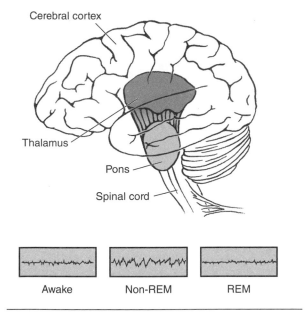

Awake   Non-REM   REM

Figure 10.2 Neurons in the pons trigger REM sleep and inhibit spinal cord neurons.

Based on Siegel 2000.

Spindles occur several times a minute throughout stages 1 to 4, whereas K complexes occur only in stage 2. Stage 3 begins later and is characterized by δ activity. Increasing δ activity denotes stage 4, or deep sleep. Sleep then becomes progressively lighter as the person reenters stage 3 and stage 2 sleep, followed by an episode of REM sleep. Rapid eye movement sleep typically begins about 80 minutes after the onset of stage 4 sleep. Beta activity, rapid eye movement, and little skeletal muscle activity occur during REM sleep.

Neurons located in the pons area of the brain stem trigger REM sleep and inhibit spinal cord neurons, leading to temporary skeletal muscle paralysis (see figure 10.2). Within the pons, the nucleus reticularis pontis oralis/caudalis (RPO/RPC) is the most important site for the production of REM sleep (see figure 10.3). Many of these neurons responsible for REM sleep use acetylcholine as the neurotransmitter. Dorsal raphe (serotonin) and locus coeruleus (norepinephrine) neurons help turn off REM sleep. Activation of the basal forebrain is a key in starting NREM sleep. It is thought that temperature-sensitive neurons in the preoptic area of the anterior hypothalamus that project to the basal forebrain are key in the control of SWS.

Common Types of Insomnia That Exercise Might Help

Sleep-onset insomnia (delayed sleep phase syndrome): The major sleep episode is delayed in relation to the desired clock time. This delay results in symptoms of sleep-onset insomnia or difficulty in awakening at the desired time.

- Psychophysiological insomnia: A disorder of somatized tension (conversion of anxiety into physical symptoms) and learned sleep-preventing association that results in a complaint of insomnia and associated decreased functioning during wakefulness.

- Transient insomnia (adjustment sleep disorder): Represents sleep disturbance temporally related to acute stress, conflict, or environmental change causing emotional agitation.

- Periodic insomnia (non-24-hour sleep–wake syndrome): Consists of a chronic (lasting a long time), steady pattern comprising 1- to 2-hour delays in sleep onset and wake times that occur on a daily basis.

- Hypnotic-dependency insomnia (hypnotic-dependent sleep disorder): Characterized by insomnia or excessive sleepiness that is associated with a tolerance of or withdrawal from hypnotic medications.

- Stimulant-dependent sleep disorder: Characterized by a reduction of sleepiness or the suppression of sleep by central stimulants and resultant alterations in wakefulness following drug abstinence.

- Alcohol-dependent insomnia (alcohol-dependent sleep disorder): Characterized by the assisted initiation of sleep onset by the sustained ingestion of alcohol that is used for its hypnotic effect.

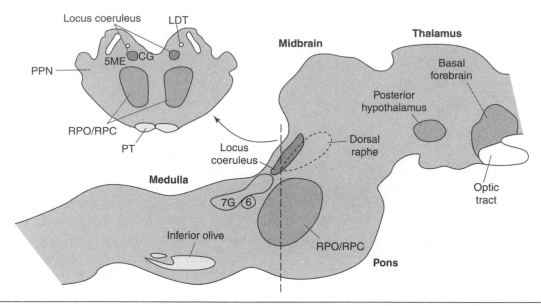

Figure 10.3 The most important site for the production of REM sleep is the nucleus reticularis pontis oralis/caudalis (RPO/RPC).

Reprinted, by permission, from E.R. Kandel, J.H. Schwartz, and T.M. Jessell, 1991, *Principles of neural science*, 3rd ed. (New York: McGraw-Hill). © The McGraw-Hill Companies.

During an 8-hour night, a sleeper without clinical disorders has four or five sleep cycles. Each lasts about 90 minutes and contains 20 to 30 minutes of REM sleep. The length of sleep stages changes throughout the night. The sleep cycle is controlled by centers in the brain stem, probably in the medulla. Slow-wave sleep, which seems to be controlled by the basal forebrain region, predominates during the first third of the night. Rapid eye movement predominates during the last third of the night and is initiated by acetylcholine released in the pons. Actions of the locus coeruleus and raphe nucleus are suppressed during REM sleep.

The most common form of the 84 types of sleep disorders is insomnia, which is defined as the subjective complaint of sleep disruption. Insomnia is characterized by difficulty in initiating or maintaining sleep, or both. It is actually a symptom and not a disorder per se. Common forms of insomnia that might be helped by exercise are defined in Common Types of Insomnia That Exercise Might Help.

MEASUREMENT

After a person has approached a physician for help with a sleep disturbance and has received

> ## Components of Sleep
>
> Sleep is described by the amount of time spent in the following states:
>
> - Stage 1
> - Stage 2
> - Stages 3 and 4 (stages 3 and 4 combined constitute SWS)
> - REM
> - REM latency
> - Wakefulness after sleep onset (WASO)
> - Sleep onset latency (SOL)
> - Total sleep time (TST)

treatment, usually pharmacological, the decision to continue sleep treatment depends on subjective ratings of improved sleep. Hence, the quality and quantity of sleep are often estimated through the use of questionnaires. However, self-assessments of sleep are often inaccurate. For example, sleep patients frequently exaggerate their loss of sleep, and treatment often involves demonstrating this overestimation to the patient. Conversely, patients who have sleep apnea (cessation of breathing during sleep) often are unaware of their disturbed sleep. Objective measures of sleep provide more accurate information on the amount and staging of sleep, which is necessary for an understanding of the biological mechanisms that govern sleep.

Sleep can be estimated using a motion sensor (i.e., an actigraph) that detects movement, especially wrist movement, during sleep. **Actigraphy** of wrist movement can determine whether someone is asleep or awake with accuracy as high as 95%. Though convenient and practical for long-term monitoring in studies of large numbers of people, actigraphy is not as accurate as **polysomnography**, which combines the use of electroencephalographic (EEG) records of brain waves; electromyographic (EMG) records of eye and chin muscle activity to detect REM sleep; strain gauge sensors on the chest and abdomen for recording respiration; and EMG electrodes on the legs for recording leg movements to determine sleep stages (see figure 10.4).

> **S**elf-assessments of the quality and quantity of sleep are often inaccurate and cannot provide information about brain waves and REM, which are measured with EEG, EMG, and other objective methods.

RESEARCH ON EXERCISE AND SLEEP

Large-scale studies on exercise and sleep have relied on self-reports of sleep and exercise, which each are limited in their value. Smaller studies have used more objective measures of sleep that provide better evidence for the effects of exercise on sleep, although the research is limited. The scientific advisory committee of the 2008 *Physical Activity Guidelines for Americans* concluded that there was only moderate evidence that physical activity improves sleep (Physical

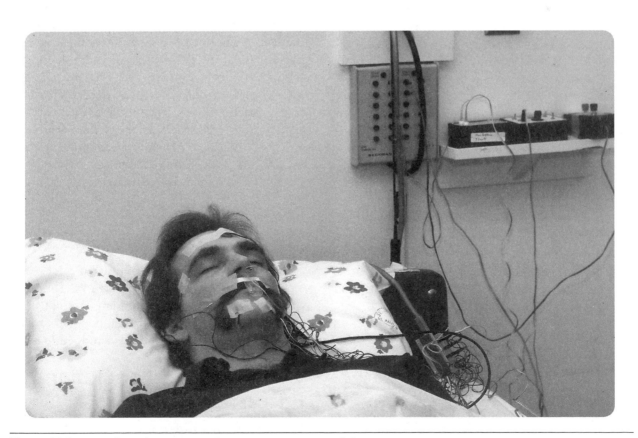

Figure 10.4 Use of a polysomnograph to measure aspects of sleep.

Activity Guidelines Advisory Committee 2008). The evidence comes from experimental studies showing that already good sleepers have small improvements in sleep as measured objectively by polysomnography after a single session of exercise, and from cross-sectional observational studies in which people who say they are physically active report sleeping better than people who say they are not active. The evidence of a positive correlation between physical activity and good-quality sleep also comes from a few randomized controlled trials of improved self-ratings of sleep quality, some corroborated by polysomnographic evidence after exercise training among people who say they have trouble sleeping or have been diagnosed with insomnia.

A Single Session of Acute Exercise

A meta-analysis of 38 studies with 211 effects from 401 participants showed that acute exercise did not alter the time it took to fall asleep or the amount of wakefulness during the nighttime sleep period (Youngstedt, O'Connor, and Dishman 1997). On average, exercise was followed by increases in total sleep time (10 min), SWS (4 min), and REM latency after sleep onset (13 min), and also a decrease in REM sleep (7 min) (see table 10.1). Those effects ranged from about 0.2 to 0.5 standard deviations, which are small to moderately large effects statistically but translate to only a few minutes of sleep, which is within people's normal night-to-night variation. The participants were good sleepers, so the effects may be underestimates of the potential efficacy of exercise among people with sleep disorders.

Contrary to previous results, this meta-analysis found that exercise that was associated with a high heat load did not increase SWS above the average effect of exercise, but high heat load was

> **A** single bout of exercise can significantly increase sleep time and decrease REM sleep, but meaningful increases in total sleep time require long-duration exercise (at least 1 hour).

Table 10.1 Effects of Acute Exercise on Sleep (Quantitative Synthesis of 38 Studies)

Variable	Effect size
Slow wave	0.19 (4.2 min)
REM	–0.49 (7.4 min)
REM onset	0.52 (13.1 min)
TST	0.42 (9.9 min)

REM = rapid eye movement; TST = total sleep time.

Based on Youngstedt, O'Connor, and Dishman 1997.

associated with increased wakefulness after sleep onset. A long duration of exercise (about 2 h) was associated with larger increases in total sleep time and larger decreases in REM, but this is of little practical importance for most people, who typically exercise 20 to 45 minutes each session.

The trivial effects of acute exercise on SWS contrast with the assumption that exercise increases SWS. Also, it is not clear that an effect of exercise on SWS means that sleep will be improved. For example, both drug treatment and exercise can increase SWS, but people don't report that they have better sleep or have less daytime sleepiness with these interventions (Landolt et al. 1998; Youngstedt, Kripke, and Elliott 1999).

In a recent study, 48 middle-aged insomnia patients (38 women and 10 men) were randomly assigned to a control group, moderate-intensity or high-intensity aerobic exercise, or moderate-intensity resistance exercise (Passos et al. 2010). Sleep was assessed by polysomnography and by a daily sleep diary. After moderate-intensity aerobic exercise, sleep-onset latency and total wake time were decreased by 55% and 30%, respectively, while total sleep time and sleep efficiency were increased by 18% and 13%. The sleep diaries also showed improvements in total sleep time (25%) and sleep-onset latency (39%), and self-ratings of anxiety were also reduced (15%).

Observational Population-Based Studies

Observational epidemiological studies have reported an association between physical activity and good sleep based on questionnaires administered to population samples, but few studies have examined the long-term effects of exercise on sleep among people with sleep disorders (Youngstedt and Kline 2006). In a survey of nearly 1,200 middle-aged men and women (ages 36-50) living in Tampere, Finland (Urponen et al. 1988), people ranked exercise first when they were asked to report, in order of importance, three practices, habits, or actions they thought were the best way to promote or improve their falling asleep quickly or their perceived quality of sleep.

Another survey of randomly selected women ($n = 403$) and men ($n = 319$) living in Tucson, Arizona, indicated that the prevalence of self-reported sleep problems and daytime sleepiness was lower among those who said that they were physically active (even among those exercising just once a week) compared to those who were sedentary (Sherrill, Kotchou, and Quan 1998; figure 10.5).

Such epidemiologic comparisons of sleep between physically active and inactive people cannot establish the direction of causality. An equally plausible hypothesis is that those who sleep better are less tired during the day and therefore more willing to engage in regular exercise (O'Connor and Youngstedt 1995). Moreover, physically active people may be more likely to engage in other healthy habits conducive to sleep, such as limited intake of alcohol and tobacco and greater exposure to bright light, all of which can improve sleep. Another explanation for anecdotal reports of better sleep after

exercise might be that people are more likely to exercise when they have more time; hence, better sleep might occur on exercise days because they already feel less stressed by other priorities (Driver and Taylor 2000).

> In epidemiological studies, exercise is associated with better sleep, but the effects may be attributable to other related factors, such as personality or participation in other health habits conducive to sleep.

Subjective ratings of sleep that are obtained in exercise studies might not be valid if participants enter the study expecting to benefit because they already believe that exercise will promote sleep. This is likely because of the folk wisdom, yet to be fully confirmed by science, that exercise helps sleep. According to this belief, the value of sleep is that it conserves or restores energy, and physical fatigue is synonymous with sleepiness.

Eleven of 13 cross-sectional studies shown in figure 10.6 that were published between 1995 and 2008 found that the chances of having insufficient or interrupted sleep are lower (mean OR = 0.73; 95% CI = 0.66-0.81) among adults who are engaged in more physical activity than among those who have less physical activity or are sedentary (Physical Activity Guidelines Advisory Committee 2008). Also, at least two population-based cross-sectional studies found that regardless of body mass index (BMI, a risk factor for sleep apnea), men and women who exercised 3 or more hours per week had lower odds of sleep apnea measured by polysomnography (Peppard and Young 2004; Quan et al. 2007).

Supportive evidence in these studies was reported for middle-aged or older men and women in the United States, Japan, Finland, Sweden, Turkey, and Australia. However, the available evidence isn't sufficient to judge whether the effects of physical activity on sleep differ according to sex, age, type of sleep disorder, or other medical conditions, which

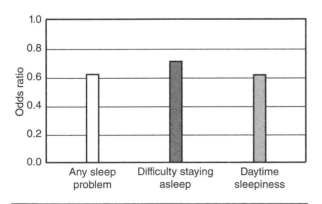

Figure 10.5 Epidemiological evidence for the relationship between exercise and daytime sleepiness.

Data from Sherrill, Kotchou, and Quan 1998.

First author	Year	Sample N
Surken	2005	409
Ohida	2001	31,260
Kravitz	2003	11,222
Phillips	2000	1,803
Kawamoto	2004	1,270
Nasermoadeli	2004	6,914
Hublin-males	2001	5,665
Ohayon	2004	8,091
Kim	2000	3,030
Akerstedt	2002	5,720
Hublin-females	2001	6,758
Sherrill	1998	722
Morgan	2003	1,042

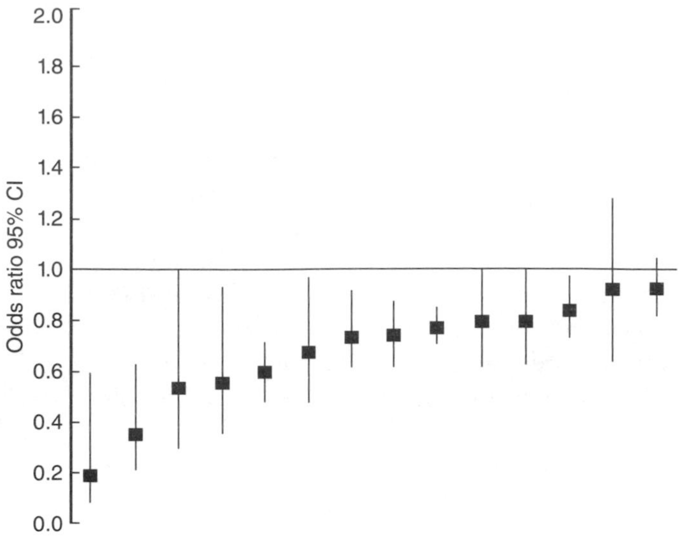

Figure 10.6 Odds ratios from population-based cross-sectional studies of physical activity and self-ratings of disrupted or insufficient sleep.

Data from Physical Activity Guidelines Advisory Committee 2008.

have been understudied. Sleep complaints were inversely related to exercise frequency in a cross-sectional study of a thousand elderly African American residents of New Orleans (Bazargan 1996).

There is also some evidence that higher levels of usual physical activity or the maintenance of physical fitness during middle age appear to be protective against incident insomnia (i.e., the development of new sleep problems) in older adults (Morgan 2003).

Nottingham Longitudinal Study of Activity and Ageing

Elderly people in the United Kingdom were originally interviewed in 1985 (n = 1,042) and later in 1989 (n = 690) and 1993 (n = 410) (Morgan 2003). Customary leisure-time physical activities (those requiring at least 2 kcal per min, performed for at least 3 min, at least weekly, for the previous 6 weeks or longer) and self-reported sleep problems (time to fall asleep and total sleep time) were assessed by interview. Insomnia cases were people who reported sleep problems *often or all the time*. There were 221 cases in 1985 and 119 incident cases between 1985 and 1993. After adjustment for age, sex, and health status, the 20% least active people had double the odds of prevalent insomnia in 1985 (OR = 2.2) and five times the odds of incident insomnia across 4 to

8 years of follow-up (OR = 5.2) when compared to the 20% most active people (Morgan 2003).

Aerobics Center Longitudinal Study

Cardiorespiratory fitness was assessed at four clinic visits, each separated by 2 to 3 years, to objectively measure cumulative physical activity exposure in 7,368 men and 1,155 women from the Aerobics Center Longitudinal Study who had not complained of sleep problems at their first clinic visit (Dishman, Sui, Church, Youngstedt, and Blair 2013). Across subsequent visits, there were 784 incident cases of sleep complaints in men and 207 cases in women. After adjustment for age, time between visits, BMI, and fitness at visit 1, each minute decline in treadmill endurance (i.e., a decline in cardiorespiratory fitness of approximately one-half MET) between ages 51 and 55 in men and between ages 53 and 56 in women increased the odds of incident sleep complaints by approximately 1% after adjustment for smoking, alcohol use, medical conditions, anxiety, and depression.

Exercise Training

Several studies have shown that physically active or fit individuals have more SWS and total sleep time. Because the comparisons were made at a cross section of time (i.e., a single point in time), these studies do not demonstrate that the improved sleep was caused by exercise rather than by other differences between the groups (e.g., healthy habits or personality); they also do not address the possibility that people who sleep well are more likely to exercise.

Although an early experimental study indicated that stopping regular exercise led to disrupted sleep (Baekeland 1970), most studies of the effects of chronic exercise on sleep have also been limited by a focus on good sleepers. Nonetheless, moderately large improvements ranging from a half to nearly a full standard deviation have been seen after exercise training: quicker SOL, less REM sleep, more total sleep time, and more SWS (see table 10.2).

Randomized Controlled Trials

The long-term effects of exercise on objective measures of sleep among poor sleepers have not been studied much. However, the results of randomized trials using physical activity as part of a sleep hygiene program (i.e., structured exercise plus exposure to outdoor bright light, efforts to keep residents out of bed during the day, the institution of a bedtime routine, and efforts to reduce nighttime noise and light in residents' rooms) (Alessi et al. 2005; Martin et al. 2007) and quasi-experimental studies (Ouslander et al. 2006) of nursing home residents or patients with sleep apnea (Yamamoto et al. 2007) have been partly favorable.

Table 10.2 Sleep Variables Most Affected by Chronic Exercise

Variable	Effect size (SD)
TST	0.94
REM	−0.57
Sleep onset	0.45
Slow wave	0.43

Results are based on a meta-analysis of 12 experiments with good sleepers. TST = total sleep time; REM = rapid eye movement.

Data from Kubitz et al. 1996.

Encouraging results have been found in randomized controlled studies with older people who complained of poor sleep. In a study of older depressed patients (mean age ~70), Singh, Clements, and Fiatarone (1997) found significantly greater improvement in self-reported sleep quality after 10 weeks of weight training ($n = 15$, 3 times per week) compared with health education training (see figure 10.7).

Likewise, randomized controlled trials conducted by King and colleagues (1997) at Stanford University have found that regular exercise training in middle-aged and older adults who had moderate sleep complaints led to improved self-reports of sleep quality (see figure 10.8).

Stanford University Studies

Self-rated sleep quality assessed using the Pittsburgh Sleep Quality Index (PSQI) and sleep diaries was evaluated in 43 healthy, sedentary men and women aged 50 to 76 who reported moderate sleep complaints (King et al. 1997). After 16 weeks of community-based, moderate-intensity exercise training (mainly 30 min of low-impact aerobics or brisk walking 4 times a week at approximately 60% to 75% of aerobic capacity), participants in the exercise training condition reported improvement in the PSQI global sleep score as well as improvements in sleep quality,

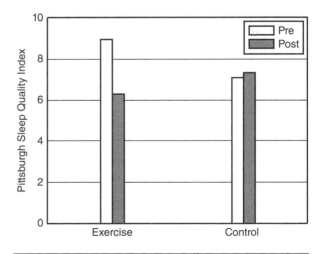

Figure 10.7 Thirty-two depressed older adults (mean age 71) were randomly assigned to a control group or weightlifting exercise (3 times per week for 10 weeks). A score greater than 5 indicates sleep problems; lower scores indicate better sleep.

Data from Singh, Clements, and Fiatarone 1997.

sleep-onset latency, and sleep duration when compared to changes reported by the wait-list control group (see figure 10.8).

In another trial, also shown in figure 10.8, 66 sedentary adults 55 years and older who complained of mild to moderate sleep problems were randomized to 12 months of a moderate-intensity endurance exercise ($n = 36$) or a health education control group ($n = 30$) (King et al. 2008). Participants in the exercise group reported improvements in PSQI sleep disturbance, minutes to fall asleep, and feeling more rested in the morning. They also had about a half standard deviation less night-to-night variability in self-rated time to fall asleep (i.e., SOL) compared to the control group (Buman et al. 2011a). Polysomnographic sleep recordings were also made while they slept in their homes to objectively measure sleep cycles. After 12 months, participants in the exercise group spent significantly less time in stage 1 sleep, spent more time in stage 2 sleep, and had fewer awakenings during the first third of the sleep period compared to the control group (King et al. 2008).

In a similar trial, 100 sedentary women aged 49 to 82 who were caring for a relative with dementia were randomized to 12 months of home-based, telephone-supervised, moderate-intensity exercise training (30-40 min of brisk walking 4 times a week at approximately 60%-75% of aerobic capacity) or to an attention-control (nutrition education) program (King et al. 2002). Exercise participants reported improved sleep quality on the PSQI, but women in the nutrition education group did not.

In a study of older sedentary adults, 15 weekly 1-hour sessions that emphasized moderate-intensity recreational sport activities (e.g., softball, dance, self-defense, swimming, and athletics) were accompanied by a small increase in self-ratings of total time spent sleeping (de Jong et al. 2006). Other studies of less vigorous exercises, such as walking or yoga, have reported smaller or statistically nonsignificant reductions in self-rated sleep (Elavsky and McAuley 2007; Gary and Lee 2007; Yurtkuran, Alp, and Dilek 2007).

Other convincing evidence that chronic exercise promotes sleep was provided by Guil-

> There is some evidence that exercise training has a positive impact on sleep in people with sleep complaints.

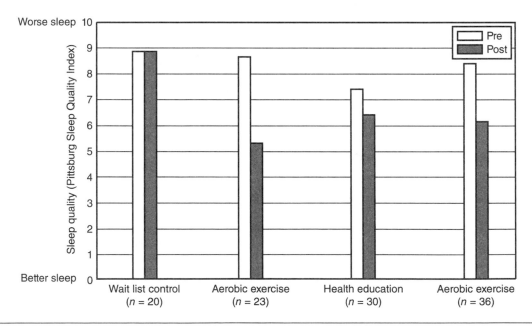

Figure 10.8 Older adults with moderate sleep problems completed 30 to 40 minutes of aerobic exercise 4 times per week for 16 weeks. The controls maintained their usual activity levels.

Based on King et al. 2008; King et al. 1997.

leminault and colleagues (1995). Thirty people (mean age 44 years) with psychophysiological insomnia were randomly assigned to three different 4-week treatments: (1) sleep hygiene education, (2) sleep hygiene combined with exercise (daily walking for 45 min), and (3) sleep hygiene plus bright light (daily 1-hour exposure of 3,000 lux). Sleep was assessed during the weeks before and after these treatments. Whereas sleep hygiene by itself resulted in a decrease in total sleep time of 3 min, the exercise treatment elicited a chronic increase in total sleep time of 17 min. However, the most impressive result of this study was that the bright light plus exercise condition increased total sleep time by nearly an hour.

Insomnia Patients

The long-term effects of exercise on polysomnographic measures of sleep among poor sleepers has only recently been studied. Sixteen women and one man ages 55 and older who were sedentary and diagnosed with primary insomnia for at least three months participated in a randomized controlled trial (Reid et al. 2010). Sleep hygiene (i.e., education and counseling about sleep-promoting behaviors) plus 16 weeks of aerobic physical activity (walking, stationary cycling, or treadmill for 30 to 40 minutes 4 times each week at 75% maximal heart rate) was compared to sleep hygiene without physical activity every other week. Those in the physical activity group improved their ratings of overall sleep quality, sleep latency, sleep duration, daytime dysfunction, and sleep efficiency (Pittsburgh Sleep Quality Index) compared to those in the control group. The physical activity group also had reductions in depressive symptoms and daytime sleepiness and increased feelings of energy compared to their scores before the intervention started.

Postmenopausal Women

Overweight or obese sedentary women 50 to 75 years of age living in Seattle who were not taking hormone replacement therapy were randomly assigned to 12 months of either moderate-intensity exercise ($n = 87$) for 45 minutes, 5 days each week (supervised and at home) or a 1-hour supervised session of low-

intensity stretching and relaxation once each week ($n = 86$) (Tworoger et al. 2003). Both stretching and aerobic exercise groups had similar improvements in self-reported sleep quality. Nonetheless, women who increased their $\dot{V}O_2max$ by more than 10% during the intervention period were less likely to have poor sleep quality, have short sleep duration, or use sleep medications at 12 months compared to women whose $\dot{V}O_2max$ stayed the same or decreased, regardless of changes in BMI or time spent outdoors.

Among women who exercised in the morning, those who got at least 225 minutes per week were 70% less likely to report trouble falling asleep compared with those who exercised less than 180 minutes per week (OR = 0.3). In contrast, evening exercisers who spent at least 225 minutes per week were three times more likely to report trouble falling asleep compared to those who exercised less than 180 minutes per week (OR = 3.3). However, those differences might have been biased because the timing of exercise sessions was self-selected, and most evening exercisers were employed, whereas the morning exercisers were mostly retired or not working.

Issues in Sleep and Exercise Research

Several characteristics of the person and of exercise can influence whether, or to what extent, exercise affects sleep. Level of fitness is a factor that could influence the effects of exercise on sleep. It is plausible that exercise might promote sleep in physically fit or active people but be stressful and hinder sleep among unfit and inactive people. However, experimental evidence indicates that fitness does not moderate the effects of acute exercise on sleep (Youngstedt, O'Connor, and Dishman 1997); this evidence agrees with surveys showing that exercise promotes sleep in the general population, which is largely sedentary (Youngstedt and Kline 2006).

Body heating from exercise as a mechanism is consistent with a proposed sleep hypothesis. The anterior hypothalamus plays an important role in regulating both heat loss and sleep. A popular hypothesis is that sleep, especially increased SWS, is improved when heat-loss mechanisms in the hypothalamus are activated by body heating (McGinty and Szymusiak 1990). Studies in which people have been immersed in hot water have supported this hypothesis by demonstrating increased SWS (Horne and Staff 1983; see figure 10.9).

One study of fit women without clinical disorders showed that increased SWS after acute exercise depends on body heating during exercise. Slow-wave sleep was increased after passive heating of the body to a level similar to that achieved during heavy exercise (Horne and Staff 1983; see figures 10.9 and 10.10). A study by Horne and Moore (1985) showed that SWS elevations following exercise could be reversed by body cooling. Since that study, sleep researchers and professionals have generally accepted that exercise helps sleep because it increases body temperature. However, a limitation of the Horne and Moore study was that body temperature was not assessed at bedtime or during sleep. Also, the exercise was performed approximately 6 h before bedtime, apparently enough time for body temperature to return to baseline levels. Meta-analysis data showing no positive moderating effects of heat load on sleep further contradict the thermogenic hypothesis (Youngstedt, O'Connor, and Dishman 1997).

Body temperature increases proportionately with exercise intensity, so sleep should be best

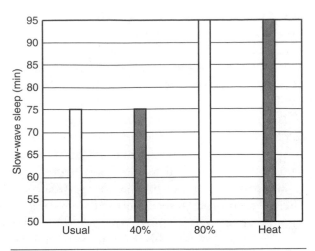

Figure 10.9 Body heating and sleep: immersing people in hot water increased their percentage of slow-wave sleep as much as exercising at 80% of aerobic capacity.

Data from Horne and Staff 1983.

helped after heavy exercise. Only about 10% of people in the general population exercise vigorously on a regular basis, so on the basis of the body temperature hypothesis, exercise should not be expected to help the sleep of most people. However, if less intense exercise is just as helpful for sleep, as evidence suggests (Youngstedt, O'Connor, and Dishman 1997), then more people may improve their sleep with exercise.

Characteristics of exercise behavior that have been examined with respect to sleep are the

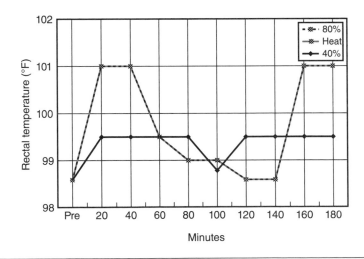

Figure 10.10 Conditions of heavy exercise (80% capacity) and passive heat produced the same body temperature. This permitted a test of whether sleep would be affected by increased body temperature during exercise.

Data from Horne and Staff 1983

duration of exercise and how long before bedtime the exercise occurs. The cumulative evidence from sleep studies indicates that as exercise duration is increased beyond 1 hour, total sleep time increases substantially (Youngstedt, O'Connor, and Dishman 1997). That observation raises questions about the practical usefulness of exercise. Most people are unlikely to exercise for the 1 hour per day found necessary to reliably improve sleep.

A common opinion of the public and of health professionals is that vigorous exercise close to bedtime will disturb sleep. Several studies have clearly contradicted that viewpoint. O'Connor, Breus, and Youngstedt (1998) found no detrimental effect on sleep of 1 hour of exercise at an intensity of 60% of aerobic capacity 30 to 90 minutes before typical bedtime. Youngstedt and colleagues (2000) found no effect on sleep of very exhaustive exercise consisting of 3 hours of cycling at 70% aerobic capacity that was completed just 30 minutes before bedtime. Myllymäki and colleagues (2011) reported no effects on sleep quality after leg cycling exercise until voluntary exhaustion 2 hours before bedtime. Moreover, a random population-based survey of Finnish adults (n = 1,190) showed that most who exercised vigorously in the evening (after 8 p.m.) reported mainly positive effects on sleep (Vuori et al. 1988). Nighttime is a practical time to exercise for many people, so unsubstantiated claims that nighttime exercise disturbs sleep might be a false barrier to exercise among people who can't find the time to exercise during the day.

> **E**xercising close to bedtime will not disrupt sleep in most people.

MECHANISMS

Understanding how exercise might influence sleep may not only have significance for clinical applications, but may also reveal important information about sleep function. However, the question of mechanisms whereby exercise may facilitate sleep remains unresolved. Body heating, discussed earlier, is one mechanism with equivocal support. Other possible but unconfirmed explanations include body restitution, energy conservation, adenosine, and increased secretion of melatonin, which helps regulate circadian sleep. This section outlines some of what we know about the mechanisms of light exposure, anti-anxiety and antidepressant effects, circadian phase shifting, and biochemical effects. Indirect evidence suggests that acute bouts of exercise are positively associated with melatonin production in women (Knight et al. 2005) and can induce circadian phase shifts (Van Reeth et al. 1994) including a phase delay in circadian melatonin rhythm (Barger et al. 2004), influence adenosine metabolism (Benington, Kodali, and Heller 1995), and activate brain neurological circuits hypothesized to help people feel less anxious and depressed (Youngstedt 2005).

Effects of Light Exposure

Low levels of illumination in the natural environment are significantly associated with depression and sleep disturbance, and bright light treatments are effective in reducing some types of depression and in enhancing sleep. The average adult receives about 20 minutes of daily exposure to bright light (i.e., more than 2,500 lux) (Espiritu et al. 1994), but can average more than 2 hours depending on location and season (Cole et al. 1995). Many people who exercise outdoors in the middle of the day (1 hour at 10,000 lux) can get 10 times the typical average, especially in the winter. Studies of acute exercise have not provided information about illumination during the exercise or throughout the day. The discrepancy between experimental evidence and anecdotal reports about exercise might be explained by the fact that many studies have been conducted inside laboratories, whereas most people who exercise do so outdoors as part of their daily routines, where light can be thousands of times brighter than normal indoor lighting. Even if bright light exposure does not mediate the effects of exercise on sleep, exposure to bright light might augment the sleep-promoting effects of exercise. Additive effects of exercise and bright light for reducing depression have been reported (Golden et al. 2005).

Anti-Anxiety and Antidepressant Effects

Anxiety disrupts sleep, and exercise can reduce anxiety for several hours in some circumstances (see chapter 6). Therefore, it is plausible that exercise promotes sleep by reducing anxiety. One study that has explored this mechanism (Youngstedt et al. 2000) was inconclusive. Although participants who exercised had significant reductions in anxiety 20 minutes after exercise compared with a sedentary control condition, there was no difference in anxiety between conditions at bedtime, which occurred 4 to 6 hours after the exercise, and there was no association between sleep and anxiety level at bedtime. Regular exercise also has antidepressant effects, so it could promote sleep indirectly by alleviating symptoms of depression, which include disordered sleep (Singh, Clements, and Fiatarone 1997).

Circadian Phase-Shifting Effects

Sleep can be disrupted when there is a desynchronization between a person's circadian pacemaker—which largely regulates sleep and wakefulness—and the sleep–wake schedule. Examples include shift work (i.e., when people work and sleep at odd hours) or jet travel across several time zones. About one-third of people aged 60 or older experience a chronic state of circadian malsynchronization that impairs sleep as much as other mechanisms underlying aging

Potential mechanisms for the effects of exercise on sleep include an indirect effect through light exposure during exercise outdoors, decreased anxiety and depression, circadian phase-shifting effects, and biochemical effects from exercise.

sleep patterns, such as sleep apnea and periodic limb movements during sleep. Correcting circadian phase can elicit dramatic improvements in sleep in older people. Evidence now suggests that exercise can elicit substantial circadian phase-shifting effects, comparable to those that occur in response to bright light (Buxton et al. 2003).

Biochemical Effects

Adenosine increases in muscles and interstitial fluids during exercise, and it is thought to facilitate the dilation of blood vessels when low levels of fuel and oxygen are detected (Radegran and Hellsten 2000). Adenosine is also believed to play an important role in the regulation of sleep (Porkka-Heiskanen et al. 1997). Youngstedt, Kripke, and Elliott (1999) found that increases in SWS after exercise were nearly three times greater after a placebo treatment compared with consumption of caffeine, which blocks adenosine neurotransmission.

SUMMARY

Acute exercise leads to a moderate delay in the onset of REM sleep, a small decrease in the amount of REM sleep, and a small increase in SWS and total sleep time—among good sleepers. Also, about a dozen observational studies have shown that physically active people have about 25% lower odds of sleep complaints than less active people. A handful of randomized controlled trials of people with insomnia or complaints of sleep problems have shown positive and large effects (more than 1 SD) of exercise training on symptoms of poor sleep and self-rated sleep quality, as well small changes in objective sleep cycles using polysomnography.

Although active people tend to say they sleep better, the vast majority of the observational studies used a cross-sectional design, which lacks the proper timing of physical activity measures. However, at least one prospective cohort study found that the least active adults had more than double the risk of incident insomnia 4 to 8 years later compared to the most active adults. Observational studies have suggested a dose-dependent association between physical activity and better sleep, but most randomized controlled trials have used low- to moderate-intensity exercise, so dose–response hasn't been well tested. One RCT and one prospective cohort study reported that lower sleep complaints were positively related to gains in cardiorespiratory fitness or inversely associated with declines in fitness during middle age. However, the minimal amount of physical activity needed to improve sleep is not known.

The biggest limitation of studies of the effects of exercise on sleep has been a focus on good sleepers. The small number of studies on chronic physical activity in sleepers without clinical disorders indicates small to moderate effects of increased SWS and TST, with decreased SOL, WASO, and REM sleep. Larger effects might be observed in people with sleep problems (Youngstedt, O'Connor, and Dishman 1997; Youngstedt 2000). Only recently has evidence appeared to confirm that acute exercise and exercise training can improve sleep measured by polysomnography in people who have been diagnosed with a sleep disorder. Until there is more research on people with disturbed sleep or on experimentally induced sleep disruption, we will not understand the potential of exercise for promoting sleep. We still have an incomplete understanding of the potential benefits of exercise on the sleep of people who have insomnia or other sleep disorders. However, we are more confident that the risks of exercise disturbing sleep are minimal; there currently is no evidence to indicate that moderate-to-vigorous leisure-time physical activity, including exercise that causes delayed-onset muscle pain (Breus, O'Connor, and Ragan 2000), will harm most people's sleep.

WEBSITES

www.sleepquest.com

http://sleep.stanford.edu

http://sleepcenter.ucla.edu

www.nhlbi.nih.gov/about/ncsdr

www.aasmnet.org/accred_centerstandards.aspx

Exercise and Pain

Exercise can create pain in a variety of ways. An 8-year-old boy falls from playground equipment and breaks his collarbone. A high school swimmer feels intense pain in the arm muscles she is using during a 100-meter free-style race. A middle-aged man experiences chest pain while jogging. A 75-year-old woman enjoys working in her garden but she feels delayed-onset muscle pain and stiffness over the next two days. Although all these types of pain can be a consequence of being physically active, acute and chronic exercise also can reduce pain. After reviewing the definition of pain, how it is measured, the scope and impact of the problem of chronic pain, and the neurobiological underpinnings of pain, this chapter examines the influence of acute and chronic exercise on pain, including its potential usefulness for patients suffering from a wide array of painful medical conditions ranging from migraines to low back pain to nerve pain resulting from chronic diabetes.

DEFINITIONS

Aristotle's views had a profound influence on science. He is credited with the doctrine of the five senses: taste, touch, sight, smell, and sound. His view of pain as solely an emotion delayed adequate attention being paid to the sensory dimension of pain (Dallenbach 1939).

Today the consensus among experts is that **pain** is always a subjective perception, and the International Association for the Study of Pain (IASP Task Force on Taxonomy 1994) defines pain as "an unpleasant sensory and emotional experience associated with actual or potential tissue damage, or described in terms of such

damage" (p. 210-213). This definition purposely avoids defining pain in terms of the stimulus causing the injury.

Although pain often is caused by injury to tissues, pain intensity ratings are not strongly linked to the magnitude of the injury. Sometimes this occurs for psychological reasons. People can falsely exaggerate pain to avoid work, obtain drugs, or fraudulently obtain financial compensation. One study of more than 33,000 legal cases estimated that 29% of personal injury, 30% of disability, and 8% of medical cases involved probable malingering or symptom exaggeration (Mittenberg et al. 2002). Biological factors also can cause an absence of a strong association between pain intensity reports and the extent of a physical injury. A stark example is the small number of people who are born with a congenital insensitivity to pain, such as those lacking functional genes for a sodium channel in nerves that convey information about tissue damage (Cox et al. 2006). People who are insensitive to pain suffer from frequent injuries of all kinds, especially in early childhood. The inability to recognize even a severe injury as unpleasant or important inhibits their ability to learn how to avoid dangerous injuries.

Much of the time, especially with regard to clinical "real-world" pain conditions, variations in psychological and biological processes simultaneously contribute to the absence of a strong association between the degree of tissue damage and the magnitude of pain intensity ratings. Well-established examples include patients who go to cardiologists complaining of chest pain but are found to have healthy coronary arteries (Kaski 2004), people without back pain but who are discovered to have objective evidence of a spine abnormality after undergoing a magnetic resonance imaging procedure (Jensen et al. 1994), and people with psychological disorders such as fibromyalgia who report widespread pain in the absence of a distinct physical cause for it (Abeles et al. 2007).

Pain is discussed, researched, and treated in part based on the duration of suffering; many have found it useful to categorized pain as either acute or chronic. Although there is no universally accepted definition of **chronic pain**, the term generally refers to that lasting beyond the typical time needed for tissue healing. Chronic pain is often the result of a chronic disease process such as osteoarthritis or cancer. Pain lasting more than three months is commonly considered chronic pain. Pain that lasts for less than three months is classified as acute pain. **Acute pain** is often the result of a single trauma such as that caused by surgery or a sport injury or physiological changes that suggest potential tissue damage such as heart muscle ischemia during exercise that provokes chest pain.

MEASUREMENT

Because pain is a subjective perception, it is usually measured through self-report. The three most commonly measured aspects of pain are location, intensity, and affect.

Pain location drawings are used to document the sensory distribution of pain (see figure 11.1). The patient can be presented with an outline of a body or a body part (e.g., knee) and asked to shade in areas that depict all the areas of the body that are in pain. The number of areas

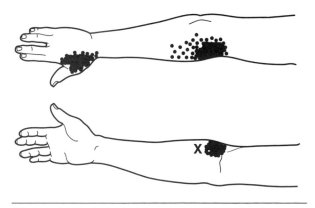

Figure 11.1 Pain location drawing of tennis elbow.

shaded often correlates with the degree of pain behaviors such as analgesic use and time spent being physically inactive.

The 0 to 10 scale is a reliable, valid, and common approach to measuring pain intensity. Patients are instructed that 0 represents *no pain* and 10 indicates the *highest possible pain intensity imaginable* (see figure 11.2). These verbal anchors are important in establishing the full range of intensities possible. Changing the verbal anchors to *no unpleasantness* and *as unpleasant as can be imagined* provides a measure of pain affect. Assessing both pain intensity and pain affect can be useful because the neurobiology underlying these aspects of pain is distinct, and pain treatments can differentially influence them. Visual analog scales (VAS) typically consist of a 10-centimeter horizontal line with verbal anchors on the left and right ends similar to those described earlier (see figure 11.3). The patient makes a mark on the horizontal line that corresponds to the pain intensity experienced. A large body of research evidence indicates that these two scales can be used to obtain reliable and valid measures of pain intensity and pain affect (Turk and Melzack 2001).

Pain can be measured in several other ways as well. Pain threshold is assessed by quantifying the minimal stimulus required to be perceived as painful. Pain tolerance is the maximal stimulus a person is willing to endure. Pain tolerance is actually pseudo-tolerance when measured for research because it would be unethical to expose people to maximally painful stimuli. For example, high mechanical pressure is used to cause pain in order to study it, but the pressure is not allowed to become so great that a bone is broken.

Multidimensional measures of pain obtain more information than just pain intensity. The most basic multidimensional measures quantify both pain intensity and affect. Others ask about a host of aspects of pain such as the quality of the pain (e.g., is it a tearing or a burning sensation?), the extent to which the pain influences activities of daily living, and how pain characteristics change over time (e.g., is the intensity greater in the morning or at night?).

Pain also can be inferred from behaviors such as the presence of a limp, guarding to protect a

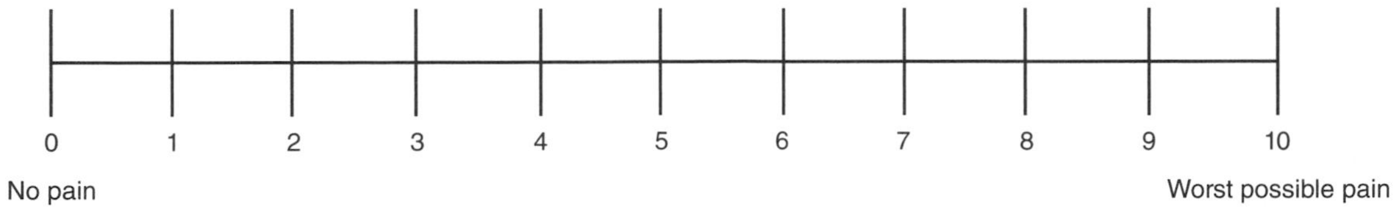

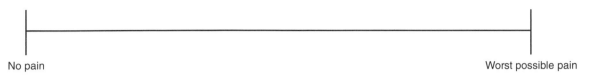

Figure 11.2   Numerical graphic 0 to 10 pain scale.

No pain   Worst possible pain

Figure 11.3   Visual analog pain scale (exactly 10 centimeters, measured in millimeters [0-100] from the left edge).

body area from being bumped, or facial expressions such as grimaces. Behavioral measures are especially useful when there are barriers to adequate linguistic communication between a patient and a therapist (e.g., with infants, non-native speakers, and people who are unconscious or have cognitive deficits). Savvy clinicians watch their patients carefully for the presence or absence of pain behaviors.

SCOPE AND IMPACT OF CHRONIC PAIN

The prevalence of chronic pain in the U.S. population is high, estimated at more than 30%, and affecting over 100 million Americans. Its prevalence is higher in women (34%) than in men (27%). Among adults, the prevalence is highest for those older than 65 (38%) and lowest for those aged 18 to 24 (12%). Chronic pain outlasts the stimulus that caused it, and its intensity often increases over time. Arthritis, low back pain, and migraine headaches are the most common types of chronic pain (Johannes et al. 2010; Manchikanti et al. 2009). Most people with low back and arthritis pain experience moderate-intensity pain daily but about one-third describe their pain as severe (Johannes et al. 2010). Countries with high incomes such as Sweden and the United States have rates of back pain that are two to four times higher than those in countries with low incomes such as Nigeria, and within a country the prevalence of back pain is higher in urban areas than in rural areas (Volinn 1997).

Childbirth is a significant source of chronic pain. The Institute of Medicine estimates that 18% of women who have Caesarean deliveries and 10% who have vaginal deliveries are in pain a year later (Institute of Medicine 2011). Up to 50% of surgical patients, depending on the type of surgery, develop chronic pain.

Chronic pain has significant economic and health consequences. In 2001, approximately 8 million people with pain were cared for at approximately 3,800 pain clinics and solo practices in the United States. Reduced performance at work resulting from chronic pain costs more than $60 billion annually (Stewart et al. 2003). More than 300 million prescriptions for analgesics are written each year in the United States, and the total cost exceeds $50 billion (Gatchel and Okifuji 2006). The vast majority of people with one type of chronic pain (up to 87%) suffer from a second (comorbid) medical condition, including other types of pain or a variety of physical (e.g., asthma, hypertension) and mental (e.g., anxiety, depression) conditions (Von Korff et al. 2005). Compared to those who are free from pain, people with chronic pain have a significantly reduced quality of life (Jensen, Chodroff, and Dworkin 2007), including disruptions in attention and working memory (Dick and Rashiq 2007), poor sleep (Smith and Haythornthwaite 2004), increased disability (Jamison 2010), social and marital problems (Flor, Turk, and Scholz 1987), and a decreased ability to retain employment (Breivik et al. 2006). Moreover, the risk of suicide is high among chronic pain patients. Two investigations showed that ~5% of those with chronic musculoskeletal pain had attempted suicide.

NEUROBIOLOGICAL BASIS OF PAIN

Pain is thought to be caused by the activation of specific circuits in the central nervous system. This can happen in the absence of tissue injury. For example, some research participants who watched movie clips of people being injured reported brief pain and showed activation of brain areas known to be involved in pain (Osborn and Derbyshire 2010). Activation of brain areas known to be involved in pain processing and concurrent feelings of pain also occur in other situations in the absence of tissue damage. Examples include people suffering from chronic pain without a medical cause such as fibromyalgia patients (Derbyshire, Whalley, and Oakley 2009) and people who imagine pain or have it induced with hypnosis (Derbyshire et al. 2004). These observations highlight the idea that pain is caused by brain neural activity, which can be independent of tissue damage.

> **E**xercise can cause and treat pain because exercise can influence the neurology that underlies pain.

Usually pain is caused by tissue damage or tissue changes portending an injury. The physiological consequences of these tissue changes activate specialized sensory receptors that respond specifically to injurious stimuli (**nociceptors**). Nociceptors then convey information about this situation via sensory afferents to the spinal cord. Within the spinal cord several ascending nerve tracts receive inputs from sensory afferents. These long **projection neurons** transmit information to subcortical brain areas, such as the thalamus, and areas within the brain's cortex. Tens of thousands of neural connections within the spinal cord can inhibit or augment the magnitude of the nociceptive signal traveling from the spinal cord to the brain. Neural circuits within the brain also can modify pain. For example, stored memories of prior injury and pain could augment pain, whereas memories of successful pain treatment or coping strategies could reduce pain. Also, neurons from the brain descend to the spinal cord and can act to inhibit or augment nociceptive activity being sent to the brain.

Acute (and chronic) exercise could increase or decrease pain by phasically (or tonically) increasing or decreasing the activity of neural circuits within the brain. Exercise also could influence pain by acutely or chronically altering the function of nociceptors, sensory afferents, spinal projection neurons, or neurons that descend from the brain and synapse on spinal projection neurons. Few experiments have been aimed at understanding the biological mechanisms by which exercise could alter pain.

Nociceptors and Sensory Afferents

This section addresses the neurology underlying muscle pain because exercise requires the activation of skeletal muscles, and exercise training most consistently improves medical conditions that involve skeletal muscle pain. Mechanical pressure and algesic biochemicals are the primary causes of skeletal muscle pain.

Nociceptors are a subset of sensory receptors in muscle that respond to **noxious stimuli**. They usually are small-diameter unmyelinated (known as either type IV or C fibers) or lightly meylinated (type III or A-δ) fibers. The majority of muscle nociceptors are type IV. High-intensity mechanical pressure, such as a 250-pound (113.4 kg) American football linebacker running at full speed into the thigh of a running back, activates type III and IV high-threshold mechanosensitive (HTM) receptors. About 60% of high-threshold mechanosensitive receptors respond to noxious pressure. Some of these nociceptors appear to be activated by high-intensity exercise, which creates high intramuscular pressure (Cook et al. 1997).

Chemicals sensitize and activate type IV polymodal nociceptors. Polymodal nociceptors respond to painfully hot and cold temperatures as well as a host of chemical stimuli that activate the nociceptive afferents. These chemical stimuli include adenosine, adenosine triphosphate (ATP), bradykinin, capsaicin, glutamate, histamine, hydrogen ions (H+), interleukins, leukotrienes, nerve growth factor, nitric oxide, **prostaglandins**, serotonin, and substance P (Mense 2009). These algesic (pain-producing) chemicals usually act on receptors on the surface of nerve cells. This can cause ion channels to open, allowing negative cations, such as sodium (Na+) and potassium (K+), to move into the cell and increase the activity of the nociceptive afferent. Muscle damage and inflammation and ischemia of either cardiac or skeletal muscle during moderate- to high-intensity exercise cause these substances to increase in concentration within the muscle. Based on experimental manipulations of individual **algesics**, the most important chemical stimulants of skeletal and cardiac muscle pain appear to be the increase in H+, bradykinin, and the actions of ATP or one of its by-products, adenosine (Birdsong et al. 2010; Mense 2009).

In the real world, these chemical stimulants act together. Exceptions can occur for those with genetic abnormalities. For example, people with **McArdle's syndrome** have a gene mutation that causes a deficiency in a muscle enzyme called myophosphorylase, which prevents them from using muscle glycogen during exercise. One consequence of the mutation is that these people have no increase in lactate during exercise. If lactate were a cause of muscle pain during exercise, then these patients should have less pain. These patients, however, are characterized by intense muscle pain that can last for several hours after exercise (Paterson et al. 1990). Clearly, and in contrast to popular belief, lactate is not a cause of muscle pain during exercise.

Other chemicals inhibit type IV nociceptors. Endogenous opioids and cannabinoids, for example, bind to nociceptive afferents and inhibit their activity. Endogenous opioids (endorphins, enkephalins, dynorphins, and endomorphins) are peptides that have biochemical properties similar to those of exogenous opiates such as heroin and morphine. Endocannabinoids (anandamide, 2-arachidonoylglycerol) are lipids

that bind to the same receptors as the active ingredient in marijuana. Moderate- to high-intensity exercise clearly increases endogenous opioid and cannabinoid levels in the periphery, where they can act to inhibit nociceptive afferent activity (Dishman and O'Connor 2009; Sparling et al. 2003).

Spinal Processing

Nociceptive afferents synapse primarily in the dorsal horn of the spinal cord. Nociceptive information is conveyed to the brain by projection neurons that make up several major tracts including the spinothalamic, spinoreticular, and spinomesencephalic tracts. The spinothalamic tract conveys information to numerous brain areas including the reticular formation, periaqueductal gray, hypothalamus, amygdala, and ventral and lateral thalamus—synapsing on cells whose axons project to numerous higher brain regions including the insular and somatosensory cortexes. The spinoreticular tract neurons project to the reticular formation at the levels of the medulla and pons before synapsing in the medial thalamus. Ultimately, neurons in this pathways synapse on key brain areas that are involved in responding to an injury including the locus coeruleus. The spinomesencephalic tract projects to numerous brain areas, and of special note are inputs to the periaqueductal gray. Cell bodies in the periaqueductal gray have axons that project to several limbic system structures including the amygdala and anterior cingulate cortex. Perhaps the key point is that because nociceptive information is critically important, it is conveyed by multiple parallel ascending pathways to a host of subcortical and cortical brain areas that coordinate an effective behavioral response (Price 2000).

Central Nervous System Processing

Within the brain, pain is processed in a widespread network of neurons. This network has many interconnections with diverse brain areas. These brain areas allow for a coordinated response to the threat presented by the noxious stimuli. For example, information is conveyed to brain areas involved in processes such as the following:

- Orientation, arousal, fear, and vigilance (examples of brain regions known to be involved in these processes include the reticular formation, locus coeruleus, periaqueductal gray, hypothalamus, and amygdala).
- Coding the intensity of the pain (e.g., primary and secondary somatosensory cortexes [SI, SII]; activity in these regions measured by fMRI is highly correlated to pain intensity ratings (Coghill et al. 1999).
- Attending to the pain (e.g., anterior cingulate cortex, orbitofrontal cortex; Bantick et al. 2002).
- The cognitive evaluation of the pain (e.g., prefrontal, parietal, and insular cortexes; Kong et al. 2006).
- Establishing a memory of the pain (e.g., hippocampus; Khanna and Sinclair 1989).
- Generating useful affective and behavioral responses to the pain (e.g., anterior cingulate, hypothalamus, amygdala, and insula; Price 2000). For example, the facial expression of pain unpleasantness can motivate helping behavior from others.

Pain Modulation

Pain can be modulated by nerve activity within the spinal cord. The activity of the projection neurons carrying nociceptive information from the spinal cord to the brain can be increased or decreased by neurons that synapse on the projection neurons.

Sensory afferents from the dermatome that is carrying non-nociceptive information converge on the dorsal horn, synapse on the projection neurons or small interneurons that synapse on projection neurons, and can modulate the activity of projection neurons. These non-nociceptive afferents are larger and faster than nociceptive afferents and carry information about light pressure, vibration, warmth, coldness, muscle stretch, and muscle force. This neuroanatomy forms the basis for treatments that reduce pain by increas-

ing the activity of non-nociceptive afferents such as the use of transcutaneous electrical nerve stimulation to treat chronic musculoskeletal pain (Johnson and Martinson 2007).

During exercise, the increased activation of sensory afferent receptors detecting non-noxious pressure, muscle stretch, and muscle force could modify muscle pain intensity. For example, generating 250 watts of power while cycling at 100 rpm would produce a greater activation of muscle stretch receptors than producing the same power output while cycling at 60 rpm. Consequently, this might allow the exercise to be perceived as less painful. Why do professional cyclists ride at a cadence between 90 and 110 rpm while most recreational cyclists ride at a much slower cadence?

The activity of the projection neurons also can be modified by other neural activity within the spinal cord. Thousands of interneurons within the spinal cord synapse on projection neurons and, depending on the neurotransmitter being released, can stimulate (e.g., glutamate, substance P, nitric oxide, calcitonin gene-related peptide) or inhibit (GABA, enkephalin, endorphin, serotonin, norepinephrine) the projection neurons.

Neurons from the brain descend into the spinal cord and can reduce pain by reducing the activity of ascending nociceptive transmission. The activation of the periaqueductal gray (PAG) is a key component of the descending pain modulation system. As illustrated in figure 11.4, the PAG receives afferent inputs not only from ascending projection neurons but from the amygdala and hypothalamus and the prefrontal, frontal, insular, and somatosensory cortexes. Activation of the PAG suppresses ascending **nociception** through its projections to the rostral ventromedial medulla (RVM) and dorsolateral pontine tegmental (DLPT) areas. Cell bodies in the RVM and DLPT areas project their axons to the dorsal horn of the spinal cord where they inhibit ascending nociceptive transmission directly or indirectly by activating inhibitory interneurons.

The descending pain modulation system is thought to account for numerous types of analgesia, including widespread cases of athletes and soldiers who report little or no pain for

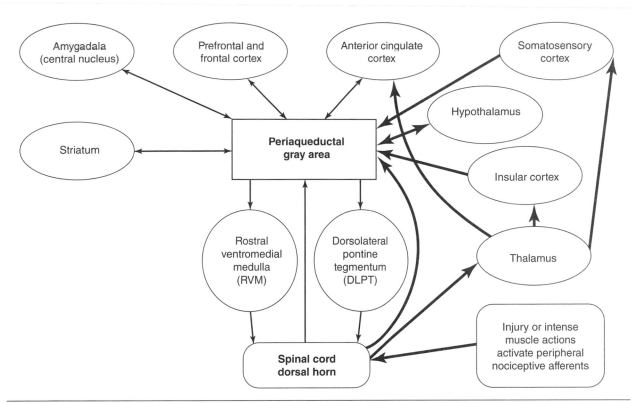

Figure 11.4 Key afferents underlying pain and the opioid pathways involved in pain modulation. Injury or intense exercise activates afferent pathways (in bold) that inform an elaborate network involved in pain. The network, including sensory and affective aspects of pain, can be modulated by an opioid-dependent system in which the periaqueductal gray (PAG) plays a central role. The PAG integrates information from several brain regions and regulates nociception via projections to the RVM and DLPT areas. These areas target nociceptive relay neurons in the dorsal horn of the spinal cord. Opioid receptors are present in the peripheral afferents and all the components of the pain modulation system.

Reprinted from *Mental Health and Physical Activity*, Vol. 2(1), R.K. Dishman and P.J. O'Connor, "Lessons in exercise neurobiology: The case of endorphins," pgs. 4-9, copyright 1998, with permission from Elsevier; Dishman et al. 1998.

several hours after a traumatic injury (Beecher 1956). Acute and chronic exercise plausibly could reduce acute and chronic pain by influencing one or more aspect of the descending pain control system. Currently there is little direct evidence that this does or does not occur.

PAIN DURING AND AFTER ACUTE EXERCISE

Painful injuries caused by participation in competitive sports are all too common. In the absence of a sport injury, many exercise bouts are pain free, but people who exercise at a high intensity or with certain medical conditions, such as arthritis or heart disease, often experience pain. This section details key aspects of pain in relation to acute exercise.

Sport-Related Injuries

Every year ~5% of recreationally active people suffer an injury while participating in sports. The prevalence decreases with age, presumably because people are less involved in sports as they get older. Researchers who obtained injury data from 100 nationally representative U.S. high schools estimated that there were 1.44 million injuries during the 2005-2006 school year (Rechel, Yard, and Comstock 2008). Studies of over 182,000 injuries and more than 1 million exposures among NCAA athletes show that the risk of injury is highest during competition and in contact sports such as football and wrestling. Combining all sports, the injury rate is highest for the lower body (accounting for more than 50% of injuries), and of these, ankle sprains are most common. Injury rates are especially high among those with a prior injury, and across all sports, men have a higher injury rate than women (Hootman, Dick, and Agel 2007). The pain and disability associated with injuries caused by participation in sports and recreational physical activities create a substantial personal and public health burden (Finch and Cassell 2006).

Skeletal Muscle Pain During Exercise

Healthy people are pain free during low-intensity exercise. During many types of moderate- to high-intensity exercise, including uphill walking or running, cycling, swimming, weightlifting, gardening and yard work, and calisthenics such as sit-ups, skeletal muscles hurt until the exercise intensity is reduced or exercise is stopped. This type of transient, naturally occurring pain is related to exercise intensity expressed relative to exercise capacity (Cook et al. 1997). For cycling exercise, thigh muscle pain threshold occurs at ~50% of peak power output and increases to a high-intensity pain at maximal exercise. These local muscle pain intensity responses to exercise can be useful for prescribing exercise intensity among some groups such as competitive athletes and people with peripheral artery disease (O'Connor and Cook 2001).

The relationship between muscle pain ratings and relative exercise intensity appears to be moderated by the absolute exercise intensity. For example, while cycling at 70% peak power output, men report higher thigh muscle pain intensity ratings than women do. The higher pain for men is likely due to the higher absolute power output at 70% because of their higher average peak power output compared to women (Cook et al. 1998). A man and woman cycling at 70% of peak power output but whose peak power outputs were 300 and 200 watts, respectively, would be cycling at quite different absolute workloads of 210 and 140 watts, respectively.

Other variables that moderate skeletal muscle pain during exercise are incompletely understood. The duration of the exercise matters. Most people run a marathon at a slow pace. Yet a survey of 1,227 marathon runners found that more than 99% reported pain during a marathon (28% reported pain by mile 13), and the average pain intensity at the primary location of pain (legs for most) during a marathon run was described as "strong." People suffering from chronic muscle pain, such as U.S. Gulf War veterans, report higher muscle pain during exercise compared to healthy controls (Cook, Stegner, and Ellingson 2010). Women with higher self-efficacy for tolerating pain reported lower muscle pain intensity during exercise (Motl, Gliottoni, and Scott 2007). College-aged African-American women with hypertensive parents reported lower thigh muscle pain during cycling compared to those with no family history of hypertension. It is known that people with hypertension, or a family history of high blood pressure, are less sensitive to several types of noxious stimuli compared to normotensives (Cook et al. 2004).

It is plausible that the unpleasantness of skeletal muscle pain during moderate- to high-intensity exercise influences the intensity at which people prefer to exercise, but little research has explored that possibility. It has been suggested that high-intensity localized skeletal muscle pain may inhibit central motor drive and reduce the ability to fully activate the muscle thereby contributing to premature muscle fatigue and reduced exercise performance (Ciubotariu, Arendt-Nielsen, and Graven-Nielsen 2007). Thus, it is not surprising that experiments have been conducted aimed at reducing muscle pain during exercise. Most of these studies have found no reduction in muscle pain during exercise, including after the consumption of codeine (Cook, O'Connor, and Ray 2000), aspirin (Cook et al. 1997), acetaminophen (Mauger, Jones, and Williams 2010), ginger (Black and O'Connor 2008), and quercetin (Ganio et al. 2010) as well as exposure to bright light aimed at influencing the brain serotonin system (O'Brien and O'Connor 2000). One dietary manipulation, however, does appear to reduce skeletal muscle pain during moderate- and high-intensity exercise: the consumption of caffeine in doses of 3 to 10 milligrams per kilogram of body weight (O'Connor et al. 2004; Motl, O'Connor, and Dishman 2003) (see figure 11.5). Caffeine also delays the onset of ischemic heart muscle pain during exercise among patients with heart disease (Piters et al. 1985).

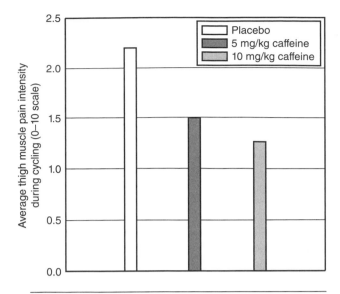

Figure 11.5 Thigh muscle pain while cycling at 60% of peak aerobic capacity is reduced after the consumption of a capsule containing either 5 or 10 milligrams per kilogram of body weight of caffeine compared to placebo capsules.

Adapted from Motl et al. 2006.

People avoid pain because it is unpleasant. Athletes, however, sometimes approach pain as a positive thing; thus the cliché "No pain, no gain." The burden of sport-related pain in the absence of a major traumatic injury would appear to be quite high in contact athletes such as American football players as well as competitive endurance athletes who expose themselves to exercise-induced skeletal muscle pain frequently. Clearly, pain need not be a barrier to performing exercise. Competitive athletes and recreationally active people who are willing to experience pain during exercise likely differ from those who shy away from such pain in numerous ways that have yet to be fully determined. Little empirical research has yet been aimed at learning whether pain during exercise is a meaningful barrier to adopting and maintaining regular exercise.

Heart Pain During Exercise

Angina, the most common symptom of coronary artery disease, is a clinical syndrome characterized by pain usually behind the sternum but also at times in the chest, jaw, shoulder, back, or arm. It usually results from a lack of oxygen to the heart muscle because of a spasm or an obstruc-

tion in one of the coronary arteries. Angina is provoked by exertion or emotional stress and is relieved by nitroglycerin. When angina occurs in response to exercise-induced increases in the work of the heart (which can be indexed by the rate–pressure product: heart rate × systolic blood pressure), it is called stable angina. Unstable angina is angina that has emerged within the last few weeks, occurs at rest, and has a crescendo pattern (increases in intensity, duration, or frequency with subsequent bouts).

The prevalence of angina is estimated at ~7% of middle-aged British men (Shaper et al. 1984). The prevalence of angina varies widely across various countries (e.g., 9.7% to 13% in Poland and below 4% in India and Switzerland). Across the world women have a ~20% greater risk of experiencing angina compared to men, and this sex-related difference is higher than average in the United States (~40% greater risk) (Hemingway et al. 2008). Approximately one in three patients with stable angina has an episode at least once per week (Beltrame et al. 2009).

Paying attention to angina is important because it is the single best predictor of heart disease. The two-year incidence of adverse events among patients with stable angina is more than 20% (Lloyd-Jones et al. 2009). Coronary artery disease patients with angina have worse outcomes than those without pain. For example, the seven-year incidence of a coronary event (e.g., death, heart attack) doubles in people with angina and electrophysiological evidence of heart disease (S-T segment depression) observed during an exercise stress test compared with those with S-T segment depression alone (Detry et al. 1985).

Exercise is one of the ABCDEs of angina treatment: aspirin/anti-anginal drug therapy, β-blockers for blood pressure reduction, cigarette smoking cessation and cholesterol-lowering drugs, diet and diabetes treatment, and education and exercise (Gibbons et al. 1999). Compared with controls without heart disease or angina but otherwise similar medically and demographically, people with stable angina are less physically active and have reduced exercise performance and quality of life (Gardner et al. 2011). Thus, these patients are prime candidates for therapeutic exercise interventions.

Early studies showed that improved symptoms after exercise training were due to a reduction in heart rate and systolic blood pressure during submaximal workloads (Clausen and Trap-Jensen 1976). More recent studies suggest that improved endothelium-dependent vasodilation of the coronary arteries also contributes to the marked reduction of myocardial ischemia and associated angina threshold during exercise (Hambrecht et al. 2004). In some patients, even maximal exercise failed to provoke angina after exercise training (Williams et al. 2006). Although exercise training can help reduce angina, its effects do not occur quickly.

Alternatives to exercise training include coronary bypass surgery and percutaneous coronary angioplasty with intracoronary stent implantation, or percutaneous coronary intervention (PCI). When PCI was compared to a one-year exercise program in patients with stable angina, PCI reduced angina more quickly than exercise did, but the more conservative exercise training treatment resulted in superior event-free survival and exercise capacity at lower costs because of reduced rehospitalizations and repeat revascularizations (Hambrecht et al. 2004).

Reduced Sensitivity to Noxious Stimuli

During moderate- to high-intensity exercise, a greater noxious stimulus is required for a person to perceive it as painful compared to what happens at rest. In one study, greater electrical current presented to the pulp of the tooth was needed for the stimulus to be perceived as painful when cycling at 200 watts (moderate) and 300 watts (high intensity), but not 100 watts (low intensity) (Kemppainen et al. 1985). This reduced sensitivity to noxious stimuli during exercise may enhance our ability to perform painful high-intensity exercise.

Experiments repeatedly have documented that people are less sensitive to noxious stimuli after exercise. This exercise-induced **hypoalgesia** effect has been shown most consistently among healthy men performing high-intensity, dynamic, large-muscle exercise, such as running or cycling, when pain intensity was assessed shortly after exercise (Koltyn 2002). This effect

has been observed with several types of stimuli including noxious pressure and heat. The effect also has been reported after brief (1.5-5 min) low-intensity (<50% of maximal voluntary contraction) isometric contractions (Umeda et al. 2010). The effect has been observed for as long as 60 minutes after exercise, but the consistency of long-lasting exercise-induced hypoalgesia has not been thoroughly tested. The cause of exercise-induced hypoalgesia is uncertain, but it could result from the fact that high-intensity exercise is itself painful. It is known that one type of pain can inhibit a second pain, which is known as conditioned pain modulation. Recent evidence shows that exercise can induce hypoalgesia through conditioned pain modulation.

The opposite effect (exercise-induced hyperalgesia) occurs in people suffering from chronic musculoskeletal pain, for instance, those with fibromyalgia (Kosek, Ekholm, and Hansson 1996). Also, Gulf War veterans with chronic pain who completed 30 minutes of submaximal exercise rated exercise as more painful and reported higher pain intensity and affect ratings in response to heat pain stimuli compared to veterans without pain (Cook, Stegner, and Ellingson 2010).

Delayed-Onset Skeletal Muscle Injury

In clinical medicine, when a large amount of muscle is rapidly injured because of exercise, it is known as exertional **rhabdomyolysis** (*rhabdo* = "striped" + *myo* = "muscle" + *lysis* = "breakdown"). High-intensity eccentric muscle actions performed by someone unaccustomed to them are the primary cause of this type of muscle and connective tissue injury. Eccentric actions occur when a muscle lengthens while producing force. For example, lowering a heavy weight using the arms requires the anterior upper arm muscles (biceps brachii) to lengthen while they produce force that resists the gravitational force of the weight.

Little pain is experienced during injurious high-intensity eccentric actions; however, immediately afterward, the ability of the injured muscles to produce force is reduced. The start of the muscle pain is delayed by about 24 hours and often lasts for several days. A dominant explanation for why the pain is delayed after intense eccentric actions is that the pain is a consequence of localized skeletal muscle inflammation (Smith 1991). The inflammation involves (1) the release of substances from the muscle cells that dilate capillaries, (2) the adhesion of leucocytes to the cell wall, (3) the migration of the leucocytes into the cell, and (4) ultimately, the repair of the tissue. The adhesion and migration steps take time and delay the onset of pain. During this process substances known to stimulate pain, such as bradykinin and prostaglandins, are released from blood-borne mast cells and muscle cells. The process also causes the swelling of muscle cells, which can increase pressure on nociceptors.

Moving the injured skeletal muscle, or pressing on it, is needed to cause pain after eccentric exercise-induced muscle injury. There appear to be no epidemiological studies documenting the prevalence of this type of pain, but anecdotal evidence suggests that the lifetime prevalence approaches 100%. Kidney failure and death can result from muscle proteins such as myoglobin being released into the blood after extensive skeletal muscle injury induced by eccentric exercise (Sayers et al. 1999). A wide variety of treatments have been tested to reduce eccentric exercise–induced pain, and small, transient improvements have been observed with some nonsteroidal anti-inflammatory drugs (NSAIDS), natural products that have actions similar to NSAIDS, and caffeine (see figure 11.6). Progressive exercise training can attenuate delayed-onset muscle injury and pain, but in many real-world situations, this is impractical. Most of the time delayed-onset muscle injury is of a low to moderate intensity and adequately managed with self-care behaviors rather than medical attention.

EFFECTS OF EXERCISE TRAINING

Sport training during youth and early adulthood can lead to chronic pain later in life. Epidemiological evidence does suggest that former competitive athletes have more degenerative changes in their joints and spine compared to nonath-

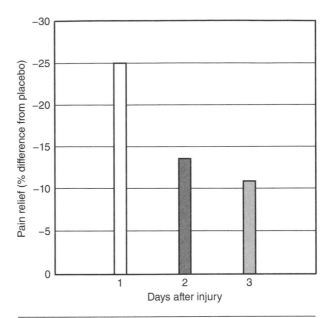

Figure 11.6 Compared to placebo, the consumption of capsules containing 2 grams of ginger for 8 consecutive days was associated with 25% less arm muscle pain after a bout of novel eccentric exercise.

Data from Black et al. 2010.

letes. These adverse consequences, however, are often countered by greater muscle function and fitness that also may be related to participation in sports (Kujala et al. 2003).

This section addresses the effect of exercise training on pain. Middle-aged adults who do not suffer from a painful medical condition frequently have minor aches and pains. Could exercise training help? One study germane to this question involved a six-month randomized controlled trial that included 430 sedentary, overweight, and obese postmenopausal women. Compared to a nonexercise control group, bodily pain scores consistent with sex and age norms at baseline were not improved by aerobic exercise training that expended 4, 8, or 12 kilocalories per kilogram of body weight each week. Those amounts of physical activity approximated 50%, 100%, and 150% of the levels recommended by the U.S. National Institutes of Health. The study confirms that exercise training has little effect on improving pain when people are experiencing few pain symptoms (Martin et al. 2009). Evidence does show that exercise training improves pain among pregnant women and other people coping with painful medical conditions as described in the remainder of this section.

Pregnancy

Regular exercise might attenuate pain related to childbirth by reducing the duration of labor. One study observed that women who exercised regularly before becoming pregnant had labor that was about eight hours shorter than that of nonexercising women. Another found that the first stage of labor was approximately two hours shorter among those who exercised during pregnancy compared to those who stopped exercising during the first trimester. A third study found that aerobic capacity measured about one month before childbirth was negatively associated with the duration of labor among 40 women who started labor spontaneously (Kardel et al. 2009). A fourth study found that women who took part in prenatal yoga reported fewer pregnancy discomforts compared to controls at 38 to 40 weeks of gestation (Sun et al. 2010). This literature, however, is mixed; about an equal number of other studies failed to find a significant association between physical activity levels and labor length (Penttinen and Erkkola 1997).

Exercise also may reduce the intensity of childbirth pain. One study tested 36 women who completed regular bouts of cycling exercise or a nonexercise control condition during their second and third trimesters. During labor, assessments of pain were made and blood was drawn and measured for several indicators of stress including β-endorphin and cortisol. Plasma β-endorphin was found to be elevated compared to controls in the women who exercised throughout pregnancy. This difference was maintained throughout labor, and pain intensity ratings during labor were lower in the women who exercised (Varrassi, Bazzano, and Edwards 1989).

Arthritis

Arthritis is the most common cause of disability in the United States. Arthritis is a disorder that involves the inflammation of the joints. Osteoarthritis and rheumatoid arthritis are the most common forms. **Osteoarthritis** is a degenerative joint disease that can affect any joint in the body but is especially common in the hips, knees, and spine. About 12% of Americans aged 25 to 74 have clinically defined osteoarthritis (Lawrence et al. 2008). **Rheumatoid arthritis** affects about

> **F**or most women, the birth of a child is a joyous occasion. Nevertheless, pain during childbirth can be intense, and for some women it can lead to chronic pain.

1% of the U.S. population and most commonly involves the wrists and finger joints. Pain and stiffness are manifestations of arthritis, and as a result, a high percentage of patients reduce their activity and become weaker and less physically fit (Mancuso et al. 2007).

Land- and water-based aerobic exercise as well as strength training appear to be safe for patients with rheumatoid arthritis. There is not strong research evidence for or against the value of hand exercise in the treatment of people with rheumatoid arthritis (Wessel 2004). At least 15 randomized controlled trials have examined the influence of whole-body exercise training in patients with rheumatoid arthritis (Stenström and Minor 2003). Ten of the 15 trials included pain as one of the outcomes. Pain improved in only 2 of the 10 trials. The available evidence indicates that exercise training is beneficial for patients with rheumatoid arthritis. It has been shown to improve strength and fitness; however, it does not consistently improve pain (Guy 2008; Ottawa Panel Members et al. 2004).

It is estimated that over 25 million Americans over the age of 25 suffer from osteoarthritis. The problem is more common in women than in men, especially for knee osteoarthritis. There is no good evidence that regular exercise increases the risk of developing osteoarthritis (Felson et al. 2007). Nonsteroidal anti-inflammatory drugs such as ibuprofen are mainstays in the treatment of osteoarthritis; however, hip or knee replacement surgery is common among these patients.

Nonpharmacological therapies for osteoarthritis such as exercise are receiving increased attention. Range-of-motion exercises that do not train the muscles appear to be ineffective therapy for osteoarthritis. Several quantitative reviews of randomized trials showed that exercise training of all types reduces the pain associated with knee and hip osteoarthritis (Fransen, McConnell, and

Bell 2002; Van Baar et al. 1999). These analyses indicate that the magnitude of the pain reduction after exercise training is modest, ranging from 0.33 to 0.50 standard deviations. Modest improvements in pain are realized from water-based exercise as well as land-based exercise especially when strength training was included (Fransen et al. 2010; Hernández-Molina et al. 2008). Combining exercise with weight loss may be an especially useful therapy. In one study the combination of exercise and 10 pounds (4.5 kg) of weight loss, but not weight loss alone, reduced pain and improved physical function in patients with osteoarthritis of the knee as compared to education about nutrition, exercise, and arthritis (Messier et al. 2004). The evidence is strong enough that exercise is recommended as an osteoarthritis treatment by several groups of experts including the American College of Rheumatology and the U.S. Department of Health and Human Services.

Low Back Pain

People between the ages of 20 and 45 are most likely to suffer from low back pain. Low back pain is the second most common cause of disability in the United States (Centers for Disease Control and Prevention [CDC] 2001b). Because many people with low back pain frequently miss work, the condition is estimated to cost between $100 and $200 billion each year. A minority of those with acute back pain develop chronic back pain, but the prevalence of chronic low back pain is increasing. Expensive treatments such as spinal injections, surgeries, and analgesic drugs are popular among people with chronic low back pain (Freburger et al. 2009). Exercise training would be an attractive alternative therapy if it were efficacious.

Several large randomized trials and systematic quantitative reviews of more than three dozen trials reveal that exercise training is more effective than usual care in reducing pain and improving physical function among people suffering from chronic low back pain (Hayden, van Tulder, and Tomlinson 2005; Liddle, Baxter, and Gracey 2004). The average magnitude of the effect on pain is clinically meaningful and moderate, and it ranges from 6 to 20 points on a 100-point pain intensity scale. The effect is well documented for several types of exercise

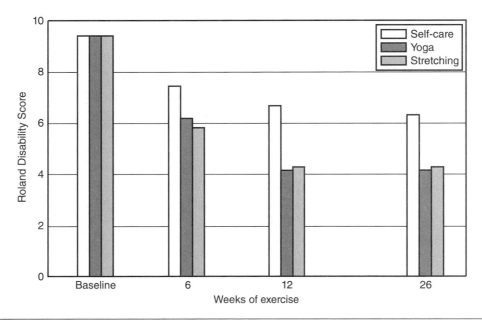

Figure 11.7 The results of a randomized trial showing mean changes in Roland disability scores, a multidimensional measure of low back pain symptoms, before, during, and after 12 weeks of yoga (n = 92 patients) or conventional stretching exercise (n = 91) compared to a self-care treatment (reading a book on back pain, n = 45) among patients with chronic low back pain. Yoga and stretching were superior to self-care for improving symptoms due to chronic low back pain.

Data from Sherman et al. 2011.

including stretching, yoga, aquatic exercise, and exercises aimed at learning how to better control the muscles of the low back (Macedo et al. 2009; Sherman et al. 2011; Waller, Lambeck, and Daly 2009) (see figure 11.7). The efficacy of strength training per se for reduced pain cannot be determined from most of the studies because strength training, when it was studied, typically was included but as one component in multidimensional rehabilitation programs. The American Pain Society and the American College of Physicians have concluded that there is good evidence of moderate efficacy for exercise in the treatment of chronic low back pain (Chou and Huffman 2007).

Migraine

Exercise training is often recommended as an aid to migraine sufferers. Cross-sectional studies with ~700 Finnish adolescents show fewer headaches among more active study participants (Kujala, Taimela, and Viljanen 1999). Until recently, there was only a limited amount of methodologically weak experimental evidence on whether exercise is an effective therapy for migraine headaches (Busch and Gaul 2008). Randomized trials have provided stronger evidence that exercise training reduces the frequency of migraine headaches (Dittrich et al. 2008; John et al. 2007; Narin et al. 2003; Varkey et al. 2011). One study compared the preventive effects of exercise training to relaxation and medication, two established migraine therapies (Varkey et al. 2011). Migraine sufferers (n = 91) were randomly assigned to three months of exercise (40 min 3 times per week), relaxation (including controlled breathing and stress management techniques), or drug treatment (**topiramate**, up to 200 mg daily). Exercise was found to be as effective in reducing migraine frequency as relaxation or topiramate. A smaller 6-week study found reduced migraine pain intensity when exercise training (45 min per session) was combined with relaxation (15 min per session) (Dittrich et al. 2008).

Peripheral Artery Disease

More than 25 million adults in the United States and Europe suffer from peripheral artery dis-

ease (PAD) (Diehm et al. 2004). PAD is usually caused by atherosclerotic blockages of arteries, and it is most common in the lower limb arteries. Most people with PAD are over age 55, and in the United States, about 20% of those with PAD report intermittent **claudication** (McGrae McDermott, Mehta, and Greenland 1999). Claudication usually involves pain in one or both calves caused by walking, and is relieved by rest.

Improvements in claudication can be realized by smoking cessation, medications that improve blood flow or lower cholesterol, and walking exercise training (Hankey, Norman, and Eikelboom 2006). An analysis of 22 randomized trials with 1,200 PAD patients showed that after walk training, maximal walking ability and walk distance improved by 150% to 200% (Watson, Ellis, and Leng 2008). Improvements appear to be best when the exercise session duration was longer than 30 minutes, the exercise occurred at least 3 times per week for at least 6 months, and the walk training was near the maximal tolerable level of calf muscle pain intensity (Leng, Fowler, and Ernst 2000). Walking behavior among PAD patients has been shown to be unrelated to the intensity of pain experienced during the exercise but dependent on psychological variables such as intention to exercise (Galea and Bray 2007). Regular supervised walk training has been found to improve maximal treadmill walking distance more effectively than medications that improve blood flow. Improvement in walking after exercise training also improves physical function and quality of life (Milani and Lavie 2007).

Neuropathic Pain

Neuropathic pain is a maladaptive pain that results from injury to the nervous system (Woolf and Mannion 1999). Patients with herpes zoster (shingles), human immunodeficiency virus, multiple sclerosis, stroke, and traumatic injury suffer from neuropathic pain that negatively affects their quality of life (Jensen, Chodroff, and Dworkin 2007).

The most common type of neuropathic pain results as a consequence of diabetes. Chronic hyperglycemia damages nerves, especially those in the foot, and this leads to loss of sensation, pain and increased sensitivity to noxious stimuli (i.e., hyperalgesia), and pain in response to stimuli that normally are not painful (**allodynia**). More than 3 million people in the United States suffer from painful diabetic neuropathy (Schmader 2002), and 60% of lower extremity amputations are performed as a result of complications from diabetes (Narayan et al. 2006). Medications such as opioid analgesics are often used to treat neuropathic pain (Dworkin et al. 2003).

Relatively little is known about whether regular exercise might be useful in reducing neuropathic pain. One randomized trial examined the influence of exercise training on the development of diabetic neuropathies (Balducci et al. 2006). A smaller percentage of participants (*n* = 31) who completed supervised vigorous treadmill walking for 4 hours per week for 4 years developed neuropathies compared to 47 controls (17% vs. 30%). The exercisers also showed increased nerve conduction velocity, a sign of healthier nerve function. Another trial with type 2 diabetics found that 12 weeks of tai chi chuan exercise improved fasting blood glucose levels and increased nerve conduction velocities (Hung et al. 2009). These observations are buttressed by positive results in several potentially relevant rodent studies. These studies, conducted with diabetic rats or rats with nerve injury, showed that exercise training reduced behavioral signs of hyperalgesia in response to light pressure and noxious thermal stimuli (Kuphal, Fibuch, and Taylor 2007; Shankarappa, Piedras-Rentería, and Stubbs 2011; Stagg et al. 2011).

With regard to pain in patients with multiple sclerosis (MS), cross-sectional studies have found less pain among physically active MS patients (Motl, Snook, and Schapiro 2008). Other analyses of cross-sectional data suggest that among MS patients, pain, fatigue, and depression represent a symptom cluster, and that physical activity behavior is moderately and negatively related to the symptom cluster (Motl and McAuley 2009). A separate analysis suggested that exercise can influence psychosocial variables such as fatigue, social support, and self-efficacy, and that changes in these variables can improve pain in MS patients (Motl and McAuley 2009). Only a small number of randomized trials involving exercise training have been conducted with MS patients (Motl and Gosney 2008), and most have not measured pain. Among those that did, the findings are mixed; some show greater improvements in pain in the exercise group (e.g., Stuifbergen et al. 2003), and others show no advantage to exercise training (e.g., Romberg, Virtanen, and Ruutiainen 2005).

Fibromyalgia

Fibromyalgia is a medical disorder that affects ~2% of people living in the United States. It is more common among women (3.4%) than among men (0.5%) (Wolfe et al. 1995). People with fibromyalgia are characterized by chronic widespread pain (affecting locations above and below the waist on both sides of the body), fatigue, sleep disruptions, and increased pain in response to tactile pressure at more than 10 of 18 possible tender points. They often have comorbid conditions, especially chronic fatigue syndrome, depression, anxiety, headaches, and rheumatoid arthritis (Weir et al. 2006). People with fibromyalgia are often physically inactive, and their physical function is reduced. More than 60% report difficulty going up one flight of stairs, walking one-half mile (0.8 km), or lifting 10 pounds (4.5 kg), and those with lower function report higher pain intensity (Jones et al. 2008).

At least 28 randomized controlled trials conducted in Europe and North America with over 1,600 patients (>95% women) have examined the influence of aerobic exercise training on pain among people with fibromyalgia. Compared to control conditions, aerobic exercise training of 6 to 24 weeks consistently improves tender point pain (Kelley 2011) and other pain dimensions among those with fibromyalgia (Hauser 2010; Ramel et al. 2009). According to experts, the average effect is clinically important, statistically significant, and moderate in size. The American Pain Society strongly recommends aerobic exercise, cognitive behavioral therapy, antidepressant drug therapy (amitriptyline), and multicomponent treatments for fibromyalgia (Häuser, Thieme, and Turk 2010). Interestingly, a large Internet survey asking fibromyalgia patients what they thought was most effective in managing their disorder found that the most popular treatments (rest, heat, antidepressants, and sleep medications) often were not the most effective (Bennett, Jones et al. 2007).

Surgical Pain

Exercise training is often recommended as rehabilitation after surgeries such as coronary artery bypass surgery, surgery for a herniated disk in the low back, and hip and knee replacement surgeries. Cardiac rehabilitation programs, which enroll numerous postsurgical patients, are consistently associated with reductions in ratings of bodily pain, and the effect is larger for the most psychologically distressed patients (Artham, Lavie, and Milani 2008). A small body of research has found mixed evidence that exercise training is helpful in reducing postsurgical back pain. In an analysis of eight well-conducted experiments involving 635 patients who underwent back surgery, the evidence was inconclusive on whether exercise training reduced back pain to an extent greater than control conditions without exercise (Rushton et al. 2011). Few studies have examined the influence of exercise training on pain as part of prehabilitation or rehabilitation associated with knee or hip replacement surgery. Uncontrolled studies show that pain is improved among exercising patients after elective knee surgery, but it is unclear whether the effect can be attributed to the exercise (Frost, Lamb, and Robertson 2002). One randomized trial examined the effect of a 4-week exercise and education program completed 2 weeks before knee surgery and found no difference in pain up to 12 months after the surgery in the exercise group (n = 65) compared to the nonexercise group (n = 66) (Beaupre et al. 2004). There is evidence that pain is a reason people refuse to comply with exercise prescribed as treatment after hip surgery (Unlu et al. 2007).

Cancer

Pain is a common symptom during cancer treatment and survivorship, and no study has reported pain prevalence of less than 14% among cancer patients (Goudas et al. 2005). Most cancer patients are willing to start an exercise program, but adherence is only about 50% (Maddocks, Mockett, and Wilcock 2009). Uncontrolled longitudinal studies show improvements in pain among breast cancer survivors who increased their level of physical activity after their cancer diagnosis (Kendall et al. 2005), but one randomized controlled trial showed no improvement in pain (Segal et al. 2001). There is insufficient evidence to show whether exercise improves pain among breast and other cancer survivors (Schmitz et al. 2005).

Promising results were found in a study that examined the effects of exercise on shoulder pain, which is a common problem after surgery for head and neck cancer. Fifty-two head and neck cancer survivors were assigned randomly to strength training or usual care exercise for 12 weeks. Usual care exercise involved stretching, postural exercises, and the use of light weights and low-resistance elastic bands. Strength training involved five to eight exercises starting at 25% of maximal strength and progressively increased to 70%. Adherence to the strength and usual care exercise programs was 95% and 87%, respectively. The strength training program significantly reduced shoulder pain and disability (McNeely et al. 2008).

Gulf War Syndrome

Military personnel who return from war have a high prevalence of chronic pain. Much of the chronic pain is explained by traumatic tissue injury, but a substantial number suffer from symptoms with no identifiable etiology. Among the most common problems are fatigue, depression, and musculoskeletal pain.

One large randomized trial (n = 1,087) compared three 12-week experimental treatments (exercise training, cognitive behavioral therapy [CBT], and a combination of exercise and CBT) to usual care. The experimental treatments showed little advantage over usual care. This trial appears to have underestimated the potential usefulness of exercise because only one supervised session of exercise per week was required and the adherence to exercise was poor. Thus, despite the large size of the trial, it is premature to conclude that pain among war veterans cannot be aided by exercise training (Donta et al. 2003).

Optimal Exercise Stimulus for Pain Relief?

Very little research to date has examined which exercise training component (mode, weekly session frequency, session duration–intensity combination, time of day), if any, most strongly affects the efficacy of exercise for pain relief. About 90% of studies have examined the effects on pain of walking, jogging, and cycling exercise modes. Although current research does not suggest a best exercise mode for pain relief across all types of chronic disease patients, evidence does suggest that pain relief is realized after all modes of exercise including yoga and strength training. A meta-analysis of studies of the effects of exercise on rheumatic diseases (mainly arthritis and fibromyalgia) found that effects on pain were not moderated by the exercise training mode (Kelley, Kelley, Hootman, and Jones 2011). This observation does not seem to be due to an inadequate number of available studies of each exercise type. For example, the efficacy of strength training for pain among patients with low back, osteoarthritis, and fibromyalgia disorders has been examined in at least five (Kankaanp et al. 1999; Mosely 2002; O'Connor, Herring, and Caravalho 2010; Rittweger et al. 2002), four (Bircan et al. 2008; Jones et al. 2002; Kingsley et al. 2005; Valkeinen et al. 2004) and eight (O'Connor, Herring, and Caravalho 2010) randomized controlled trials, respectively. With regard to yoga, 9 of 10 randomized trials found significantly greater pain relief after yoga compared to the control interventions (Posadzki et al. 2011).

SUMMARY

Exercise and pain are common companions. Participating in sports and exercise often leads to acute injuries and pain, and for some, these injuries lead to chronic pain. Pain in the active skeletal muscles occurs during moderate- to high-intensity exercise. For some, this type of pain may inhibit maximal exercise performance. Chest pain during exercise is common among those with heart disease and provides useful information to both the patient and the therapist. Novel eccentric exercise causes transient muscle pain that is delayed in onset. This type of injury is often mild, but when it is severe, it can be mortal.

Exercise is also used in the treatment of a variety of painful conditions. The strongest evidence that exercise training is useful in relieving pain comes from studies of patients with low back pain, osteoarthritis, peripheral artery disease, and fibromyalgia. A limited amount of promising research suggests that exercise training may improve pain among pregnant women, migraine sufferers, and patients with neuropathic pains resulting from diabetes and multiple sclerosis.

WEBSITES

http://health.nih.gov/topic/pain

www.ampainsoc.org

www.theacpa.org

Self-Esteem

Exercise can affect mental health through multiple social and psychobiological mechanisms; but regardless of how the change comes about, the outcome is manifest, at least partly, in attitudes, beliefs, and feelings about the self. Exercise has great potential for changing self-perceptions, and anecdotal accounts of why people exercise often include reports of improvements in self-concept and self-esteem. However, experimental evidence for increases in self-esteem that can be directly attributed to an independent effect from exercise is limited.

This chapter delineates the relationship between how people feel about themselves and their levels of physical activity. Theories and models of self-concept and self-esteem are presented to lay the foundation for understanding the interaction between exercise behavior and self-perceptions. The measurement of physical self-concept and self-esteem is described in some detail to shed light on some of the issues in conceptualizing and measuring **attitudes** and **beliefs** about the self. The ways self-esteem is defined and assessed with respect to exercise have affected the scope and quality of research in this area. This chapter reviews the literature examining the relationship between self-perceptions and exercise behavior to summarize what we know and illustrate issues inherent in studying exercise and self-esteem.

Positive self-esteem is one of the key indicators of good mental health and a significant correlate of life adjustment.

Effects of Positive and Negative Self-Esteem

A positive assessment of oneself can enhance mood and support healthy behaviors, whereas negative self-esteem can lead to depressed mood and disadvantageous behaviors.

- High self-esteem is associated with independence, leadership, adaptability, and resilience to stress (Wylie 1989).

- Low self-esteem is associated with depression, anxiety, and phobias (Baumeister 1993).

- Low self-esteem in adolescence increases the risk for adjustment problems and poor mental and physical health in adulthood (Trzesniewski et al. 2006).

- Self-esteem may moderate the stress–illness relationship by influencing the appraisal of stress and subsequent physiological responsivity (Rector and Roger 1997).

THE SELF-SYSTEM

The self is a complex system of constructs that has been organized by theorists into a directing and organizing self and a composite of attributes and characteristics that make up the self in action (Harter 1996). The directing self organizes the self in action into a coherent structure, which is commonly termed *self-concept* by social psychologists or *identity* by clinical psychologists and psychiatrists (Fox 2000). **Self-concept** is an organized configuration of perceptions of the self that are within conscious awareness. It is multidimensional, and it includes many subcomponents, or domains, such as the academic self, the social self, the spiritual self, and the physical self. Self-concept is a critical factor in mental health. A stable and coherent framework of self is necessary for making sense of the world.

The concept of a unidimensional core identity has expanded to intuitively appealing and practical multidimensional models of the self (e.g., Marsh 1997; Shavelson, Hubner, and Stanton 1976). Figure 12.1 presents an example of a multidimensional hierarchical model. Imagine the self-concept system as a pyramid, with global self-concept at the apex and general constructs at the next-lower level. Specificity increases downward, with the most situation-specific self-perceptions at the base. Higher-order constructs are dependent on lower-order components. For example, how we define ourselves socially depends on our relationships with family, coworkers, and friends. Changes in specific components (i.e., communications with siblings) affect these more general constructs and influence global self-concept. Self-esteem in this model is a result of the personal assessment of how we are doing with respect to the constructs that are highly valued and considered important.

The **self-schemata** is a cognitive structure that represents people's knowledge of themselves and their attributes, and is thought by some theorists to guide how people retrieve, select,

> **"THE WAY** in which to increase self-esteem, and to overcome a feeling of being inferior to one's fellows is to develop one's native abilities . . . . A good outlet . . . in boys and girls is sports and games, in which they can learn to perform well and to take real pleasure. Accomplishment builds confidence, which helps to overcome the feelings of diffidence and inferiority" (Rathbone et al. 1932).
>
> *Josephine Langworthy Rathbone, 1932, cofounder of the American College of Sports Medicine in 1954.*

and organize information about themselves. Kendzierski (1994), applying the self-schemata concept to exercise, proposed three types of people: exercise schematics, nonexercise schematics, and aschematics. Exercise schematics describe themselves as exercisers and hold physical self-constructs as important to their self-image. Nonexercise schematics have a self-schema for not exercising. Aschematics might be irregularly active, but being physically active is not important to their self-image. Exercise schematics are more likely to follow through on intentions to exercise and have an easier time overcoming a lapse in an exercise routine than aschematics do. Experience is part of schemata development, but the development of the exercise schemata depends on events and activities including, but not limited to, exercise experiences.

A common understanding of **self-esteem** is that it refers to how much one likes or values

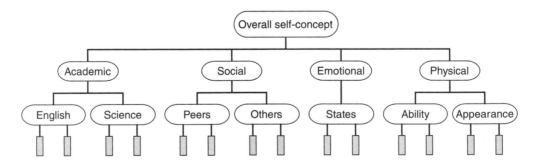

Figure 12.1 A multidimensional hierarchical model of the self; specificity increases from the apex (overall self-concept) to the base.

R.J. Shavelson, J.J. Hubner, and G.C. Stanton, 1976, *Review of Educational Research* 46(3): 407-441, "Self-concept: Validation of construct interpretations," copyright © 1976. Reprinted by permission of Sage Publications.

oneself, and there is an intuitive association between positive self-esteem and good mental health. In the social sciences, self-esteem, a hypothetical construct, is the evaluation of the self-concept and includes feelings associated with that evaluation. It is the summary judgment of how well the self is doing in specific areas and overall based on one's personal value system and standards. Self-esteem can thus be quantified as the sum of evaluations of various attributes of oneself. Other terms used to describe self-esteem are *self-worth, self-regard, self-respect,* and *self-acceptance* (Blascovich and Tomaka 1991).

Self-esteem was initially conceived as a global construct, but the conceptualization has expanded into one that is more multidimensional. Facets of self-esteem (e.g., judgment of physical capabilities) contribute to global self-esteem to the extent that those attributes are important to a sense of self (see figure 12.2). Thus, to understand self-esteem, we must consider the dominant culture and the individual's internalization of the culture's values and ideals. For example, if the cultural ideals include a lean body and a person has a high percentage of body fat, physical self-esteem will be low to the extent that the person values physical self-concept and accepts cultural ideals. If the dominant culture elevates family and social relationships above physical appearance and other subcomponents of physical self-concept, body size will have less influence on self-esteem.

Although some researchers distinguish between self-concept and self-esteem, others (e.g., Sonstroem 1998) consider facets of self-concept to be components of global self-esteem. This integration is based on the idea that we cannot describe the self without some evaluation and an affective response. For example, in the Exercise and Self-Esteem Model (Sonstroem and Morgan 1989), one of the domains of global self-esteem is physical self-worth. Physical self-worth is influenced by physical competence and physical self-acceptance in several subdomains, such as strength and aerobic endurance. Physical competence is what we think we can do and is similar to self-concept. Self-acceptance is what we feel about what we can do, and indicates how satisfied we are with our level of competence. This level of satisfaction represents a component of general self-esteem.

> **S**elf-concept is an objective accounting of who we are. Self-esteem is how we feel about who we are.

Self-esteem has a clear link to psychological well-being, but it also serves to direct behavior. This motivational feature of self-esteem guides behavior through the desire for self-enhancement. The **self-enhancement hypothesis** is based on the premise that people do things that they expect will result in positive feelings of competence and esteem (Biddle 1997). They act as they perceive themselves to be and engage in behaviors they think will lead to success

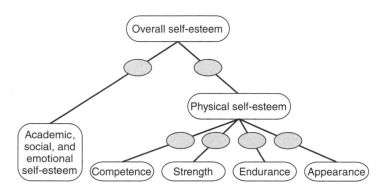

Figure 12.2 Different people emphasize different facets of themselves in forming their self-esteem.

Reprinted, by permission, from K. Fox and C.B. Corbin, 1989, "The physical self-perception profile: Development and preliminary validation," *Journal of Sport & Exercise Psychology* 11(4): 408-430.

and enhancement of the self. Thus, behavioral choices are influenced by the need to increase or sustain positive evaluations of self-concept. The concept of self-efficacy is useful in this model in that people are more likely to engage in a behavior if they are confident that they will be successful and will thus be able to enhance their sense of self. This model can be used to predict future behavior. For example, a person with high self-efficacy for swimming but little confidence in his ability to in-line skate would be more likely to take a date to a pool than to a roller rink.

THEORIES AND MODELS

The exercise and self-esteem model developed by Sonstroem and Morgan (1989) that incorporates physical self-concept and self-esteem to explain how exercise might influence global self-esteem was expanded to include physical self-worth (Sonstroem, Harlow, and Josephs 1994). This model is hierarchical and multidimensional with global self-concept and self-esteem at the apex and psychosocial perceptions progressing down from the general to the specific. Specific physical criteria, such as the time it takes to run a mile, interact with specific exercise self-efficacy, which is a component of the subdomain physical condition. Positive changes in the physical consequences of specific activities (e.g., increased endurance, decreased body fat) lead to enhanced self-efficacy, which was proposed to mediate the effects of changes in physical consequences and subdomain self-perceptions on global self-perceptions. Some evidence points to the effects of self-efficacy on global self-esteem that are parallel with physical activity outcomes, mediating effects through the subdomains self-esteem and physical self-worth (McAuley et al. 2005). Physical self-worth is expected to mediate the effects of physical condition self-concept and self-efficacy on self-esteem. This model offers a cognitive link between higher-order constructs of the self and actual behaviors.

McAuley, Mihalko, and Bane (1997) tested this model in a 20-week training study with 41 male and 42 female sedentary middle-aged adults. They found significant increases in global self-esteem, physical self-worth, and physical condition. There were no changes in global self-esteem when the investigators controlled for physical self-worth, a result that supports this model of exercise and self-esteem. Elavsky (2010) applied this model to 143 middle-aged women over a 2-year period and found that changes in self-perceptions relative to physical condition and body attractiveness mediated the effects of physical activity, self-efficacy, and body mass index (BMI) on changes in physical self-worth and global self-esteem. Increases in self-perceptions relative to an attractive body were also significantly associated with increases in physical self-worth and subsequently global self-esteem. Resistance exercise training also increased physical self-worth and self-esteem in a hierarchical manner among college students (Moore et al. 2011).

Fox and Corbin (1989) presented a conceptual model of the physical self via the development of the Physical Self-Perception Profile shown in figure 12.3. This model also includes physical self-worth, along with sport competence, attractiveness, physical condition, and strength. Because perceptions of the self-concept are influenced by how someone values a particular domain, Fox and Corbin stressed the relationship between physical competencies and importance, and included a measure of importance (Perceived Importance Profile) (Fox 1990).

Who people think they are affects their self-esteem and guides their behavior. They process information and make decisions via the self-schemata so that their behavior and the outcomes of their behavior are consistent with goals and a personal theory of the self (Fox 1997). Thus, the self is an active agent in self-concept development and maintenance, and the degree of success is reflected in self-esteem. In addition to maintaining consistency, the self directs behaviors that serve to enhance the self.

> **S**elf-concept is multidimensional and hierarchical, and self-perception can vary from level to level.

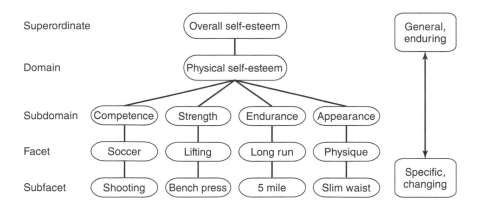

Figure 12.3   Structure of physical self-esteem.
Based on Fox 1990.

Self-esteem is influenced by demographic characteristics, the physical body, sensory input, psychosocial dynamics, and the social and cultural environments.

According to the self-enhancement hypothesis, specific activities to enhance the self are directed by a need to feel competent, worthy, and loved by others. People are motivated, then, to act in order to feel connected to others and to experience a sense of self-determination. Fox (1997) described several self-enhancement strategies that are summarized in table 12.1.

FACTORS INFLUENCING SELF-ESTEEM

Demographic characteristics, such as sex and age, influence self-concept. Numerous studies have found more favorable self-concept and self-esteem scores in males than in females across age groups. Self-concept seems to be stable in adulthood in respect to the effects of age. Hirsch and Lykken (1993) looked at self-concept factors in 678 monozygotic and 547 dizygotic twin pairs (aged 27 to 86) and concluded that self-concept crystallizes early in adulthood and reflects a strong genetic influence. In general, self-esteem follows a trajectory similar to self-concept. Orth, Trzesniewski, and Robins (2010) assessed

self-esteem in 3,617 adults aged 25 to 104 four times over 16 years and found that self-esteem increased during young and middle adulthood, peaked at about age 60, and declined in old age, likely due to changes in socioeconomic status and health.

Various malleable physical, psychological, and social variables can contribute to the evaluation of self-concept. Changes in the body's structure and function influence self-perceptions. Adolescence, pregnancy, weight loss and gain, injury, menopause, disease, and aging are examples of events that alter the physical self and have an impact on self-perceptions. One way physical changes can influence self-esteem is through the modulating effects of sensory input on self-evaluation. The muscle strain experienced in a weightlifting class by someone recovering from an injury, and the joint stiffness an older woman feels getting out of an automobile, are examples of sensations that can contribute to poor physical self-esteem.

The physical body provides a substantial interface between the individual and the world and influences self-esteem. Appearance is a means of communication and an expression of status and sexuality. Judgment of the physical self influences global self-esteem, but the importance of the physical self in self-esteem is greater when the other self components are less developed or when physical condition is highlighted, such as from disease or injury. The lack of a complex sense of self has been presented as one reason exercise can have a more potent influence on self-esteem in children than on people of other

Table 12.1 Self-Enhancement Strategies

Behavioral strategy	Example
Choose behaviors that have a high probability of success and positive affect.	George rowed for his college crew team, so he decides to buy a kayak and attend a few roll sessions.
Act in ways to maximize social approval and support.	George gives the novices in his class tips he learned from crew, and they help each other load the kayaks at the end of class.
Withdraw from activities that tend to result in failure, lack of success, and negative affect.	Folks from the roll class organize a trip to a bike trail to go in-line skating on Sunday, but George bows out. In high school he fell several times trying to learn how to roller skate and does not want to make a fool of himself in front of his new friends.
Psychological strategy	**Example**
Discount the importance of activities that do not result in success and positive affect.	George thinks that in-line skating is dangerous for other people cycling and running on the bike trails.
Shape attributions for events to present the self-concept in the best light.	George believes he helps the roll class go more smoothly by helping out when the instructor is busy. He thinks they are making faster progress and benefiting from his knowledge and skills.
Engage in self-affirmation and self-verification when the self-concept is threatened.	Some of the folks in the roll class reject George's advice and ignore his comments, saying, "This is not the same as crew." George gets a book on kayaking and identifies skills kayaking shares with rowing. He pays attention to the classmates who ask him for help.

ages. Exercise can also positively affect the self-perception of patients with chronic diseases, such as cardiovascular disease and breast cancer, through improving physical function.

The physical body had a significant role in self-identity and self-esteem in 20th-century society, and will likely continue to have a strong influence. Sparks (1997) discussed the concept of the "socially constructed body" and referred to a theme for framing the body based on "the *mechanical body* and the *body beautiful*" (p. 87). Advances in medical technology have made it possible to reshape and rebuild physical attributes. Cosmetic surgery and a range of ergogenic aids have expanded the limits of the possible in physical appearance and performance. The increased perception of control over appearance and function has been supported by the media and by product promotion. The body has been redefined as a symbol of health, success, and wealth. The physical self has become an item of social currency.

The view of the body as malleable also promotes self-regulation and individual responsibility for our health and wellness. However, there can be negative effects on self-esteem when unrealistic cultural ideals for shape and size are adopted and used to judge one's appearance, especially given that typical correlations between perceived attractiveness and physical self-worth have been about $r = .70$ (Fox 1997). Self-esteem is threatened when there is a discrepancy between competence and importance, such as when high importance is attached to body image but the competence to make necessary changes to fit

> **S**elf-esteem is influenced by characteristics of the physical body and the interaction between self-perceptions and the ideals of popular culture.

the ideal is low. According to cognitive discrepancy models, adopting unrealistic ideals leads to poor self-concepts even when accomplishments are otherwise good. Marsh (1999) tested this model in a study in which 793 high school students indicated their actual, ideal, future, and potential body images by selecting from 12 silhouettes that varied along an "obese–skinny" continuum. Marsh found support for a cognitive discrepancy model in that more demanding, increasingly slender ideal body images had a significant negative impact on self-concept. Inasmuch as unrealistic ideals for the female body are promoted in the United States and other industrialized societies, the lower physical self-esteem in females across the life span is not surprising.

Psychological dynamics also influence self-esteem. For example, Ryan and Deci's self-determination theory (Deci et al. 1991), which evolved from cognitive evaluation theory (Deci and Ryan 1980) contributes the concepts of contingent versus true self-esteem and self-determination to understanding how self-esteem is influenced. Motivation for behavior exists on a continuum that ranges from amotivation through four levels of extrinsic motivation to one true motivation. Contingent self-esteem is based on meeting external standards; there is no personal control over reinforcement, and behavior is not self-determined. True self-esteem is based on meeting personally defined standards, and behavior is internally regulated. True, or intrinsic, motivation is integrated into self-identity, and self-esteem is enhanced through mastery or self-determination, which supports feelings of independence and confidence. The successful resolution of self-identity developmental tasks—which include separating the self from the environment and others, discovering personal causation, testing the environment, and learning about the self from the responses of others (Sonstroem 1998)—can be viewed from the standpoint of a self-determination model as the internal regulation of behavior.

Self-concept is developed in part through the establishment of internal standards for the self. Internal standards are established by evaluating personal behavior (i.e., mastery, degree of improvement, goal achievement, and objective performance). Self-concept, however, develops in a social environment, and the influences of society and cultural values are strong. The perspective of a core identity that develops through interactions between the self and society ("socially constructed self"; Sparks 1997) highlights the challenge of maintaining a coherent self-identity in response to changing roles and social expectations.

Cross-cultural studies demonstrate the power of society in defining what is acceptable. For example, judgments about physical size and shape are matched against cultural ideals; African-American women with lower socioeconomic status who are heavy do not have a poor body image, whereas white women who are heavy aspire to a thin, lean ideal (Davis 1997). Gender also plays a role in the cultural messages about the ideal body. Self-esteem, BMI, and perception of weight status were measured in 13,000 16-year-old adolescents participating in the National Longitudinal Study of Adolescent Health (Wave II) (Perrin et al. 2010). Twenty-five percent of normal-weight girls and 8% of normal-weight boys perceived themselves as overweight. There were ethnic differences in the misperception of overweight as well; the lowest proportion occurred in black males, and the highest in Asian females. Low self-esteem was associated with increased odds of misperceiving overweight status by white girls regardless of actual BMI, in black girls and white boys above the 20th BMI percentile, and in Asian girls above the 60th BMI percentile. Low self-esteem was not related to misperceived weight status by black and Asian boys in any weight category.

Social and cultural factors influence self-concept development and evaluation through the application of external standards to the self. External standards include referred appraisals and social comparisons (Sonstroem 1998). **Referred appraisal** is how we think significant others perceive us. From this perspective, self-concept is formed by our appraisals of what significant others think about us. Most of us are familiar with the idea of a self-fulfilling prophecy, which has been demonstrated countless times in the classroom and on athletic fields when teachers and coaches have high expectations of students who end up meeting those expectations.

External standards also influence self-concept development through social comparison, which involves observing others and comparing ourselves to them. A middle-aged mother of four may acknowledge her physical ability to carry her 3-year-old child around during a day trip to an amusement park (internal standard based on objective performance), but she may not consider herself physically strong if she compares herself to friends who lift weights at a gym (external standard based on social comparison).

The setting and peer group used for social comparisons can have a significant impact on self-evaluations. For example, a recreational weightlifter who identifies himself as the strongest man at the local gym in his small town may discover that he is not as strong as most of the men working out at a gym in Los Angeles. Marsh and colleagues (1997) demonstrated this "big fish/little pond" effect in a study of physical self-concept in 1,514 elite high school athletes and nonelite students. Physical self-concepts were higher in the elite group than in the nonelite group, as would be expected. However, nonelite athletes in the athletically selective high school whose comparison group was the elite athletes scored lower than general students (nonathletes) from a nonsports high school on several physical self-concept variables. Self-perceptions are also dynamic in that the response to achievement or failure in performance may result in a change in the standards to which one judges oneself. For example, after winning his first road race, a runner might not compare himself to novice recreational runners anymore; he may, instead, change his reference group and his self-perceptions.

Fox summarized the characteristics of people with low self-esteem (1997). For example, those with low self-esteem have a less defined sense of self and less self-knowledge. They are thus more susceptible to external cues and events that can threaten self-esteem. Their self-concept is composed of simpler and fewer components, which offer fewer opportunities to self-affirm when their self-concept is threatened. There is also a mismatch between their level of perceived competence and the importance they attached to those competencies. For example, someone with low self-esteem may define herself primarily

Psychosocial Contributions to Self-Esteem

- Perceived competence
- Self-approval
- Perception of power
- Self-acceptance
- Sense of self-worth

From Fox 1997.

through physical attractiveness and define what is ideal based on infomercials promoting expensive exercise equipment or dietary supplements. She may be unaware of the realistic limits her stocky body shape places on her. Her ongoing failure to make the desired changes in her body fosters low self-efficacy for achieving a highly valued slim, muscular body and will perpetuate low self-esteem.

MEASUREMENT

The nature of self-esteem as a hypothetical construct contributes to issues in measurement because there are no objective criteria to validate measures against. Instead, researchers must use **convergent validation** (strength of association with established scales that measure other similar variables and constructs) and **divergent validation** (lack of association with scales that measure dissimilar constructs) strategies, or evaluate the scale's face validity (the consonance of the scale items with accepted definitions of the concept to be measured).

Self-esteem and self-concept are multidimensional constructs and are difficult to assess unless instruments are also multidimensional.

Measurement of Variables of Self

The measurement of psychological constructs is discussed in some depth in chapter 2, and the issues and strategies presented in that chapter also apply to the development of instruments to measure self-perceptions. For example, instruments need to be based on some theory of the self, and the target population should be considered in creating scale items. Fox (1998) described additional issues in self-perception scale development, such as the clarity of the item format.

The level of subscale specificity is complicated by a lack of knowledge about the range of physical activity and sport experience of the population. For example, it is hard for people to rate their confidence in tennis if they have never picked up a racket. Some address this issue by phrasing items so that respondents judge their ability in different sport and exercise areas on their own terms of reference, and researchers also use specific scales for specialized populations. For example, items associated with competence in general skills, such as agility, would allow the respondents to come up with their own frames of reference, such as tennis or soccer. However, a scale with items addressing specific tennis competencies could be used to determine differences between males and females who join a tennis club.

Determining the reliability of self-perception instruments depends on the theoretical perspective on the stability of the construct. Global self-esteem is viewed by many as traitlike, and

Self-Esteem as a Hypothetical Construct

Self-esteem is a hypothetical construct that is quantified, for example, as the sum of evaluations across salient attributes of one's self or personality (Blascovich and Tomaka 1991, 115).

thus should demonstrate good test–retest reliability. Constructs closer to the base of a hierarchical model, such as strength self-esteem, are more mutable. Thus, differences in scale values between administrations may be due to actual change, confounding the ability to measure the stability of the instrument over time. Researchers developing instruments to measure physical activity also have a dilemma in determining the temporal stability of a questionnaire (see chapter 13 on correlates).

Contemporary self-concept and self-esteem models are hierarchical and multidimensional. Thus, scales developed based on these models must undergo validation of the scale as a whole and of the individual components. External construct validation involves administering the scale in conjunction with established instruments and measuring the degree of association. Marsh (1997) described a method of external validation called between-network validity. A measure of self-concept would be compared with other constructs according to a theoretically based, logical pattern of relationships. The scale should be significantly related to some scales and not to others as predicted by theory. A self-concept instrument based on the Shavelson, Hubner, and Stanton (1976) multidimensional hierarchical model should have distinct multidimensional components (i.e., academic, social, physical, emotional, spiritual) that are not correlated. Each component should have specific subcomponents (physical includes performance and appearance), which can each also have specific components (performance includes strength, endurance, coordination, flexibility, etc.). The statistics for determining the within-network validity of self-concept instruments include factor analysis and multitrait–multimethod analysis (Marsh 1997), which were introduced in chapter 2.

Instruments to Measure Self-Perception

Valid and reliable ways to measure self-perceptions are necessary for understanding the relationship between physical activity behavior and self-concept and self-esteem discussed earlier. Several instruments have been developed since the 1950s to measure self-perceptions relevant to physical activity and are described in the following sections. Early research in physical self-concept was dominated by studies evaluating body image and its relationship with global self-esteem (Marsh 1997). Thus, because of the historical significance as well as the importance of body image in self-esteem and in exercise motivation, we begin with selected instruments that measure body image.

Body Image

Body image has been assessed using a variety of methods, including distortion techniques, silhouette and photograph rating, computer-generated reproductions of perceived body shape and size, and paper-and-pencil questionnaires (see figure 12.4), and more than 50 measures are available (Thompson 2004). One of the first scales to measure body image was the Body Cathexis Scale, developed by Secord and Jourard in 1953. Body cathexis is defined as "the degree of feeling satisfied or dissatisfied with various parts or processes of the body" (Secord and Jourard 1953, 343). The respondent rates 46 body parts and functions on a 5-point scale ranging from *have strong feelings and wish change could somehow be made* to *consider myself fortunate,* and the scores are summed. Body image scores are based on affect rather than perception. A limitation of the Body Cathexis Scale is its assessment of body image as a unidimensional concept (i.e., a single score derived from a sum of responses). The Body Esteem Scale was developed by Franzoi and Shields in 1984 based

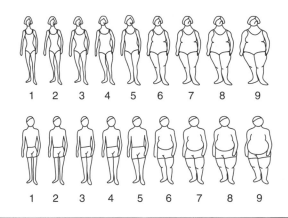

Figure 12.4 Perception of body size can be assessed by asking a respondent to mark which one of the figures shown is most like him- or herself.

on the Body Cathexis Scale. This revised scale is divided into three sex-specific factors measured by 32 items. For males, subscales include physical attractiveness, upper-body strength, and physical condition. Subscales for females measure sexual attractiveness, weight concern, and physical condition.

Measurement of body image can be unidimensional or multidimensional, but there is general agreement that body image is a multidimensional psychological construct. Although body image has been conceptualized to include several elements, the two constructs that appear consistently in the literature are evaluation or appraisal of the body and expression of satisfaction with the body (Rowe, Benson, and Baumgartner 1999). For example, the Body Areas Satisfaction Scale (BASS) is a standardized assessment of evaluative body image that is part of the Multidimensional Body-Self Relations Questionnaire Appearance Scales (MBSRQ-AS) (Cash 2000). The MBSRQ-AS contains 34 items and includes additional subscales for appearance evaluation, appearance orientation, overweight preoccupation, and self-classified weight. Body image scales have been developed for specific populations, such as the Body Image and Relationships Scale (Hormes et al. 2008), which has been used to assess changes in attitudes about appearance, health, physical strength, sexuality, relationships, and social functioning following treatment for breast cancer.

Self-Concept

Early scale-development research was guided by a unidimensional conceptualization of self-concept. As with the Body Cathexis Scale, the sum of responses to several items was used to compute a single, global self-concept score. This approach assumes equal weight for items representing various aspects of the self, such as academic and physical self-concepts. Specific scales to measure the physical self were limited by this conceptual framework (e.g., Body Cathexis Scale) until the emergence of multidimensional models (e.g., Shavelson, Hubner, and Stanton 1976) and self-perception profiles (e.g., Harter 1982) in the late 1970s and early 1980s. The inclusion of a hierarchical model provided an organization that fostered scale development research and testable hypotheses, as well as subscales that assessed self-concept in specific domains.

The Tennessee Self-Concept Scale (original: Fitts 1965; Roid and Fitts 1994) was the first multidimensional self-concept scale in which self-concept was composed of general and specific factors. Separate scores are generated for physical self, moral-ethical self, personal self, family self, and social self domains. For each domain, identity (e.g., description of physical self), self-satisfaction (degree of satisfaction with physical self-image), and behavior (participation in physical activities) can be computed (Blascovich and Tomaka 1991). Although designed to measure self-concept, this scale has been used as a general measure of self-esteem in many studies (Blascovich and Tomaka 1991).

The Self-Description Questionnaire (SDQ) (Marsh, Smith, and Barnes 1983) was developed to test the Shavelson, Hubner, and Stanton (1976) model in children younger than adolescence. The SDQ measures self-concept based on a multidimensional hierarchical self. It includes measures of a general sense of self, more specific facets, or domain self-concepts, and even more specific skills and abilities within each domain. The two domains are academic and nonacademic. The nonacademic domain consists of physical abilities, appearance, relationship with peers, and relationship with parents. Marsh also developed two other versions of this scale to use with adolescents (SDQ-II; Marsh, Parker, and Barnes 1985) and older adolescents and adults (SDQ-III; Marsh and O'Neill 1984).

Physical Self-Concept

The two multidimensional physical self-concept scales described next were developed on the basis of a structural model of self-concept. Advances in computers and multivariate statistical techniques have been applied to these newer scales and have enabled researchers to enhance the quality of these physical self-concept assessments.

In the late 1980s, Fox and Corbin (1989) developed the Physical Self-Perception Profile (PSPP) to measure physical self-concepts based on work by Harter (1985, 1986) and the Shavelson, Hubner, and Stanton (1976) model. Content validation was undertaken by extensive reviews of previous research and interviews with college students regarding important components of the physical self. The PSPP has five subscales (see Physical Self-Perception Profile Subscales). Each scale has items that reflect perception about product (competency/adequacy), process (acquisition/maintenance), and perceived confidence (self-presentation). A global physical self-worth subscale is also included. The format of the items, structured-alternative, was chosen to reduce social desirability responding, but may be confusing. The Perceived Importance Profile (PIP) was developed to accompany the PSPP to measure the importance placed on each subdomain with regard to more global self-worth, but support for its value in models of physical self-concept and esteem is mixed (Fox 1998; Marsh 1997).

The factorial validity of a revised version of the PSPP-R was recently tested using confirmatory factor analysis on samples of university students from Sweden, Turkey, and the United Kingdom (Lindwall, Asci, and Hagger 2011). First-order four-factor models, including correlated factors of sport competence, physical conditioning, body attractiveness, and physical strength, were supported, as were second-order factor models in which the four factors were subordinate to a general factor of physical self-worth.

The Physical Self-Description Questionnaire (PSDQ) was developed based on the Marsh/Shavelson hierarchical model of self-concept (Marsh 1990). Respondents rate each of the 70 statements on a 6-point true–false response

Physical Self-Perception Profile Subscales

- Sport competence
- Physical condition
- Body attractiveness
- Physical strength
- Physical conditioning

From Fox and Corbin 1989.

scale, and scores for 11 scales are generated from the responses (see Physical Self-Description Questionnaire). The process by which the PSDQ was validated is a model for scale construction in the social sciences: using 14 field criteria of physical fitness to establish criterion-related validity (Marsh 1993), establishing convergent and discriminant evidence for construct validity judged against existing instruments (Marsh et al. 1994), and testing the invariance of the scales with people in four age groups who completed the PSDQ four times during a 2-year period (Marsh 1998).

A meaningful comparison of physical self-concept among groups of people who might view self-concept differently (e.g., racial or ethnic groups) requires that the measurement instruments have equivalent measurement properties. The factorial validity and invariance of the Physical Self-Description Questionnaire (PSDQ) among American black (n = 658) and white (n = 479) adolescent girls in the 12th grade were examined in one study (Dishman, Hales, Almeida, et al. 2006). Construct validity was examined by estimating correlations between PSDQ subscales and external criteria (physical activity, physical fitness, BMI, and participation in sports). The hypothesized 11-factor model demonstrated adequate overall fit that was equivalent in both groups. Convergent and discriminant evidence for construct validity was supported by the pattern of correlations with the external criteria. The results indicate that a meaningful comparison of PSDQ scores can be made between black and white girls in the 12th grade and that valid inferences from PSDQ scores can be made about specific aspects of physical self-concept. Despite lower levels of physical activity, sport participation, and fitness, and higher BMI, black girls had similar self-esteem and higher physical self-concept and perceived appearance compared to white girls.

A shortened form of the PSDQ with 40 of the original 70 items retained the original structure of 11 correlated factors. The PSDQ-S was cross-validated in samples of 708 Australian adolescents, 349 Australian elite-athlete adolescents, 986 Spanish adolescents, 395 Israeli university students, and 760 Australian older adults (Marsh, Martin, and Jackson 2010).

Physical Self-Description Questionnaire

Global Subscales

- Physical self-concept
- Global self-esteem

Physical Self-Concept Subscales

- Body fat
- Strength
- Activity
- Endurance/fitness
- Sport competence
- Coordination
- Health
- Appearance
- Flexibility
- Self-esteem

Self-Esteem

Self-esteem was initially thought to be a global construct. The most frequently used self-esteem scale—and the standard that has been used in subsequent self-esteem scale development—is the Rosenberg Self-Esteem Scale (Rosenberg 1965). It is global and unidimensional and consists of 10 items that have strong internal consistency and test–retest reliability. The Coopersmith (1967) Self-Esteem Inventory (SEI) is another popular unidimensional measure of self-esteem. It was originally developed for children and has been adapted for adults. Although the revision to this scale (SEI Form B; Coopersmith 1975) was thought to measure positive self-regard unidimensionally, subsequent analyses have found different factor structures, indicating multidimensionality; but no stable interpretable pattern has been determined (Blascovich and Tomaka 1991).

The conceptualization of self-esteem has expanded into one that is more multidimensional through the influence of Shavelson, Hubner, and Stanton (1976)—that is, that facets of self-esteem contribute to more-global self-esteem. For example, how you judge your ability to run a mile influences the esteem you hold for your physical capabilities. The Janis-Field Feelings of Inadequacy Scale (FIS) (Janis and Field 1959) was adapted by Fleming and Watts (1980) and Fleming and Courtney (1984) to use in a multidimensional fashion. Five factors were found to contribute to global self-esteem: social confidence, academic ability, emotionality, physical appearance, and ability.

The Physical Estimation and Attraction Scales (PEAS; Sonstroem 1978) includes two global components defined as estimation (self-perceptions of physical ability) and attraction (measured interest in physical activity). The PEAS was derived from a forerunner of the Exercise and Self-Esteem Model (Sonstroem and Morgan 1989) to measure estimation and attraction, which were defined as mediating variables in physical ability, physical activity participation, and self-esteem relationships. Use of the PEAS has declined, but it is an example of an early attempt to go beyond unidimensional measurements and to combine instrument development with model building.

Global self-esteem is rather stable, and its value as an outcome variable in exercise research is limited because meaningful changes in self-esteem from physical activity are difficult to detect. Global scales may lack the necessary sensitivity, although researchers persist in using global scales to measure changes after exercise interventions. Targeting self-evaluations of very specific attributes is one way to overcome this problem, and it is an approach that is supported by a hierarchical multidimensional model of self-esteem.

Hierarchical models require that researchers address two issues in scale construction (Marsh 1998). First, items should be relevant; that is, they should be applicable to what the researcher is interested in measuring. For example, the statement *I can bench press twice my body weight* would not be as predictive of entering a 5K road race as the statement *I can exercise for a long time without getting winded*. Second, items should be at the same level of specificity

as the construct being measured. The statement *I am physically fit* would not assess the subdomain of strength self-concept as well as the statement *I am strong* would. Tracking changes in the physical strength subscale of the Body Image and Relationships Scale in breast cancer survivors over the course of a strength training program is an example of using a measure that is at the same level of specificity as the intervention. Researchers would be more likely to detect changes in this specific relevant subscale than in a global score derived from this scale.

EXERCISE AND SELF-ESTEEM

The body of research on exercise and self-esteem is not as extensive as that addressing the relationship between exercise and other psychological variables, such as depression and stress responsiveness. The overall evidence for effects of exercise on global self-esteem is mostly positive, but mixed (Fox 2000; McAuley 1994). Ambiguous results may reflect limitations in the study design and instrumentation as well as the trait-like nature of self-esteem, which renders it less likely to be changed by interventions. Although the cumulative evidence points to changes in self-esteem as a result of participation in exercise programs, most of the studies lacked control for confounding variables, such as perceived task demands, response distortion, and expectancy for self-esteem changes (Sonstroem 1998).

The next section addresses research that has addressed the relationship between exercise and self-esteem. It is organized into summaries of meta-analyses and reviews, examples of correlational and longitudinal studies, and a discussion of research with special populations.

Meta-Analyses and Reviews

Compared to the literature dealing with exercise in relation to other mental health areas, there have been few reviews of research on exercise and self-esteem or self-concept. Gruber (1986) surveyed the literature on interventions exploring the relationship between physical activity and self-esteem development in children. He found 84 intervention studies and conducted a meta-analysis with the 27 studies that reported adequate data for the analysis. The average effect size (ES) supporting positive effects of exercise on self-esteem was 0.41. The development of global self-esteem was influenced by participation in directed play or physical education (or both) in elementary school children, and more benefits were found in children low in self-esteem and in those from special populations (see figure 12.5). Greatest gains from exercise for self-esteem were for children with disabilities, with a 0.57 ES. Benefits from fitness-type activities (ES = 0.89) were greater than those from participation in creative activities (ES = 0.29), sports (ES = 0.40), and motor skill activities (ES = 0.32). However, confidence intervals were not provided for these differences, which often were based on very few studies and may not represent true differences in effects.

Also, results from this meta-analysis should not be taken as strong evidence against improvements in children's self-esteem from playing sports. Almost all of the studies in Gruber's meta-analysis used global measures of self-esteem, which may not reveal changes in specific physical self-evaluations. Research that has included scales to measure specific subcomponents of self-esteem, such as sport-related self-esteem (e.g., Anshel, Muller, and Owens 1986), has

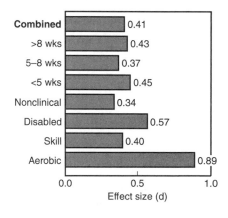

Figure 12.5 Meta-analysis of 27 longitudinal studies in children. There was no effect for the length of training; effects were larger for children who were disabled and from aerobic activities.

Data from Gruber 1986.

shown increases from sport participation. A later meta-analysis of physical activity and mental health studies found five cross-sectional and two prospective population-based studies of physical activity and mental health in a total of 14,823 youths ages 3 to 18, but just two randomized controlled trials of 50 youths (Strong et al. 2005). Table 12.2 shows the effects of exercise on components of self-concept from uncontrolled and controlled trials.

A subsequent meta-analysis of eight randomized, but poorly controlled, trials examining the effects of mainly aerobic exercise or sport training on children and youths indicated a moderate (0.49 SD; 95% CI = 0.16-0.81) effect of physical activity (Ekeland et al. 2004). However, the small number of diverse studies didn't provide information on the modifying influences of various types of exercise or settings.

Lirgg (1991) conducted a meta-analysis of 35 studies to examine the magnitude of the effect of gender differences on self-confidence to perform various physical activities. Men were found to be significantly more confident than women, although all but one of the tasks were "masculine" (i.e., strength focused, competitive) or gender neutral. Women were significantly more confident than men in the one study that used a "feminine" task (i.e., expressive, graceful). The magnitude of the gender differences was not affected by the level of competitiveness of the task situation.

Fox (2000) conducted a qualitative review of 37 randomized and 42 nonrandomized controlled exercise intervention studies that measured the effects of exercise on self-esteem and physical self-perceptions. The description of the studies sheds light on the difficulty in producing an organized review of the literature. Outcome variables were a variety of constructs measured with several instruments. Only a few of the more recent studies were based on theoretical models and used instruments with sound psychometrics and subscales to measure multidimensional physical self-concepts. General conclusions, even considering the weakness and scarcity of the research, were positive. Almost 80% of the studies indicated significant changes in physical self-worth and other physical self-perceptions after exercise training, but only half of the results

Table 12.2 Effects of Exercise Training on Self-Concept and Self-Esteem in Youth

Outcome	Effects (K)	Effect (SD)	95% CI
**Self-esteem	29	0.51	0.31, 0.71
Sport competence	5	0.77	−0.10, 1.64
*Social self-concept	9	0.25	0.007, 0.484
Academic self-concept	6	0.27	−0.36, 0.90
* $p < .05$ ** $p < .01$			

Reprinted from *Journal of Pediatrics*, Vol. 146(6), W.B. Strong et al., "Evidence based physical activity for school-age youth," pgs. 732-737, copyright 2005, with permission from Elsevier.

> **P**ositive associations between exercise and self-esteem have been found, but effects are stronger for people who are initially lower in self-esteem.

were significant for positive changes in self-esteem. Positive effects were found for men and women, but greater benefits were measured in those initially lower in self-esteem. Both aerobic and weight training positively influenced self-esteem, but there was some indication that the short-term effect is greater for weight training. A later meta-analysis of about 50 mostly small randomized controlled trials reported an average increase in self-esteem of about 0.25 standard deviation among adults (Spence, McGannon, and Poon 2005).

People's physical self-esteem tends to improve more after fitness training than after participating in competitive sports, in which success and feelings of accomplishment are less assured (Spence, McGannon, and Poon 2005). Self-esteem is increased among adults (Spence et al. 2005) and youths (Strong et al. 2005) when physical fitness is increased, more so than when the physical activity setting and study outcomes are focused on motor skills. However, the study designs used have not clarified the importance of the social context of the physical activity settings relative to features of physical activity, exercise,

and fitness. Thus, it remains unclear whether it is exercise itself that increases self-esteem, or something in the social context of the exercise setting, including people's expectations of benefits (Desharnais et al. 1993). The greatest gains in self-esteem can be expected in people with low initial levels, and in those for whom physical attributes have a relatively high value as a part of global self-concept.

Correlational Evidence

Physical self-concept is influenced by the level of physical activity and has consistently shown moderately strong correlations with global self-esteem across the life span (Fox 2000), although more so with physical self-esteem (see figure 12.6). Thus, correlational evidence suggests that participation in physical activity and exercise could play a meaningful role in physical self-esteem through effects on physical self-concept.

Longitudinal Studies

Several studies have documented favorable changes in self-concept and self-esteem after participation in aerobic and strength conditioning

> **E**xercise has more potent effects on physical self-concept and self-esteem than on general self-perceptions.

	Correlations	
	Overall self-esteem	Physical self-esteem
Physical self-esteem	0.62	
Sports competence	0.32	0.49
Condition	0.33	0.65
Body appearance	0.48	0.72
Strength	0.24	0.43

Figure 12.6 Evaluations of appearance and physical function are more strongly related to physical self-esteem than to overall self-esteem (n = 1,191 college females and males).

Data from Fox and Corbin 1989.

programs. A meta-analysis of exercise interventions targeting body image also showed positive effects regardless of exercise mode (Campbell and Hausenblas 2009). Correlational studies reveal stronger evidence for changes in physical self-worth and other physical self-perceptions than for global self-esteem (Fox 2000; Sonstroem 1998).

Most studies of children that have been conducted since Gruber's 1986 meta-analysis have continued to find positive effects of exercise on changes in self-esteem (e.g., Boyd and Hrycaiko 1997), and effects have been found in children as young as 3 years old (Alpert et al. 1990). However, not all of the studies of exercise training and self-esteem in children have demonstrated significant effects. Faigenbaum and colleagues (1997) did not find differences in self-concept or self-efficacy after an 8-week strength training program implemented with 15 children aged 7 to 12, although there were significant changes in physical strength measures. Effects on self-perceptions after a 13-week aerobics training program were also not demonstrated in 67 children in grades 3 through 5 (Walters and Martin 2000). Discussions in both studies suggest that ceiling effects for the self-perception measures contributed to the lack of significant findings. High initial scores left little room for improvement after exercise. Self-esteem is inversely related to BMI in youths, and thus the effects of physical activity may be more easily detected in overweight children. For example, Goldfield and colleagues (2007) found significant

improvements in perceived physical condition, body satisfaction, and overall physical self-worth in 30 overweight and obese children after an 8-week intervention to increase physical activity and decrease sedentary activities, even without significant changes in BMI.

Self-esteem is closely tied to body esteem in females, particularly white females (Calhoun 1999). Females are at greater risk of developing eating disorders, and the precipitating and escalating distortions in body image and negative effects on self-esteem have likely contributed to the interest in the potential benefits of exercise training on self-perceptions in women. There is evidence that participating in regular exercise has positive effects on body esteem in women. Bartlewski, Van Raalte, and Brewer (1996) examined the effects of aerobic exercise on body image concerns of female college women. Significant increases in body esteem and decreases in physique anxiety were found for female students in an aerobics class, but not for those in a comparison academic class, from the beginning to the end of an academic term. Positive effects of exercise on body perceptions were also found for older women in a study by McAuley and colleagues (1995). Physique anxiety was prevalent in a cross-sectional sample of middle-aged and older women, but participation in a 20-week aerobic exercise program resulted in a decrease in physique anxiety for those middle-aged women who also had a favorable change in body composition.

Improvements in self-esteem among females have been demonstrated for various exercise modes, such as walking (e.g., Palmer 1995), strength training (Brown and Harrison 1986), strength training and aerobic exercise (Caruso and Gill 1992), and yoga (Elavsky 2010). Significant improvements in physical self-concept have also been demonstrated in college students after strength training classes (Van Vorst, Buckworth, and Mattern 2002), as well as after strength training classes compared to the aerobic exercise of swimming and a no-exercise control condition (Stein and Motta 1992).

Studies with middle-aged and older men and women have shown effects for changes in self-perception with physical activity, as well. For example, McAuley, Mihalko, and Bane (1997) measured changes in domain and global levels of self-esteem after a 20-week walking exercise program in sedentary middle-aged men and women. The participants showed significant increases in global self-esteem, physical self-worth, and physical condition. There is also some evidence that positive changes in self-perceptions after an aerobic training program are maintained after the program is over. Opdenacker, Delecluse, and Boen (2009) measured changes in global self-esteem, physical self-perceptions, self-efficacy, BMI, aerobic capacity, and physical activity (accelerometer and self-report) after an 11-month intervention and 1 year later in 186 older adults. Participants were randomized to control, lifestyle, or structured exercise groups. Compared to the control group after the intervention, both exercise groups showed greater improvements in self-perceived physical condition and sport competence, and the lifestyle group had greater increases in body attractiveness and physical self-worth. At a 1-year follow-up, the increase in body attractiveness remained significant for the lifestyle group, with the addition of significantly better scores on global self-esteem. Increases in self-perceived physical condition and sport competence remained significant for the structured group, and increases from pretest to follow-up on body attractiveness were also significantly greater than those in the control group.

Special Populations

The strongest effects for the influence of exercise on self-esteem are for those initially lower in self-esteem (see figure 12.7; McAuley 1994). It follows that people who have experienced threats to their self-esteem could benefit from improvements in physical self-concept. We look now at research on exercise and self-esteem in a number of special populations, from women during pregnancy to people with developmental disabilities to people diagnosed with cancer, among other conditions.

Exercise can have specific beneficial effects on self-esteem in women during and after pregnancy through an impact on body image and through improved endurance and other physiological adaptations. Evidence from some studies indicates that exercise can help with premenstrual syndrome and dysmenorrhea and that physically active women have better moods across the menstrual cycle than sedentary women do (Mutrie 1997). Exercise can also help maintain or enhance self-esteem during menopause, although little specific research has been conducted in this area.

It is well established that physiological adaptations as a result of exercise training contribute to significant improvements in activities of daily living in older adults (American College of Sports Medicine 2009). There is growing evidence for psychological benefits of regular exercise, such as the alleviation of depression symptoms and an improved sense of personal control and self-efficacy. For example, low-income older adults who participated in physical activity as part of the Community Healthy Activities Model Program for Seniors (CHAMPS) improved self-esteem, and those who adopted and maintained physical activity over the six-month intervention period had improved scores for anxiety, depression, and overall psychological well-being (Stewart et al. 1997).

Exercise and sport have positive effects on self-esteem and other psychological variables in children, adolescents, and adults with devel-

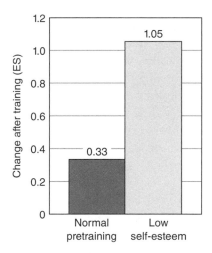

Figure 12.7 Self-esteem appears to increase the most after exercise training among those with low self-esteem. Change in self-esteem after two separate 8-week aerobic exercise training programs (effect size) is shown.

Normal: Data from Wilfley and Kunce 1986; Low: Data from Ossip-Klein et al. 1989.

opmental disabilities (Bartlo and Klein 2011). Participation in exercise and sport is associated with reduced maladaptive behavior, along with improved physical fitness, self-esteem, and social competence in this population. Participation in Special Olympics has resulted in higher social competence and more positive self-perceptions compared with those of people similar in age and IQ who do not participate (Dykens and Cohen 1996). People with physical and mental disabilities are likely to experience psychological gains from exercise, such as an increase in self-esteem, but well-controlled experimental studies are needed to determine the optimal programs for specific benefits in specific disability groups (Rimmer et al. 2010). Schmitz and colleagues (2010) reviewed the literature on the effects of exercise training on cancer survivors and found consistent positive effects from exercise on physical and functional well-being, as well as beneficial effects on psychological functioning, including improved self-esteem in breast cancer survivors.

The physical self plays a role in the development of the whole self, but the level and impact of physical activity and concomitant physical changes in self-esteem depend on a variety of factors, such as the value the person places on aspects of physical self-concept and initial self-perceptions. Detecting effects from exercise on self-perceptions depends on the quality of the measurement instruments, the sample population, and the ability to measure the level and type of exercise during the observation period. Given the conceptual examination of self-esteem and self-concept, it is not surprising when studies that use global measures of self-esteem, such as the Tennessee Self-Concept Scale and the Rosenberg Self-Esteem Scale, do not show effects from exercise training programs. Many studies examining the effects of exercise on self-concept and self-esteem have also been limited in design by the self-selection of subjects to various exercise modes. Controlled research designs and the application of psychometrically sound instruments based on a multidimensional and hierarchical model of self-concept will certainly make meaningful contributions to what we know about the effects of exercise on self-esteem in various populations.

By and large, observational population studies have not included measures of self-esteem and social support to determine whether they confound or mediate the lower rates of depressive symptoms found among physically active people. Also, most randomized controlled trials did not examine whether reduced depression after exercise training was mediated by enhanced self-esteem (Motl et al. 2005), nor did they use the proper comparison groups to demonstrate that reduced depression after exercise was independent of social support. Nonetheless, such cognitive and social factors deserve further study, especially self-esteem. Self-esteem is a cornerstone of mental health and behavior, and depression is often associated with low self-esteem. Because body image is related to general self-concept, an improvement in body image or physical skills can contribute to improvements in general self-esteem in people who place a high value on physical attributes relative to the other aspects of self-concept (Sonstroem 1998) and might reduce the primary or secondary risk of depression.

Correlational evidence suggests that physical activity and sport participation might reduce depression risk among adolescent girls by positively influencing physical self-concept, which increases self-esteem independently of girls' fitness, BMI, and perceptions of sport competence, body fatness, and appearance (Dishman, Hales, Pfeiffer, et al. 2006). Cross-sectional relations between physical activity and sport participation with depression symptoms were tested among 1,250 girls in the 12th grade. There was a strong positive relation between global physical self-concept and self-esteem and a moderate inverse relation between self-esteem and depression symptoms. Physical activity and sport participation each had an indirect, positive relation with global physical self-concept that was independent of objective measures of cardiorespiratory fitness and body fatness (see figure 12.8).

Although causal mediation cannot be inferred from cross-sectional relations, the use of structural equation modeling allowed us to estimate the relations among variables simultaneously, test group differences, and compare alternative, direct models to the hypothesized mediational

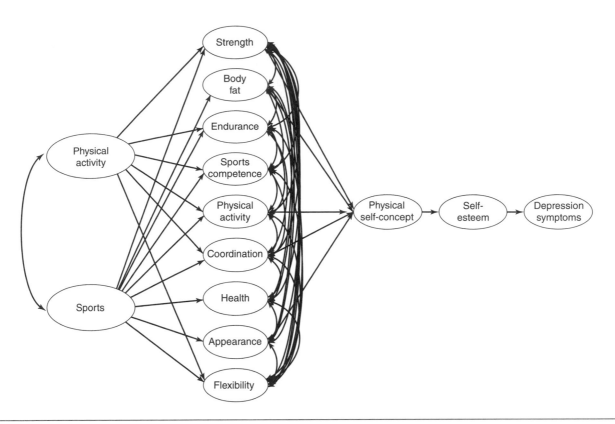

Figure 12.8 Physical self-concept and self-esteem mediate cross-sectional relations between physical activity levels and depression symptoms in adolescent girls.

Adapted, by permission, from R.K. Dishman et al., 2006, "Physical self-concept and self-esteem mediate cross-sectional relations of physical activity and sport participation with depression symptoms among adolescent girls," *Health Psychology* 25(3): 396-407.

model. The findings suggest aspects of physical self-concept that, if changed, might have the greatest effect on global physical self-concept, self-esteem, or depression symptoms. Physical activity interventions might include aspects that emphasize strength and coordination as well as general physical activity. Also, body self-concept (i.e., appearance and body fat) seems to play an important role in the development of physical self-concept and self-esteem in adolescent girls, regardless of whether the primary outcome of physical activity might be an improvement in depression symptoms. Longitudinal studies describing the natural course of change in self-concept exist (Cole et al. 2001; Marsh and Yeung 1998), but there seems to be no information on the mechanisms for this change or how it relates to other variables commonly associated with self-concept. A key to understanding how physical activity, sport participation, physical self-concept, self-esteem, and depression symptoms relate lies in how these variables change

with respect to each other over time or as the result of an intervention.

MECHANISMS

Mechanisms for changes in anxiety and depression from exercise training have been the topic of numerous studies, with some support for psychobiological effects. There has been considerably less research to determine how exercise may change self-esteem. The relatively stable nature of self-esteem, particularly in adults, obviously makes the detection of changes more difficult; and the lack of clinical criteria for self-esteem instruments prevents the identification of a practical amount of change. Although alterations in fitness are readily perceived and provide a concrete, tangible basis for self-evaluation, self-concept changes in adults after aerobic or strength training programs often do not track closely with changes in fitness variables (see figure 12.9). Thus, biological mechanisms for

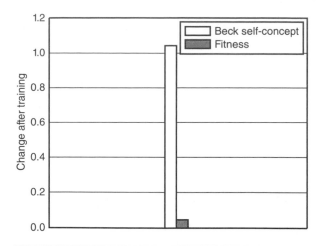

Figure 12.9 Changes in self-esteem are not necessarily dependent on changes in fitness. Change after training (effect size) in 40 mildly depressed college women: self-esteem increased 1.05 SD, but fitness (estimated from a submaximal exercise test) did not change after 8 weeks of jogging.

Data from Ossip-Klein et al. 1989.

changes in self-perceptions do not easily come to mind.

Identifying mechanisms is also complicated by the influences of possible mediating factors, such as group dynamics, situation factors, exercise history, personality characteristics, self-efficacy, and health status. However, several psychologically based mechanisms have been proposed.

Other factors related to social influence or personal expectancies might artificially influence a person's rating of self-esteem. Desharnais and colleagues (1993) approached the question of mechanism from a rather novel perspective. They hypothesized that motivated individuals in an exercise program would have psychological benefits simply because they expect they will. In other words, these researchers proposed a strong **placebo effect**. In the study, men and women were randomized to an experimental or

a control exercise class. The two classes received the same training and both groups had increased fitness, but the participants in the experimental class were told initially and throughout the training program that it was designed to improve physical and psychological well-being. Self-esteem as measured by the Rosenberg Self-Esteem Scale increased significantly for the treatment but not the control class, supporting the presence of a placebo effect for improvements in self-esteem from exercise training (see figure 12.10). This study is also interesting because of the significant differences in global self-esteem.

DISTORTED BODY IMAGE AND EXERCISE

In addition to evidence that physical activity and exercise can have a positive influence on physical self-esteem, there is evidence from clinical studies that some people who are highly physically active also have psychiatric disturbances

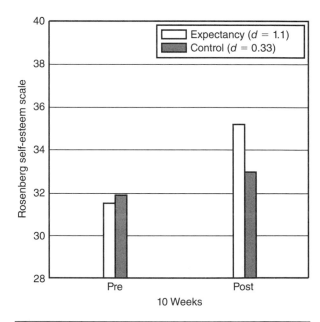

Figure 12.10 Participants in one group (expectancy) were told that training would "improve their psychological well-being," whereas those in the control group (control) were not explicitly told to expect this. The greater increase in self-esteem after 10 weeks of training illustrates a placebo effect.

Data from Desharnais et al. 1993.

> **T**he positive effects on self-esteem from exercise are likely due to psychosocial rather than biological mechanisms.

Psychosocial Factors Influencing Self-Concept and Self-Esteem After Exercise

- Exercise-induced improvements in perceptions of competence or appearance
- Improved sense of autonomy and control over the body
- Improved sense of self-acceptance

- Sense of well-being
- Sense of belonging and significance through social contact from exercise in a group or a social setting

What Is a Placebo?

In research, a **placebo** is any treatment given to a control group that is meant to have no effect and is used in comparison to the treatment that is being tested. In therapy, it is a treatment that is deliberately used for nonspecific, psychological, or psychophysiological effect on the assumption that there is no specific activity for the condition being treated.

that are associated with distorted body image (Davis 2000). That has led to some concern among health professionals that exercise training might carry some risk for psychopathologies related to eating disorders, substance abuse, and social adjustment problems. The epidemiological experiments and controlled clinical trials that are necessary to determine the prevalence of these disorders and the extent exercise is an independent, causal risk factor for their development have not been conducted. Nonetheless, it is important to acknowledge that exercise may present such a risk and that these topics are worthy of clinical attention and scientific investigation.

Eating Disorders

Results from a clinical study (Yates, Leehey, and Shisslak 1983) suggested that excessive exercisers, particularly runners, present symp-

toms analogous to anorexia nervosa: a common family history; similar socioeconomic class and pressures; a preoccupation with food and leanness; and personality traits of anger suppression, asceticism, denial of medical risk, introversion, and perfectionism. Although exercise is promoted as a healthy alternative to restrictive dieting among weight-conscious females, the possibility that exercise commitment could lead to anorexia or bulimia for some people who have a risky personality or history is a concern.

Although there are undoubtedly anorexics or bulimics who are compulsive exercisers, controlled research (Blumenthal, Rose, and Chang 1985; Dishman 1985) has indicated that in most cases, exercise commitment and anorexia nervosa are separate entities. In fact, case reports describe an effective treatment of anorexia that uses a combination of psychotherapy and running. Although anorexics often boost the impact of food restriction by hyperactivity, their fitness ($\dot{V}O_2$peak) is very low compared to that of committed exercisers (Einerson, Ward, and Hanson 1988), and stress-hormone profiles differ between the groups. Anorexics often have elevated scores on standard tests of psychopathology, whereas habitual runners usually score in the normal range of the same tests and show mood profiles that indicate positive mental health (Blumenthal, Rose, and Chang 1985). Table 12.3 lists shared and unique characteristics of anorexic and athletic females.

Some studies with small samples of elite ballerinas, gymnasts, and wrestlers found higher-than-expected rates of eating problems.

Table 12.3 Anorexic Versus Athletic Female

SHARED FEATURES
Dietary faddism
Controlled calorie consumption
Specific carbohydrate avoidance
Low body weight
Resting bradycardia and low blood pressure
Increased physical activity
Amenorrhea or oligomenorrhea
Anemia (may or may not be present)

DISTINGUISHING FEATURES	
Athlete	**Anorexic**
Purposeful training	Aimless physical activity
Increased exercise tolerance	Poor or decreasing exercise performance
Good muscular development	Poor muscular development
Accurate body image	Flawed body image (believes herself to be overweight)
Body fat level within defined normal range	Body fat level below normal range
	Biochemical abnormalities if abusing laxatives, diuretics, or both

Based from McSherry 1984.

However, it has not been established how long the eating problems persist in these populations, and whether they represent goal-appropriate behaviors for the sport, rather than medical or psychological pathology (Dishman 1985). *Anorexia athletica* has been proposed as a subclinical syndrome of anorexia nervosa (Sundgot-Borgen 1994), and 21% of a sample of more than 500 elite Norwegian female athletes were judged at risk for an eating disorder (Sundgot-Borgen and Torstveit 2004). However, the prevalence of disordered eating and the independent, causal risk of sport and exercise have not yet been established by controlled epidemiological and clinical studies. In most cases, the eating behaviors of athletes do not appear to signal anorexia nervosa or bulimia (O'Connor and Smith 1999).

Muscle Dysmorphia

Harvard-affiliated researchers proposed a form of body dysmorphic disorder, which is categorized under obsessive-compulsive and related disorders in the *DSM-IV* (Phillips et al. 2010). Their term **muscle dysmorphia** describes a condition in which both men and women develop a pathological preoccupation with their muscularity (Phillips, O'Sullivan, and Pope 1997). They presented case studies that supported an association between muscle dysmorphia and severe subjective distress, impaired social and occupational functioning, and the abuse of anabolic steroids and other substances (Gruber and Pope 2000; Pope et al. 1997).

Their investigation of muscle dysmorphia was continued in a test of the hypothesis that men in Western societies would desire to have a leaner and more muscular body than they had or perceived (Pope et al. 2000). The height, weight, and body fat of college-aged men in Austria ($n = 54$), France ($n = 65$), and the United States ($n = 81$) were measured. Next, the men chose pictorial body images that they believed represented (1) their own body, (2) the body they ideally would like to have, (3) the body of an average man of their age, and (4) the male body they believed women would prefer. The men's actual fat and muscularity were compared with that of the four images chosen. Despite modest differences between measured body fat and the amount of fat of the images chosen, men from all three countries chose an ideal body that was 28 pounds (12.7 kg) more muscular on average

Diagnostic Criteria for Body Dysmorphic Disorder

A. Preoccupation with an imagined defect in appearance. If a slight physical anomaly is present, the person's concern is markedly excessive.

B. The preoccupation causes clinically significant distress or impairment in social, occupational, or other important areas of functioning.

C. The preoccupation is not better accounted for by another mental disorder (e.g., dissatisfaction with body shape and size in anorexia nervosa).

Reprinted, by permission, from American Psychiatric Association, 1994, *Diagnostic and statistical manual of mental disorders*, 4th ed. (Washington, DC: American Psychiatric Association), 468.

than themselves. The men also estimated that women preferred a male body about 30 pounds (13.6 kg) more muscular than themselves, even though women in fact said they preferred an ordinary male body. The investigators speculated that the wide discrepancy between men's ideal body image and actual muscularity might help explain muscle dysmorphia and some anabolic steroid abuse.

Another study reported comparisons on psychological and behavioral variables between 24 men classified as having muscle dysmorphia and 30 comparison weightlifters without clinical disorders recruited from gymnasiums in the Boston area (Olivardia, Pope, and Hudson 2000). Men with muscle dysmorphia scored higher on body dissatisfaction; risky eating attitudes; the prevalence of anabolic steroid use; and a lifetime prevalence of *DSM-IV* mood, anxiety, and eating disorders. These men also frequently reported that they experienced shame, embarrassment, and impaired function at work and in social situations. McFarland and Kaminski (2009) surveyed 304 college men and found that, compared to

normal, high symptoms of muscle dysmorphia were associated with obsessive-compulsive symptoms, hostility, and paranoid ideation, as well as more dieting, the use of diet pills, and vomiting as a method of weight management. Similarly, several cases of body dysmorphia were also reported among 75 female bodybuilders recruited from Boston-area gymnasiums (Gruber and Pope 2000). Poor psychosocial functioning can also persist over time in men and women with body dysmorphic disorder (Phillips, Quinn, and Stout 2008).

Exercise Abuse

Separate from cases of eating disorders and muscle dysmorphia are case reports of compulsive involvement with or dependence on exercise training. Morgan (1979b) described eight cases of "running addiction," defined as when a commitment to running exceeded prior commitments to work, family, social relations, and medical advice. Similar cases have been labeled *positive addiction, runner's gluttony, fitness fanaticism, athlete's neurosis, obligatory running,* and *exercise dependence* (Dishman 1985; Sacks and Sachs 1981). We understand very little about the origins, diagnostic validity, or mental health impact of abusive exercise, but some researchers are beginning to look at physiological similarities to substance abuse, such as blunted cardiovascular and cortisol reactivity (Heaney, Ginty, Carroll, and Phillips 2011).

Although for most people, the benefits of exercise exceed the risks of abuse, emotional or social adjustment problems may be present when a person is unable or unwilling to interrupt or taper an exercise training program, or to replace a preferred form of exercise with an alternative despite a medical exigency or vocational or social responsibilities. The few studies that show psychopathology in habitual runners also indicate that an exaggerated emphasis on exercise roles or fitness abilities (as can happen in other areas of life) can reflect a preexisting proneness to an imbalanced and insecure self-concept (Davis 2000; Dishman 1985). There is also evidence for obsessive exercise as a secondary condition to eating disorders (e.g., Zmijewski and Howard 2003).

Exercise Dependence Diagnostic Criteria Based on *DSM-IV* Diagnostic Criteria for Substance Dependence

Clinically significant impairment or distress, as manifested by three or more of the following:

1. Tolerance: defined as either a need for increased amounts of exercise to achieve the desired effect, or diminished effect with continued use of the same amount of exercise

2. Withdrawal: as manifested by either the characteristic withdrawal symptoms for exercise, or the same (or a closely related) amount of exercise is engaged in to relieve or avoid withdrawal symptoms

3. Intention effects: exercise is often taken in larger amounts or over a longer period than was intended

4. Lack of control: there is a persistent desire or unsuccessful effort to cut down or control exercise

5. Time: a great deal of time is spent in activities necessary to obtain exercise

6. Reduction in other activities: social, occupational, or recreational activities are given up or reduced because of exercise

7. Continuance: exercise is continued despite knowledge of having a persistent or recurrent physical or psychological problem that is likely to have been caused or exacerbated by the exercise (e.g., continued running despite injury)

Reprinted, by permission from H.A Hausenblas and D. Symons Downs, 2002, "How much is too much? The development and validation of the exercise dependence scale," *Psychology & Health* 17(4): 387-404.

SUMMARY

Self-esteem is an important concept in the social sciences and in everyday life. It is determined through a combination of personal convictions and internalized values from the dominant culture and selected subcultures, and consists of the evaluation of the various aspects of self-concept. Most people would agree that positive self-esteem is associated with good mental health, so linking exercise with improvements in physical self-concept and thus with better self-esteem offers another reason for adopting and maintaining a physically active lifestyle. Obviously, though, things are not that simple.

This chapter included a discussion of how self-esteem and self-concept are related; it also presented models for understanding how exercise can influence self-perceptions. The physical self, which includes the physical body and the way the body is valued and judged, is an important component of self-esteem and

seems to be critical in Western societies. Thus, changes in structure, function, and physical self-concept with exercise can have a significant impact on self-worth. Self-esteem also influences behavioral choices as a function of expectations about how the behavioral outcomes will affect self-perceptions. According to self-enhancement theory, people choose activities in which success is likely over those with the likelihood of failure. And there is good evidence that behavior can affect self-esteem. For example, people make more positive judgments about the self after successfully completing a difficult task (e.g., mastery experiences).

Generally, the effects of exercise on self-esteem are strongest for those lowest in initial self-esteem. Effects from physical activity or exercise are specific; they influence perceptions of physical performance ability, for example, but not academic self-esteem. The careful measurement of self-concept and self-esteem is critical, and the sensitivity gained through the use of a multidimensional hierarchical model of the self will help us detect and explain the effects of exercise on the self in various populations over time. Intuitively, body image influences self-esteem, particularly in societies in which appearance is highly valued, and it is a construct that we should measure when exploring the relationship between exercise and self-esteem.

Finally, it is also important to consider that risks to mental health or social adjustment may be associated with an extreme dedication to exercise or a preoccupation with fitness or physique. Concepts such as anorexia athletica, muscle dysmorphia, and exercise abuse are not recognized as psychiatric diagnoses related to distorted self-image. Nonetheless, their appearance in the clinical and scientific literatures illustrates that their measurement, prevalence, health consequences, and relationships with exercise warrant study.

WEBSITES

www.self-esteem-nase.org

www.mentalhelp.net (search on the word *self-esteem*)

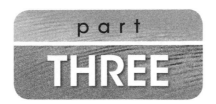
The Psychology of Physical Activity Behavior

Part II focused on the psychological benefits of exercise and increased levels of physical activity. Given the evidence for improved mood as well as the public perspective that exercise is good for us, the low rates of participation in leisure-time physical activity in developed nations with market economics are perplexing. Interventions to promote long-term increases in leisure-time physical activity have also had modest, although encouraging, results (Conn, Hafdahl, and Mehr 2011; Dishman and Buckworth 1996b). Apparently, there are considerable impediments to enhancing physical and mental health through the promotion of physical activity. This problem, like other contemporary concerns of exercise psychology, is not new. English-born Robert Jeffries Roberts, director of physical education in the late 1880s at the Young Men's Christian Association in Springfield, Massachusetts, stated, "I noticed when I taught slow, heavy, fancy, and more advanced work in acrobatics, gymnastics, athletics, etc., that I would have a very large membership at the first of the year, but that they would soon drop out" (Leonard 1919, pp. 123-124).

This part of the book explores the dynamics of exercise behavior that are relevant for addressing the problems of inactivity and nonadherence. The next three chapters offer insights into why people do or do not participate in regular physical activity in their leisure time. The chapters present the evidence of likely determinants of exercise adherence and lifestyle physical activity (chapter 13), theories of behavior change (chapter 14), and interventions to increase exercise adoption and adherence (chapter 15). A final chapter on perceived exertion (chapter 16) brings home our perspective that exercise is a behavior with intrinsic physiological features. Our perceptions of the immediate physiological sensations from physical activity determine how we think about our identity with respect to exercise, and these perceptions can influence our subsequent behavior choices.

Descriptive research that identifies the correlates of physical activity behavior and exercise is useful for characterizing groups, tracking trends in the relationships among variables, and stimulating further research. However, the application of theoretical models is necessary for explaining and predicting behavior, as well as for creating viable hypotheses and developing interventions. In most cases, research on interventions to increase physical activity has done a poor job of verifying that the intervention changed the theoretical mediators of physical activity (Rhodes and Pfaeffli 2010); but this could be a result of an inadequate application of theory to research, or of problems in measuring behavioral outcomes and psychosocial variables. The following chapters present summaries of what we know about exercise behavior. They also provide critiques of the research on the determinants of exercise and physical activity, the application of theories, interventions to change physical activity behavior, and perceived exertion.

Correlates of Exercise and Physical Activity

Considerable research has been conducted to identify factors that increase or decrease the likelihood that someone will adopt and maintain an active lifestyle. Most of these studies have been cross-sectional or prospective. Few controlled studies have involved the experimental manipulation of variables presumed to operate as determinants, and it is likely that multiple factors interact together to "cause" exercise adoption and maintenance. Determinants or causes of physical activity behavior are determined using mediation analyses, as discussed in chapter 2 and illustrated in chapter 15, and few studies have tested for mediation. This chapter focuses on correlates, or variables, for which there are established reproducible associations or predictive relationships, rather than cause-and-effect connections, although you may occasionally see the term *determinant* used in the literature and in this chapter.

Knowing the correlates of exercise and physical activity has several practical implications. Theories guide research, but evidence from well-designed studies can be used to support or refute the application of specific theories to exercise behavior. Many theories of behavior have been applied to exercise promotion, as you will see in chapter 14, and they have yielded mixed results in describing and predicting physical activity behavior. Thus, identifying the correlates of physical activity can promote revisions and improvements in theoretical models used in exercise research and interventions. For example, there is no consistent association between physical activity behavior and perceived social pressure to exercise (i.e., a sub-jective norm). This weak relationship presents a challenge to the application of the theory of reasoned action to physical activity because a subjective norm (i.e., normative beliefs) is one of the key variables this theory proposes for understanding and predicting behavior. On the other hand, exercise self-efficacy (i.e., confidence in one's ability to engage successfully in a specific behavior) has differed significantly among sedentary people, people interested in beginning regular exercise, novice exercisers,

Benefits From Studying Exercise Correlates

- Defining correlates promotes the design and application of better theoretical models.
- Inactive segments of the population can be identified, and resources for promoting exercise adoption and maintenance can be properly allocated.
- Discovering modifiable variables that influence behavior change will result in more effective interventions that target those variables.
- Identifying determinants of exercise adoption and maintenance in special populations will enable the creation of more personalized interventions.

and those who have maintained regular exercise. This relationship between exercise self-efficacy and levels of physical activity and motivation to exercise strengthens the application of stage or process models that include self-efficacy.

Knowing the correlates of exercise and physical activity can also help to identify inactive segments of the population and guide the allocation of resources to increase exercise adoption and adherence in these high-risk groups. In the United States, the degree of urbanization is associated with people's levels of physical activity. The highest prevalence of physical inactivity is found in the rural South. Given that sex (female) and income are other established determinants of physical inactivity, the funding of intervention programs targeting low-income southern women who live outside of urban centers would be warranted.

Determining malleable variables that influence behavior change can direct interventions to target those variables and increase the efficacy of those interventions. Modifiable variables consistently associated with physical activity include motivation, social support, self-efficacy, perceived barriers, perceived benefits, enjoyment of activity, processes of change, intention to exercise, and lower intensity of exercise. These are examples of variables that should be tested in intervention research to see whether changes in them will result in changes in behavior—rather than investing time and money in variables that are inconsistently or weakly related to physical activity, such as exercise knowledge.

Finally, expanding our understanding of characteristics that influence physical activity in specific populations will foster the creation of personalized interventions that are more likely to meet the needs of the target group, and thus increase the probability of maintaining the behavior change. Although some variables, such as self-efficacy, motivation, and perceived barriers, operate across a range of populations, the strength of specific correlates probably varies among population subgroups. For example, social support may influence exercise behavior more in women than in men, and the type of social support for exercise (e.g., from family or friends) may vary in importance as a function of sex. Identifying specific correlates associated

with adoption, early adherence, and maintenance can inform the selection of strategies to implement at different times in a long-term intervention.

CLASSIFICATION OF CORRELATES

The social cognitive theory provides a convenient framework for organizing the myriad variables that have been studied along with level of physical activity. One useful aspect of the social cognitive theory is a dynamic interacting structure that organizes determinants into characteristics of the person, the environment, and the target behavior. In this chapter, correlates of exercise and physical activity are organized and described under three general categories: past and present characteristics of the person, past and present environments, and aspects of exercise and physical activity. See table 13.1 for a summary of correlates and their associations with physical activity.

Identifying correlates that reside in the person is of practical importance because this allows us to distinguish population segments that are responsive or resistant to physical activity interventions. For example, cigarette smoking and low income can be markers of underlying habits and circumstances that reinforce sedentary behavior. Identifying environmental influences can give insight into real and perceived barriers to exercise adoption and maintenance. Addressing correlates at the environmental level also demonstrates the need to implement interventions beyond the individual and small group to include facility and policy planning at the community and national levels. More researchers are evaluating the effects of the constructed environment on behavior; for example, some are conducting studies to determine the influence of the layout of neighborhood roads (i.e., community structure) on residents' walking patterns (see figure 13.1). Aspects of physical activity itself, such as intensity and mode, can have significant effects on adoption and maintenance. For example, a sedentary person would be more likely to join a walking program than a high-intensity aerobics

Table 13.1 Associations of Correlates With Physical Activity in Adults

Correlate	Associations with activity in supervised program	Associations with overall physical activity*
DEMOGRAPHIC AND BIOLOGICAL FACTORS		
Age	0 0	– –
Blue-collar occupation	– –	–
Education	+	+ +
Sex (male)		+ +
Genetic influences		+ +
High risk for heart disease	0	–
Injury history		+
Income/socioeconomic status		+ +
Overweight/obesity	0	– –
Race/ethnicity (nonwhite)		– –
PSYCHOLOGICAL FACTORS		
Attitudes	0	0 0
Perceived barriers to exercise	–	– –
Enjoyment of exercise	+	+ +
Outcome expectancy values (expect benefits)	+	+ +
Health locus of control	0	0
Intention to exercise	+	+ +
Knowledge of health and exercise	0	0 0
Perceived lack of time	– –	–
Perceived health or fitness		+ +
Poor body image		–
Mood disturbance	–	– –
Normative beliefs	0	0 0
Self-efficacy	+ +	+ +
Self-motivation	+ +	+ +
Self-schemata for exercise (self-image as an exerciser)		+ +
Stage of change	+ +	+ +
Stress		0
Value of exercise outcomes		0

(continued)

Table 13.1 *(continued)*

Correlate	Associations with activity in supervised program	Associations with overall physical activity*
BEHAVIORAL ATTRIBUTES AND SKILLS		
Activity history during childhood/youth		+
Activity history during adulthood	+ +	+ +
Dietary habits (quality)	0 0	+ +
Past exercise program	+ +	+ +
Processes of change		+ +
School sports	0	0
Skills for coping with barriers		+
Smoking	– –	–
Sports media use		+
Decision balance sheet	+	+
SOCIAL AND CULTURAL FACTORS		
Class size	–	
Exercise models		0
Group cohesion	+	
Past family influences		0
Physician influence		+ +
Social support from friends/peers	+	+ +
Social support from spouse/family	+ +	+ +
Social support from staff/instructor	+	
PHYSICAL ENVIRONMENT FACTORS		
Access to facilities: actual	+	+
Access to facilities: perceived	+	+
Climate/season	–	– –
Cost of program	0	0
Disruptions in routine	–	
Home equipment	+	+
Enjoyable scenery		+
Frequent observations of others exercising		+
Adequate lighting		+

(continued)

Correlate	Associations with activity in supervised program	Associations with overall physical activity*
PHYSICAL ENVIRONMENT FACTORS *(continued)*		
Heavy traffic		0
High crime rates in the region		0
Hilly terrain		+
Neighborhood safety		+
Presence of sidewalks		0
Satisfaction with facilities		+
Unattended dogs		0
Dog ownership		++
Urban location		–
PHYSICAL ACTIVITY CHARACTERISTICS		
Intensity	– –	–
Perceived exertion	– –	– –

Key: + + = repeatedly documented positive associations with physical activity

+ = weak or mixed evidence of positive association with physical activity

0 0 = repeatedly documented lack of association with physical activity

0 = weak or mixed evidence of no association with physical activity

– – = repeatedly documented negative associations with physical activity

– = weak or mixed evidence of negative association with physical activity

Blank spaces indicate no data available.

Adapted from Dishman, Sallis, and Orenstein 1985; Trost et al 2002.

dance class; and adherence would be better in a low- to moderate-intensity physical activity program than in a vigorous program (Dishman and Buckworth 1996b; Perri et al. 2002). There are also differences in the determinants of level of physical activity and exercise behavior, as well as of participation in supervised and unsupervised programs (Dishman, Sallis, and Orenstein 1985).

No single variable explains and predicts physical activity and exercise behavior. The signifi-

cance of specific correlates must be considered in the context of other personal, environmental, and behavioral factors and from the perspective of **reciprocal determinism**, which is a component of social cognitive theory that provides a practical slant on studying correlates. Reciprocal determinism describes a mutually influencing relationship among two or more factors (see figure 13.2). Thus, correlates of physical activity are not isolated variables. They interact dynamically to influence behavior, and the pattern of this interaction among variables will change over time; the types of determinants and the strength of their influence will change over the course of the behavior (i.e., adoption, early adherence, long-term maintenance) and the developmental stage of the individual.

> **N**o single variable explains and predicts physical activity and exercise.

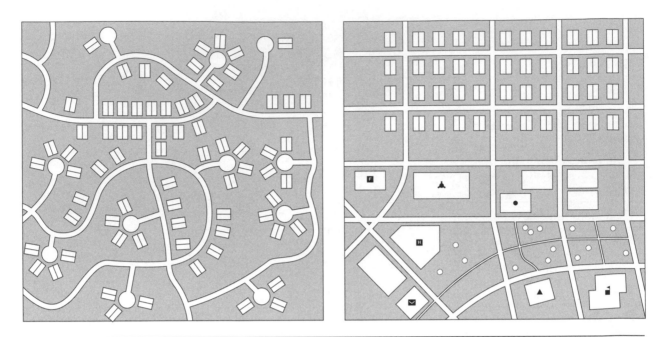

Figure 13.1 Researchers are making more efforts to evaluate how elements of the constructed environment influence patterns of physical activity.

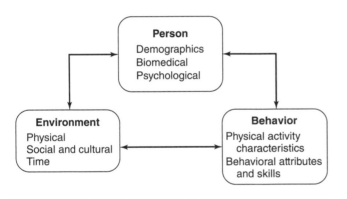

Figure 13.2 Correlates of exercise behavior.

Characteristics of the Person

Important factors that influence decisions and actions reside, or originate, within the person. Many variables, such as decision-making skills and perceptions of exercise benefits and barriers, are targets of behavior change interventions. Other characteristics of the person related to the level of physical activity are not amenable to change (e.g., age and sex), but must be identified and considered in the design of exercise promotion programs and interventions. The characteristics of the person that have been considered in correlates research have been organized into demographic and biological factors;

Example of an Interaction Between Exercise History and Environment

A woman who has just started exercising might be motivated to walk in her neighborhood when the weather is nice regardless of whether she is alone, but when it is cold, she may walk only if friends come along. After regular exercise has become an established behavior, external support becomes less important and walking does not depend on the company of others regardless of the weather.

psychological, cognitive, and emotional factors; and behavioral attributes and skills.

Demographic and Biological Factors

Demographic variables that are consistent correlates of physical activity are sex, age, ethnicity, education, income, and occupation. Males are more likely to be active than females are. The sex difference in exercise and level of physical activity is consistent among various racial and ethnic groups. Higher levels of physical activity in male children may be related to the differential development of motor skills, differences in body composition, and gender socialization toward sport and physical activity (Kohl and Hobbs 1998). In adolescents and adults, sex differences in the level of physical activity vary based on the exercise mode and physical activity intensity.

Accelerometer data from participants ages 6 to over 70 in the 2003-2004 National Health Interview Survey in the United States ($N = 6,329$) were analyzed to determine gender-specific, age-related changes in physical activity patterns (Troiano et al. 2008). Activity counts were consistently higher for males than females for all ages except in the 60-to-69 age group, in which they were similar. Activity counts declined with age, especially from childhood through adolescence. When accelerometer data were categorized into moderate and vigorous activity, males aged 6 through 11 spend the most time in vigorous activity (~10-16 min per day), whereas adults spent less than 2 minutes per day at this intensity. Children younger than age 16 obtained more than 1 hour a day of moderate- or high-intensity activity, but this dropped to 33 minutes for males and 20 minutes for females ages 16 to 19. From

that point, activity remained fairly stable until a progressive decline beginning with the 50-to-59 age group. According to accelerometer data for minutes of activity, 48.9% of boys and 34.7% of girls aged 6 through 11 met their public health recommended level of physical activity. This proportion was lower for adolescents ages 12 to 15 (boys: 11.9%; girls: 3.4%).

A count of bouts of activity revealed that only 3.8% of American men and 3.2% of American women met the adult recommendations. These estimates contrast with prevalence based on self-reports of exercise and physical activity (see figures 13.3 and 13.4). Factors that likely contribute to these discrepancies are self-reported overestimates of intensity and duration, a time period of accelerometer data that does not capture usual activity, or participation in activities not captured by accelerometers, although the low self-report participation in activities such as swimming weakens the latter explanation.

Overall, self-reported participation in physical activity decreases with increasing age, although age has less of an impact on moderate-intensity activity. Middle adulthood (30 to 64 years) is associated with lower levels of regular vigorous activity and strengthening activities, but the pattern of activity is relatively stable until retirement, when there is some improvement until

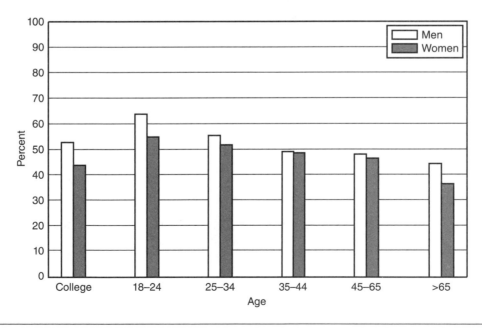

Figure 13.3 Participation in recommended levels of physical activity among males and females by age.

Data from Behavioral Risk Factor Surveillance 2008; College Health Risk Behavior Survey 2010.

the final period of life (Caspersen, Pereira, and Curran 2000). Certainly, age effects interact with other influences on the level of physical activity. For example, a longitudinal analysis of physical activity and retirement showed that activity increased after retirement from a sedentary job, but decreased after a more physically demanding job (Chung et al. 2009).

Level of physical activity declines with age, but the age at which the decline begins and the pattern of decline are not clear (Stone et al. 1998). However, accelerometer data from National Health and Nutrition Examination Survey (NHANES) collected in 2003-2004 indicated a significant decrease in the proportion of youths who met the moderate-intensity physical activity recommendation after age 11, regardless of race (see figure 13.5) (Whitt-Glover et al. 2009). Results from the Youth Risk Behavior Surveillance from 1999 to 2007 indicate that the prevalence of moderate and vigorous physical activity, participation in daily school physical education, and being physically activity in physical education classes did not change significantly over time (Lowry et al. 2009). A decline in activity from 9th through 12th grades occurred overall, but 11th-grade students experienced a significant increase in activity over time, although their

levels were still below Healthy People 2010 goals for this population.

Several studies examined the determinants of physical activity in younger age groups. Sallis, Prochaska, and Taylor (2000) reviewed 108 studies published between 1970 and 1999 on the determinants of physical activity in children (ages 3 to 12) and adolescents (ages 13 to 18). For children, positive associations were found for sex (male), healthy diet, physical activity preferences, intentions to be active, previous physical activity, access to programs or facilities, and time spent outdoors. Negative associations were found for general barriers to exercise. Variables positively associated with physical activity in adolescents were sex (male), ethnicity (European American), achievement orientation, intention, perceived competence, community sports, sensation seeking, siblings' participation in physical activity, previous physical activity, parental support, support from significant others, and opportunities to exercise. Negative associations for adolescents were age, depression, and being sedentary after school and on weekends.

Other reviews have indicated that exercise self-efficacy and social support are significant factors in the level of physical activity for both children and adolescents (e.g., Sallis and Owen

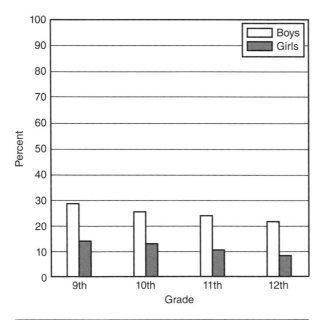

Figure 13.4 Self-report participation in recommended 60 minutes of physical activity every day: male and female adolescents.

Data from Youth Risk Behavior Surveillance System 2009.

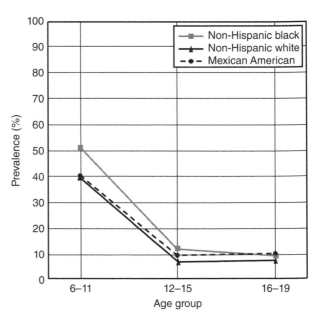

Figure 13.5 The estimated prevalence of meeting the moderate-intensity physical activity recommendation is not as great based on accelerometer data.

Data from Whitt-Glover et al. 2009; NHANES 2003-2004.

1999; U.S. Department of Health and Human Services [USDHHS] 2010; Van Der Horst et al. 2007). There are also mixed associations between parents' activity levels and the activity levels of their children. The relationship is stronger for females but less significant for adolescents in general (Kohl and Hobbs 1998). For adolescents, peer pressure is a stronger social determinant of physical activity level than family support is, although in youth (Sallis et al. 1992) and college students (Wallace et al. 2000), family support for exercise is more important for females and peer support is more important for males. Environmental influences positively associated with physical activity among children and adolescents include the presence of sidewalks, having a destination or walking to a particular place, access to public transportation, low traffic density, and access to neighborhood or school play areas or recreational equipment (USDHHS 2010).

In terms of ethnic influence, non-Hispanic whites are generally more active than other racial or ethnic groups regardless of age. Results from the 2007 Youth Risk Behavior Survey showed that non-Hispanic white students (66.3%) were more likely to participate in vigorous physical activity than Hispanic (63.2%) and African-American students (57.8%) (Lowry et al. 2009). The effects of ethnicity were similar for moderate-intensity activity. Fewer African-American (23.1%) and Hispanic (23.0%) youth participated in moderate-intensity activity compared to non-Hispanic whites (27.6%).

Although there are some associations between exercise and ethnicity, evidence that this relationship is independent of social class is inconclusive. Crespo and colleagues (2000) analyzed physical inactivity and indicators of social class (i.e., education, family income, occupation, employment, poverty, and marital status) among Caucasians, African Americans, and Mexican Americans completing the Third National Health and Nutrition Examination Survey between 1988 and 1994. The authors found that in each category of social class, women and minorities showed a higher prevalence of leisure-time inactivity than Caucasian men did. Among youth, there is some evidence for different correlates based on racial or ethnic group; self-reported television viewing, enjoyment, and parental encouragement were more strongly correlated with physical activity among blacks than among other groups, and self-efficacy was more strongly related to activity in non-Hispanic whites (Whitt-Glover et al. 2009).

Income is a component of socioeconomic status (SES), which has a strong inverse relationship with sedentary lifestyle for both sexes and every race and ethnic group (USDHHS 1996). For example, African-American males in poverty are three times more likely to be sedentary than African-American males with a high family income. Socioeconomic status is also positively associated with physical activity in children and adolescents. For children and adolescents, higher SES means more access to physical activity programs in and out of school. Transportation to facilities and events influences accessibility and represents an important form of direct support from parents and responsible adults that can influence exercise participation.

Longitudinal population studies that evaluate concurrent changes in physical activity and changes in purported determinants can provide stronger evidence for the role of specific personal variables in exercise adoption and adherence. Education and income are positively associated with physical activity and have been associated with increased activity in prospective studies. For example, people with similar aerobic capacities in high school had significantly higher aerobic capacities eight years later if they were civil servants, white-collar workers, or students compared to those who were in blue-collar jobs or unemployed (Anderson 1996). Adoption of vigorous physical activity by sedentary people has been predicted by age (inverse), self-efficacy, and neighborhood environment for males and by education, self-efficacy, friend social support, and family social support for females (Sallis et al. 1992).

Other prospective studies have shown associations between declines in physical activity in adults and social isolation, lower education, low income, blue-collar occupation, marital status (unmarried), depression, low levels of life satisfaction, and less-than-excellent perceived health (Kaplan et al. 1996; Schmitz, French, and Jeffery 1997). Occupation effects are more difficult to identify because most studies comparing occupation to physical activity have been cross-sectional and can be influenced by seasonal differences in activities (e.g., landscaping, construction). In addition, the variability in job demands is large, especially for blue-collar jobs that have the possibility of mechanization.

A variety of factors have been correlated with lack of adherence to structured exercise programs (Franklin 1988). Personal factors include smoking, blue-collar occupation, low self-esteem, low motivation, overweight or obesity, depression, anxiety, and low ego strength. Characteristics of the program that are related to dropping out are excessive cost, inconvenient time or location, lack of exercise variety, exercising alone, lack of positive feedback or reinforcement, and poor leadership. Other factors related to nonadherence are lack of time, lack of spousal support, inclement weather, rural residency, excessive job travel, injury, medical problems, and job change or move.

> **A**ge, ethnicity, education, income, occupation, and biology are personal characteristics that influence exercise behavior and level of physical activity.

Most of the research on determinants of physical activity has focused on cognitive, social, and environmental variables. However, intrinsic biological influences may significantly affect the level of physical activity. Rowland (1998) proposed an anatomical–physiological entity that regulates the amount of daily physical activity that is analogous to brain centers controlling behavioral–physiological processes such as hunger and temperature regulation. The biological regulation of physical activity is one of the interacting mechanisms for the regulation of energy balance, along with caloric intake and energy expenditure in the form of resting metabolic rate.

Evidence for the role of genetics in physical activity behavior has been established in part by studying monozygotic (MZ; identical) and dizygotic (DZ; fraternal) twins. Stubbe and colleagues (2006) reviewed data on exercise par-

Genes or Environment (or Both)?

If physical activity levels are more similar between monozygotic (MZ; identical) twins, who share all the same genes, than between dizygotic (DZ; fraternal) twins, who share only half their genes, then there is a genetic component to physical activity. If the correlation of physical activity levels between twin pairs is similar for MZ and DZ twins, then common environmental factors shared by the twins seem to explain the variation in physical activity, regardless of genes. Because MZ twins share the same environment and the same genes, a correlation in pairs of MZ twins that is less than perfect (i.e., less than 1.0) indicates that unique environmental experiences not shared by the twins explain the variation in physical activity.

ticipation in 85,198 MZ and DZ twins ages 19 to 40 participating in the GenomEUtwin project. The mean heritability of exercise participation was 62%, although there was a range of 27% to 70% across the seven countries in the study. The contribution from unique environmental factors on exercise was also significant for all countries, although that from common environmental factors was significant only for Norwegian men. Genetic contributions may also be involved in variations in the level of spontaneous activity, and there is some evidence that the genetic influence is stronger at younger ages (Lightfoot 2011). The literature on the genetic determinants of sport participation, daily physical activity, and resting metabolic rate has shown small to moderately high contributions to interindividual variations in daily physical activity; researchers have attributed the range in heritabilities to differing methods and design. The genetic contributions to exercise adherence warrant closer examination.

Physiological adaptations to exercise training also have a genetic component. There is evidence for high-, low-, and no-responder genotypes in regard to exercise training. Wilmore and colleagues (1997) described individual responses to training with respect to aerobic capacity, plasma lipoprotein, insulin response, skeletal muscle enzyme activity, and adipose tissue metabolism that ranged from a low of 0% to highs of 50% to 100% of pretraining values. There was significant variation in the response to exercise training with respect to the level and rate of change, even considering effects from age, sex, and prior exercise experience. Research is needed to explore the effects of responder **genotype** on psychological variables, such as self-efficacy and self-motivation, that are relevant for exercise adherence.

Other physiological variables can play a critical role in behavior and interact significantly with psychosocial constructs. For example, physical discomfort has been negatively correlated with self-reports of physical activity, and those who perceive their health as poor are unlikely to adopt and adhere to an exercise program.

Psychological, Cognitive, and Emotional Factors

Cognitions, such as attitudes, beliefs, and values, are personal characteristics that researchers have studied as potential influences on physical activity behavior. The cognitive variable that has been consistently associated with physical activity in almost every study that included it is **self-efficacy**, which is the belief in one's ability to engage successfully in a specific behavior with a known outcome. Self-efficacy is similar to level of confidence and is based on judgments of capabilities. Self-efficacy is central to Bandura's social cognitive theory, in which it is designated as the most powerful determinant of human behavior. Self-efficacy develops from (1) actual success, (2) watching others like oneself succeed, (3) being persuaded by someone, and (4) emotional or perceived signs of coping ability (e.g., lowered perceived exertion after increasing fitness; Bandura 1997).

Self-efficacy, by definition, is task and situation specific. For example, a recreational swimmer can be confident that she can easily swim a mile in the 50-meter indoor pool (high self-efficacy) but have no faith in her ability to water-ski

(low self-efficacy). Thus, the more specific the measure of self-efficacy, the better the potential to predict the behavior. There are also various types of self-efficacy, such as task (confidence in one's ability to run 5K in less than 25 min) and barrier (confidence in one's ability to fit in a workout the week before final examinations), which can have different degrees of influence on exercise over time (Ashford, Edmunds, and French 2010; Blanchard et al. 2007). Of course, self-efficacy is not a major influence on behavior when goals or incentives are not present. That is, believing that you can accomplish something is not important when you have no reason to try.

Longitudinal studies with different populations have shown that exercise self-efficacy increases as one moves from an established sedentary lifestyle to the long-term maintenance of regular exercise, and that the level of self-efficacy predicts subsequent physical activity. Exercise self-efficacy can be both a determinant and a consequence of exercise (see figure 13.6; McAuley and Blissmer 2000). Self-efficacy influences the choice of activities, the amount of effort expended, and the degree of persistence. Research on exercise and self-efficacy supports a greater role for self-efficacy in the adoption of and during the early stages of an exercise program, but it may also be important in maintenance, depending on the type of self-efficacy (e.g., self-efficacy to overcome barriers or to make time to exercise; Blanchard et al. 2007) and physical activity (e.g., maintenance of vigorous exercise; Sallis et al. 1986). Significant improvements in exercise self-efficacy after exercise training have been demonstrated in a variety of

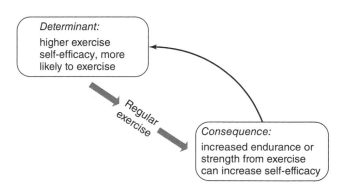

Figure 13.6 Exercise self-efficacy can be both a determinant and a consequence of physical activity.

> The cognitive variable that has the strongest consistent relationship with exercise is self-efficacy.

populations such as men infected with HIV-1 (human immunodeficiency virus-1; Lox, McAuley, and Tucker 1995) and older adults (McAuley, Lox, and Duncan 1993). Moreover, interventions have been designed to enhance exercise self-efficacy as a strategy to effect behavior change (Ashford, Edmunds, and French 2010).

Another theory-based cognitive variable related to physical activity and exercise is **behavioral intention**, which is the key proximal determinant of voluntary behavior according to the theory of planned behavior. Behavioral intention can provide an indication of motivation, such as how much effort someone is willing to put into a particular activity, although intentions must be maintained over time to sustain behavior and achieve behavioral goals. Most research that has tested the effects of intention on exercise has found strong relationships between intention and overall physical activity. Godin (1994), examining 12 studies of exercise and intentions, reported correlations between behavioral intention and exercise that ranged from $r = .19$ to $.82$ with a mean of $r = .55$.

Self-motivation, which is the generalized tendency to persist in the long-term pursuit of behavioral goals, is also positively associated with supervised and overall physical activity. Successful endurance athletes have consistently scored high on self-motivation, and self-motivation has discriminated between adherents and dropouts across a wide variety of settings including adult fitness programs, cardiac rehabilitation, commercial spas, corporate fitness programs, and college campuses (Daly et al. 2002; Knapp 1988; Sonstroem 1988). Self-motivation is associated with physical activity in adolescent boys (Biddle et al. 1996) and girls (Motl et al. 2002), exercise adherence in older adults (André and Dishman 2012), and initial exercise adherence in patients with COPD (O'Shea, Taylor, and Paratz 2007).

Motivation, defined as the internal forces that produce the initiation, direction, intensity, and persistence of a specific goal-directed behavior, is another psychological correlate of physical activity. Two general types of motivation have been studied in respect to levels of physical activity. Initial motivation to exercise is associated with more extrinsic motives (a focus on outcomes of behavior, such as weight loss), but over time, persistence is fostered by intrinsic motivation (e.g., enjoyment, pleasure in the behavior itself) (Rodgers et al. 2010). For example, in a sample of 220 healthy college students, intrinsic motivation to exercise was high in students in the maintenance stage of change and lowest in those in the contemplation stage (Buckworth et al. 2007). After 10 weeks, intrinsic motivation was greater than extrinsic motivation in the students who maintained physical activity, but decreased over time in those in the continually inactive group.

Other cognitive variables that have been positively associated with supervised and overall physical activity are enjoyment of exercise (Motl et al. 2001), expectations of benefits (Dishman et al. 2002; Motl et al. 2000), self-schemata (e.g., seeing oneself as an exerciser; see chapter 12), and exercise stage of change. For example, enjoyment of activity was an independent predictor of meeting moderate or vigorous physical activity recommendations for African-American men and meeting strength training recommendations for African-American women (Bopp et al. 2006). Exercise stage of change is a classification based on current and previous exercise behavior and motivational readiness to become and remain physically active. Exercise stage has been positively associated with supervised and overall physical activity, and has been used frequently in studies to predict the adoption and maintenance of regular exercise.

Perceived barriers to exercise are negatively associated with supervised and overall physical activity in adults and children. Lack of time has a stronger inverse association with participation in structured programs than with overall physical activity. A perceived lack of time is also the principal and most common reason given for dropping out of supervised clinical and community exercise programs and for inactive lifestyles. For many, however, reporting a lack of time may reflect a lack of interest in or commitment to physical activity—that is, saying there is not enough time to exercise is more socially acceptable. Thus, lack of time may be a true determinant, a perceived determinant, the reflection of poor behavioral skills such as poor time management, or a rationalization for a lack of motivation to be active.

Lack of time and caregiving duties were the most frequently reported barriers to physical activity in a sample of 2,912 middle-aged and older women in the United States (King et al. 2000). The other most frequently reported barriers to physical activity were lack of energy, being too tired, and lack of a safe place to exercise. When the data were analyzed across racial and ethnic groups, there were differences in barriers that correlated with being sedentary. For example, being tired was strongly associated with less physical activity for Hispanic women, but not for people in other racial or ethnic groups. Caregiving duties were associated with less activity only for African-American women. Some of the results from this study do not mirror what we think would support or hinder physical activity, such as the positive association between physical activity and unattended dogs for African-American women. This finding may reflect more opportunities to observe dogs in the surrounding neighborhood as a result of being outside walking or working in the yard, for example, and may be a marker of getting outside more to observe such events. Another issue is a concern with the validity of traditional instruments for measuring physical activity for minority women. In any case, these results provide important information and illustrate the need for additional research to clarify associations between barriers and physical activity in specific population groups.

Several psychological variables that have weaker relationships with physical activity and exercise are attitudes, control over exercise, psychological health, and poor body image. Although some studies have shown weak relationships between exercise and personality variables, there is consistent evidence that neuroticism is negatively related and extroversion is positively related to exercise behavior (e.g.,

Courneya and Hellsten 1998). Several studies have also reported associations between conscientiousness and exercise. Research has shown no consistent associations between supervised or overall physical activity and health locus of control, normative beliefs, stress, susceptibility to illness or seriousness of illness, valuing exercise outcomes, and knowledge of health and exercise.

Knowledge alone does not seem to be enough to change behavior, but clear, relevant information about the benefits of physical activity and ways to become more active may be a factor in motivating people to consider adopting regular exercise. For example, in a random telephone survey of 2,002 American households in the 48 contiguous states and the District of Columbia, 94% of respondents were aware of traditional physical activities that provide a health benefit, but only 68% to 71% were aware of specific exercise guidelines and lifestyle physical activities that benefit health, regardless of age, race or ethnicity, or education (Morrow et al. 2004). Knowledge was not related to physical activity behavior enough to result in a health benefit.

Behavioral Attributes and Skills

Activity history during adulthood and participation in an exercise program in the past are positively associated with supervised and overall physical activity. Dietary habits (positive), processes of change (transtheoretical model; see chapter 14), and smoking (negative) are also associated with participation in supervised programs. There is also some evidence for a relationship between physical activity and decisional balance (i.e., weighing the costs vs. the benefits of exercise), skills for coping with barriers, and a type A behavior pattern. Activity history during childhood and youth, use of alcohol, participation in school sports, and sport media use have had mixed associations with supervised or overall physical activity. There is growing evidence that being active when young can influence the level of physical activity later in life. For example, data on 7,794 participants who completed questionnaires about physical activities at age 14 and again at age 31 indicated that frequent participation in sports after school were associated with a high level of physical activity later in life (Tammelin et al. 2003). Other longitudinal studies have found a decreased risk of inactivity in adulthood among people who were very active in adolescence (e.g., Huotari et al. 2011). However, the lack of a consistent relationship between physical activity and sport in childhood and youth and adult levels of physical activity points to the need to examine the characteristics of youth activity that are more likely to foster sustained active lifestyles. Many models for physical education in the public schools are based on teaching and fostering sport or activity skills that can be carried over into adulthood, but the competitive nature of school sports may overshadow the implementation of this philosophy and confound long-term effects.

> Lack of time is one of the most frequently reported reasons for not exercising and for dropping out of an exercise program.

Researchers have investigated the associations between the level of physical activity and other health behaviors, such as dietary habits and smoking. Pate and colleagues (1996) examined associations between physical activity and other health behaviors from the 1990 Youth Risk Behavior Survey. Data from over 11,000 youths aged 12 to 18 indicated that little or no involvement in physical activity was associated with cigarette smoking, marijuana use, poor dietary habits, television watching, failure to wear seat belts, and a perception of low academic performance. Level of physical activity was not associated with cocaine use, sexual activity, physical fighting, or self-perception of weight. Steptoe and colleagues (1997) assessed the prevalence of physical activity and other health habits over the previous two weeks in 7,302 males and 9,181 females aged 18 to 30 in 21 European countries. For the whole sample, physical inactivity was significantly associated with smoking, unsatisfactory sleep time, no desire to lose weight, low social support, and depression. Knowledge was not a determinant of physical activity in this population, but there was evidence that knowledge had a positive influence on beliefs in the health benefits of physical activity. Relationships between physical activity and alcohol consumption were inconsistent.

Behaviors that require little energy expenditure (i.e., sedentary activities) have been examined in respect to physical activity. Time spent watching television has an inconsistent association with level of physical activity, but it has been used as an indicator of how sedentary someone is. Watching television is only one of several media or screen-based activities, such as computer use, that require minimal energy expenditure, and television watching may not be a useful marker of inactivity. For example, researchers discovered a negative correlation between television time and other sedentary activities in 1,484 adolescents in the United Kingdom (Biddle, Gorely, and Marshall 2009), and in another sample of 450 adolescents, time watching television during the week was similar for active and inactive boys and girls, but more computer use during weekdays predicted higher physical activity levels (Santos, Gomes, and Mota 2005). High levels of physical activity are not necessarily correlated with low levels of sedentary behaviors, and we need to partial out the effects for various types of activities that require little energy expenditure.

Television watching and other sedentary behaviors are typically viewed as part of the continuum of physical activity, with MET values between 1 and 1.5 (Owen et al. 2000). Dietz (1996), Owen and colleagues (2000), and others have proposed an independent and interactive relationship between sedentary behaviors and physical activity behaviors, and sedentary behavior has been proposed to be a specific class of behaviors with unique determinants and health consequences (Owen, Healy, Matthews, and Dunstan 2010). Too much sitting is different from too little exercise and may have negative health consequences independent of the level of exercise. Thus, identifying determinants of sedentary behaviors may have practical implications in view of some of the research showing that interventions to decrease participation in sedentary behaviors are efficacious in increasing level of physical activity (e.g., Epstein et al. 1997).

Environmental Determinants

Exercise physiologists have been accused of dealing with the body while ignoring the mind, and psychologists have been charged with treating the mind and disregarding the body. Exercise psychologists should incorporate the strengths of these two disciplines to consider the entire person, but we need to take another step and study the person–environment interaction. (Even the most committed cyclist pauses before he takes his bike out in a snowstorm!) A strength of the social cognitive theory is the inclusion of environmental factors in a model of behavioral influences. Environmental determinants of exercise behavior and physical activity can be divided into the human environment and the physical environment.

Human Environment

The human environmental can have a strong impact on behavior through shaping norms, providing or impeding opportunities and resources, and presenting models of behavior. For example, the social environment was the strongest independent predictor of being physically active in a cross-sectional study of 3,342 adults from six European countries (Ståhl et al. 2001). Social support includes companionship; encouragement; assistance or information from friends, family members, and others; tangible aid and service from the community; and advice, suggestions, and information from professionals. Social support also varies in frequency, durability, and intensity (Courneya and McAuley 1995; McNeill, Kreuter, and Subramanian 2006). Social influences in the form of social support and prompting typically have strong positive associations with physical activity, and social isolation has shown negative associations.

In a meta-analysis of social influence and exercise, Carron, Hausenblas, and Mack (1996) examined the separate effects of social influence variables on exercise behavior, cognition, and affect (satisfaction and attitude). Overall effect sizes were small to medium, but effects of 0.62 to 0.69 were found for family support and the support of important others on attitudes about exercise, and for family support and task cohesion on exercise behavior. Social support

from family and friends is consistently related to physical activity in cross-sectional and prospective studies, and increased group cohesion in exercise classes leads to increased exercise adherence (Estabrooks 2000). Support from a spouse appears also to be reliably correlated with exercise participation, and better exercise adherence has been found for people who join fitness centers with their spouses than for married people whose spouses do not join.

Social support has a consistent association with physical activity in children and adolescents. A meta-analysis of 30 cross-sectional studies found positive but small associations ($r =$ ~.10 to .20) of parental encouragement ($r = .21$), modeling (i.e., parents being physically active; $r = .10$), and instrumental behaviors (e.g., providing transportation or buying sports equipment; $r = .17$) between child and adolescent physical activity levels (75% used self-reports by parents or children) (Pugliese and Tinsley 2007). However, there is little evidence for the effectiveness of intervention methods to increase family involvement for promoting physical activity in children (O'Connor, Jago, and Baranowski 2009).

The impact of social interactions and social influences on exercise appears to be different for males and females. For example, adherence to a structured exercise program was predicted by women's perceptions that they received adequate guidance and reassurance of worth, but social provisions did not predict adherence in men (Duncan, Duncan, and McAuley 1993). In a longitudinal study of 903 university students, initial lower levels of social support for physical activity were associated with lower physical activity for women only (Molloy et al. 2010). A study of college students revealed that social support for exercise from family members was related to the level of physical activity for females, but support from friends was more significant for males (Wallace et al. 2000).

The relationship between social support for exercise and sex may be different over the course of contemplating, adopting, and maintaining exercise. Results from a cross-sectional study of healthy middle-aged adults indicated that perceived expectations to be physically active and motivation to comply with perceived expectations were greater for inactive women

Social support is related to physical activity, but this influence is modified by gender.

than for inactive men (Troped and Saunders 1998). Men and women who were adopting or maintaining exercise were similar on motivation to comply. Thus, social support for exercise may be a more important influence for women in the early stages of exercise adoption and should be considered in the development of interventions that target sedentary women.

In general, participation in supervised exercise programs is weakly associated with class size and social support from staff or instructors. No consistent associations have been found for exercise models or past family influence with exercise participation or physical activity. However, support for physical activity from four-legged friends may be important (Epping 2011). Studies have reported consistent relationships between dog ownership and level of physical activity. A positive association between physical activity and unattended dogs was reported by King and colleagues (2000) in a sample of 2,912 middle-aged and older racially mixed women. The authors speculated that spending more time outside and thus observing more dogs was responsible for this result, but the association between dog ownership and more physical activity, especially walking, is more straightforward.

Recreational walking was associated with the number of registered dogs within a 0.8-kilometer (0.5-mile) radius of the respondents in a study of 1,215 residents of Queensland, Australia (Duncan and Mummery 2005), and dog owners in a sample of 984 residents of San Diego, California, were more likely to meet physical activity guidelines. Brown and Rhodes (2006) found significantly more walking per week in dog owners (300 min) than in people without dogs (168 min) in a sample of 351 Canadian adults. They also found that a sense of responsibility or obligation to maintain the health and well-being of one's dog mediated dog walking. Dogs can also have a beneficial effect on physical activity in children. In a sample of 2,065 children ages 9 and 10, those with family dogs had significantly

more accelerometer-measured activity counts and steps per day than did those in families without dogs (Owen et al. 2010).

Physical Environment

Climate and season are the only characteristics of the natural physical environment that have a strong and consistent association with the overall level of physical activity. In children and adolescents, activity levels are lowest in the winter and highest in the summer. Observational studies suggest that time spent outdoors is one of the best correlates of physical activity in preschool children (Kohl and Hobbs 1998; Sallis and Owen 1999). Time spent outdoors during cooler months was associated with objectivity-measured physical activity in 380 10- to 12-year-old children (Cleland et al. 2008). Opportunities for being physically active outdoors also decrease for adults during the winter, and this can affect physiological markers of physical activity. One study that compared exercise classes conducted in autumn and spring found that six-month follow-up measures of aerobic capacity were significantly lower at the follow-up after winter (autumn class) than after summer (spring class) (Buckworth 2001). In addition, aerobic capacity significantly increased for those retested after summer. However, students who had participated in strength training classes during the same measurement periods demonstrated no seasonal effects for measures of strength, suggesting that weather is not as great a barrier to participation in strength training as it is to engaging in aerobic activities.

Disruptions in routine have a weak negative association with participation in supervised programs, and costs of programs and home exercise equipment show no consistent associations with supervised or overall physical activity. Access to exercise facilities has been found to influence participation, although the relationship is complicated. Access can be considered in terms of environment (i.e., geography), economics, and safety (e.g., running in some New York City neighborhoods is risky because of air pollution and high crime rates). However, access can also be considered in terms of perception. When access to facilities has been measured by objective methods (e.g., distance), access typi-

> **S**eason and climate have a strong and consistent association with the level of physical activity.

cally has been related to both the adoption and maintenance of supervised and overall physical activity. However, perceived access is associated only with participation in supervised programs.

Raynor, Coleman, and Epstein (1998) considered the interaction between accessibility and the reinforcing value of the alternatives in a study of 34 sedentary adult males. Accessibility was operationalized as physical proximity to physically active and sedentary alternatives. The amount of time out of a possible 20 minutes that participants spent exercising was compared among four conditions that varied as a function of accessibility to both active and sedentary alternatives (see figure 13.7). The most time (20 min) was spent exercising when the active alternatives were near (in the same room) and the sedentary alternatives were far (5 min walk away). Regardless of the accessibility of the active alternatives, if the sedentary alternatives were near, less than 1 minute on average was spent exercising. Participants were active 42% of the time when both alternatives were less accessible. The researchers concluded that sedentary adult males would be more physically active if the physical activities were more convenient and the sedentary activities were less convenient.

The effects of the natural and constructed environment on levels of physical activity can vary based on age. A systematic semi-quantitative review of 150 studies on environmental correlates of physical activity among children and adolescents found significant associations between variables of the home and school environments and children's physical activity. Factors that influenced the physical activity levels of children 3 to 12 years old were the degree to which their fathers were physically active, time spent outdoors, and school policies about physical activity. Those most influential for adolescents ages 13 to 18 were support from significant others, their mothers' education levels, family income,

and nonvocational school attendance (Ferreira et al. 2007). Low crime rates were characteristic of the neighborhood environment associated with higher levels of physical activity in adolescents 13 to 18 years old. Overall, however, only 176 of 497 comparisons among children (35%) and 215 of 620 comparisons among adolescents (35%) were statistically significant, and not just because most studies had samples too small to detect small effects. In addition, most of these studies used self-ratings of environmental features and physical activity and cross-sectional designs.

A systematic review of 47 studies of social and physical environmental factors and physical activity among adults concluded that the availability of physical activity equipment was convincingly associated with vigorous physical activity and sports and that the connectivity of trails was associated with active commuting (Wendel-Vos et al. 2007). Other possible but less consistent correlates of physical activity were the availability, accessibility, and convenience of recreational facilities. No evidence was found for differences between men and women. Among studies that used an objective measure of the environment, only 33 of 129 comparisons (26%) showed a positive association between a feature of the environment (usually the access to or convenience of a physical activity opportunity) and physical activity levels. Ten inverse associations were found.

Only 3 of the 47 publications used longitudinal data to study the environmental determinants of physical activity, and only one of those used an objective measure, which showed no association. However, at least one experimental study suggests that interventions can overcome perceived environmental barriers to walking. Inactive adults (aged 30-65, 85% women) completed one of three conditions in a three-month randomized controlled trial: a single mail-out of a self-help walking program ($n = 102$); that program plus a pedometer ($n = 105$); or a no-treatment control group ($n = 107$). Adjustments were made for baseline walking, social support, self-efficacy, intention to change behavior, and sociodemographic characteristics. Among people who perceived their walking environment to be unpleasant, those in the self-help plus pedometer group were more likely than controls to increase their total walking time and to undertake regular walking (OR = 5.85; 95% CI = 2.60-12.2) (Merom et al. 2009).

Some characteristics of the physical environment have consistent relationships with physical activity for children, adolescents, and adults, but a literature review of 31 studies on the environment and physical activity in older adults found inconsistent associations (Van Cauwenberg et al. 2011). There were only three prospective studies, which are necessary for speculation about causal relationships. Other weaknesses in studies with older adults were the failure to address specific types of activity and specific environmental characteristics concurrently, and missing assessments of both the actual and perceived environment.

Features of the built environment have been measured in three main ways: (1) people's perceptions obtained by telephone interview or by questionnaires, (2) observations by raters (e.g., neighborhood audits) (Colabianchi et al. 2007), and (3) archival data sets (e.g., census records) linked with geographic information systems (GIS; Brownson et al. 2009). GIS blends cartography with database technology and statistical analysis to measure, manage, analyze, and model data about geographic locations. GIS provides an objective method for geocoding (i.e., finding geographic coordinates using latitude and longitude) from other geographic data. Other data

from satellite global positioning system (GPS) measurements that can be used to understand the built environment and physical activity include people's place of residence and neighborhood (e.g., census street addresses linked with street segments and postal zip codes), street connectivity (i.e., number and directness of travel route options), and distances to schools, physical activity facilities, and other places for various physical activities (e.g., parks and trails).

The comprehensive measurement of the built environment is important because of evidence that the physical environment (which includes population density; the quality of the pedestrian environment; and the composition of the neighborhood with respect to retail, service, and community facilities) influences commuting behavior and incidental physical activity (see figure 13.1). For example, in a sample of 449 Australian adults aged 60 and older, environmental factors that were significantly associated with being physically active were believing that footpaths were safe for walking and access to local facilities (Booth et al. 2000). Environmental influences may differ based on the purpose of walking. Saelens and Handy (2008) reviewed reviews and research on characteristics of the built environment and walking for transportation versus recreational walking. Proximity to destinations is a consistent correlate, but density and mixed land use may be more important for utility walking than for walking for exercise.

The degree of urbanization and geographic region are environmental characteristics that are also associated with the overall level of leisure-time physical activity in the United States (see figure 13.8). Data from the 2001 Behavioral Risk Factor Surveillance Survey indicate that the overall prevalence of physical inactivity is lowest in central metropolitan areas (14.6%) and in the West (11.2%; Reis et al. 2004). Physical inactivity is highest (24.1%) in rural areas, particularly in the southern United States (17.4%). The inverse relationship between degree of urbanization and physical inactivity is relatively consistent when data are stratified by age, sex, level of education, and household income. When looking specifically at associations between physical activity and environmental factors in rural residents, pleasant aesthetics, trails, safety from crime,

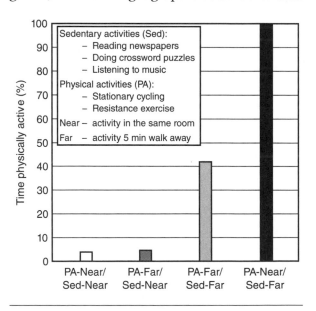

Figure 13.7 Participation in physical activity as a function of accessibility and behavioral alternatives.

Based on Raynor, Coleman, and 1998.

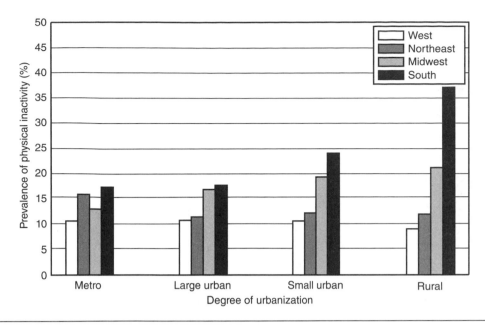

Figure 13.8 Nonoccupational leisure-time physical inactivity by degree of urbanization and geographic region of the United States: 2001 BRFSS.

Data from Reis et al. 2004.

Physical Activity Characteristics

Characteristics of exercise (i.e., mode, intensity, duration, and frequency) are possible determinants of physical activity. A recent meta-analysis of adherence in 27 randomized exercise trials concluded that the effect of prescribed frequency ($d = 0.08$), intensity ($d = 0.02$), duration ($d = 0.05$), and mode of activity (d ranged from 0.03 to 0.10) were small or trivial (Rhodes et al. 2009). However, most of the trials manipulated only a single feature of exercise exposure and used very different definitions of adherence (e.g., attendance at supervised sessions, maintenance of heart rate within a prescribed intensity range, exercising for the prescribed duration, and weekly frequency according to personal diaries). Only a few of the trials defined adherence according to whether people dropped out, which has been the hallmark definition of exercise adherence for the past 35 years. One trial reported 85% attendance, but 42% of the participants had dropped out! In fact, studies that reported only dropout rates were excluded

from the review. Half the trials lasted less than six months, which has been the standard time frame used to define maintenance of an exercise program. The dropout rate averaged 18% (522 of 2,829 participants), ranging from 0% in a home-based program that relied on people's diaries to verify adherence to 30% to 40% in some six-month and two-year trials. Only 25% of the trials adjusted their adherence measure for the number of people who dropped out. Finally, a number of the trials actively used behavior modification approaches to improve overall adherence, thus confounding a true test of whether features of physical activity modify adherence rates.

Another recent review of studies that targeted short bouts of physical activity (i.e., ≤10 min) integrated into the daily routine of organizations (particularly schools and workplaces) concluded that the results had been modest but consistently favorable for promoting feasible and sustainable increases in physical activity that are more appealing to segments of the sedentary population (Barr-Anderson et al. 2011). However, of the 40 studies evaluated, just 5 studies in schools and 2 studies at workplaces were randomized controlled trials that used a measure of physical activity as an outcome. Just one 3-year trial of the five school-based trials (the others lasted 5 to

> **L**ow- and moderate-intensity activities generally have better adherence than higher-intensity activities.

20 months) and two of the workplace trials lasting 10 to 12 weeks reported a significant increase in physical activity.

Exercise mode can also be a factor in adherence, but interactions with characteristics of the person are likely, such as age, sex, skills, enjoyment of the activity, and access. For example, adherence was similar for 116 older women randomized to six months of supervised swimming or walking followed by six months of unsupervised exercise (Cox et al. 2010), and 32 overweight and obese men and women randomized to 16 weeks of circuit training completed more than the prescribed amount of exercise compared to those randomized to traditional resistance training, who consistently did less of the prescribed exercise (King et al. 2010).

Generally, exercise intensity has an inverse relationship with the adoption and maintenance of exercise programs (Perri et al. 2002; Pollock et al. 1991; Sallis et al. 1986), but personal variables should be considered when assessing this relationship. For example, initially sedentary adults who had high levels of past exercise had better adherence to higher-intensity compared to moderate-intensity exercise training over six months (Anton et al. 2005). Although adherence was similar in a one-year randomized exercise trial with middle-aged adults assigned to low or high exercise intensities (King et al. 1991), each group selected intensities during the year that regressed toward a moderate intensity. Basing exercise prescriptions on preferred intensities is a strategy worth examining for increasing adherence to exercise programs.

Numerous studies have assessed physiological and psychological responses to acute exercise of varying intensities, including preferred and self-selected, but we found only one intervention that compared adherence to a prescribed and a preferred exercise program. Forty-three women with symptoms of depression were randomized to supervised exercise at their preferred exertion level or in accordance with national guidelines for 30 minutes, three times per week for four weeks (Callaghan, Khalil, and Morres 2009). Dropout rates were similar, and adherence was greater in the preferred group (66% vs. 50%). In addition, depression scores decreased significantly in the preferred group but not in the prescribed group. Although better outcomes were found for the preferred training group, they also received 15 to 20 minutes of motivational support each session, whereas the prescribed group received healthy lifestyle education for an equal amount of time. Effects on adherence and psychological outcome could not be attributed solely to exercising at a preferred intensity.

Injury appears to have a strong influence on maintaining or abandoning regular physical activity, and a well-documented dose–response relationship exists between physical activity and orthopedic injuries (Macera et al. 1989). Injuries from high-intensity, high-volume exercise can end an exercise program, but participants' subjective responses to injury can influence the probability that they will adopt an alternative exercise mode when injured.

Characteristics of physical activity influence exercise behavior, but factors moderating the adoption and maintenance of various intensities and modes of exercise are probably different. However, few studies have examined the differences in the determinants of the adoption and maintenance of various exercise modes (e.g., walking vs. weight training).

ISSUES IN RESEARCH

The more than 400 published studies of physical activity correlates (e.g., Sallis and Owen 1999; Trost et al. 2002) should give some general indication of what is and what is not related to participation in exercise programs and overall level of physical activity. Several variables have already been described that have consistent associations with physical activity (e.g., age and income). However, physical activity behavior is complicated and dynamic, and it is not surprising that no single variable can reliably describe and predict level of physical activity. Indeed, variables are likely different for different people, and the level of influence and specific key factors change during the natural history of the behavior and as a function of developmental periods. For example, some correlates of physical activity are similar for children and adolescents (e.g., self-efficacy), but many more personal, social, and environmental influences are different (Sallis, Prochaska, and Taylor 2000).

The accurate measurement of suspected determinants is a primary issue in physical activity research. The assessment of some demographic variables, such as sex and age, is fairly consistent across studies. However, several instruments can be used to measure the same psychosocial construct. For example, two studies on the influence of enjoyment on exercise maintenance yielded opposite results, but they used different instruments to measure enjoyment. There are also different ways to measure environmental factors (e.g., actual and perceived) that can muddle the ability to compare study results.

Drawing conclusions about the relationship between exercise and purported determinants is complicated by the variety of instruments used to measure the same psychosocial construct and by the specific nature of some psychological variables. For example, there is a general acceptance of exercise self-efficacy as an exercise determinant, but global exercise self-efficacy measures may not present a true picture of the relationship between self-efficacy and exercise. By definition, self-efficacy is situation specific, and measures of self-efficacy should be specific to the study design and hypotheses. Specific self-efficacy scales, such as barrier, coping, resisting relapse, task, and making time to exercise, will help tease out the relationship between self-efficacy and the process of exercise adoption, maintenance, relapse, and resumption. Self-efficacy for resisting relapse would also be

> There is no consensus for measuring physical activity, and potential psychosocial and environmental correlates of exercise have been assessed using a variety of instruments and methods.

less relevant than task self-efficacy for someone learning a resistance training routine, whereas self-efficacy for making time to exercise would be more useful in discriminating level of physical activity in a cross-sectional design. A global measure of self-efficacy would not be as sensitive as specific measures of exercise self-efficacy would be under these conditions.

Research on exercise correlates is also limited by an absence of uniform standards for defining and assessing physical activity. There are considerable challenges in accurately measuring physical activity that can affect our ability to identify exercise correlates (see chapter 2). Self-reports of physical activity are less accurate for people who exercise irregularly. Activities at moderate and low intensities are easily forgotten and difficult to measure, making it hard to discover the factors that control the adoption of and adherence to these types of physical activity. It is also difficult to get accurate estimates of levels of physical activity in children, and *how* children engage in activity is a further complication. Children may have many short (less than 1 min) bouts of high-intensity exercise throughout the day, making it hard to quantify the volume of activity and their energy expenditure.

SUMMARY

Determinants of exercise and physical activity are variables that have shown consistent correlations with level of activity. Age, sex, education, income, motivation, self-efficacy, perceived barriers, enjoyment, self-schemata, lack of time, exercise history, social support, and season are some of the variables that have shown repeated associations with physical activity and exercise. However, complex multiple interactions among exercise determinants change over time. Making sense of inconsistencies in the research is challenging, but identifying factors that are significantly associated with level of physical activity and the adoption and maintenance of regular exercise is a valuable line of research with practical benefits. Understanding the personal and environmental factors associated with sedentary lifestyles and low rates of adoption and adherence can help identify high-risk groups to which programs can be directed. Identifying modifiable variables that have strong and consistent associations with adoption and adherence can focus the direction of interventions on multiple levels, including changes in the structured environment. However, too few studies are available on children, people who are elderly, those who are physically challenged, and ethnic and minority groups. Moreover, direct comparisons of variables affecting exercise behavior in males and females are limited, as are studies specific to exercise mode. Issues in the measurement of physical activity and purported determinants must be considered in evaluating and designing research in this area.

WEBSITES

www.cdc.gov/nchs/nhis.htm

www.cdc.gov/brfss

www.cdc.gov/HealthyYouth/yrbs/index.htm

chapter 14

Theories of Behavior Change

Throughout the centuries philosophers, and more recently psychologists, have tried to understand why people behave the way they do. Many attempts have been made to organize information about people and the world around them that can be used to explain and predict human behavior. However, countless individual and contextual variables interact in patterns to influence behavior, and these patterns change over time. This complex abundance of information has been reduced and made more manageable through the application of theories.

Exercise psychology has applied several theories from the social, psychological, and biological literatures to explain and predict the effects of physical activity on mental health. Various theories have also been applied to explain and predict the adoption and maintenance of an active lifestyle. In chapter 15 on interventions, you will see how various theoretical perspectives that are used to reach the same goal can result in different treatments and different interpretations about what influenced the outcome. This chapter focuses on the major theories that have guided exercise psychology research. We discuss basic definitions and core concepts and provide examples of how the theories have been applied.

A theory is a type of model (see table 14.1). Models are generalized, simplified representations that are used to organize vast amounts of information. Models guide our thoughts and actions by defining which of myriad variables to focus on and which to ignore in a given situation. They help us explain and predict the world around us. Models allow us to interpret information in similar ways. Even the novice computer user knows that the small picture of a printer on the computer screen can be used to control the printer's functions. The picture of a printer is an iconic model. **Iconic models** are models with two or three dimensions that look like what they represent but are smaller or larger. **Analogue models**, such as graphs and maps, use a set of properties to represent the actual set of properties of the idea or event using transformational rules (e.g., 1 in. = 1.5 miles [2.4 km]). Conceptual models are diagrams of proposed causal linkages among a set of concepts that are believed to be related to a particular research question or are the focus of an intervention. Conceptual models are informed by theories and empirical findings, and can include elements from multiple theories conceptualized at multiple levels. Sometimes components are included that are not part of the established theory (e.g., personality) but represent empirical findings or the experience of professionals.

Theories are symbolic models that are used to guide the design, execution, and interpretation of research. A theory is the formulation of underlying principles of certain observed phenomena that have been verified to some degree. Theories of human behavior provide assumptions about behavior and specify relationships among key variables that are necessary for explaining and predicting behavior. Theories allow us to predict what will occur beyond empirical evidence; they allow us to go beyond what we already know. For example, the theory of behaviorism emphasizes antecedents and consequences of a target behavior to predict the frequency of that behavior. If we know that Jeff likes to spend time with Mary, we can predict that he will run more if he runs with Mary, who exercises regularly.

Theories of behavior change are models that represent human behavior. Over the years, several theories have been developed to order all the things that could influence what people do

Table 14.1 Types of Models

Model type	Description
Iconic	A two- or three-dimensional model that looks like what it represents, but is larger or smaller. Examples include photographs and sculptures.
Analogue	An actual set of properties of an idea or event represented in two or three dimensions using transformational rules that can represent change or a process. Examples include maps and graphs. For example, attendance in an aerobics class over 12 weeks can be presented in a graph, with the time in weeks on the x-axis and the percentage of participants attending each week on the y-axis.
Conceptual	A graphic or pictorial representation of constructs and their relationships to represent a specific hypothesis, context, relationship, problem, or topic. Examples include a visual representation of a theory (see figure 14.3) and a framework for organizing and integrating information (see figure 2.1).
Symbolic	Intrinsically meaningless symbols that represent ideas, events, or things and are not at all like what they represent. Examples include scripts and mathematical models. Theories are linguistic or mathematical models that guide the design, execution, and interpretation of research. The exercise and self-esteem model in figure 12.3 has been tested in several research studies.
Mixed	A combination of models that represent large and complex amounts of information. Examples include websites and books. The 2008 Physical Activity Guidelines for Americans can be viewed on a website at www.health.gov/paguidelines.

and why they do it. These theories represent various **ontological** assumptions (about what things are made of) and **cosmological** assumptions (about how things are organized and how they change). For example, behaviorism is based on a **materialistic** perspective on the nature of reality that reduces the mind to the functioning of the nervous system and biochemical and electrical processes. Behavior is described through linear chains of cause-and-effect relationships in which a stimulus and response are linked through learning. Cognitive psychologies stem from **idealism**, in which reality is seen as the expression or embodiment of the mind. What we do, how we feel, and how things affect us are presumed to be influenced by learned

associations among thoughts, affects, actions, and contexts. Thus, theories influence the ideas we accept and the actions we perform. They enable us to interpret and organize information in a logical and consistent format. Theories also spur research to support or refute that they are correct in the way they view behavior.

BEHAVIORISM

In the early part of the 20th century, John B. Watson (1919) wrote *Psychology From the Standpoint of a Behaviorist,* in which he asserted that psychology should be a science of behavior and not of the mind. Watson was followed by B.F. Skinner, whose first important book, *The Behavior of Organisms,* was published in 1938. Skinner and his colleagues conducted numerous carefully controlled laboratory experiments over the next 40 years in their search for observable facts that affect learning. They developed empirically derived principles of behavior that include a central role for environmental determinants. Behaviorism, also known as learning theory, is based on the assumptions that psychology is

> Theories are principles and assumptions that are used to explain and predict; theories of behavior change are models of human behavior.

about behavior and that a true account of behavior should not consider mental states, which are not open to direct observation and cannot be measured independently. Personality is seen as the sum of an individual's observed responses to the external world.

Using behaviorism as a theoretical foundation involves focusing on the quantitative relationships between **independent** (cause, stimulus) and **dependent** (effect, response) **variables**. Key variables and predictions center on the relationships among stimulus, response, and consequences. As already mentioned, the emphasis is on looking at linear chains of cause-and-effect relationships in which the stimulus and response are linked through learning. Empirical research, which assumes that encounters with objects and events yield objective knowledge, provides the foundation for approaching the explanation and prediction of behavior. Change or learning is assumed to work the same way for all people.

> **K**ey variables in behaviorism to explain and predict behavior are the observable antecedents and consequences of the behavior.

Classical conditioning and **operant conditioning** provide the framework for understanding and modifying behavior through associative learning. Classical conditioning entails learning to associate two stimuli and is based on the work of Ivan Pavlov, whose ideas played an important role in the development of behaviorism. An **unconditioned** (or reinforcing) **stimulus** that is capable of eliciting a reflexive response is paired with a neutral stimulus. You may be familiar with the example of the pairing of food, which elicits salivation in the dog, with the ringing of a bell. Eventually, the dog salivates when the bell rings even though no food is present. The bell has become a **conditioned stimulus** and will continue to elicit the salivation in the dog (now a conditioned response) unless the bell is never paired with the food again. In this case, the salivation response will diminish and eventually disappear, a process called extinction.

Behaviorism

Stimulus → *Learning* → Response → Consequences

Operant conditioning involves pairing a reinforcing or punishing event with a voluntary response to change the rate of responding. In this case, the respondent learns to associate a response with its consequences. To enhance the response rate, a **reinforcing stimulus** (e.g., a reward) should occur in the presence of another stimulus when a specific response occurs. The rat that got a food pellet when it pressed the bar received a reinforcer (food) when the voluntary behavior of pressing the bar occurred. Eventually, the response (operant behavior) may be emitted in the presence of the other stimulus, or in this case, when the rat encounters the bar. A **discriminative stimulus**, or prompt, is an environmental cue about the nature of a behavioral consequence. Cheese bubbling on a pizza (discriminative stimulus) indicates a very good chance that eating the pizza (behavior) will result in a burned mouth (behavioral consequence).

Obviously, stimuli and the reinforcing events are critical variables for understanding and predicting behavior when one uses behaviorism as a theoretical foundation. Events and situations coming before (**antecedents**, stimulus, cues) and after (**consequences**, **reinforcement**, rewards, punishments) a specific behavior are identified to explain the behavior. Consequences that will explain the behavior should be related directly, either concretely or symbolically, to that behavior. Changes in the consequences will increase or decrease the frequency of the behavior. For example, feeling relaxed and in a good mood after jogging will increase the frequency of this behavior. If jogging, now a conditioned behavior, no longer results in reinforcement (e.g., hot weather makes the jogging stressful), the behavior tends to occur less often and will eventually be extinguished if consequences continue to be unpleasant.

Antecedents and Consequences

Concrete antecedent: dog barking until you take her out for a walk

Concrete consequence: fatigue after a vigorous exercise session

Symbolic antecedent: coupon for a free aerobics class

Symbolic consequence: certificate for completing an exercise program

Behavior theory has been useful in conceptualizing the types of antecedents and consequences that can influence exercise adoption and maintenance (see table 14.2). **Latency**, the amount of time that passes between the stimulus and the response, can be used to identify antecedents and consequences as **proximal** (close in time to the target behavior) or **distal** (occurring long before or after the target behavior). For example, a notice that the swimming pool will be closed in two weeks is a distal antecedent to attending aerobics classes or jogging while the pool is closed. Clear and cool weather when a jogger wakes up can be a proximal antecedent for running that morning. Being late for class after completing an additional two sets of strengthening exercises is a proximal consequence of that exercise session. Losing or

maintaining weight is a distal consequence of regular exercise.

Many earlier research studies on exercise adherence were based on the principles of behaviorism and used reinforcement control and stimulus control to increase physical activity. It was presumed that behavioral patterns are sustained because they are cued and reinforced. Thus, exercise was viewed as a behavior that can be modified (acquired and maintained) by changing the antecedents, the behavior itself (skill development, shaping), and the consequences (rewards, reinforcement) of the behavior. For example, several studies reported using contingency contracting, in which subjects received specific rewards after meeting predetermined criteria for exercise frequency and duration. Little or no attention was given to cognitive processes, affect, or motivation.

COGNITIVE BEHAVIORISM

The early work of Donald Meichenbaum, one of the founders of the "cognitive revolution" in psychotherapy, laid the groundwork for extending behavior modification to include cognitions and thus for developing cognitive behaviorism. In one study, the behavior of impulsive first- and second-grade children was altered by training them to talk to themselves first overtly and then covertly to increase self-control (Meichenbaum and Goodman 1971). Subsequent research in clinical populations indicated that traditional behavior modification strategies supplemented

Table 14.2 Types of Antecedents and Consequences Predicted to Influence Exercise Behavior

Type	Examples
Environmental	Weather, commercials, media, air quality, access to facilities, safety, time
Social	Modeling (in media and face-to-face), friends, family
Cognitive	Thoughts, attitudes, beliefs, values; emotions; self-efficacy, self-concept; motivation
Physiological	Health, fitness, ability
Personal	Exercise history, health history, education, income, personality, traits
Perceptual	Fatigue, pain, vigor

with self-instructional training resulted in better and more sustained outcomes (Meichenbaum and Cameron 1994). This led to the conclusion that what the person says to him- or herself, rather than environmental consequences of behavior, is of primary importance in modifying maladaptive behaviors.

Cognitive behaviorism is a theoretical perspective that shares some assumptions with behaviorism. The stimulus and the response are central to explaining behavior, but a significant difference from behaviorism is that cognition is defined as the critical mediating variable. Whereas behaviorism contends that matter is the only reality and that reality is understood though the physical sciences, cognitive behaviorism is based on an interactive dualistic perspective. This perspective in turn is based on the assumption that we are made up of both material and nonmaterial phenomena (dualism). The nonmaterial phenomena include sensations, perceptions, thoughts, and feelings that interact with and influence the material self.

A wide range of dysfunctional or maladaptive behavior results from faulty cognitions and beliefs that have an effect on behavior through the resulting emotional response. Learning or insight can restructure, augment, or replace faulty thoughts with behaviorally effective beliefs and cognitive skills. Simply put, cognitions cause behavior, and cognitions can be changed. Thus, the key to changing behavior is to change thoughts. A popular strategy based on this model is **cognitive restructuring**. Cognitions are identified that limit the likelihood of positive action by eliciting a negative emotional response, such as a sense of futility ("I can never stick with an exercise program"). The faulty statement is reframed to be more realistic and supportive of the potential for change ("I have not been able to maintain regular exercise yet"). A number of strategies that have emerged from cognitive

> **C**ognitive behaviorism holds that cognitions determine behavior and that cognitions can be changed.

behaviorism, such as self-monitoring and goal setting, have been used frequently in exercise behavior change interventions (see chapter 15).

SOCIAL COGNITIVE THEORY

Social cognitive theory evolved from social learning theory, which proposes that the majority of behaviors are learned through social interaction. Social cognitive theory was formalized in the mid-1980s through the work of Albert Bandura. Walter Mischel is a contemporary of Bandura's who emphasized cognitive and situational variables in understanding human behavior, and contended that intra-individual cognition was an important influence on behavior. Bandura built on the idea of intra-individual cognition and extended his own work on observational learning and self-regulation. Bandura's *Social Foundations of Thought and Action: A Social Cognitive Theory* (1986) describes the conceptual framework of this theory.

Social cognitive theory uses cognitions in the context of social interactions and behavior to explain human action, motivation, and emotion. Important concepts in social cognitive theories are described in table 14.3. Basic assumptions of social cognitive theory are that behavior is founded in cognitive activity, is purposeful action, and is under the direct control of the individual—that is, individuals are capable of self-reflection and self-regulation. **Self-reflection** refers to an ability to symbolize and thus anticipate and plan for future events. Something that a person anticipates will occur in the future becomes a mental formulation in the present time and can motivate current behavior. Behavior is thus controlled and regulated in anticipation of symbolized future events.

Another assumption within social cognitive theory is that self-regulating processes mediate the effects of most environmental influences. Cognitive mechanisms that support **self-regulation** (e.g., how people modify their own behavior) include personal goal setting, efficacy expectations, outcome expectations, and outcome values. The ability to symbolize and conceptualize a future helps to guide the development of goals, which are devised according

Table 14.3 Key Variables in Social Cognitive Theory

Variable	Explanation
Outcome expectancies	Outcomes are what is expected to happen externally and to oneself as the result of a behavior. Benefits (desired outcomes) and costs (undesired outcomes) can have various influences depending on their relationship to the behavior (proximal or distal) and the individual's perceived vulnerability.
Outcome value	The outcome can have varying degrees of reinforcement value or incentive value, and can be something one wishes to obtain or to avoid.
Intention	Intention is the strength of readiness to perform a behavior.
Self-efficacy expectancy	Self-efficacy is a cognition. It is a belief in one's ability to engage successfully in a specific behavior with a known outcome.

Assumptions of Social Cognitive Theory

1. People have symbolizing capabilities.
2. Behavior is purposive or goal directed and is guided by forethought. This is dependent on the capability to symbolize.
3. People are self-reflective; they can analyze and evaluate their own thoughts and experiences.
4. People are capable of self-regulation. They can alter their own behavior and their environment, and they adopt personal standards for their behavior and use those standards to guide behavior and motivate themselves.
5. Environmental events, inner personal factors (cognition, emotion, and biological events), and behavior are mutually interacting influences (triadic reciprocality.

to standards whose achievement will elicit positive self-evaluation. Goals are set that represent valued and desired objectives and point out a discrepancy between *actual* behavior and the *target* behavior. The discrepancy provides negative feedback that stimulates the direction and intensity of actions to reduce the incongruity.

For example, Joe believes that running a 5K road race (target behavior) will demonstrate that he is a good runner, and he values this self-concept. However, Joe can run only 3K without stopping (actual behavior). The discrepancy between how far he *wants* to run and how far he *can* run helps to direct his training program. Thus, goals provide direction and motivation in support of self-regulation.

Self-efficacy is the degree to which people believe they can successfully engage in specific behaviors in particular situations with known outcomes. Self-efficacy is a learned belief that is developed through experiences and modeling. It includes three domains: strength, generality, and level. Strength refers to the perceived ability to overcome common barriers to engaging in a behavior *(Can I make time during lunch to go for a walk?)*. Generality is the ability to generalize the behavior to other similar behaviors *(If I can play tennis, can I also play racquetball?)*. Level is the degree to which a behavior can be engaged in successfully *(If I can run 3 miles with friends, can I run in a 5K race? Can I train for and run in a 10K race?)*. The significance of self-efficacy in behavior change is further developed in Bandura's self-efficacy theory.

Outcome expectation is the perception that a given behavior will lead to a certain outcome. Outcomes are what one expects to happen to oneself and to the external situation as a result of a behavior. The influence of benefits (desired outcomes) and costs (undesired outcomes) on the behavior depends on a variety of factors, such as whether they are proximal or distal to

According to social cognitive theory, behavior is the outcome of social learning, and characteristics of the person, environment, and behavior itself interact to influence behavior.

Triadic Reciprocality (Example)

The likelihood that a young woman will participate in vigorous exercise depends on what benefits she expects from exercising and the value she places on that outcome (person variables), access to a safe place to exercise and peer influences (environmental variables), and the level of intensity and type of exercise (characteristics of the behavior). Having a safe place to play basketball could influence the perceived benefits of someone who knows she will need an athletic scholarship to attend college, but a peer making fun of the way she dribbles can affect her perception of benefits versus costs, the intensity of her practice, or both.

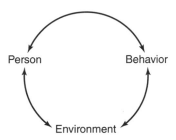

Triadic reciprocality

Assumption: environmental events, inner personal factors (cognition, emotion, and biological events), and behavior are mutually interacting influences.

the behavior. For example, if Sue walks for an hour after work 5 days a week, she believes she will lose weight (distal desired outcome), but she will have less time to spend with her family (proximal undesired outcome).

Outcome value refers to the incentive value or reinforcement value of the outcome. Value is determined in part by the extent to which the outcome will affect the person's sense of welfare and self-esteem. Thus, the outcome can be something one wants to obtain or avoid, and the strength of the value will influence effort and persistence. For example, Brad entered a new high school in the fall, and the boys in his class had been lifting weights for several years. Brad started working out with weights every day after school. Increasing muscular strength and size is very important to Brad because he wants to be more like his new friends and fit in.

A central assumption of social cognitive theory is that people also influence the environment, and this influence is bidirectional (e.g., reciprocal determinism). It is proposed that behavior change operates through mutually interactive effects among aspects of the person, the environment, and the behavior itself. This concept of a dynamic reciprocal interaction, called **triadic reciprocality**, was applied in chapter 13 to frame the relationships among physical activity correlates. Exercise correlates have been organized into three categories—person, environment, and behavior—but research to test the dynamic interactions among them has been limited.

BANDURA'S SELF-EFFICACY THEORY

Bandura's self-efficacy theory is a competency-based theory that has been applied extensively to exercise behavior in healthy adults (Ashford, Edmunds, and French 2010), children and adolescents (Lubans, Foster, and Biddle 2008), older adults (Netz et al. 2005), and clinical populations (Artinian et al. 2010). An assumption of this theory is that the primary mediator of all behavior change is the cognitive mechanism called self-efficacy, which has been described as an important variable in social cognitive theory and in the transtheoretical model of behavior change. According to Bandura's self-efficacy theory, self-efficacy expectancy, outcome expectancy, and outcome value are three basic cognitive mediating processes that determine behavior (see

Cognitive Mediating Processes That Determine Behavior). Adoption and persistence in behaviors are determined by expectations about one's skills and capabilities to engage successfully in the specific target behavior in particular situations, as well as expectations about the outcomes and the value placed on those outcomes.

The higher the self-efficacy, the higher the goals one sets and the more persistence one exhibits toward reaching those goals. People dissatisfied with their current exercise or fitness

Cognitive Mediating Processes That Determine Behavior

- *Self-efficacy expectancy:* Beliefs and expectations about how capable one is to perform the necessary behaviors to achieve an outcome. Self-efficacy is specific to a situation and behavior, but it can generalize to other similar situations and behavioral demands. High self-efficacy for following an aerobics routine increases the likelihood someone will enroll in an aerobics class, but might not generalize to confidence in beginning weight training.

- *Outcome expectancy:* The estimation of the probability that a behavior will produce a specific outcome or result. Desired outcomes can be extrinsic (tangible) or intrinsic (self-respect or self-satisfaction). The outcome expected is related to the efficacy for a specific behavior. For example, one might believe that swimming is one of the best modes for achieving overall fitness but have low confidence about swimming enough on a regular basis to increase fitness.

- *Outcome value:* The reinforcement value or incentive value of the desired outcome. If increased fitness is highly valued, the effort and persistence to follow a fitness regimen are greater than if fitness is not valued.

Self-Efficacy Expectations (Example)

At his medical exam, Matt weighed 10 pounds (4.5 kg) more than his target weight. This information motivates him to seek strategies to achieve his goal weight. Self-efficacy expectations will determine his choice of goals, strategies, effort, and persistence and the affective responses he has to his level of performance. If Matt is confident that he can fit a walking program into his schedule but has always had problems sticking with any diet, he will be more likely to control his weight by exercising than by changing his eating habits unless his expectations about diet change. The adoption of a behavior follows from self-initiated reactions that are stimulated by a discrepancy between personal goals or standards and knowledge of personal achievement.

levels who adopt challenging goals and are confident (i.e., have high self-efficacy) that they can attain their goals will presumably have optimal motivation for maintaining exercise (Dzewaltowski 1994). People with high self-efficacy who fail often will attribute the failure to insufficient effort and are likely to persist. Those with low self-efficacy may attribute failure to low ability and be more likely to give up.

Self-efficacy expectations are developed from performance accomplishments (i.e., mastery experiences), vicarious experiences (i.e., modeling or observing others), verbal persuasion (i.e., encouragement or positive feedback), and the interpretation of physiological or psychological arousal (e.g., anxiety, perceived exertion). Performance accomplishments provide the most potent influence on efficacy expectations. Self-efficacy increases when one masters difficult or previously feared tasks. Skills are developed and refined and coping mechanisms are developed through personal experiences. Vicarious experiences are experiences in which people learn by observing events or people. Observing someone similar to oneself succeeding through effort and being rewarded increases one's efficacy to also perform that behavior. Verbal persuasion can take the form of self-talk or encouragement from significant others. High physiological arousal during the performance of a task can impair performance and decrease efficacy expectations. Strategies to change behavior based on self-efficacy theory focus on manipulating these sources of efficacy information to increase exercise self-efficacy.

THEORY OF PLANNED BEHAVIOR

The theory of planned behavior (TPB) evolved from the theory of reasoned action (TRA), which was developed by Fishbein and Ajzen to explain and predict social behavior in specific contexts (e.g., Ajzen and Fishbein 1974). A basic assump-

tion is that people make rational decisions about their behavior based on information and beliefs about the behavior and its consequences, what they expect, and the value they place on the outcome. These beliefs and attitudes are influenced by individual and environmental factors, such as personality, education, past behavior, and cultural factors. However, the most important predictor of behavior is the intention, or readiness, to perform or not perform the behavior (see figure 14.1).

Intention is a person's estimate of the likelihood he or she will perform a specific behavior. It is a function of the attitude toward the behavior, the attitude toward the social norms regarding the behavior, and **perceived behavioral control**. The attitude toward the behavior is a function of the beliefs about the consequences of engaging in the behavior and an evaluation of those consequences (cost–benefit analysis). People can have many beliefs about a behavior and evaluations of the consequences related

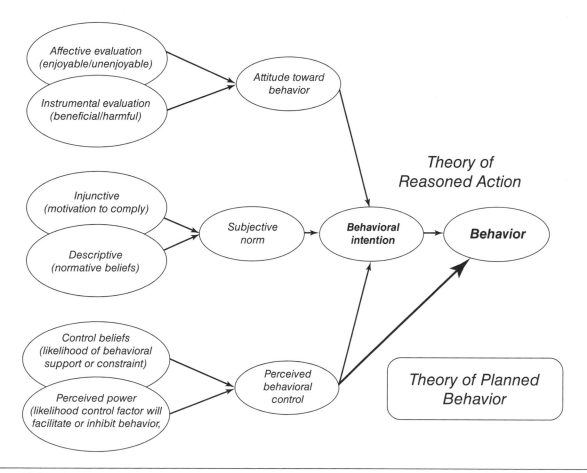

Figure 14.1 The theory of reasoned action and the theory of planned behavior.

to each belief—that is, the overall evaluations of performing the behavior. For example, Jim may believe that exercise can help him lower his serum cholesterol, but maintaining a regular exercise program will take time away from writing his dissertation. Subjective norms (i.e., perceived social pressure to perform the behavior) consist of perceptions of what other people think about the behavior (Jim's best friend Bob enjoys competing in triathlons) and the person's motivation to comply with others' expectations (Bob wants Jim to bike with him this weekend, and Jim wants to spend time with Bob). Perceived behavioral control is the perception of how easy or difficult the behavior will be based on an evaluation of the barriers and resources. Perceived behavioral control can influence the target behavior directly and can also be mediated by intention.

More than 200 exercise studies have been published using TPB, and consistent strong associations have been found between intentions and level of physical activity, as well as between exercise intention and perceived behavioral control, and between exercise intention and attitude (Rhodes and Nigg 2011). Perceived behavioral control can influence behavior directly (see figure 14.2) to the extent that perceptions of control include actual behavioral influences, such as the skills necessary for carrying out the behavior, opportunities, and resources (e.g., Rhodes and Courneya 2003). However, associations between subjective norms and exercise intentions typically have been weak (Fishbein 2008; Rhodes and Nigg 2011). In addition, this model gives a static profile of beliefs and attitudes and does not account for changes in cognitions over time.

Applications of TPB to exercise behavior research have typically involved measures that are specific to the behavior, context, and goal in question (e.g., Hausenblas, Carron, and Mack 1997; Kimiecik 1992). Fishbein (2008) emphasizes the importance of defining a target behavior in terms of action in a specific context directed at a target at a certain point in time. This is valuable when helping someone come up with a clear plan to exercise, and when measuring intentions and behavior. For example, a scale to measure exercise intentions could include the statement *I intended to do strength training*

> **S**elf-determination theory is based on assumptions that people are motivated to engage in behaviors to meet three basic human needs and that motivation varies in the degree of self-regulation on a continuum.

every other day for the next two weeks rated on a 7-point scale from 1 (*strongly disagree*) to 7 (*strongly agree*). This specificity in measurement is a major strength of TPB given the wide variety of exercise behaviors and settings.

SELF-DETERMINATION THEORY

Historically, researchers have examined motivation in terms of volume or amount, but in the 1980s, Edward Deci and Richard Ryan proposed that the type and quality of motivation would be more important in predicting behavior, and they developed the self-determination theory (SDT) of human motivation. SDT is a broad theory that addresses personality development; self-regulation; psychological needs; life goals and aspirations; energy and vitality; nonconscious processes; relations of culture to motivation; and the impact of the social environment on motivation, affect, behavior, and well-being (Deci and Ryan 2008). The four subcomponents that constitute SDT are the basic needs theory, cognitive evaluation theory, organismic integration theory, and causality orientation theory (see Ryan and Deci 2002).

The assumption that autonomy, competence, and relatedness are basic psychological needs is a key aspect of SDT. The degree to which these needs are fulfilled or thwarted is the basis for individual differences in motivation. Exercise psychologists can thus analyze a behavioral strategy or environmental factors with respect to its effect on meeting these needs. For example, running alone at a time you choose satisfies autonomy needs, but running a challenging course with a good friend can satisfy the needs for competency and relatedness. If we can set

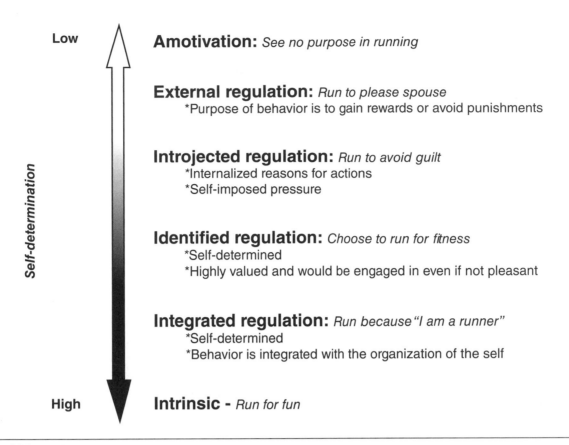

Low

Amotivation: *See no purpose in running*

External regulation: *Run to please spouse*
  *Purpose of behavior is to gain rewards or avoid punishments

Introjected regulation: *Run to avoid guilt*
  *Internalized reasons for actions
  *Self-imposed pressure

Identified regulation: *Choose to run for fitness*
  *Self-determined
  *Highly valued and would be engaged in even if not pleasant

Integrated regulation: *Run because "I am a runner"*
  *Self-determined
  *Behavior is integrated with the organization of the self

High

Intrinsic - *Run for fun*

Self-determination

Figure 14.2 Self-determination continuum.

up a situation in which exercise addresses these basic needs, motivation will be stronger and adherence will be more likely. In fact, several physical activity interventions based on SDT have used strategies that foster a sense of control over the exercise routine, offer mastery experiences, and promote social support (see chapter 15).

Motivation has been classified as intrinsic (e.g., exercise for enjoyment) or extrinsic (e.g., exercise for reward or to avoid negative consequences separate from behavior) based on goals or reasons for the behavior. Generally, when the purpose of exercise is more intrinsic, it is more likely to be sustained. Often, exercise for extrinsic reasons (e.g., to lose weight) is discontinued when the external goal is met because exercise was just a means to an end. SDT extends the idea of motivation and describes a continuum of motivation based on level of autonomy from autonomous (intrinsic) to controlled (extrinsic) motivation (Deci and Ryan 2008; see figure 14.2).

Autonomous motivation is developed through the ongoing satisfaction of basic needs and involves choice or a self-endorsement of one's

action. Autonomous motivation has the highest level of self-determination and is associated with intrinsic motivation. Valuing or enjoying the activity underpins intrinsic motivation and is contrasted with engaging in the activity because of self-imposed pressure or the promise of rewards separable from the behavior itself (extrinsic motivation). More extrinsic regulatory styles involve external and internalized regulations of behavior that arise from external rewards or punishments, or from internal pressures (e.g., Mark bicycles to class because it is better for the environment than driving a short distance, even though he would really rather drive). External regulations of motivation can foster contingent self-esteem, approval motives, and avoidance of feelings of guilt and shame. For example, Mary exercises only because she wants to lose weight, and she feels good about herself when she follows her weekly exercise plan. If she misses a day of exercise, she feels guilty.

In general, autonomous motivation leads to better psychological health and long-term persistence in the motivated behavior (Deci and Ryan 2008). Studies have also shown associations between more intrinsic regulation of exercise behavior and psychological well-being. Cross-sectional studies have found that different types of motivation are associated with different levels of exercise; that is, people who have more intrinsic motivation for exercise also exercise more than those with more externally regulated motivation (e.g., Edmunds, Ntoumanis, and Duda 2006). Moreover, longitudinal studies indicate corresponding changes in level of exercise and more intrinsic motivations (Rodgers et al. 2010). Researchers have also examined the role of goal content (what) and motives (why) and found that more intrinsic goal content is associated with more sustained exercise (Wilson, Mack, and Grattan 2008). However, it is important to address both goal content and motives because, for example, someone can exercise to be healthy (an intrinsic goal) and be motivated to do so out of guilt (introjected regulation), whereas someone else can walk to lose weight (an extrinsic goal) because he enjoys walking (intrinsic regulation). The application of SDT in interventions, such as applying strategies to enhance autonomy, competence, and relatedness, is covered in chapter 15.

Some researchers are beginning to study the pattern and process of motivational regulation development in respect to exercise, which is important in the development and application of SDT. Rodgers and colleagues (2010) examined results from six studies that measured motivational regulations (external, introjected, identified, and intrinsic motivation; see figure 14.2) and exercise. Two studies were cross-sectional assessments of adults reporting regular exercise ($n = 202$; $n = 1,054$), and four were intervention studies (n range = 38-160) that lasted from 10 to 24 weeks. Although participants at the end of the interventions became more autonomous in their motivation to exercise, they were still lower on all types of self-regulation compared to regular exercisers in the cross-sectional samples. More controlled (extrinsic) regulation did not change much after the interventions. However, identified regulation changed faster than intrinsic motivation, which implies that although exercise may not be inherently enjoyable for many people, it can be valued. From

this, the researchers speculated that substantial changes toward self-regulated motivation can occur early in an exercise program, but levels for these exercisers are still not as high as those for regular exercisers even after six months of training. Rodgers and colleagues (2010) propose that self-determined forms of motivation are not well developed enough after six months of regular exercise to sustain behavior, calling to question the six-month marker proposed in some research and theory (e.g., the transtheoretical model described later).

STAGE THEORIES

The general paradigm for predicting behavior in the early development of behavior change theories was based on order, stability, and equilibrium. Theories of causality, such as behaviorism, evolved from a mechanistic view in which fixed-sequence pathways were said to link events in patterns of cause-and-effect relationships. The view was that the elements necessary for change and their interactions were not modified by their relationships or history, and that change was predictable and controllable.

The influence of **field theory** led to a broadening of the concept of change to include the proposition that events are a function of the nature and organization of *all* conditions in which they are embedded. Most of the theories presented so far have conceptualized behavior change as an event that is influenced by a number of variables in a linear pattern. People are placed on a continuum of probability of change according to their scores on multiple predictor variables. Newer models have been influenced formally and informally by quantum theory, nonlinear thermodynamics, and chaos theory to consider the contributions of instability, diversity, multiple dimensions and levels of effect, nonlinear relationships, and temporality in explaining change. The latter concept—that

Stage models of behavior reflect the dynamic, nonlinear process of behavior change.

of a temporal dimension—has been included in some of the newer and more promising stage models of behavior change.

Stage theories assign each individual to one of a limited number of categories, or stages. Those in the same stage are similar to each other with respect to specific characteristics, such as level of physical activity, and those in different stages demonstrate substantial differences in these characteristics. Stage theories may also include parameters for how long people stay in a particular stage and for the usual sequence of movement from stage to stage. People typically spend a certain amount of time or accomplish specific tasks in stage A before they are ready to move to stage B. However, movement through the stages of health behavior change is not inevitable or progressive. For many people, behavior change does not follow an orderly, predictable pattern. Often, people trying to change a health behavior get stuck in a stage or cycle through stages out of sequence or at varied rates of progression. Stage models allow for the process to go forward, go backward, cycle, or stop, providing a context for describing relapse and readoption.

In addition to the concept of irregular progression, stage theories define barriers to change that are similar among people in specific stages and are important for progression to the next stage. Because there are different barriers in each stage and specific tasks that must be accomplished to move to the next stage, stage models imply stage-specific interventions. For example, the health action process approach developed by Schwarzer (1992) distinguishes between motivational (decisional) and volitional (action) phases of health behavior change. People develop an intention to act in the motivational stage based on self-efficacy, perception of risk, and the pros and cons of action. Strategies to help people decide to start regular exercise could involve enhancing task self-efficacy, identifying the risks of inactivity, and pointing out the benefits of an active lifestyle. In the volitional stage, action planning is necessary for fostering the initiation of the goal behavior by specifying when, where, and how to act (e.g., after supper, go to the gym and walk around the track for 30 min), whereas coping planning involves identifying situations that put engaging in the behavior at risk and developing suitable coping responses (e.g., when there is an evening PTA meeting, get up 45 minutes earlier and walk before breakfast).

The **transtheoretical model of behavior change (TTM)**, also known as the stages of change model, is a general model of intentional behavior change that includes a temporal component as a critical factor in describing and predicting behavior. It is the stage model most frequently applied to exercise (see table 14.4). In the late 1970s, Prochaska and DiClemente, observing smokers trying to quit without professional intervention, found that these self-changers passed through specific stages as they tried to decrease or eliminate this health-related behavior. Prochaska and DiClemente developed transtheoretical therapy in the late 1970s and early 1980s based on this research and a transtheoretical analysis of 18 leading systems of psychotherapy (see Prochaska 1979; Prochaska and DiClemente 1982, 1983). The principles and mechanisms of transtheoretical therapy were

Table 14.4 The process of adopting and maintaining regular exercise is described through specific stages of behavior change.

Stage	Intention to exercise	Exercise
Precontemplation	No	None
Contemplation	Yes (within 6 mo)	None
Preparation	Yes (within 30 d)	Irregular < criterion amount*
Action	Yes	Regular ≥ criterion amount for <6 mo
Maintenance	Yes	Regular ≥ criterion amount for >6 mo

*Usually >20 min on 3 or more days/wk, at least moderate intensity.

Stage Theories: Stages and Possible Patterns of Behavior Change

Stages of Behavior Change

A (not engaging in the target behavior)

B (not engaging in the target behavior but having strong intentions to do so)

C (recent adoption of the target behavior)

D (established participation in the target behavior)

Examples of Possible Patterns of Change

Progressive order: A →B →C →D

Backward: A →B →C →B →A

Cycle: A →B →A →B→A

then used to construct the transtheoretical model of behavior change.

The transtheoretical model describes health behavior adoption and maintenance as a process that occurs through a series of behaviorally and motivationally defined stages (see figure 14.3). Although the model was developed to describe changes in addictive behavior, it was expanded to include the adoption of preventive health behaviors and the use of medical services. Dishman in 1982, Sonstroem in 1988, and Sallis and Hovell in 1990 promoted the concept of a dynamic model of exercise behavior that included stages, and in the early 1990s, Marcus and others applied the transtheoretical model to exercise behavior (e.g., Marcus et al. 1992; Marcus and Simkin 1993). Since then, more than 100 studies have applied the transtheoretical model to exercise and physical activity.

The transtheoretical model includes three levels: stage of change, constructs hypothesized to influence behavior change, and level of change. Level of change has not been addressed in the exercise literature, and many studies applying or testing the transtheoretical model with exercise use only the first level of this model—that is, stage of change. Stage is the temporal dimension

in which change unfolds. Empirical analysis has established five distinct stages that are relatively stable but open to change. A six-month time period is typically used to define stages, assuming that six months is about as far in the future as people can anticipate making changes. A sixth stage, *termination,* represents a point at which there is 100% confidence in the ability to maintain the behavior change and there is no risk of a relapse to previous stages, although this last stage is not often used in exercise studies and is likely more appropriate for cessation of an unhealthy behavior.

The number and descriptions of exercise stages of change have been varied. For example, some researchers do not include a time frame for the intention to begin exercise (e.g., within 30 days) as a criterion for classification in the preparation stage. Others have divided preparation into two stages, characterized by some exercise but distinguished by the intention to adopt regular exercise. Physical activity stages of change have also been applied in research studies and interventions that address the U.S. Centers for Disease Control and Prevention and the American College of Sports Medicine's recommendations for daily physical activity.

The second level of the transtheoretical model includes three constructs that are hypothesized to influence behavior change. They are self-efficacy to overcome barriers, incorporated from social cognitive theory (see the discussion earlier in this chapter); **decisional balance**, which is the evaluation of the pros and cons of the target behavior; and **processes of change**, which are the strategies used for changing behavior. Several studies have examined exercise stage and self-efficacy for exercise; and in general, self-efficacy is lowest in the early stages (e.g., precontemplation) and higher in each adjacent stage, with the highest exercise self-efficacy seen in the maintenance stage. There is some longitudinal evidence that exercise self-efficacy increases as one moves from an established sedentary lifestyle to long-term maintenance of regular exercise (Dishman, Vandenberg, Motl, and Nigg 2010; Marcus et al. 1994; Plotnikoff et al. 2001). However, these data cannot tell us whether people are more active because they have higher self-efficacy, or if they have higher self-efficacy because of past success

Exercise Stages (Example)

- *Precontemplation stage:* People are inactive and have no intention to start exercising. They are not seriously thinking about changing their level of exercise within the next six months, or they deny the need to change.

- *Contemplation stage:* People are also inactive, but they intend to start regular exercise within the next six months.

- *Preparation stage:* People are active below a criterion level (typically defined as at least 3 times per week for 20 min or longer), but intend to become more active in the near future (within the next 30 days).

- *Action stage:* People have engaged in regular exercise at the criterion level for less than six months. Motivation and investment in behavior change are sufficient at this stage, and the perceived benefits are greater than the perceived cost. However, this is the least stable stage. People in the action stage are at the greatest risk of a relapse.

- *Maintenance stage:* People have been exercising regularly for more than six months. Exercise behavior is more established than in the other stages, and the risk of a relapse is low.

with exercise so that their experience is the true determinant of their current behavior.

Decisional balance is another construct from the transtheoretical model that is believed to influence exercise behavior. Based on the decision theory of Janis and Mann (1977), perceived costs and benefits to oneself and significant others are considered important influences on behavior change. There is good evidence that two constructs (i.e., pros and cons) are adequate for exercise. The relationship between the pros and cons of exercise and exercise stage typically shows that pros increase and cons decrease with movement to each subsequent stage. Most of the evidence for exercise also indicates that the crossover between pros and cons occurs during the contemplation or preparation stage; this is consistent with several other health behaviors.

The processes of change are strategies associated with movement along the stages and are divided into cognitive/experiential and behavioral. Cognitive/experiential processes are defined as the set of processes through which people gather relevant information on the basis of their own actions or experiences. An example of a cognitive process is self-reevaluation, in which people reappraise their values regarding inactivity. Behavioral processes are the set of processes in which the information is generated by environmental events and behaviors, such as stimulus control and reinforcement control.

Temptation is a factor in the TTM that is applicable to cessation behaviors. Temptation represents the urge to engage in an unhealthy behavior (e.g., smoking) in challenging situations and should decrease as one progresses through the stages (Prochaska and Velicer 1997). Although not applied to exercise as frequently as other TTM constructs, the temptation to refrain from exercise is associated with an affective component and the perception of competing demands. However, affect and competing demands were weakly related to physical activity levels measured repeatedly across two years (e.g., Dishman, Vandenberg, Motl, and Nigg 2010).

The level of change dimension is the context in which the problem behavior occurs. These levels include symptom/situational, maladaptive cognitions, current interpersonal conflicts, family/systems conflicts, and intrapersonal conflicts. Although not typically applied in exercise research, identifying the level of the problem could be used to guide interventions. For example, the level of change for someone who wants to begin strength training but does not have access to a fitness center would be situational. Setting up a home exercise program would have more efficacy for this person than targeting her cognitions.

Despite its appeal as a model for exercise behavior change and its application in several intervention studies, some uncertainty remains about whether the stages and processes of the transtheoretical model are applicable to understanding exercise behavior change, as Bandura argued in 1997. Recall that theories of behavioral change should be considered provisional, subject to change, improvement, and eventual replacement. Thus, scholars continue to test the application of the transtheoretical model to exercise behavior.

Longitudinal studies support earlier cross-sectional findings that people appear to use both cognitive/experiential and behavioral processes when they attempt to increase or maintain their levels of physical activity. Both cognitive and behavioral processes of change predicted 12-month physical activity status in a randomized controlled trial to promote physical activity, although processes of change assessed at 6 months did not predict the adoption or maintenance measured at 12 months (Williams, Dunsiger, Ciccolo, et al. 2008).

In a multi-ethnic cohort of 500 adults living in Hawaii who were observed at six-month intervals three or more times for two years, people who maintained or attained the Healthy People 2010 physical activity guidelines were more likely to retain higher scores on self-efficacy and both experiential and behavioral processes of change across the two years of observation (Dishman, Vandenberg, Motl, and Nigg 2010). However, the stages were not useful for predicting change in physical activity (Dishman, Thom, Rooks, et al. 2009). Stage was more likely to falsely classify people as meeting the guideline than to falsely classify them as not meeting it. Probabilities of predicting six-month transitions were about 50% for the stable class of meeting the guideline each time and just 25% for transitions between meeting and not meeting the guideline, which was worse than a chance prediction.

The TTM assumption that interventions matched to the person's stage would be more effective than those that were not has also been examined in a few studies with mixed results. For example, a stage-matched intervention group was more successful than a mismatched and control group after 16 weeks of a physical activity intervention, but was not more effective than standard care (Blissmer and McAuley 2002) and control groups.

OTHER THEORIES APPLIED TO EXERCISE AND PHYSICAL ACTIVITY

The theories reviewed so far are the prominent models in exercise behavior research, but several other models have also been applied to exercise, with varying success.

Health Belief Model

The health belief model was developed by Rosenstock and others in the 1950s to explain poor compliance with immunization and tuberculosis screenings. The health belief model explains health behavior at the level of individual decision making regarding the adoption or cessation of behaviors related to risk or control of a disease. The model centers on perceptions of how much of a personal threat the disease is and how effective the behavior change will be in reducing the threat. The likelihood of taking action is influenced by a cue to action (internal or external) and demographic and sociocultural variables. The readiness to adopt a health behavior depends on motivation, an evaluation of the threat of illness resulting from not changing behavior, and the perception that the behavior in question will reduce the threat. Modifying factors include demographics, structural factors (cost, complexity), attitudes, interaction factors (between patient and care provider), and enabling factors (social pressure, past experiences). Social support and self-efficacy have been added to the original model, which should enhance its predictive utility.

The health belief model appears more useful for preventive health behaviors and compliance

The word *ecology* stems from the Greek *oikos* ("household") and *logos* ("knowledge"). The term was first used by Ernst Haekel in 1866 to describe "the comprehensive science of the relationships of the organism to the environment."

Health Belief Model: Beliefs That Influence Exercise Behavior

- Perceived susceptibility to developing health problems because of inactivity (e.g., coronary heart disease, obesity)
- Perceived impact of the health problems on quality of life (perceived severity)
- Belief that adopting an active lifestyle will be beneficial
- Extent to which the benefits of exercising exceed the cost of exercising (perceived cost–benefit ratio)

Social ecological models are grounded in Lewin's equation:

$$B = \rightarrow(P, E)$$

where B = behavior, P = person, and E = environment.

with medical regimens, and less useful when applied to exercise. It is, essentially, an illness avoidance model. In fact, some studies indicated that perceived susceptibility was inversely associated with exercise adherence. It may be that physical activity and exercise are not perceived by some as health behaviors. People exercise for social interaction, enjoyment, mastery, and competition, as well as to enhance health; and motivation for exercise can change.

Social Ecological Models

Social ecological models have evolved from the seminal work of Kurt Lewin, the father of modern social psychology, whose field theory (1935) formally introduced the idea that behavior is a function of both the individual and the environment. The "field" contains the person and his or her dynamic psychological environment (e.g., perceptions), and behavior was proposed to depend on the current field rather than past or future environments. Subsequent scholars expanded on the nature of the environment and the relationship among the person, the behavior, and the environment (Sallis, Owen, and Fisher 2008). For example, in 1968 Roger Barker introduced the idea of a "behavioral setting," consisting of social and physical situations in which behavior occurs. In the late 1970s and early

1980s, Rudolf Moos and Urie Bronfenbrenner categorized environmental factors and influences to explain behavior, drawing attention to natural and built environments, organizational settings, sociocultural characteristics, and social climate (e.g., Moos 1979) and various levels of systems: micro (interactions among family and work groups), meso (e.g., family, school work settings), and exo (economics, culture, politics) environments (e.g., Bronfenbrenner 1979).

Ecological models contrast with other theories discussed in this chapter, which focus on the individual (e.g., attitudes, beliefs, cognitions, behavioral skills, and experiences) and more local social influences such as family and friends. Social ecological models consider the broader community, organizations, culture, and policies, as well as the constructed and natural environments, to explain behavior and guide interventions. One assumption is the interdependence among people, their behavior, and the environment, with multiple levels of influence that affect the adoption and maintenance of behavior. Intrapersonal, interpersonal, community, environmental, and organizational resources are thus considered when designing behavior change interventions, and multilevel modeling (see chapter 2) is applied to analyze intervention effects. Another assumption common to social ecological models is that effects across and between levels interact, and at each level of analysis specific resources are identified that can be "leverage points" that can have a greater impact on behavior (see figure 14.3). According to Sallis, Owen, and Fisher (2008), the basic principles of ecological perspectives are that (1) multiple levels of factors influence behavior, (2) influences interact across levels, (3) multilevel interventions should be most effective, and (4)

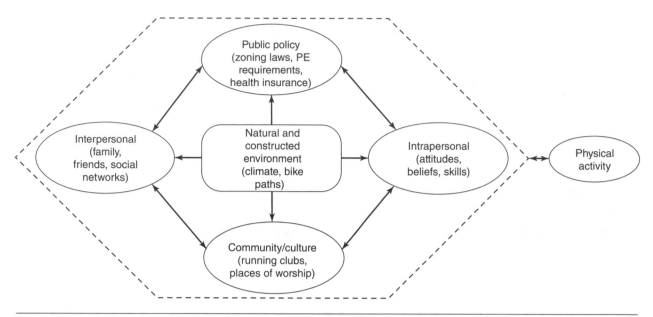

Figure 14.3 Interrelationships among social ecological components.

models are most effective when they are behavior specific.

Fleury and Lee (2006) conducted a descriptive review from a social ecological perspective of 23 studies on correlates of physical activity in African-American women that illustrates the range of factors considered with this model. Results were organized into intrapersonal, interpersonal, community and environment, and organizational influences. Low motivation (e.g., perceived lack of willpower, low self-efficacy) was an important intrapersonal barrier to physical activity. Moderate intrapersonal correlates were functional ability (fatigue from exercise, the perception that exercise is "hard work," health concerns, and comorbidities), socioeconomic status, and education. A low association was found for employment. Interpersonal factors were particularly important for African-American women, especially social support through encouragement and the opportunity to spend time with family and friends, as well as instrumental support such as aid with caregiving to free up time to be active. Observing others being active (a reflection of social norms) and participating in organized religious activities were also consistently associated with more physical activity. The community and environment factors that were barriers included a lack of safe places to exercise, culturally specific physical activities, sidewalks, and streetlights.

Increased activity was associated with community coalitions that incorporated the development of leadership skills and resources. Although few studies examined the role of organizational and policy resources, Fleury and Lee (2006) found that African-American women identified strong and supportive community organizations and partnerships as important for fostering increased physical activity.

Relapse Prevention Model

Most of the theories described in this chapter can be applied to the adoption and maintenance of behavior change. The **relapse prevention** model, which was derived from social learning theory, focuses on the maintenance of voluntary self-control efforts and the cyclical nature of long-term behavior change. The goal in the application of the model is to help people who are attempting to modify their behavior cope effectively with situations that could tempt them to return to the old, undesired behavior pattern. Marlatt and Gordon (1985) originally designed the model to enhance maintaining abstinence from a high-frequency, undesired behavior—that is, addictive behavior. Maintenance of behavior change is described in the context of the person's ability to cope with relapses cognitively and behaviorally.

Relapse begins with a **high-risk situation**, which is a situation that challenges one's confidence in adhering to a desired health behavior. For exercise, high-risk situations can include boredom, bad weather, negative mood, social situations, and lack of time. An adequate coping response to a high-risk situation leads to increased self-efficacy and a decreased probability of relapse. Inadequate coping or no coping leads to decreased self-efficacy and possibly positive expectations of what will happen if the desired health behavior is skipped (e.g., "I can go to the football game if I don't go to the gym today"). The more rigid the rule for meeting the target behavior, the more likely the deviation will be perceived as a slip. For example, if the "rule" is to exercise at the gym on Saturdays at 1:15 p.m. for 35 minutes, going to the game instead can be a slip (an acute, isolated missed exercise session), but starting 10 minutes late can also be perceived as a slip. A perception of slipping may lead to the abstinence violation effect, or in the case of exercise, the *adherence* violation effect. One of the characteristics of this effect is the experience of cognitive dissonance—an incongruity between thoughts or feelings and behavior. For example, the slip behavior (i.e., missing one exercise class or not meeting a specific rigid exercise plan) does not match the self-concept of being in control of exercise behavior. Another cognitive component of the abstinence or adherence violation effect is all-or-nothing thinking, such as defining oneself as either a success or a failure, which is also a risk for increased mental stress (see chapter 4). The emotional components of an abstinence or adherence violation include a sense of failure, self-blame, lowered self-esteem, guilt, and perceived loss of control, which can set the stage for relapse.

A lifestyle imbalance in which "shoulds" exceed "wants" also predisposes a person to relapse. People who spend more time doing what they *should* do at the expense of doing what they *want* to do feel deprived, and the desire for indulgence or self-gratification increases. For example, Bill has been exercising each weekend since his blood pressure was found to be elevated at his last physical. He has missed several fishing trips because of his exercise program, and he feels frustrated and left out when his friends talk about how much fun they had. Positive expectations of not adhering to the behavior change make relapse more attractive, as well. If he skipped his workout this weekend, Bill could try out his new fishing rod on a trip to the coast with his friends.

Conceptually, the relapse prevention model seems useful for exercise adherence, given that ~50% of those who begin a regular exercise program drop out within the first six months, most within the first three months. However, the model was developed for maintaining the cessation of high-frequency undesired behaviors, and in the case of exercise, the goal is to maintain a low-frequency, desired behavior that requires considerable repeated effort. It is clear when someone relapses from smoking cessation, but it is hard to identify when a lapse from regular exercise becomes a relapse. Some researchers have defined a lapse as no exercise for a week, but it may be difficult for exercisers to identify a lapse for themselves or to deal with a lapse in time to forestall relapse.

One component of relapse prevention training that may not be effective with exercise is a planned relapse, in which the person voluntarily returns to the undesired behavior, in this case inactivity, for a short period of time under controlled conditions. Planned relapse may not be a good strategy for acquisition behaviors in general, particularly in the early stages of behavior change (Marcus and Stanton 1993).

Other strategies for relapse prevention, such as identifying high-risk situations and planning for them, and setting flexible goals (rules), have been applied to exercise with some success. In one study, acute high-risk situations, components of the relapse prevention model relevant to slips, and exercise outcomes at three-month follow-ups were examined in 59 adults participating in regular exercise for an average of five years (Stetson et al. 2005). The average number of high-risk situations over the measurement periods was 3.5; the most common were bad weather,

> **H**igh-risk situations and rigid rules increase the risk of relapse.

inconvenient time of day, being alone, negative mood, and being physically tired. Exercising in spite of a high-risk situation was associated with positive cognitive coping strategies, such as task-oriented problem solving and positive reappraisal, although there were no reports of using social support as a coping strategy. Women were twice as likely as men to miss an exercise session in response to a high-risk situation, but this might have reflected a greater tendency for women to report slips. Although there are limitations in relying on retrospective recall, this study illustrates that high risk-situations do not guarantee slips and relapse, as well as the importance of the way exercisers cope with a challenging situation in fostering adherence.

Habit Theory

A habit is defined as a goal-directed behavior that has been performed repeatedly and has become automatic. It is thus performed without conscious thought or decision in which at least one other course of action is considered. A habit is a thing done often, and thus, according to habit theory, easily (Ronis, Yates, and Kirscht 1989). Habit theory proposes that automatic cognitive processes are set in motion by situational cues, so conscious thought is not required. Situational consistency contributes to habit formation; therefore, vivid, numerous, and consistent cues support behavior change maintenance. Another supposition of habit theory is that the simpler and more discrete the behavior, the more likely it will be to become habitual and be elicited by situational cues. Thus, components of an exercise routine can be examined, and parts of the routine can be identified as potential habits. For example, putting running clothes out the night before, driving to the gym after work, and stopping work at noon to walk with friends are behavioral candidates for control by automatic cognitive processes.

Aarts, Paulussen, and Schaalma (1997) developed a model of physical exercise and habit formation to describe the process by which exercise habits are formed. This model contains several of the components of habit formation just discussed. The development of a physical activity habit begins with an initial contemplative decision process in which the need to exercise is evaluated based on perceptions of desirability, social pressure, and behavioral control. A positive evaluation leads to intentions and the actual exercise behavior. If the consequences of the behavior are pleasant, the recurrence of exercise depends on the opportunity to perform the behavior under similar circumstances. Over time, the contemplative decision process becomes less complex. As the behavior is repeated, it is automatically activated by the situational features that precede exercise. Exercise becomes a habit that no longer needs reasoned consideration. The development of lifelong exercise habits depends on overcoming several obstacles, such as a lack of positive immediate consequences and difficulty in repeating the same behavior in similar circumstances (i.e., disruptions in exercise routines as a result of changes in work schedules, social obligations), which impedes the repetition that is important in habit formation.

Strength of habit (subjective experiences of repetition and automaticity) has been measured with the Self-Report Habit Index (Verplanken and Orbell 2003), and the strength of exercise habits has been associated with level of exercise in several studies. For example, Rhodes and colleagues (Rhodes, de Bruijn, and Matheson 2010) tested the role of habit in predicting physical activity within the theory of planned behavior in 153 college students and found that habit accounted for an additional 7% of variance in physical activity beyond intention. However, a strong exercise habit even along with an intention to exercise is not a guarantee that someone will be physically active (e.g., de Bruijn 2011).

Physical Activity Maintenance Model

The physical activity maintenance model (PAM) developed by Nigg, Borrelli, Maddock, and Dishman (2008) assumes that predictors of adoption are different from predictors of maintenance. This model adds to our understanding of exercise behavior by incorporating triggers for physical activity relapse, integrating individual and environmental variables important for maintenance, and conceptualizing physical activity maintenance as an active process. This model is multilevel and considers intrapersonal factors, but also social environment and community structures, proposing a reciprocal relationship between the environment and the person, as does the social ecological model (see figure 14.4).

PAM mediators include goal setting, self-efficacy, and motivation. Goal setting operates through commitment and achievement and influences the direction, regulation, and persistence of effort. Goal setting serves as a mechanism to build mastery experiences through goal attainment and influences self-efficacy. Barrier and relapse self-efficacy are most relevant to this model, in which self-efficacy is proposed to have direct and indirect effects on behavior through motivation and goal setting. Motivation is considered from an intrinsic perspective, that of self-motivation, which is a disposition to persist independently of context-specific beliefs and extrinsic expectations of the pros and cons of maintaining regular physical activity. Goal setting, self-efficacy, and motivation are interrelated and integral and have reciprocal influences in this model. For example, motivation to keep running during a long, hot summer can lead to goal modification, and achieving these new goals can enhance self-efficacy to maintain exercise.

The environment and life stress are considered contextual influences on PAM mediators. These contextual influences can be opportunities and affordances that are filtered by perceptions, cog-

nitions, and motivation, and they are moderated by existing conditions. An important contribution of this model is the inclusion of life stress as a critical contextual element to explain patterns of physical activity—specifically as a potential trigger of relapse. Life stress affects behavioral maintenance because stress decreases and redirects personal resources away from physical activity; distracts from setting goals; increases negative affect, depression, and anxiety; and thus decreases motivation for physical activity. In addition, chronic stress can compromise the immune system, leading to increased fatigue and physical weakness.

ISSUES IN THE APPLICATION OF THEORIES OF EXERCISE BEHAVIOR

Just as there is no single determinant of exercise and physical activity, no single theory seems to be adequate for describing and predicting exercise behavior. The theories we have presented are all reasonable models of human behavior and contain many of the variables related to exercise behavior that research on exercise correlates has revealed. The three most popular theories in exercise psychology are social cognitive theory or self-efficacy theory, the theory of planned behavior, and the transtheoretical model (Biddle

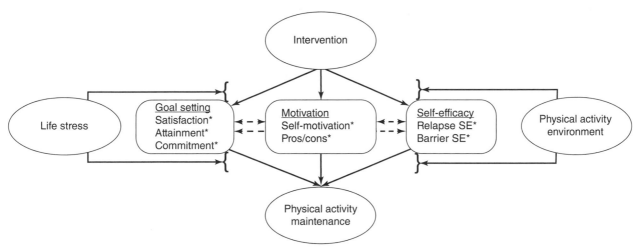

*Constructs specific to maintenance of PA, which may be correlated to each other.

Figure 14.4 Physical activity maintenance model.

Reprinted, by permission, from C.R. Nigg et al., 2008, "A theory of physical activity maintenance," *Applied Psychology* 57(4): 544-560 and Fuchs 2009; Rhodes and Nigg 2011). The self-determination theory and social ecological approaches are being applied with greater frequency, and in European research, the health action process approach (HAPA; Schwarzer 2008) has figured prominently. However, many of these theories have been applied to exercise incompletely, and more studies are needed that empirically test the application of specific theories to exercise behavior and address exercise maintenance explicitly (e.g., the physical activity maintenance model).

In a review of exercise behavior change interventions in 1998, Baranowski, Anderson, and Carmack argued that interventions work through mediating variables, but that current theoretical models used to select mediating variables often do not account for substantial amounts of variability in the targeted outcome. The authors recommended more basic behavioral and social science research to understand physical activity behavior, which would include the examination of theoretical constructs. Meeting this charge would help to clarify the role of personal, environmental, and behavioral variables and their relationships in predicting and explaining patterns of physical activity.

More researchers are taking on this challenge to address the insufficient body of literature on the accuracy of individual theories to explain and predict physical activity. Those who are should consider the research issues addressed in chapter 2, such as the measurement of psychosocial constructs. Theory testing in physical activity behavior has been limited by cross-sectional or short-term (e.g., two weeks) prospective studies. Temporal sequencing is critical to test theoretical constructs and requires experimental or natural longitudinal research. Data analysis to verify the theoretical constructs and their interrelationships requires multivariate statistical techniques. These points can be incorporated into the criteria for applying theory to physical activity behavior research (see table 14.5) proposed by Nigg and Paxton (2008), who also called for guidelines such as the CONSORT statement (see chapter 15) for reporting the theoretical foundations of behavioral interventions.

Certainly, the design, implementation, and interpretation of research on exercise behavior must be based on theory. In addition to the theories described in this chapter, many other theories of human behavior are available that can be used to understand and predict exercise behavior. The selection of a theory should be guided by the evidence for its application to the unique characteristics of exercise and the relationships between theoretical constructs and exercise behavior. Some researchers have addressed this issue by developing theories specific to exercise (e.g., Aarts, Paulussen, and Schaalma 1997; Nigg et al. 2008), whereas others have advocated integrating theories across multiple domains of the social, behavioral, and biomedical sciences (Epstein 1998) or adding specific components to existing theories to increase the amount of variance in physical activity that can be explained.

Table 14.5 Criteria for the Appropriate Application of Theory to Physical Activity Behavior Research

1. Theory identification
2. Entire theory description
3. Translating all of the theory components into the intervention
4. Implementing all of the intervention components
5. Assessing all of the theory components
6. Ensuring congruency between theoretical variables and outcome
7. Ensuring fidelity of the intervention protocol
8. Appropriately assessing change in outcome

Adapted from Nigg and Paxton 2008.

SUMMARY

Behaviorism considers behavior change to be the result of modifications in antecedents and consequences and their cuing and reinforcing strength. Cognitive behaviorism defines intra-individual factors as the key to behavior change. The application of social learning–based theories to exercise behavior involves describing exercise and physical activity as volitional behavior influenced by conscious decision making, and emphasizes the roles of self-efficacy, attitudes, beliefs, motivation, and intentions to varying degrees. Although attitude models in general account for no more than 35% of the variance in exercise behavior, these models are primarily concerned with decision making, which is a predisposing factor in terms of actual behavior change. Enabling factors (accessibility, the availability of resources, environmental factors) and reinforcing factors (rewards and incentives) add to the explanation of exercise adoption and maintenance, and should be considered in a comprehensive model of exercise behavior that includes a biological component.

Psychosocial, physiological, and environmental factors change over time, and thus their contributions to exercise behavior are dynamic. The inclusion of a temporal dimension in a model of exercise behavior, such as that described by stage and relapse prevention models, expands our ability to understand how people change and has implications for improving the effectiveness of interventions. Although some argue for developing new theories, we have yet to establish a sufficient body of literature from studies that used theories appropriately and mapped theoretical mediators to behavior change strategies and approaches.

WEBSITES

www.bfskinner.org/BFSkinner/Home.html

www.nacbt.org

www.des.emory.edu/mfp/bandurabio.html

www.uri.edu/research/cprc/TTM/detailedoverview.htm

www.psych.rochester.edu/SDT

Interventions to Change Physical Activity Behavior

Anyone who has tried to change a health-related behavior knows that doing something as simple as drinking more water each day is not easy, even though we know it is good for us and we feel better for doing it. Exercise is good for us, and we feel better when we exercise on a regular basis, but it is not a simple behavior. Without intervention, there is a 50-50 chance that someone who has started an exercise program will stop within 6 months. The aims of this chapter are to describe models and strategies used to get people to start and stick with regular exercise and to describe interventions that have been implemented in various populations; we hope also to offer some insight into why the efforts to keep people physically active have not been successful.

OVERVIEW

The primary goals in exercise behavior change research are to get sedentary or irregularly active people to adopt regular exercise habits or increase their levels of lifestyle physical activity and to keep physically active people active on a regular basis. Decisions about what to change and which strategies to use are based on the procedural model guiding the intervention. Procedural models define what should be done, when, and under what conditions to produce a specific outcome. They are derived from propositional models or theories, such as behaviorism, which were discussed in chapter 14. For example, if the theoretical foundation of the intervention is behaviorism, then the assumptions about how changes in behavior occur are

based on the relationships among antecedents, consequences, and the target behavior. The procedural model derived from behaviorism would involve strategies such as stimulus control (modifying the antecedents) and reinforcement control (modifying the consequences), and the goal would be defined in terms of changing the rate of responding (i.e., increase or maintain the frequency of exercise). The choice of which theory-based variables to target should be based on factors that have been documented to mediate exercise behavior—which is another reason to study the correlates of physical activity. Another consideration is the target population, which can dictate the types and constraints of intervention designs and strategies.

> **T**he goal of exercise interventions is to increase the number of people who adopt and maintain a physically active lifestyle.

We need to keep several points in mind when considering the various approaches used to promote the adoption and maintenance of a physically active lifestyle. First, changing the level of physical activity is not like changing most other health behaviors. With physical activity, the goal is to adopt and maintain a positive health behavior, rather than to give up or stop a negative health behavior, such as smoking cigarettes. Second, physical activity is unique in that it is a biologically based behavior with interactions between physiological and psychosocial antecedents and consequences. For example, soreness is a possible physiological consequences of a bout of exercise that can be interpreted cognitively as lack of capability and lead to lower self-efficacy. Illness and disease can contribute to fatigue, which can reduce the motivation to be physically active.

Third, keep in mind that physical activity is a complicated behavior. Walking the dog, attending an aerobics class, and taking the family to the park are all preceded by chains of cognitive, behavioral, and social events that involve multiple decisions and actions. Some of these activities, such as getting the family to the park for a Saturday fitness event, have many links, whereas taking the stairs instead of the escalator may simply involve noticing a sign promoting physical activity and walking to the stairs. Decisions and subsequent actions are influenced by personal characteristics, physiological responses and adaptations, social factors, and environmental conditions.

Fourth, exercise is a dynamic behavior, as illustrated by the application of stage and adherence models to exercise (see chapter 14). A variety of factors influence the adoption, early adherence, long-term maintenance, and resumption of exercise after a period of inactivity. This last point concerns the targeted quality and quantity of physical activity. The type of regimen should match the objectives of an exercise program and the resources and motivation of the target population. Swimming 5 days a week for an hour each time will facilitate weight loss, but access to a pool and the willingness to spend that much time exercising are necessary for adoption and adherence.

Maximizing adherence to an exercise program is critical for achieving the desired outcome, but also for testing the efficacy of the intervention to increase the level of physical activity or improve physical or mental health. We need participants to follow the prescription and complete all the assessments so we can determine the effects of the intervention on outcome variables, as well as the aspects of the intervention that mediated the outcome. In addition, Consolidated Standards of Reporting Trials (CONSORT) guidelines (see chapter 2) state that all participants' data should

---

Characteristics of Exercise as a Target Behavior

- The goal is to adopt and maintain a positive health behavior.
- Exercise is a biologically based behavior.
- Exercise is preceded by chains of psychological, behavioral, and social events that require multiple decisions and actions.
- Different combinations of factors mediate the adoption, early adherence, long-term maintenance, and resumption of exercise after relapse.
- The quality and quantity of exercise vary as a function of purpose.

---

be included regardless of adherence, increasing the motivation for researchers to emphasize adherence so they can gather as much actual data as possible and minimize the imputation of missing data.

INTERVENTION CONTEXT

This section presents the context for describing interventions to change physical activity behavior in terms of characteristics of the person (i.e., the target group), the setting, and the level of the intervention. Characteristics of the target group, such as age, living situation, and income, should be considered in selecting interventions. For example, a program for increasing physical activity in overweight middle school children will be very different from a program to increase the number of factory workers who adopt regular exercise. The setting, which can range from a high school physical education class to an urban recreation facility, presents a variety of resources and limitations. Interventions can be applied on an individual, group, community, or societal level, and this will also influence the choice of strategies. Numerous approaches have been

A comprehensive model of exercise interventions requires a consideration of the characteristics of the target group, the intervention setting, and the level of the intervention to guide program goals and strategy selection.

used to influence physical activity. This chapter provides descriptions of several interventions applied to various populations and their potential for changing physical activity behavior. We end with a discussion of issues involved in the development and implementation of exercise behavior change interventions.

Characteristics of the Person

It is becoming increasingly evident that interventions applied in general, without consideration of the unique demands of the population, have limited impact. *One size does not fit all.* Information about the client or target group enables us to select the best strategy, the most appropriate setting in which to implement the strategy, and the level of intervention that will have the greatest impact. Exercise stage, demographic characteristics, cognitive variables (e.g., knowledge, attitudes, and beliefs), and self-regulation skills (e.g., goal setting, self-monitoring) are some of the personal characteristics that have been considered in the development and implementation of exercise interventions.

Exercise Stage of Change

Determining exercise stage of change as described by the transtheoretical model of behavior change (TTM; see chapter 14) is useful because different goals and strategies are necessary based on whether the person is currently active and the person's intentions to begin or maintain regular exercise (see table 15.1). Although there is some evidence that current stage based on the TTM is not useful for predicting changes in physical activity (Dishman, Thom, et al. 2009), a person's current and past levels of physical activity and motivational readiness

(behavioral intention) can be useful in selecting goals and strategies. For example, the health action process approach (HAPA; Schwarzer et al. 2007; Schwarzer et al. 2008) distinguishes among nonintentional, intentional, and action stages and recommends corresponding strategies. Motivational interventions are applied to someone in the nonintentional stage, and action planning (e.g., specifying when, where, and how the activity will be performed and overcoming anticipated barriers to action) is applied to someone in the intentional or action stage. Stage-matched strategies based on HAPA were tested in an Internet-based intervention by Lippke and colleagues (2010), in which significantly more members of the group receiving the stage-based intervention moved forward to the action stage than did those in the control condition.

Traditional strategies will not work with someone who is not ready to change. For example, people in the precontemplation, or nonintentional, stage may be resistant to recognizing or modifying a problem. Auweele, Rzewnicki, and Van Mele (1997) examined factors in the adoption of exercise in 133 male and 132 female sedentary middle-aged adults in Belgium. They found a significant group of indifferent sedentary adults for whom exercise was irrelevant (60% of the total sample). These people did not include exercise as part of their lives or self-concepts and did not see exercise as a way to achieve desired goals. The authors proposed that some people may simply not be receptive to any intervention.

The stages of the TTM have often been used to categorize participants before selecting intervention strategies. Contemplators are aware of the problem and are thinking about changing, but they have not made the commitment to change. At this point, the costs of exercising are perceived to be greater than the benefits. Cognitive factors to consider are the perceived barriers to starting an exercise program, outcome expectations, outcome values, and psychosocial variables, such as exercise self-efficacy. Exercise history can affect self-efficacy in that those who have had positive experiences with exercise will have more confidence in their ability to exercise again.

People in the preparation stage have already begun to change their behavior. They intend to begin regular exercise within a short period of time and may already be exercising, but below a criterion level. Setting goals that are based on capabilities, values, resources, and needs is important. Accomplishing challenging goals will increase a sense of mastery, which will also enhance exercise self-efficacy.

Most people who start an exercise program drop out within the first six months. Therefore, the first few months after someone has adopted regular exercise (the action stage) are critical. Establishing a regular exercise routine involves a significant commitment of time and energy. According to habit theory (chapter 14), most of the behaviors necessary for engaging in exercise still require conscious consideration and active decision making in the early adoption period. Action planning is critical in early adoption

according to HAPA. Other strategies such as those in table 15.1 can support the new behavioral patterns while exercise becomes a more established, automatic routine.

Maintaining regular exercise is the goal for novice and long-term exercisers. People who have been regularly active for more than six months (maintenance stage) have a decreased risk of relapse. However, permanent maintenance is not guaranteed, and there remains the potential for lapses in an exercise routine as a result of relocation, family commitments, travel, medical events, or other disruptions. The physical activity maintenance model (PAM; see chapter 14) examines the individual psychological and contextual variables that support or impede long-term maintenance. For example, because PAM

Table 15.1 Exercise Stages, Goals, and Sample Behavior Change Strategies

Exercise stage	Goal	Strategies
Precontemplation	To begin thinking about changing	Providing information about the role of exercise in good health Strengthening the actual and perceived personal benefits of exercise Reducing or countering the actual and perceived costs of and barriers to exercise Fostering a personal value for exercise
Contemplation	To adopt regular exercise	Creating marketing and media campaigns with accurate, easy-to-understand guidelines for beginning an exercise program Offering activities to increase exercise self-efficacy, such as mastery experiences Evaluating the pros and cons of exercise
Preparation	To adopt regular exercise at an appropriate target level	Creating a thorough physical and psychosocial assessment (self-monitoring) Establishing realistic and reasonable goals Evaluating environmental and social supports and barriers and addressing barriers accordingly
Action	To establish exercise as a habit	Creating behavior modification strategies, such as shaping, stimulus control, reinforcement control, and self-monitoring Developing and implementing plans to overcome barriers Planning when, where, and how to exercise Addressing relapse prevention
Maintenance	To maintain lifelong regular exercise	Reevaluating exercise goals Planning ways to cope with risk situations and potential lapses Introducing variety into the exercise routine

identifies stress as a potential trigger of relapse, stress management would be one technique for promoting exercise maintenance.

Demographics

Demographic variables, such as age, sex, ethnicity, and education, are not targets for change. However, demographic variables often function as moderators. As noted in chapter 2, a moderator is a variable that affects the direction or strength (or both) of the relationship between the independent variable and the outcome variable. Moderators always function as independent variables (Baron and Kenny 1986) and can be represented by an interaction, such as better adherence for men than women to an exercise intervention that promotes competition (see figure 15.1).

Demographic characteristics can influence the receptiveness to interventions and the exercise behavior itself. Obviously, the presentation of the intervention and the materials must suit the educational level and developmental stage of the target group. Behavior change strategies and physical activities that will appeal to elementary school children are not the same as those that will motivate college students. Demographic characteristics also yield important information about structuring an intervention so that it is more enticing to participants. For example, older adults as compared to younger people find health and fitness motives more salient for adopting and maintaining an active lifestyle. Women are more likely than men to adopt exercise for weight loss (e.g., McAuley et al. 1994), but this may not be the case with African-American women (see chapter 12). Appearance and social

interaction may also be more important in an exercise program for women than for men, who may find competitiveness a greater incentive to exercise (Markland and Hardy 1993). Interventions that have been effective with minority populations have tailored strategies to be sensitive to cultural beliefs, values, language, literacy, and customs (Artinian et al. 2010).

Cognitive Characteristics

Identifying attitudes and beliefs about physical activity provides important information for designing and implementing behavior change strategies. For example, we would not expect a sedentary middle-aged woman who believes she is active enough in her job to respond to a sign-up sheet for a work site aerobics program, but she may be ready to listen to compelling information in a media campaign about the benefits of physical activity for women like herself. Knowledge is not enough to change behavior, but clear, relevant information about the personal benefits of physical activity and practical suggestions for ways to become more active can influence attitudes, beliefs, and expectations.

Exercise self-efficacy is frequently studied as a correlate of exercise behavior and is a key mediator of behavior change according to several theoretical models. The relationship between self-efficacy and exercise adoption is fairly consistent, but the role of self-efficacy in maintenance depends on the type of self-efficacy. Oman and King (1998) and McAuley, Courneya, and colleagues (1994) examined the relationship between self-efficacy and exercise and found good evidence for effects of self-efficacy on adoption but not on adherence. However, Garcia and King (1991) examined the relationship between self-efficacy and exercise adherence in a middle-aged community sample and found a positive correlation between self-efficacy and adherence for months 1 to 6 and months 7 to 12.

Better evidence for the role of self-efficacy in exercise and physical activity behavior has been found in intervention studies applying mediation analysis. In 2004, Dishman and colleagues evaluated the effects of the Lifestyle Education for Activity Program (LEAP), a comprehensive school-based intervention, on self-efficacy and other variables derived from social cognitive

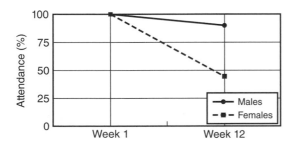

Figure 15.1 Sex moderates the effects of the intervention on attendance. This graph shows attendance at the beginning and end of a competition-based exercise intervention.

theory as mediators of change in physical activity among black and white adolescent girls. The multicomponent intervention emphasized the enhancement of self-efficacy to overcome barriers to physical activity and the development of behavioral skills by using curricular activities within physical education classes and health education instruction. Latent variable structural equation modeling indicated that (1) the intervention had direct effects on self-efficacy, goal setting, and physical activity; and (2) self-efficacy partially mediated the effect of the intervention on physical activity. This study provided the first evidence from a randomized controlled trial that the manipulation of self-efficacy results in increased physical activity among adolescent girls.

Blanchard and colleagues (2007) also found that barrier self-efficacy was important in exercise maintenance. They analyzed data from the Physical Activity Counseling Trial and found that task and barrier self-efficacy mediated the effects of the intervention on physical activity during the intervention. The effects for task self-efficacy were greater during the intervention and faded at follow-up, whereas barrier self-efficacy stayed strong as a mediator throughout the follow-up.

Cognitive processes of change from the TTM are important in motivating people to change their levels of physical activity, but there is good evidence that people use both cognitive and behavioral strategies when they attempt to increase and maintain physical activity.

> **C**ognitive and behavioral strategies may both be effective in establishing and regulating a new behavior.

Motivation is another cognitive characteristic that can affect the utility of interventions. Motivation can have different contributions to behavior according to how it is conceptualized. According to achievement goal theory, motivation is influenced differently for people with ego versus task orientations (Duda and Nicholls 1992). **Ego orientation** refers to motivation based on winning or being better than someone

else, whereas **task orientation** indicates motivation to persist to master the task. The point of reference for someone with a task orientation is not the behavior of someone else (winners and losers) but past personal performance. This person's goal is self-improvement, although motivational orientations are somewhat dynamic. For example, Joe might have started a 5K road race to achieve his personal best time, but he shifts to an ego orientation when he realizes after 4K that he is close to the fastest runner. At this point his motivation shifts to winning the race. Some studies indicate that men are more likely than women to have an ego orientation and thus might be more likely to participate in physical activities that provide opportunities for competing against others.

Self-motivation is a generalized tendency to persist in the long-term pursuit of behavioral goals and interacts with self-efficacy and goal setting in maintaining a behavior change. Someone with lower self-motivation might need more support for both adopting and maintaining regular exercise. Motivation can also be conceptualized as on a continuum from amotivation to intrinsic motivation (see the discussion of self-determination theory in chapter 14). There is good evidence that motivation to exercise may be more extrinsic at the beginning of an exercise program, but become more intrinsic over time. Some studies have even found that extrinsic rewards or motives for exercise early in a program can hamper the development of intrinsic reasons to exercise (e.g., Frederick and Ryan 1995).

Intervention Settings

Settings in which interventions can take place include the home, medical care facilities, schools, work sites, and the community. Different settings

> **T**he setting of the intervention presents different specific supports and barriers to physical activity depending on the target populations and goals.

present different real and perceived barriers and supports for physical activity depending on the target group.

Home-Based Programs

Home-based programs can offer accessibility and convenience to those limited by family commitments, finances, location, health, or transportation. A home-based program should include initial instruction in self-management strategies and appropriate exercise prescriptions, particularly for those just beginning to exercise because the bulk of the intervention is unsupervised. Support for exercise that can occur in group programs may be lacking in home-based programs, but regular mailings, phone contacts, and contact via the Internet and mobile technology from providers can supply some social support and feedback.

Studies that have compared adherence rates for home-based programs to those for programs in traditional exercise facilities have generally indicated positive results for the home-based interventions (e.g., Ferrier et al. 2011). The strengths of home-based programs include privacy, low cost for the participant and provider, and the opportunity for participants to personalize the intervention, such as choosing the time to exercise and the type of activity. More contemporary randomized clinical trials (RCTs) for exercise promotion that use a home-based model combine supervised and unsupervised exercise (Courneya 2010). For example, participants meet several times on site individually or in groups for instruction in exercise and behavioral supports for adherence (e.g., goal setting, barrier identification and management) before they exercise on their own. With the increase in the length of interventions and the inclusion of long-term follow-up in many RCTs, more strategies such as initial supervision are necessary to support retention and adherence. Booster activities such as phone, mail, or Internet follow-up can facilitate long-term adherence (Müller-Riemenschneider et al. 2008).

Health Care Facilities

Health care facilities have great potential as settings in which to promote exercise, particularly for women, who are more likely than men to visit their physicians. The promotion of exercise in this setting is being championed by the Exercise is Medicine (EIM) campaign, whose goal is to make exercise a standard part of medical care (see chapter 1). Time constraints, lack of training in medical school regarding exercise behavior, and lack of reimbursement for preventive services have limited the implementation of exercise promotion programs in hospitals, community clinics, and private practices, although support and materials from EIM professionals are making inroads to target some of these barriers.

PACE (Physician-Based Assessment and Counseling for Exercise) is a program developed in the 1990s for medical settings that addresses time constraints on a physical activity intervention using stage-matched materials (e.g., Bolognesi et al. 2006; Calfas et al. 1996). The general format involves administering a short questionnaire to determine the patient's exercise stage before meeting with the physician. The patient receives a stage-matched written program with specific recommendations, which the patient and physician then review. Some type of follow-up, such as booster calls by the health educator or another staff member, is used to monitor progress and answer questions. Tailoring materials to patients' exercise stage to promote exercise in this setting has had mixed results, though. Bull, Jamrozik, and Blanksby (1998) tested the effects of verbal advice from a physician, combined with standard or stage-matched supportive written material on exercise, in initially sedentary patients at 1, 6, and 12 months after the office visit. Compared to a control group that received no materials or advice, more patients who received an intervention were active 1 and 6 months later, regardless of the type of intervention. On the other hand, Kirk and colleagues (2009) implemented stage-matched interventions (in-person and written) in patients with type 2 diabetes. There was no change in physical activity over 6 and 12 months regardless of receiving standard care or initial stage-matched physical activity consultation in person or in writing. However, a subgroup analysis of patients with a baseline count of fewer than 5,000 steps per day found significant increases in physical activity for the in-person group, no change for the in-writing group, and a decrease in the standard care group. These results remind us to consider additional factors such as baseline physical activity, which can moderate the effects of an intervention.

Schools

Schools are a critical setting for the development of health behaviors. More than 70% of states in the United States require that schools follow national or state physical education standards or guidelines (Lee et al. 2007). As a result, school-based physical education interventions have the potential for increasing physical activity among a large population of youth (Kahn et al. 2002).

In 2011, the Division of Adolescent and School Health (DASH) of the U.S. Centers for Disease Control and Prevention (CDC) released *School Health Guidelines to Promote Healthy Eating and Physical Activity.* There are nine guidelines that emphasize and address policies and programs at multiple levels with associated strategies. These guidelines are timely because most physical education classes do not teach the cognitive or behavioral skills necessary to increase activity out of class or to maintain exercise upon graduation. In addition, some school staff are allowed to used physical activity as a punishment. Nationwide, 32.2% of schools allow the use of activities such as running laps and doing push-ups to punish students for bad behavior in physical education, whereas only 8.9% of schools discourage this practice (Lee et al. 2007).

There is some evidence for moderate effects of comprehensive school-based health promotion programs when a randomized design and extensive interventions are used and measurements are valid and reliable (Stone et al. 1998). The Child and Adolescent Trial for Cardiovascular Health (CATCH) is an example of a multicenter randomized controlled community trial that targeted children in grades 3, 4, and 5 (Luepker et al. 1996) and sought to produce changes in dietary and physical activity behaviors. The intervention, which was based on social cognitive theory and organizational change, was implemented in class, with the family, and through policy changes in schools randomized into experimental (56 schools) and control (40 schools) groups. Participants in the CATCH pro-

gram increased moderate to vigorous physical activity in class and vigorous activity out of class, and these changes were maintained three years postintervention.

Four recent reviews on school-based interventions and 11 RCTs and 9 controlled trials published in 2007-2010 were systematically reviewed by Kriemler and colleagues (2011). They found good support for the benefits of school-based interventions on physical activity. The evidence was consistently positive for increased physical activity in school and out of school. In addition, three of the four studies that reported objectively measured physical activity showed increases in total physical activity. Using multicomponent intervention strategies was the most consistently positive strategy.

Most of the studies implementing interventions in the schools have targeted upper-elementary-age students; few have been done in high schools. Unfortunately, there is a disturbing national trend toward reduction in required physical education classes with increasing grade. In 1991, 42% of U.S. high school students participated in a physical activity class each day, but participation decreased to 31.5% overall in 2011, with significant decreases from the 9th (41.3%) to the 12th (24.2%) grades (Centers for Disease Control and Prevention [CDC] 2012). Data indicate no compensatory increase in physical activity out of class. In addition, children are sedentary the majority of the time during physical education classes.

Because physical activity significantly declines in adolescents, more community opportunities for recreational activities and sports should be considered. Other directions for interventions through the schools could include curricula that target the behavioral skills necessary for lifelong physical activity, the integration of physical activity into other academic classes (such as having students compute target heart rate zone in math class or write essays in English class on making exercise fun), noncompetitive inclusive after-school recreation programs, and programs that include parental involvement. Programs that have included some of these strategies with success are the Middle School Physical Activity and Nutrition (M-SPAN) intervention (Sallis et al. 2003), and two programs for sixth- and eighth-grade girls, the Trial of Activity in Adolescent Girls (TAAG) (Webber et al. 2008), and the LEAP trial (Pate et al. 2007).

College physical education can have an important role in the primary prevention of inactivity-related diseases (Sparling 2003). According to data from the American College Health Association, in 2010, 52.3% of men and 43.6% of women in U.S. colleges and universities met physical activity guidelines. These less-than-optimal rates are related to the lifestyle of college students, which includes prolonged sedentary activities such as sitting in a classroom, reading and studying, and doing computer-based work. A pattern of sedentary activity developed and reinforced in college can be sustained after graduation, and health behavior patterns established during college and young adulthood create future habits that are difficult to amend (Nelson et al. 2008). Maintaining sedentary habits during and after college can have significant health repercussions in view of the heart disease risk factors already present in some college students (Sparling, Snow, and Beavers 1999), especially those who are inactive (Sacheck, Kuder, and Economos 2010). And college students make up a large portion of the population. According to the U.S. Census, 19.7 million students were projected to be enrolled in colleges and universities in the United States in 2012 (U.S. Census Bureau 2012), and about 68.1% of the high school graduates in 2010 were enrolled in college in 2010 (Division of Labor Force Statistics 2011).

Studies of U.S. college alumni have shown that a conceptually based physical education program and more required hours of physical education produced alumni with better attitudes toward exercise who also reported more physical activity (Brynteson and Adams 1993). Additionally, according to these studies, required physical education in college was associated with better health knowledge; more positive attitudes toward exercise, diet, and smoking; and exercise postgraduation (Pearman et al. 1997). In 2000, 33% of responding U.S. colleges and universities required conceptually based fitness and wellness classes for all undergraduates (Hensley 2000), and this proportion increased to 44% in 2009 (Kulinna et al. 2009). This trend may be enhanced with the promotion of Exercise is Medicine on Campus program (see http://exerciseismedicine.org/campus.htm).

Work Sites

The work site is another setting for exercise interventions with a captive audience for 40 (plus or minus) hours per week. Programs vary widely with respect to facilities available, activities offered, target audiences, costs to employees, and incentives. In general, work site fitness programs have had equivocal success. On-site fitness facilities may be convenient to some; but they may be a barrier to those whose work hours conflict with scheduled programs, those who rely on others for transportation home, or those who simply do not want to spend more time at the work site. Issues in work site programming include documenting a favorable cost–benefit ratio for employee fitness programs, selecting goals and a target audience, developing ways to institutionalize a fitness program that will sustain corporate culture changes, implementing rewards and incentives, and recruiting and retaining participants.

A meta-analysis of 26 studies published between 1972 and 1997 found a small (0.25 SD) effect size for work site interventions increasing level of physical activity (Dishman et al. 1998). A similar small effect (0.21 SD; 95% CI = 0.11-0.31) was reported in a more recent meta-analysis of the effects of work site programs on physical activity (Conn et al. 2009). Although Taylor, Connor, and Lawton (2011) also found a small effect (0.21 SD; 95% CI = 0.17-0.26) in their meta-analysis of work site programs, interventions using theory more explicitly were more effective in increasing physical activity (0.34 SD; 95% CI = 0.23-0.45).

Two work site–based studies that illustrate the role of policy and environmental approaches in promoting physical activity are the Los Angeles Lift-Off (Yancey et al. 2004) and Move to Improve (Dishman et al. 2009). Los Angeles Lift-Off was a physical activity promotion program that integrated a single 10-minute exercise break into regularly occurring meetings and events during work time at the Los Angeles County Department of Health Services work sites. The unique characteristics of this study were the "minimal" environmental change and the fact that it targeted underserved populations. The results indicated that more than 90% of meeting attendees participated in the exercises.

Move to Improve was a multisite group randomized controlled trial consisting of a 12-week intervention to increase moderate to vigorous physical activity among employees at 16 work sites of a large retail company. It targeted features of the workplace environment as well as employee motivation using personal and team goal setting. The proportion of participants who met the Healthy People 2010 recommendation for regular participation in either moderate or vigorous physical activity remained near 25% at control sites during the study but increased to 51% at intervention sites.

Communities

The settings for physical activity interventions in communities are diverse (e.g., places of worship, private and nonprofit fitness centers, and city or county recreational departments), and the types of intervention can range from exercise classes to mass media campaigns. Programs in places of worship can be faith placed (secular programs using the facilities) or faith based (programs integrating religious beliefs with health promotion), but both types can provide the impetus to begin exercising and the social support and encouragement to stay active. Places of worship are community anchors for many minority groups and can promote exercise by providing positive role models, peer-led exercise classes, and information about exercise through church channels.

For-profit and nonprofit fitness centers, such as YMCAs and YWCAs, Boys and Girls Clubs, and sport leagues, have been traditional sites for exercise promotion and fitness programs. Comprehensive facilities, flexible hours of operation, classes for beginners, and low-cost or complimentary child care are features that have been included to increase accessibility to more people.

Many city and county recreational departments have neighborhood recreational centers. About 80% of the population make some use of municipal facilities, and a smaller but substantial percentage use park programs and services (Godbey et al. 2005). The effectiveness of their physical activity programs depends on a number of factors, such as safety, privacy, hours of operation, transportation, and child care availability.

Entire communities have been the site of several long-term multicommunity interventions. These campaigns represent large-scale, high-intensity, high-visibility programming and often use TV, radio, newspaper, and other media to raise program awareness, disseminate targeted or segmented health messages, and reinforce behavior change. This strategy often employs multicomponent, multisector, and multisite interventions. The Stanford Five-City Project (Young et al. 1996) and the Wheeling Walks intervention (Reger et al. 2002) are examples of effective community-wide campaigns.

Cooperation among community organizations can enhance the effectiveness of exercise promotion programs. For example, the National Recreation and Park Association has partnered with the National Heart, Lung, and Blood Institute on the Hearts N' Parks program, whose goal is to promote physical activity in parks to reduce the occurrence of chronic diseases. Active Community Environments (ACEs) is another good example of a model for encouraging environmental and policy interventions at a community level to increase physical activity and improve public health. ACEs is a CDC-sponsored community intervention to promote walking, bicycling, and developing accessible recreation facilities. The goals are (1) to encourage the development of pedestrian- and bicycle-friendly environments, (2) to promote active forms of transportation such as walking and bicycling, and (3) to disseminate information about the program. However, studies of multicomponent community-wide interventions to increase physical activity have produced inconsistent findings. A *Cochrane* review published in 2011 examined the weaknesses in these intervention studies and concluded that these types of interventions do not effectively increase population levels of physical activity (Baker et al. 2011).

Virtual Environment

Advances in Internet infrastructure and accessibility have supported a greater use of technology to provide interventions partly or entirely in a virtual environment using mobile and wireless technologies and applications. The Internet is used by 79% of American adults, 83% of whom use it to look for health or medical information

(Pew Internet and American Life Project 2011b). Worldwide, there are more than 5 billion wireless subscribers (Barak, Klein, and Proudfoot 2009; World Health Organization [WHO] 2011). The increase of interventions in a virtual environment was highlighted in the August 2009 issue of the *Annals of Behavioral Medicine,* which was dedicated to articles on the science of Internet interventions. Computer-based health promotion interventions previously limited to desktop and laptop computers (i.e., e-health) have evolved along with advances in mobile technology (i.e., mHealth) and corresponding high penetration. The number of wireless subscribers in the United States increased from 207.9 million in December 2005 to 302.9 million in December 2010, with a penetration of 96% (number of active wireless units divided by the total U.S. and territorial population) (Blumberg and Luke 2011).

Terms to describe these virtual intervention methods include *m-health, e-health, web-based interventions,* and *telehealth.* WHO defines m-health as a component of e-health that is supported by mobile devices, such as mobile phones and patient-monitoring devices. Web-based interventions can be educational interventions that are self-guided, human supported, or some combination of the two (Barak, Klein, and Proud-

foot 2009). This medium has distinct advantages, such as timeliness, accessibility and convenience, and the ability to personalize messages.

Interventions using mobile technology have the advantage of interacting with people more frequently and in the context of the target behavior (Riley et al. 2011). Delivery can be through voice, text, applications on mobile devices, or mobile web. Thus, interventions can be personally and temporally tailored to real-time psychological, behavioral, and environmental conditions. For example, participants can log an exercise session and answer brief questions about their state affect on a handheld mobile device and receive real-time feedback with a wireless connection.

Level of Intervention

Interventions can take place at various levels within each setting. There are one-on-one programs (e.g., PACE) and programs for small groups, such as a strength training classes and walking clubs. The intervention can also be applied on a broader level—on the community level (e.g., EIM, ACES [All Children Exercise Simultaneously]), via legislation supporting increased physical activity (e.g., requiring the construction of bike paths), or nationwide through federal health promotion agencies. In 2006, Americans from government, nongovernment, private industry, and nonprofit organizations dedicated to physical activity and public health began developing the National Physical Activity Plan (NPAP), a comprehensive set of policies, programs, and initiatives that aim to increase physical activity in all Americans. Launched in 2010, NPAP programs include comprehensive multilevel strategies promoting physical activity in schools; at work sites and parks; and through sports, transportation, and advocacy.

With respect to duration, programs can range from one-time events to broad-based interventions spanning several years to ongoing programs, such as NPAP and EIM. Community-based fun runs or walks supporting a local charity may happen only once a year, but they can be opportunities for people who primarily want to help the organization to start thinking about exercise for its own sake. How long an intervention

Examples of Health Services

- Health call centers
- Mobile telemedicine
- Appointment reminders
- Community mobilization and health promotion
- Mobile patient records
- Patient monitoring
- Health surveys and data collection
- Health surveillance
- Health awareness raising
- Decision support systems

Based on WHO 2011.

needs to be to increase adherence has not been established. Studies that have measured exercise stage of change imply that those who have been regularly active for more than six months are at a reduced risk of relapse. However, results from our meta-analysis of exercise interventions indicate that effects were unrelated to the number of weeks the intervention lasted or the length of the follow-up period (Dishman and Buckworth 1996b). Many RCTs of exercise interventions last from one to two years (Courneya 2010), but dropout typically increases and the level of physical activity decreases along with the length of the intervention and follow-up.

Interest is growing in more ongoing interventions at the community, or societal, level that entail environmental engineering, community action, and legislation to support active lifestyles (e.g., NPAP). Local governments and health agencies can develop safe, accessible facilities for exercise with well-equipped buildings and competent staff. Actions can be taken to ensure safe neighborhoods for walking, jogging, and bicycling through lighting improvements and the construction of sidewalks and bike paths. Making the environment more conducive to physical activity is a goal of Active Community Environments Initiative, a program of the U.S. Department of Health and Human Services and the Centers for Disease Control and Prevention, and is one of the target areas for NPAP. Efforts include a collaboration with the National Park Service's Rivers, Trails, and Conservation Assistance Program to promote the development of parks and recreational areas close to population concentrations, as well as a collaboration with public and private agencies to promote National and International Walk to School Day.

A multidimensional perspective is necessary for understanding physical activity behavior and guiding intervention development at the level of the environment. Sallis and Owen (1999) proposed an ecological model that uses the "behavioral setting" to explain and predict influences on physical activity. The behavioral setting includes intrapersonal, social environmental, and physical environmental factors (see table 15.2). This framework can be used to identify behavioral settings in which people are more likely to be physically active, and to determine where more potent interventions can be implemented. For example, bike paths, downtown walkways, and attractive visible stairs are aspects of the constructed environment that should foster increased activity in urban settings.

Using ecological models expands our ability to identify barriers to physical activity, which are also defined on different levels (see table 15.3). Personal barriers can be psychological, such as low exercise self-efficacy or a perceived lack of time, and physical, such as past injuries or fatigue. Barriers can also be interpersonal—for example, peers may provide support and encouragement for sedentary behaviors. Environmental barriers are natural (e.g., inclement weather) and constructed (e.g., lack of transportation to an exercise facility, unsafe neighborhoods). A culture that promotes thinness and associates it with fitness fosters another barrier to exercise. Introducing a temporal dimension to this model

Characteristics of Communities That Support Physical Activity

- Sidewalks
- On-street bicycle facilities
- Safe and convenient street crossings
- Multiuse paths and trails
- Parks
- Recreational facilities

- Public facilities, such as schools, available for recreation services
- Mixed-use development and a connected grid of streets (allowing homes, workplaces, schools, and stores to be close together and accessible to pedestrians and bicyclists)

Recommendations From the Task Force on Community Preventive Services Regarding the Use of Selected Interventions to Increase Physical Activity Behaviors and Improve Physical Fitness

Informational Approaches to Increasing Physical Activity

- Community-wide campaigns: These large-scale, highly visible, multicomponent campaigns direct their messages to large audiences using a variety of approaches, including television, radio, newspapers, movie theaters, billboards, and mailings. *Recommended with strong evidence.*

Behavioral and Social Approaches to Increasing Physical Activity

- Individually adapted health behavior change programs: These programs are tailored to a person's specific interests or readiness to make a change in physical activity habits. Teaching behavioral skills such as goal setting, building social support, self-rewards, problem solving, and relapse prevention, the programs help people learn to incorporate physical activity into their daily routines. *Recommended with strong evidence.*

- School-based physical education (PE): This approach seeks to modify school curricula and policies to increase the amount of time students spend in moderate to vigorous activity while in PE class. Schools can accomplish this either by increasing the amount of time spent in PE class or by increasing students' activity levels during PE classes. *Recommended with strong evidence.*

- Social support interventions in community contexts: The goal of this approach is to increase physical activity by creating or strengthening social networks. Examples include exercise buddies, exercise con-tracts, and walking groups. *Recommended with strong evidence.*

Environmental and Policy Approaches to Increasing Physical Activity

- Creating or improving access to places for physical activity combined with informational outreach: Examples include building walking or biking trails or making it possible for people to use exercise facilities in community centers or in the workplace. Informational outreach includes activities such as providing training on equipment, seminars, counseling, risk screening, and health forums and workshops. *Recommended with strong evidence.*

- Point-of-decision prompts to encourage stair use: These signs are placed by elevators and escalators and encourage people to use nearby stairs instead. *Recommended with sufficient evidence.*

- Community-scale urban design land use policies and practices: Examples involve the efforts of urban planners, architects, engineers, developers, and public health professionals to change the physical environment of urban areas of several square miles or more in ways that support physical activity. *Recommended with sufficient evidence.*

- Street-scale urban design and land use policies: Examples involve the efforts of urban planners, architects, engineers, developers, and public health professionals to change the physical environment of small geographic areas, generally limited to a few blocks, in ways that support physical activity. *Recommended with sufficient evidence.*

Reprinted from CDC, 2001, "Recommendations and reports, increasing physical activity: A report on recommendations of the Task Force on Community Preventive Services," *Morbidity and Mortality Weekly Report* RR18: 1-16.

Table 15.2 Factors in the Behavioral Setting That Influence Physical Activity

Factor	Categories	Examples
Intrapersonal	Demographics Biological Cognitive and affective Behavioral	Age, health status, self-efficacy, self-regulation skills
Social environmental	Supportive behaviors Social climate Culture Policies governing incentives for activity and inactivity Policies governing resources and infrastructures related to activity and inactivity	Recreational habits of friends and family, work site fitness programs, mall walker groups
Physical environmental	*Natural* Weather Geography	Relative humidity and temperature, grade of hills
	Constructed Urban or suburban Architectural Transportation Entertainment and recreation	Population density, road maintenance, community budget for streetlights, environmental lobbies, high school physical education requirements

Adapted from Sallis and Owen 1999.

Table 15.3 Barriers to Physical Activity

Factor	Examples
Intrapersonal	Nonexerciser self-schemata, low exercise tolerance, poor time management skills, lack of time, low income
Social environmental	Sedentary peer group, unsafe neighborhood, culture that does not value physical activity
Physical environmental (natural and constructed)	Extended periods of high temperatures and humidity, urban congestion, lack of parks

addresses the impact of life transitions such as graduation, marriage, childbirth, and divorce on an established exercise routine, along with seasonal variations in opportunities for physical activity.

SPECIFIC STRATEGIES

The tools for helping individuals, groups, and communities become and stay regularly activity have been studied extensively in various popula-tions, and a wide variety of strategies are available. Deciding what works best and with whom can be informed by recommendations from health promotion organizations. For example, the Task Force on Community Preventive Services is an independent, nonfederal panel consisting of 15 members, including a chair, appointed by the director of the CDC. The *Guide to Community Preventive Services* (popularly called the *Community Guide*) is a periodic report that provides public health decision makers with recommendations about population-based interventions for the promotion of health and the prevention of disease, injury, disability, and premature death for use by communities and health care systems. The task force reviewed and assessed evidence on the quality and effectiveness of community-based interventions for increasing physical activity (Kahn et al. 2002), and made some recommendations for interventions.

Insight into effective strategies can also be gained from quantitative and qualitative reviews. Two meta-analyses to determine the efficacy of interventions to increase exercise adherence and factors that moderate and mediate their success, published 15 years apart, both found the most robust effects for behavior modification strategies (Conn, Hafdahl, and Mehr 2011; Dishman and Buckworth 1996b). A review of 74 studies published between January 1997 and May 2007 on diet or physical activity interventions was conducted to provide evidence-based recommendations to promote physical activity and dietary changes; the purpose of these changes was to reduce cardiovascular risk factors in adults (Artinian et al. 2010). Goal setting, self-monitoring, follow-up after the intervention is over, feedback and reinforcement, self-efficacy enhancement, and motivational interviewing implemented individually or in groups were found to be effective strategies, and teaching behavioral skills to support behavior change was also recommended.

A review of 18 theory-based interventions to foster weight loss through diet and exercise found that self-efficacy was the most frequently targeted variable, and offering opportunities for social comparison was the most common strategy (Bélanger-Gravel et al. 2010). Providing instruction and teaching self-monitoring were also used regularly. Other common strategies were prompting practice, identifying barriers, and prompting intention formation; when used in combination, these produced a significant between-group effect on physical activity at posttest and follow-up in overweight and obese people. Again, the most effective single strategy to promote physical activity and weight loss was behavior modification, but this was mostly in the short term; long-term effects were inconclusive.

A review of 22 theory-based physical activity interventions in adult nonclinical populations published from 1998 to 2008 indicated that half of the interventions failed to show an effect on physical activity (Rhodes and Pfaeffli 2010). The remaining studies reported that interventions had impacts on proposed mediators, but only six of them examined the mediating effects. The researchers concluded that self-regulation constructs may have the most effect on changes in physical activity and that the mediating effects of self-efficacy and outcome expectation constructs were shown to be trivial, but in limited studies.

A wide variety of strategies are used to promote the adoption and maintenance of regular physical activity, but similar terms do not always mean similar techniques, which may account for some of the mixed results regarding the effectiveness of strategies reported earlier. This section provides general descriptions of some of the strategies used in practice and research to increase exercise adoption and adherence. Health education, exercise prescriptions, behavior and cognitive behavioral management, and motivational interviewing have been used in a variety of settings. The use of technology in everyday life has increased exponentially, and likewise technology has been incorporated into behavior change interventions. Stage-matched interventions have been applied in community and medical settings and can increase the success of exercise programs. Aspects of relapse prevention training are important in fostering exercise adherence. Environmental approaches are taking on a more important role as we recognize the impact of situational and social factors on behavior change and maintenance.

Health Education

Interventions described as **health education** generally treat exercise as a disease prevention or health promotion behavior and target changes in cognitive variables. Programs using health education approaches have had little impact on exercise adherence (Dishman and Buckworth 1996b). However, such programs can increase knowledge and influence attitudes and beliefs about exercise to help inactive people consider beginning an exercise program. They can also provide concrete information about exercise classes and programs, which is useful for novice exercisers. Examples of health education applied to exercise include health screenings and health risk appraisals, mass media campaigns, and marketing strategies.

Health Screenings and Health Risk Appraisals

According to social cognitive theory, goals are developed when there is a discrepancy between actual and desired behaviors or characteristics. Health screenings and health risk appraisals, by documenting the fitness characteristics of an individual in relation to healthy norms, can make information personally relevant and enhance motivation to become more active. However, controlled studies using health risk appraisals and fitness test information as interventions have shown little or no effect on behavior. Attitudes and intentions may be affected, but not behavior. Generally, programs to increase knowledge may have short-term effects, but they result in no lasting change.

Mass Media

The mass media can promote health behavior change by introducing new ideas, reinforcing old messages to maintain behavior change, promoting attention to existing programs, and supplementing community-based interventions (Flora, Maibach, and Maccoby 1989). The goals of media campaigns vary according to the target group's behavior and readiness to change. A media campaign directed to people in the precontemplation stage should capture people's attention and motivate them to contemplate becoming more active. For those who are already considering participation in an activity program, the desired outcome is to motivate them toward action by increasing the personal relevance of the behavior change and decreasing the perceived barriers to exercise. Mass media are probably most useful in promoting exercise adoption. The usefulness of a media campaign is diminished for people who are already exercising. One can expect better results from mass media interventions that apply concepts from social marketing, such as integrating models of consumer behavior and

considering the attributes of the target population (e.g., media habits, education) in developing and disseminating intervention materials.

Mass media campaigns that are linked to specific community programming can be particularly effective in influencing levels of physical activity. This approach is exemplified by the VERB campaign, which targeted a cohort of 2,729 "tweens" (young people ages 9 to 13) in communities across the United States with mass media efforts, Internet links, and community events and programs designed to increase and maintain physical activity (Berkowitz, Huhman, and Nolin 2008). This exemplary quasi-experimental intervention was characterized by the use of multiple-media, segmented messages and links to community programming (Berkowitz, Huhman, and Nolin 2008). After one year, 74% of the children surveyed were aware of the VERB campaign, and subgroups of these children (9 and 10 years of age, girls, children whose parents had less than a high school education, children from urban areas that were densely populated, and children who were low active at baseline) engaged in more median weekly sessions of free-time physical activity than did children who were unaware of VERB. The average 9- to 10-year-olds who were aware of the VERB campaign engaged in 34% more free-time physical activity sessions per week than did 9- to 10-year-olds who were unaware of the campaign (Huhman et al. 2005).

Exercise Prescriptions

Exercise prescriptions have been used to increase exercise adoption and adherence, but have not been effective when used as a single strategy. The intensity of the exercise and the structure of the regimen are barriers to some sedentary people, whose reluctance to become more active may be tied to a misperception that the traditional structured prescription is their only option (Pate, Pratt, et al. 1995). Evidence from large-scale studies of physical activity and aerobic fitness was examined in the early 1990s, and research concluded that health benefits could be gained from minimal increases in activity and fitness. These findings and the low prevalence of exercise adherence provoked a reconsideration of the traditional exercise prescription and a modification of recommendations in 1995 to accumulate 30 minutes or more of moderate intensity exercise in shorter bouts of 8 to 10 minutes on most days of the week. American College of Sports Medicine (ACSM) guidelines for level of physical activity have been further revised (see table 15.4), retaining the flexibility of accumulating physical activity and offering options of meeting the guidelines with different levels of intensity. The recommendations of the American Heart Association (AHA) and the ACSM are consistent with the guidelines published by the U.S. Department of Health and Human Services in 2008 and include modifications for children and adolescents (i.e., accumulate ≥60 minutes of physical activity each day) and older adults (e.g., use relative intensity to determine level of effort). Recommendations for special populations (e.g., preschool children and pregnant women) are also available.

Characteristics of Lifestyle Physical Activity

- Duration: accumulate at least 30 minutes
- Frequency: most days of the week
- Intensity: at least moderate
- Mode: leisure, occupational, or household
- Planned or unplanned
- Self-selected activities

Adapted from *American Journal of Preventive Medicine,* Vol. 15(4), A.L. Dunn, R.E. Andersen, and J.M. Jakicic, "Lifestyle physical activity interventions. History, short- and long-term effects, and recommendations," pgs. 98-412, copyright 1998, with permission from Elsevier.

Table 15.4 American College of Sports Medicine Exercise Prescription Recommendations for Adults

Year	Intensity ($\dot{V}O_2$max)	Duration (minutes)	Frequency (days/week)	Key points
1990	50-85	20-60	3-5	Stressed developing and maintaining fitness, body composition; recommended guidelines for muscular strength and endurance
1991	40-85	15-60	3-5	Encompassed activities that may enhance health without having a major impact on fitness
1995*	Moderate	30 or more; at least 8 each bout	Near daily	Emphasized the important health benefits of moderate physical activity
2008**	Vigorous	20	3	Option to do an equivalent mix of moderate and vigorous aerobic activities
	OR			
	Moderate	30	5	
	AND			
	Strength training		2	8 to 12 repetitions of 8 to 10 exercises covering all major muscle groups

* Centers for Disease Control and Prevention and American College of Sports Medicine recommendations.

** American Heart Association and American College of Sports Medicine recommendations.

Data from Pate et al. 1995.

Lifestyle physical activity has been the target of several interventions. Jakicic and colleagues (1999) were the first researchers to compare the effects of prescribing multiple short bouts of exercise to accumulate a target duration with a single bout of exercise for the desired duration on change in weight, adherence, and fitness. Women who were overweight were randomized to 5 days per week of (1) progressive programs of continuous sessions, (2) multiple 10-minute bouts at convenient times throughout the day, and (3) multiple 10-minute bouts with exercise equipment (e.g., motorized treadmill) provided to their homes. Fitness and leisure-time physical activity improved in all three groups during the 18 months of the intervention, with less decline in adherence in the short-bout group that had the home equipment compared to the short-bout group without equipment.

Dunn and colleagues (1997, 1999) added support for lifestyle physical activity by comparing a group-based lifestyle physical activity program (1995 CDC/ACSM recommendations) to a traditional structured exercise program in Project Active. The effects of the two 6-month intervention programs on modifying the risk of cardiovascular disease in sedentary people were examined in 235 initially sedentary men and women. After 24 months, aerobic capacity was significantly higher than at baseline for both groups. Both groups had significant decreases in blood pressure and percentage of body fat, and most subjects in both groups were meeting the 1995 CDC/ACSM criteria.

These and other studies that have targeted lifestyle physical activity support the effectiveness of a lifestyle approach to changing physical activity and reducing health risks. (See Dunn 2009 for a review of lifestyle interventions to reduce cardiovascular disease.) Effectiveness studies have demonstrated that lifestyle physical activity interventions can be delivered in medical clinics, at work sites, in communities, and in homes using a variety of methods, such as in-person, telephone, and Web based. The lifestyle approach to increasing and maintaining the level of physical activity increases the options for sedentary people less inclined to participate in structured exercise programs. The flexibility of a lifestyle-based approach to physical activity may reduce perceived barriers to participation, such as time and effort, and make regular physical activity more psychologically accessible to the general population. A woman who is sedentary and overweight might not have considered regular exercise when the traditional prescriptions were promoted, but would consider the active lifestyle recommendation, especially if she is already walking at some level.

We need to keep in mind, however, that the lifestyle recommendation is not the solution for all health concerns. For example, weight loss is fostered by greater caloric expenditure compared to intake, and evidence points to the need to include both aerobic and strength training activities in physical activity programs. However, there is support for lifestyle activity to promote weight loss by substituting physical activities for less active behaviors, such as walking instead of riding in a car and taking the stairs instead of the elevator. These behaviors could be useful in increasing caloric expenditure and easier for overweight and obese people to fit into their daily lives than structured exercise.

> **E**xercise prescriptions must be based on the individual's capabilities and goals.

Behavioral Management

Behavioral management approaches encompass a wide range of strategies typically applied to individuals and small groups. Stimulus control, reinforcement control, and contingency contracting are based on behaviorism. These strategies are rooted in the traditions of behavior modification and cognitive behavioral modification therapies and generally target the antecedents (cues) and consequences of exercise behavior. Antecedents and consequences are related directly, or concretely (e.g., a friend asks you to go in-line skating, or you have a sharp muscle cramp after a maximal treadmill test), or symbolically (e.g., a high school bowling trophy or a picture of you finishing a swim competition) to the target behavior. Antecedents and consequences are also considered with respect to their temporal

> **B**ehavior modification has one of the best track records for increasing exercise adherence. The key is targeting critical antecedents and meaningful consequences.

association with the target behavior—that is, proximal (close in time) or distal (occurring long before or after).

Stimulus Control

Stimulus control involves manipulating antecedent conditions, or cues, that can prompt behavior *or* the decision to engage in a behavior (e.g., seeing the weather report for rain all week is a cue to decide about alternatives to running outside). Antecedents can be cognitive (e.g., reading a flyer from a new fitness facility in your neighborhood), physiological (e.g., feeling stiff from studying all day), or external (e.g., your dog approaches you with the leash in her mouth). Stimulus control can include strengthening cues for the target behavior and minimizing cues for competing behaviors. Competing behaviors are activities that impede engaging in the target behavior. Eating a hamburger and watching television are competing behaviors for jogging in your neighborhood. Keeping the computer turned off when you get home can minimize the cue for a sedentary activity that would compete

with an afternoon jog. Cues for exercise are strengthened when they are repeatedly linked with the target behavior—for example, exercising at the same time in the same place each day. Environmental stimuli, such as posters, phone calls, text messages, and adhesive notes, can serve as cues to prompt exercise. Stimulus control is often used as part of an intervention to complement and prompt the use of other strategies (e.g., receiving a text message reminder to self-monitor that day's exercise).

Stimulus control is frequently used with individuals and small groups, but it can be applied on a community level. Point-of-decision informational prompts can serve in a variety of settings to encourage people to walk or bicycle instead of driving and to use the stairs instead of the elevator. A classic study by Brownell, Stunkard, and Albaum (1980), which was replicated by Blamey, Mutrie, and Aitchison in 1995, successfully used a point-of-decision cue to increase physical activity. A poster encouraging people to take the stairs was placed near the escalator and stairs in a public building. During the intervention in both studies, significantly more people used the stairs than before or after the poster was displayed.

Reinforcement Control

Motivation to exercise depends on anticipated future benefits (outcome expectations). However, the more distal the desired outcome is from the behavior, the less power it has as a motivator. More immediate rewards must be provided to

Two Behavioral Management Strategies

Strategy	Definition	Examples
Stimulus control	Modifying conditions or cues that come before the target behavior	Adhesive notes, exercise equipment in visible locations, social support, telephone prompts, posters, radio and television ads
Reinforcement control	Modifying a desired condition or event during or after the target behavior to increase the frequency of the behavior on which the reward is contingent	Verbal praise, T-shirts, certificates

support the behavior. **Reinforcement control** increases the frequency of a target behavior by presenting something positive (positive reinforcement) or by removing something negative (negative reinforcement) during or after the behavior (see table 15.5). Examples of negative reinforcement for exercise are a decrease in psychological stress and an improvement in injury recovery during a rehabilitation program. However, positive reinforcement is used more often with exercise. A positive reinforcer, or reward, can be intrinsic (i.e., a direct result of the behavior, usually affective or cognitive) or extrinsic (i.e., a tangible reinforcement for the behavior). Intrinsic rewards can be a sense of satisfaction, achievement, enjoyment, enhanced self-esteem, or muscle relaxation. Examples of extrinsic rewards are certificates, T-shirts, coupons, and items with personal saliency, such as football tickets.

Reinforcement can involve providing the reward during or after the target behavior or pairing a low-preference behavior with a high-preference behavior (i.e., contingency reinforcement). An example of contingency reinforcement is setting up an exercise program so that the person must complete an aerobics routine before watching a favorite television show.

It is important to combine both extrinsic and intrinsic rewards for exercise, especially early in a program. The discussion of self-determination theory in chapter 14 points out that helping people develop intrinsic motivation fosters adherence better than having primarily extrinsic rewards does.

Reinforcement is crucial in the early stage of exercise adoption because the longer someone has been inactive, the longer it will be before the exercise behavior itself becomes reinforcing. Immediate feedback from exercise for novices can be pain and fatigue, which can be punishing. Immediate, positive rewards can counter this, such as praise and encouragement. Reinforcement control can also be used to change the contingencies or consequences that support or maintain a sedentary lifestyle. Some consequences of exercise that encourage inactivity are fatigue, muscle soreness, anxiety about time, perceived negative attention from more fit people, and shame or embarrassment about one's body or performance. Ways to counter these consequences are to set appropriate exercise prescriptions to reduce perceived physical strain and to offer exercise classes exclusively for beginners and less fit people.

Contingency Contracts

Contingency contracts (behavioral contracts) use reinforcement strategies to reward a specific behavior. Elements of contracts include objective measures of success, specific consequences of meeting and not meeting mutually agreed-upon objectives, a time frame, and the involvement of at least one other person. Written contracts have several benefits: the person participates in developing the behavior change plan; the written outline of expected behaviors serves as a reference over time; the terms of the contract are incentives to gain rewards or avoid **punishment**; and there is a formal commitment between the participant and another person to make specific changes. An example of a behavioral contract is shown in figure 15.2.

Table 15.5 Reinforcement and Punishment

Type	Objective	Positive	Negative
Reinforcement	*Increase* the frequency of the target behavior	*Add* something positive: Charting the number of miles or kilometers walked on the gym achievement board after each walking class	*Remove* something negative: Stretching after a jog to decrease muscle tightness
Punishment	*Decrease* the frequency of the target behavior	*Add* something negative: Muscle cramps after long walks	*Remove* something positive: Missing supper with the family on the nights the swimming class meets

Figure 15.2 Example of a behavioral contract, also known as a contingency contract.

Cognitive Behavioral Modification Techniques

Cognitive behavioral modification techniques are based on cognitive behavioral theory and social cognitive theory. These strategies for initiating and maintaining behavior change focus on the individual and include decision making, self-monitoring, goal setting, self-efficacy enhancement, and relapse prevention training, which are also considered self-regulation strategies. They incorporate many of the characteristics of reinforcement control and stimulus control, but the targets of the interventions are the cognitive variables assumed to be the mediators of behavior. The goal for the cognitively based strategies is to teach participants the cognitive and behavioral skills they need to control the conditions that prompt and reinforce behavior. Client participation in the change process is stressed. For example, self-reinforcement involves participants' establishing their own rewards and the specific criterion levels of the target behaviors necessary for achieving the rewards. The strategies we consider next, along with self-reinforcement and contingency contracting, are cognitive behavioral approaches.

> The focus of cognitive behavioral modification is on the individual. The goal is to teach cognitive and behavioral skills so that the individual can modify the conditions that prompt and reinforce behavior.

Decisional Balance

Decision making, or decisional balance from the transtheoretical model, is a behavior change strategy in which participants write down all anticipated short- and long-term consequences of the behavior change. Through this process, people become aware of benefits of the new behavior and receive help in finding ways to avoid or cope with anticipated negative consequences. Evaluating the costs and benefits of exercise is an important strategy for people contemplating the adoption of exercise because the perceived costs, or cons, of exercise likely outweigh the perceived benefits. This strategy can be used to point out benefits of exercise that the person might not have considered. Decision making can also be effective in identifying potential barriers to behavior change that can then be dealt with proactively. For example, someone who plans to exercise at 6 a.m. during the week may not have considered how getting up that early will affect a spouse who works the late shift.

Self-Monitoring

The strategy of **self-monitoring** is used in smoking cessation and other health behavior change programs to identify the cues and consequences of the target health behavior. Thoughts, feelings, and aspects of the situation before and after successful and unsuccessful attempts at the target behavior are recorded and reviewed. The effectiveness of self-monitoring on influencing behavior increases when participants monitor with greater frequency, detail, and proximity to the behavior being monitored. Self-monitoring is a practical way to collect information about behavior patterns that can be used to identify cues and barriers to exercise, and self-monitoring has been associated with successful exercise adherence and maintenance of weight loss. Internal and external cues that inhibit and prompt exercise can be determined, and the consequences of exercise can be examined in terms of their reinforcing properties. Information from self-monitoring can also help to identify the best times in a person's schedule for an exercise routine and any accommodations that will be necessary, such as having supper an hour later to accommodate exercising after work. Self-monitoring may be particularly useful for people who have been active in the past as a strategy to identify factors that contributed to their lapse in regular exercise. Electronic notebooks and calendars, computer programs, graphs, and charts can be used to record daily or weekly progress. Electronic devices (e.g., mobile phones) used for self-monitoring also open up the opportunity for prompting behavior. Periodic evaluation of behavioral records by fitness professionals can provide meaningful positive feedback and help the person monitor goals.

Goal Setting

A basic assumption of many cognitively based theories is that motivation is regulated by conscious goals. **Goal setting** is an effective strategy for supporting exercise behavior change, and goal setting is generally effective in increasing physical activity (Shilts, Horowitz, and Townsend 2004; Shilts, Townsend, and Dishman 2013). Recall that we set goals when there is a discrepancy between actual and desired behaviors or characteristics and we acknowledge a need for change. Functions of goal setting are then to provide direction, determine the level of effort to be expended, foster persistence, and support the search for strategies to achieve the goal.

For goals to be realistic and achievable, a comprehensive psychological and physiological assessment is necessary. For example, someone who wants to decrease the time it takes to jog 3 miles (4.8 km) has to know her present 3-mile jog time. Exercise testing can provide baseline fitness information for designing a safe and personalized exercise program that is less likely to result in punishing physical consequences, such as muscle soreness or injury, and more likely to be the type of routine that will meet the person's specific goals. Test results can be motivating when people compare their results to healthy norms or their own previous results. Repeated testing can also provide feedback for evaluating and revising goals.

A psychosocial assessment yields valuable information about attitudes, beliefs, expectations, and past experiences that can be barriers or supports to goal achievement. Reviewing previous attempts at change can show what worked and what did not, decreasing the likelihood of repeating past mistakes. Identifying psychological barriers, such as low exercise self-efficacy, helps shape goals that can address the needs of the whole person in his or her social context.

A large body of research on goal setting in sport indicates several characteristics of goals that enhance performance (e.g., Kyllo and Landers 1995). Many of these also enhance exercise behavior. Flexible, specific goals that are consistent with people's capabilities, values, resources, and needs are more effective than general, nonspecific goals. A combination of short-term and

Characteristics of Good Goal Setting

- Reasonable
- Realistic
- Does not depend on someone else
- Specific
- Measurable
- Challenging
- Time frame
- Flexible
- Meaningful
- Motivating
- Short term and long term
- Includes timely and specific feedback
- Considers social and physical environment
- Addresses physiological factors (e.g., health, fitness)

Examples of Exercise Behavior Goals

General	Behaviorally Specific and Measurable
To get more fit	To increase by 10% how long I can run for my next graded exercise test
To exercise regularly	To walk 4 or 5 days this week for 20 to 30 minutes each day
To get stronger	To bench press 125% of my body weight by June 5

long-term goals is better than long-term goals only. Because self-efficacy increases with mastery experience, initial goals should be challenging but realistic to foster confidence.

Self-Efficacy Enhancement

Self-efficacy is one of the most consistent psychosocial determinants of exercise adherence and a key variable in several theories (e.g., social cognitive theory, TTM). Belief in our capabilities influences our behavior, affect, and cognitions. The acquisition of new behaviors, the effort we expend on a task, the length of time we persist despite obstacles, our emotional reactions, and our thought patterns are affected by self-efficacy. There are four sources of information relevant to self-efficacy (i.e., mastery experience, vicarious experience, verbal persuasion, and physiological or affective states; see table 15.6), so it makes sense to target them in an intervention. Several studies have implemented interventions specifically designed to enhance exercise self-efficacy as a method of promoting behavior change.

• Mastery experiences may be the most potent method for increasing self-efficacy; people who are successful at meeting challenging tasks acquire and refine skills and develop coping strategies that foster confidence in their ability to repeat the task or similar tasks (generality dimension of self-efficacy). One way to facilitate

> **T**he most powerful way to enhance self-efficacy is through mastery experiences.

mastering a challenging task is to divide the task into manageable components and arrange them in logical order from easy to hard. Novices who attend an advanced aerobics class can be discouraged by the fast-paced, complicated steps, whereas those who enroll in a beginners' class can learn the routine one step at a time and increase their confidence in their ability to follow more complicated patterns.

• Social modeling can take the form of mastery models or coping models. In both cases, modeling is more effective if the model is similar to the participant; for example, an older woman watches other women in her age group successfully lifting weights. Mastery modeling entails watching someone succeed at a task; coping modeling presents someone having difficulty with a task but eventually succeeding. The latter strategy is useful in demonstrating effective problem-solving strategies relevant to the task and the target group. Exercise interventions to enhance self-efficacy have used mastery modeling (for example, having participants watch videos of people with similar characteristics engaging in exercise at various levels of progress).

Table 15.6   Sources of Self-Efficacy Information

Source	Exercise examples
Mastery accomplishments	Swimming 1/2 mile (0.8 km) for the first time; increasing weights in a strength training program; getting a hole in one after taking golf lessons; learning a new dance step successfully
Social modeling	Disabled people attending Special Olympics; adolescent girls watching the U.S. women's soccer team play; a retired physical education teacher taking a group from a senior citizen center on a walk in the park
Verbal persuasion	Your jogging partner tells you that you are setting a faster pace than before; your spouse tells you your exercise is paying off in how trim you look; your fitness coordinator comments on your good form during a bench press
Interpretation of physiological states	Being able to keep up a conversation after walking up a steep hill; being reminded that sweating a lot after exercising on a hot day is how your body cools you down; identifying how the sensation of muscle strain relates to the amount of weight lifted and the number of repetitions

• Verbal persuasion can enhance self-efficacy through the provision of encouragement and support from significant or powerful others. Verbal persuasion applies timely and specific feedback about exercise behavior and can be thought of as a form of positive reinforcement. Feedback is more effective if it comes from a credible source and is specific and meaningful. A student volunteer telling a cardiac rehabilitation patient, "You did a good job today," as the patient walks out of the clinic is not as effective as the rehabilitation director telling him, "Congratulations. You were able to walk an additional half mile today," as he steps off the treadmill. Information from self-monitoring can be used to teach self-persuasion. Negative self-talk surrounding exercise bouts is identified ("I just can't walk more than two miles") and reframed to encourage positive patterns of cognitions regarding exercise ("Six months ago I couldn't walk around the block. I am making steady progress").

• Interpretations of physiological and emotional responses can hamper self-efficacy—for example, feeling anxious before a test and interpreting your emotional response as a sign that you are not prepared. Novice exercisers often view the normal physiological responses to exercise (i.e., increased respiration and heart rate, sweating, and muscular sensations) with some anxiety or discomfort. Interventions have addressed this component of self-efficacy by informing participants about the normal physiological responses to exercise and ways to interpret these responses.

Relapse Prevention

Chapter 14 included a discussion of relapse prevention as a model of behavior. Relapse prevention as an intervention was initially implemented with people who had decreased or eliminated an undesired high-frequency behavior, such as smoking. Exercise behavior is a low-frequency, health-promoting or -enhancing behavior; nevertheless, applying components of relapse prevention to exercise adherence has proven successful to some extent. Several studies have tested the relapse prevention model with exercise and have found increased adherence when this model was used as part of broader cognitive behavioral modification programs.

The basic format for relapse prevention interventions involves identifying high-risk situations and developing effective coping strategies. High-risk situations are circumstances that challenge one's confidence in maintaining the desired behavior change. High-risk situations for maintaining regular exercise are events or situations that are incompatible with exercise, such as eating, drinking, overworking, and smoking. Some other relapse antecedents for exercise are boredom, lack of time, laziness, vacation, bad weather, inconvenient time of day, being alone, negative mood, being physically tired, and illness (Simkin and Gross 1994; Stetson et al. 2005).

> **H**igh-risk situations for exercise relapse are boredom, lack of time, laziness, vacation, and illness.

Knapp (1988) described the application of relapse prevention to exercise in detail. First, participants learn about the processes of relapse. Next, they identify high-risk situations for themselves. Self-monitoring is a useful strategy for obtaining this information. On the basis of identified high-risk situations, participants receive skills training to improve their coping responses. Strategies include assertiveness, time management, and stress management training; guidance in seeking emotional or instrumental support; and training in positive reappraisal, positive self-talk, and problem solving. Expecting positive outcomes from not exercising (e.g., watching a favorite television show while skipping aerobics class) increases the risk of relapse, so the positive outcome expectations of not exercising are identified and addressed (e.g., recording the television show and watching it as a reward after going to the aerobics class). Participants learn how to plan for slips by setting aside backup times for exercise and alternate modes and places to exercise (e.g., walking on a treadmill if the pool is closed). For example, if snow in the forecast puts an evening walking routine at risk, an aerobics tape can offer an alternative way to work out.

Flexible goals (walk *or* do aerobics 3 or 4 times a week) can provide protection from potential slips and the all-or-none thinking that increases the risk of relapse. People who think they have "blown it" by missing one exercise session are especially at risk of relapse. Rigid goals that are difficult to meet ("I will run at 12:10 each day for 45 minutes") also set people up for relapse. Another relapse prevention strategy is to correct a lifestyle imbalance in which "shoulds" outweigh "wants." One can reframe exercise as a desired, pleasurable activity instead of an obligation by setting up activities that are fun and by including rewards for exercising.

Motivational Interviewing

Motivational interviewing (MI) is a behavior change technique that Miller and Rollnick developed in the 1980s as a counseling method for the behavioral treatment of alcohol problems. The foundation of this technique is an empathic person-centered style that emphasizes evoking and strengthening the client's own verbalized motivations for healthy change. Training in MI involves knowledge and skills in four areas: (1) expressing empathy, (2) developing discrepancy to help the client realize the gap between values and problematic behavior, (3) respecting clients' resistance as normal, and (4) supporting the clients' self-efficacy (Rollnick, Miller, and Butler 2007).

An MI counselor helps clients identify the pros and cons of exercise, work through the barriers and ambivalence to change, and develop strategies for beginning and sticking with an exercise program. MI is often implemented in one 30- to 60-minute one-on-one session followed by several brief telephone support calls, although it can be adapted to different settings and consist of shorter sessions (Rollnick, Miller, and Butler 2007). MI can be used for a range of problems, including exercise, and shows potential to enhance intentions and engagement, increase self-efficacy to change, and foster change in less time than traditional interventions (Lundahl et al. 2010). MI has compared well to standard treatments for increasing physical activity in people with chronic heart failure (Brodie and Inoue 2005), long-term cancer survivors (Bennett et

al. 2007), and people who are overweight and obese (Van Dorsten 2007).

Telehealth

Interventions provided through the Internet and mobile technologies can provide a large volume of efficient, interactive, and tailored content that can be easily updated. These interventions range from semi-self-guided to fully self-guided. Benefits include reducing barriers to traditional on-site interventions, such as scheduling, transportation, and conflicts with other commitments, and can thus increase adherence and reduce treatment time and cost. Although few technology-based interventions have focused exclusively on physical activity as the outcome variable, effects are generally similar to those of traditional methods (Marcus, Ciccolo and Sciamanna 2009). Also, there is good evidence that interventions that use the telephone primarily are effective for increasing people's levels of physical activity (Eakin et al. 2007).

Mobile technology has promise as an intervention method. Riley and colleagues (2011) reviewed health behavior interventions that used mobile technology, defined as computer devices designed to be carried on the person throughout the day. They found 12 studies that reported using mobile technology for weight loss, diet, and physical activity interventions, four delivered via PDAs and the rest using mobile phones, mostly through text messaging. Some of the interventions were auto-adjusted; others were manually adjusted. Overall, they found modest but significant weight loss and related outcomes with mobile interventions. In addition, this technology affords innovative approaches, such as providing music on a mobile phone at a tempo that encourages an appropriate walking pace (Liu et al. 2008). Automated sensors, such as resident GPS and accelerometers, can expand the data available from mobile devices for measurement and intervention, and graphic displays of progress charts, animation, video, and games can enhance the quality of user feedback. Virtual training programs can also provide structure, support, and prompting, and electronic social networks can link people to a community of other exercisers. Technology-based interventions also offer a unique opportunity to provide just-in-time interventions, which are adjusted based on data gathered during the intervention and can provide a tailored response when a problem first appears (Intille et al. 2003). Traditional interventions, on the other hand, usually have a lag between input and intervention response.

Although technology offers exciting opportunities for creative interventions, it can pose unique challenges in assessing the intervention fidelity. Whereas engagement can be assessed in a face-to-face intervention by the facilitator (qualitative) and attendance (quantitative), web page viewing frequency may be a function of the web page architecture. For example, participants may have to view a certain page to go to other pages, inflating the hits for the gateway page. Additionally, web-based interventions can be semi-self-guided to fully self-guided, which should also be taken into account to assess adherence and engagement. Another limitation of Internet interventions is the high attrition, more than 50% in some studies (Danaher and Seeley 2009). Access to high-speed Internet is another issue. Only two thirds of American adults have high-speed broadband connection at home, although rates are significantly higher for urban, high-income, nonminority groups (Pew Internet and American Life Project 2011a).

ENVIRONMENT AND POLICY–BASED INTERVENTIONS

Psychological and behavioral theories have been applied to induce behavior change on a large scale at the organizational (e.g., community recreation centers, church-based fitness programs, diffusion strategies through schools), environmental (e.g., facility planning, construction of bike paths), social (e.g., family interventions), and policy (e.g., statewide physical education requirements) levels. Cost-effective and pragmatically convenient avenues, such as mail, telephone, e-mail, and websites, have been used to reach large numbers of people for whom traditional clinically based interventions are not accessible or acceptable.

Examples within this domain of physical activity promotion include creating or enhancing existing walking and biking trails or exercise facilities and increasing access to existing facilities by reducing barriers (e.g., increasing safety, enhancing affordability). These efforts often include personnel and participant training; social support; and the further integration of these structures, facilities, and programs into participants' communities. An exemplary intervention of this type, described by Linenger and colleagues (1991), included new infrastructure (i.e., bike paths), access to facilities (e.g., expanded hours of operation, lighted and integrated paths), and improved programming on a residential U.S. naval base (Linenger et al. 1991). Recent studies have documented that developing such infrastructure is reasonable from a cost perspective (Wang et al. 2004).

An emerging strategy involves placing physical activity on the public policy agendas of communities, emphasizing the promotion of physical activity guidelines, providing organizational incentives, addressing institutional and environmental barriers, and using media effectively (Hoehner et al. 2008). An example of this promising intervention approach comes from the work of Gomez, Mateus, and Cabrera (2004) with Muvete Bogotá, a community-based physical activity program in Bogotá, Colombia.

Increasing physical activity in a school setting can also be at the level of the environment. One study evaluated the impact of a playground redesign intervention across time on children's recess physical activity levels using combined physical activity measures (Ridgers et al. 2007). Fifteen schools located in economically depressed areas in a large city in England each received 20,000 pounds (about $33,000 U.S. in 2003) from a national Sporting Playgrounds Initiative to redesign the playground environment using multicolor playground markings and physical structures. Eleven schools served as matched socioeconomic controls. Physical activity levels during recess were quantified using heart rate telemetry and accelerometry at baseline and again 6 weeks later and 6 months after the playground redesign intervention. Statistically significant intervention effects were found across time for moderate-to-vigorous and vigorous physical activity.

> ## Examples of Legislation to Promote Physical Activity
>
> - Alter the environment to encourage physical activity for transportation. Close streets in cities to cars; create convenient bike paths and footpaths.
> - Revise building codes. Make stairs easy to find, centrally located, attractive, and safe.
> - Fund facilities for recreation. Create more parks and recreation centers that are safer and more convenient to low-active seg-
>
> ments of the population; provide adequate personnel for programs and security.
> - Create tax incentives. Provide tax incentives for companies with work site fitness programs.
> - Modify health insurance regulations. Reduce insurance premiums for heath behaviors such as regular physical activity.

WHY CAN'T WE KEEP PEOPLE ACTIVE?

MEDIATORS AND INTERVENTION EFFECTIVENESS

The United States saw little progress in Healthy People 2010 physical activity and fitness goals from baseline (1997) to the final assessment in 2008 (National Center for Health Statistics [NCHS] 2011). Adult participation in regular moderate or vigorous physical activity stayed at 32%, and regular vigorous activity increased from 23% to 24%. There were significant desired changes in no leisure-time activity (40% to 36%), regular muscle strengthening activity (18% to 22%), and walking for transportation (17% to 21%). More adolescents watched less than two hours of television per school day (57% to 67%), and more children and adolescents walked for transportation (31% to 36%). However, there were significant declines in percentage of senior high schools that required daily physical education for all students (5.8% to 2.1%) and bicycling for transportation for both children and adolescents (2.4% to 1.5%). Wide-ranging interventions have been implemented over the past 35 years to increase the adoption of and adherence to regular exercise, while at the same time a 50% dropout rate from exercise programs has persisted. Moreover, none of the Healthy People

2010 physical activity and fitness objectives were met (NCHS 2011). Physical, social, and political environments are receiving more attention as targets for interventions, and multilevel interventions using technology may prove to be more effective than more traditional approaches.

We attempted to address the questions *What works best, under what conditions, and with whom?* in our meta-analysis of exercise intervention studies, and found the strongest effect for behavior modification strategies (Dishman and Buckworth 1996b). Behavior modification also had the strongest effect in a meta-analysis of physical activity intervention studies with adults published between 1960 and 2007 (Conn, Hafdahl, and Mehr 2011). Only about 20% of the studies reviewed in our 1996 meta-analysis reported a follow-up to the intervention, and those studies typically showed that increases in physical activity or fitness associated with the interventions diminished as time passed after the end of the intervention. A *Cochrane* review of interventions promoting physical activity published in 2005 (Hillsdon, Foster, and Thorogood 2005) likewise found only 19 studies that reported follow-up data from 6 months or more that revealed a moderate effect on self-reported physical activity and fitness. However, heterogeneity in the characteristics of the interventions and inadequate detail limited the ability to draw conclusions. Thus, there are major issues in discovering how people adopt and maintain regular physical activity, which we discuss next.

Application of Theories

Chapter 14 addresses several theories that have been used to describe and predict levels of physical activity, but which theories will provide the best models for interventions promoting behavior change and maintenance? To understand the reasons for our limited success in getting people to adopt and maintain regular physical activity, we need to take a closer look at *how* interventions have been developed and implemented. Many interventions have been developed without a theoretical model or with only selected components of a model. Without a theoretical framework, the choice of variables cannot be well justified and the ability to interpret results is limited. An important step in answering which theories provide the best models is standardizing the reporting of how theories have been operationalized in interventions and providing details about methods and strategies. In fact, Masse and colleagues (2011) recommended the development of guidelines for reporting the theoretical foundations of behavioral interventions similar to the CONSORT statement for reporting randomized clinical trials. We also need long-term intervention studies and repeated follow-up assessments to track the process of adherence and relapse in theory-based interventions.

Literature reviews of physical activity interventions are now attending to the quality of the studies in respect to theory and mediator analysis. For example, Bélanger-Gravel and colleagues (2010) reviewed 18 studies published between 1980 and 2008 to investigate the long-term impact of theory-based interventions on physical activity among overweight and obese people. The theories most often applied were traditional behavior modification and social learning and social cognitive theories, used alone in eight interventions and with other theories in six interventions. However, only eight of the theory-based interventions specified which theoretical variables were targets. Specific techniques that were used in studies showing a between-group effect on physical activity at posttest and follow-up included prompting practice, barrier identification, and prompting intention formation. The most effective strategy was behavior modification, but this was mostly in the short term; long-term effects were inconclusive. Consistent increases in physical activity were found over time regardless of group, and few studies showed a superior effect of the intervention at follow-up. This lack of group difference may be related to the failure of most interventions to change theoretical mediators compared to the control group. Only one study performed appropriate mediation analysis, and self-efficacy was found to mediate the effects of the intervention on physical activity.

Implementation of Behavior Change Strategies

Ideally, exercise interventions should change the variables that are, according to a theory, responsible for changes in the outcome. Testing the intervention to make sure these key variables are actually changed (i.e., construct validation of the intervention) is becoming more common. One limitation to this is the lack of standardized definitions of the behavior change techniques. Self-monitoring, goal setting, or other strategies may be listed as part of exercise interventions, but implemented differently. Often, articles have page limits that lead to brief mentions of intervention components; without these details, it is difficult to faithfully replicate effective interventions. Identifying the specific techniques that contribute to effectiveness across interventions is thus also limited.

Abraham and Michie (2008) and Michie and colleagues (2008) developed a theory-linked taxonomy of 26 generally applicable behavior change techniques that correspond with changing key determinants of behavior. Their selection of techniques was partially based on reviews of interventions designed to increase physical activity and healthy eating. For example, "prompt-specific goal setting" is defined as involving "detailed planning of what the person will do, including a definition of the behavior specifying frequency, intensity, or duration and specification of at least one context, that is, where, when, how, or with whom" (Abraham and

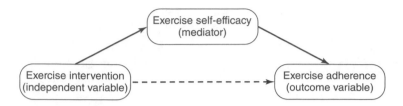

Figure 15.3 Self-efficacy mediates the effects of the intervention on exercise adherence when there are significant relationships between the intervention and self-efficacy, and between self-efficacy and exercise adherence (solid lines). Additionally, the relationship between the intervention and exercise adherence is not significant when the effects of self-efficacy are removed (dotted line).

Reprinted, by permission, from R.M. Baron and D.A. Kenny, 1986, "The moderator-mediator variable distinction in social psychological research: Conceptual, strategic, and statistical considerations," *Journal of Personality and Social Psychology* 51: 1176.

Michie 2008, 382). Time will tell whether these definitions are accepted and applied in exercise interventions.

Analysis of Mediators

Strategies should be designed to change suspected theoretical mediators, but the next step, mediation analysis, is often not taken. Chapter 2 defined *mediator* as the variable that accounts for the relationship between the independent variable and the outcome variable. For example, an intervention (independent variable) to increase exercise adherence (outcome variable) using Bandura's self-efficacy theory would aim to increase exercise self-efficacy (the mediator) (see figure 15.3). Baron and Kenny (1986) published a seminal article that distinguished between moderators and mediators of behavior change and social psychological outcomes. Using their model, three conditions must be met for exercise self-efficacy to be a mediator in our example. First, there must be a significant relationship between the intervention and exercise self-efficacy. Second, there must be a significant relationship between exercise self-efficacy and exercise adherence. Simply put, the intervention should increase self-efficacy, and increases in self-efficacy should be related to better adherence. Finally, to support the mediator role of exercise self-efficacy, the effects of the intervention on adherence should not be significant when one controls for the relationship between the intervention and self-efficacy *and* the relationship between self-efficacy and adherence. Thus, there is evidence that self-efficacy accounts for the relationship between the intervention

and the outcome because removing it weakens or eliminates the intervention's effect.

In a review and meta-analysis of techniques used to change exercise self-efficacy (Ashford, Edmunds, and French 2010), the most effective interventions used feedback and vicarious experiences; persuasion, graded mastery, and barrier identification were less effective in changing self-efficacy. As described earlier, to determine whether self-efficacy mediates exercise behavior change, the intervention must first change both self-efficacy and the target behavior before testing for mediation. Twenty-seven intervention studies published between 1966 and 2009 were included in another meta-analysis (Williams and French 2011) to identify strategies that changed both physical activity self-efficacy and physical activity in healthy adults. Strategies included in interventions that successfully changed physical activity and self-efficacy were action planning, reinforcing effort or progress toward behavior, and providing instruction. Interestingly, interventions that included setting graded tasks and relapse prevention were associated with lower physical activity and self-efficacy. It may be that the application of these strategies was not the same in each study considering that lack of details about interventions is a weakness in this literature. Additionally, some strategies are more effective at different points in time and with different populations. For example, relapse prevention may not be appropriate during the establishment of an exercise routine.

Deciding which theories and strategies have the best chance of increasing exercise adherence requires a careful analysis of the effects of the intervention on the theoretical mediator variables and the effects of the purported mediators on behavior. One example of a study that illustrates the clear application and testing of a theoretically based intervention was published by Silva and colleagues in 2011. They conducted a one-year RCT with a two-year follow-up with 221 overweight and obese women who were randomized to an intervention based on self-determination theory or a control group. The intervention group participated in 30 sessions that targeted communication skills, stress management, exercise, diet, and self-care, with a focus on a style that would increase autonomous regulation for exercise and weight control: providing structure and choice options, supporting autonomous decisions, encouraging personal treatment goals, limiting external contingencies and controls such as outcome-based rewards or praise, and monitoring externals such as behaviors and body weight. The goal was to help the participants develop a sense of ownership and mastery within a social framework. They found that maintenance of moderate and vigorous exercise was important in mediating the effects of the intervention on weight loss. Autonomous regulations measured at the end of the intervention were also related to exercise at the two-year follow-up, and this effect was fully mediated by autonomous regulation measured at the follow-up, showing a theoretically supported link between increased autonomous motivation and exercise and long-term maintenance of weight loss.

SUMMARY

Interventions must be based on the characteristics of the target group, the limitations of the setting, and a consideration of potential personal and environmental barriers to participation. There is good evidence for the effectiveness of strategies based on behavior modification.

However, there is no consensus on guidelines for interventions to increase and maintain physical activity, and gaps remain in what we know about the long-term maintenance of regular exercise. Traditional interventions have not addressed the cyclical or dynamic nature of exercise behavior, and the dropout rate from structured exercise programs has remained at 50% for the past 35 years. Intervention research has focused on implementing behavior change strategies and measuring the subsequent change in levels of physical activity. Few studies have tested the construct validity of the intervention by determining whether the intervention changed the selected mediators and whether the mediators changed the target behavior.

Future research should be directed toward testing the validity of theories for exercise behavior and testing the construct validity of interventions. Controlled longitudinal studies with specific populations are needed to establish what works and with whom. There is also the need to implement interventions at the level of the social and physical environment and explore the opportunities technology innovations present. Environments that prompt increased activity, offer accessible facilities, remove real and perceived barriers, and reward physical activity are likely prerequisites for the adoption and long-term maintenance of an active lifestyle.

WEBSITES

www.cdc.gov/healthyyouth/npao/strategies.htm

www.cdc.gov/nchs/healthy_people/hp2010/hp2010_final_review.htm

www.cdc.gov/physicalactivity/professionals/index.html

http://paceproject.org

www.thecommunityguide.org/pa/index.html

chapter 16

Perceived Exertion

Perceived exertion, sometimes called effort sense, is a person's subjective judgment of effort during physical activity. It results in part from a perceptual integration of sensations (the afferent neural inflow to the central nervous system [CNS]) that arise from the neural, physiological, and chemical signals associated with muscular force production. In this way, people can notice an increase in exercise intensity when it is imposed on them (e.g., during an incremental exercise test). Perceived exertion can also depend on central motor commands (the efferent neural outflow from the CNS) that activate skeletal muscle, the heart, breathing muscles, and other organs during exercise. It is accepted that copies of those motor commands are sent to sensorimotor regions of the central nervous system to provide a memory of expected sensations of movement, which seems to provide the main or only sense of effort when sensations of movement are impaired or absent. In this way, people say they are aware of increased effort during willed muscle contractions even when they have lost some limb sensations after anesthesia or trauma. Peripheral signals and sensations that occur during exercise are also compared with expected ones based on central motor commands. In this way, people can detect, possibly at different levels of consciousness, when effort is less or more than expected. This allows the motor system to make adjustments in force during weightlifting (e.g., when something is heavier than expected) or in pace during running or cycling (e.g., when a grade steepens without advance warning) to match performance intentions.

Perceived exertion is a **gestalt**—*gestalt* being a German word that, roughly translated into English, means "a pattern, a segregated whole, or a totality." Thus, a person's overall judgment about exertion represents something other than merely the sum of its parts (i.e., specific sensations during exercise; see figure 16.1). Nonetheless, it is important to understand the specific sensations that contribute to the whole perception. Those sensations arise from physiological strain, which differs according to the type and intensity of exercise and the person's level of fitness or training. Examples include sensations of force from contracting muscles during limb movements and during breathing, and sensations of temperature, sweat, and other factors that change in proportion to how energy expenditure varies during heavy exercise. Feelings of pain and discomfort, though separate from the sense of effort, can nonetheless add to a person's overall ratings of perceived exertion during intense, prolonged exercise. The relative importance of sensations and motor commands to perceived exertion can differ according to the type, intensity, and duration of physical

Components of Perceived Exertion

Motor command: Corollary copies of neural outflow from the motor system sent to the sensory system; provides a memory of expected sensations of muscular exertion. Peripheral signals: Neural inflow to the sensory system during force production; provides sensory consequences of muscular exertion.

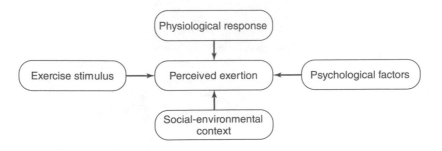

Figure 16.1 Perceived exertion as a gestalt.

exertion. Regardless of its precise origins in varying circumstances, perceived exertion is a useful concept for understanding people's responses to exercise and a usual tool for helping them regulate their exercise behavior.

Because the brain filters sensations, personality or mood might also affect perceived exertion—directly by influencing the quantity or quality of perceptions, or indirectly by influencing how people report perceived exertion to others. How people rate perceived exertion can be influenced by external cues in the exercise setting, including distractions or factors that motivate people to consciously or subconsciously raise or lower the ratings they report to others to make a good impression.

Fifty years of research on perceived exertion has led to a large body of information supporting its endorsement by the American College of Sports Medicine (ACSM) as a practically important component of exercise testing and prescription (ACSM 2009). Studies also suggest that perceived exertion is an important factor influencing whether people choose to be physically active and how vigorously they perform physical activity. This chapter reviews the history of perceived exertion and presents the basics of (1) how the methods of psychophysics have been used to determine the growth of perceived exertion during exercise; (2) how exercise professionals without training in psychophysics can use practical rating scales to measure perceived exertion during exercise; (3) the physiological, psychological, and social environmental factors that influence perceived exertion, in addition to the actual physical work being done; and (4) practical applications of perceived exertion for exercise testing, prescription, and monitoring exertion during exercise.

A BRIEF HISTORY

Debates about the existence of a **"muscle sense"** were common among physiologists and psychologists in Europe during the mid-to-late 19th century. The Scottish physician and anatomist Charles Bell proposed that a person's judgment of willed muscular force arose from sensory nerves from the muscle but not motor nerves to the muscle (Bell 1826). Building on Bell's idea, the French neurologist Guillaume Duchenne is credited as the first to draw a distinction between a muscle sense resulting from movement and a central, muscular consciousness of voluntary movement (Duchenne 1867, cf. Clarac 2008). In his 1886 treatise "Optik," the German neurophysiologist Hermann von Helmholtz then laid the foundation for the view that the perception of force comes from the central motor command (Southall 1924). Von Helmholtz noted that when the eye is moved manually without using the eye muscles, people perceive that their visual field has moved when it has not. He reasoned that this occurs because the predicted eye position has not been updated by the sensorimotor efference copy of the motor command sent to the eye muscles.

Henry Bastian preferred the term *kinesthesia* to *muscle sense* because some of the sensory afference during movement came from structures other than muscle, including tendons, joints, and skin (Bastian 1887-1888). Charles Sherrington later distinguished "proprioception" (awareness of movement from the senses of muscle, tendon, and joint) from "interoception" (senses from internal organs) and "exteroception" (senses outside the body) (Sherrington 1906). By the turn of the 20th century, it was commonly accepted that muscle sense had both central (i.e., motor command) and peripheral (i.e., kinesthesia) origins.

About 50 years later, research on coordination using insects, fish, and frogs by the German zoologist Eric von Holst (von Holst and Mittelstaedt 1950) and the American neuropsychologist Roger Sperry (Sperry 1950) provided the basis of the present-day concepts of kinesthesia, which include comparators between the internal feedforward of the central motor command to sensorimotor brain centers (efference copy, or corollary discharge) and the external feedback from peripheral senses (Crapse and Sommer 2008; Gandevia 1996; McCloskey 1978). The idea of an efference copy connotes a single, actual copy of the motor command to muscles sent also to sensory areas. However, a copy from the motor system to the sensory system would need to occur at many levels in the nervous system to account for reflexes and willed movements that differ in accuracy, precision, force, and timing. The idea of corollary discharge is that signals from the motor system can originate from almost all levels of the motor pathway and can target any level of the sensory processing stream (Crapse and Sommer 2008). This is discussed in more detail later in the chapter.

In 1892, American psychologist James McKeen Cattell, a student of Wundt and longtime owner-publisher of the journal *Science,* reported what appears to have been the earliest scientific study of perceived exertion when he and a colleague sought to determine whether men could accurately produce a handgrip force that they perceived to be twice or half that of a standard force (Fullerton and Cattell 1892). The next study of perceived handgrip force didn't appear until 1959 (Stevens and Mack 1959), and it was not until the 1960s that the concept of perceived exertion, as we now know it, emerged. Swedish psychophysicist Gunnar Borg became interested in people's perceptions of physical work after being informed by his medical colleagues that some of their patients who complained of having lost capacity for work actually had normal working capacities during cycling exercise. That indicated to Borg that the patients had underestimated their actual level of fitness. Later, Borg developed the first rating scales that could be used to measure perceived exertion, stimulating the development of perceived exertion as a field of scientific study and application (Borg 1962).

"IN STANDING, walking, and running, every effort of the voluntary power, which gives motion to the body, is directed by a sense of the condition of the muscles, and without this sense we could not regulate their actions . . . . it does not seem possible that a motor nerve can be the means of communication of the condition of the muscles to the brain."

Charles Bell 1826, 167-168

Swedish psychophysicist Gunnar Borg developed the first rating scales for the measurement of perceived exertion, and coined the term *rating of perceived exertion* (RPE).

Types of Perception

Perceptions of physical stimuli can be judged by quality or quantity. According to early Harvard psychophysicists Stevens and Galanter, quality, such as the hue or position of a light or the pitch of a sound, exists along a metathetic continuum, whereby "discrimination behaves as though based on a substitutive mechanism at the physiological level." In contrast, quantity, such as the brightness of light or the loudness of sound, exists along a prothetic continuum, whereby "discrimination appears to be based on an additive mechanism by which excitation is added to excitation at the physiological level" (Stevens and Galanter 1957, 377).

Perceived exertion is a perception of quantity more than of quality. Observations that people's judgments about the quantity of a physical stimulus might be distorted by their perceptions were first described and organized into lawlike postulates by psychophysicists during the first

> **J**udgments by people about the intensity of a physical stimulus do not necessarily grow linearly as the stimulus grows linearly. Determining how perceived exertion increases with the increasing intensity or duration of exercise is fundamentally important for prescribing and monitoring exercise.

half of the 20th century. It is now known that judgments by people about the intensity of a physical stimulus do not necessarily grow linearly as the stimulus grows linearly. Determining the pattern of increase in perceived exertion with the increasing intensity or duration of exercise is fundamentally important for prescribing and monitoring exercise among the public. Exercise professionals usually give their clients recommendations about the proper amounts of exercise based solely on physiological responses or adaptations to exercise that increase in a mainly linear pattern. If people perceive the amount of exercise in a nonlinear way, or perceive the amount to be less or more than physiological indicators of strain suggest, their comfort, fitness, or health may suffer.

PSYCHOPHYSICS AND PERCEIVED EXERTION

Researchers in the field of **psychophysics** study psychological judgments of physical stimuli. Those judgments are based on a sensation (a passive process defined as the stimulation of sensory nerve fibers by a stimulus) and a percep-

> **S**ensation is the stimulation of sensory nerves by a stimulus or signal. Perception is the cognitive interpretation of sensations. Perceived exertion is the rating of such perceptions during exercise.

tion (an active process defined as the cognitive interpretation of sensations). The study of psychophysics is based on standardized methods of manipulating physical stimuli and measuring the perceptual response to the stimuli. Just as those methods have been used to measure perceptions of specific physical stimuli (e.g., the brightness of light; loudness of sound; and speed, length, or passage of time), they can be used to measure perceived exertion during exercise.

Classical Psychophysics

Three common methods employed by classical psychophysicists are the method of limits, the method of adjustment, and the method of constant stimuli. The **method of limits** involves judging the magnitude of stimuli presented in a series across a range of intensities in ascending and descending orders. This method allows one to determine the lower and upper thresholds for perception. The lower threshold is called the stimulus threshold, which corresponds to the minimal intensity of the stimulus that someone perceives as just noticeable; stimulus intensities below the stimulus threshold are not perceived. The higher threshold is called the terminal threshold, which corresponds to the maximal intensity of the stimulus that someone can perceive; stimulus intensities above the terminal threshold are not perceived.

The **method of adjustment** involves making judgments of equality between two stimuli. A person is presented with a stimulus having a standard, objectively measured intensity and is then asked to adjust a comparison stimulus until he or she perceives it to be of the same magnitude as the standard stimulus. The **method of constant stimuli** also involves the presentation of a standard stimulus and a comparison stimulus. In this case the task for the person judging the two stimuli is to indicate whether the comparison stimulus is perceived and, if so, whether it is different from the standard stimulus. The comparison stimulus that is first perceived to be different from the standard stimulus 50% of the time is referred to as the **just noticeable difference (j.n.d.)**. The j.n.d. represents the smallest amount of change in the intensity of the stimulus required to perceive it.

Researchers in the 1960s developed **signal detection theory** (SDT) (Green and Swets 1974), which departed from classical psychophysical theory by emphasizing that a person's likelihood of reporting a change of signal strength is due to two interacting factors: **perceptual sensitivity-added** (d'), which reflects the person's capacity to discriminate changes in signal strength; and **bias** (β), or response criteria, which is a decision rule based on factors such as past experiences, instructions, and the expected cost and benefits. SDT, when applied to the **receiver operating characteristic (ROC) analysis** developed by radar engineers during World War II to detect the enemy, provides a method of assessing the balance between correct decisions (true positives and true negatives) and errors of commission (false positives) to quantify the contributions of perceptual processing and bias during human decision making. This is similar to test sensitivity, specificity, and predictive value described in chapter 2.

An ROC curve is a plot of the sensitivity or true positive rate versus the false positive rate (i.e., 1-specificity) to yield a binary (yes–no) classification system as the discrimination threshold (d') is varied (e.g., below or above 50%). The area under curve (AUC) is the probability that a randomly presented positive case (e.g., an increase in exercise intensity) will be judged higher than a randomly presented negative case (e.g., a decrease in intensity or no change). That probability should be ≥50% for a j.n.d. Because every point on a given ROC curve arises from the same value of the discrimination threshold being used, ROC curves can quantify not only a person's judgment of a standard exercise intensity but also how that judgment may be altered by specific conditions (e.g., indoors versus outdoors, alone or in the presence of others, or in varying temperatures). For example, later in the chapter, we'll see that people tend to rate perceived exertion lower when asked by a member of the opposite sex. Their actual perceptual abilities didn't change, but their willingness to give a true rating was likely altered by a social exchange.

The j.n.d. for various types of dynamic exercise has not been examined using signal detection theory, but early studies of cycling exercise showed that healthy people could sense random changes in work of at least 150 kg force m/min or about 25 watts (Morgan 1973; Skinner et al. 1973). The j.n.d during prolonged exercise is unknown (e.g., Dishman et al. 1994) but has potential relevance for pacing decisions that athletes make during training and competition and for understanding levels of preferred exertion during activities of daily living and leisure-time exercise in nonathletes.

> **A** just noticeable difference (j.n.d.) is the smallest amount of change in the intensity of the stimulus required to perceive it.

Classical psychophysicists were interested in scaling physical stimuli to determine the shape of the relationship between the physical growth of a stimulus and the perceived growth of the stimulus, averaged across people. Good examples are judgments of sound or the brightness of light. A whisper is easily heard in a quiet room but is inaudible in a cheering crowd. The beam of a car's headlights can be blinding in a rearview mirror but so dim in daylight that it is easy to forget to turn the headlights off. Mathematical laws that describe such perceptions more precisely provide a good start for understanding the growth of perceived exertion.

Common experience can make the mathematical laws of psychophysics easier to understand. For example, when humans hear linear increases in sound pressure level or wattage generated by an electrical amplifier, they do not perceive sound as increasing linearly. Rather, the judgment of sound grows mostly as a logarithm of light intensity, such that a 200-watt stereo amplifier is not perceived to be twice as loud as a 100-watt amplifier, which is not perceived to be twice as loud as a 50-watt amplifier.

The first mathematical equation describing the growth of human perception of physical stimuli was proposed by German physiologist Ernst Heinrich Weber. In his 1834 book, *De Tactu [About Touch]*, Weber reported his findings that sensations have stimulus and terminal thresholds and presented his most widely recognized concept, the j.n.d. On the basis of his theoretical work on the perception of weight, temperature, and pressure, Weber proposed that the j.n.d. was a ratio of the magnitude of the stimulus, rather than an absolute amount. For example, a greater weight must be added to 100 pounds (45 kg) than to 50 pounds (22.7 kg) for the person lifting it to notice that any weight has been added. Weber's law states that the amount of change in the stimulus necessary to produce a j.n.d. grows at a constant (k) linear percentage of the magnitude of the physical stimulus (S). For example, if

the j.n.d. during cycling exercise were 10 watts at an exercise stimulus of 100 watts, k would be .10 (i.e., 100 / 10). At 200 watts, the j.n.d. should be 20 watts (i.e., 200 × 0.10), and at 300 watts it should be 30 watts. Thus, according to Weber's law, each stepwise increment in exercise intensity would be perceived to have less quantity than the previous increment because the absolute value of each j.n.d. would increase.

However, Weber's law is not congruent with what humans typically experience during exercise. Perceived exertion during moderate intensities generally increases in proportion to increases

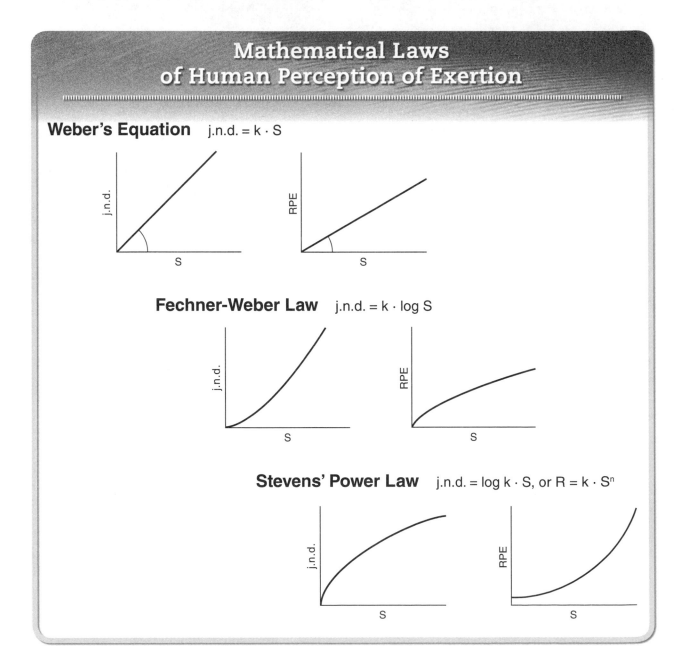

Mathematical Laws
of Human Perception of Exertion

Weber's Equation   j.n.d. = k · S

Fechner-Weber Law   j.n.d. = k · log S

Stevens' Power Law   j.n.d. = log k · S, or $R = k \cdot S^n$

in exercise intensity. And, as people approach maximal exertion, the j.n.d. for increased power output becomes smaller, making increases in intensity more easily noticed.

The scientist who first determined that Weber's ideas did not hold for all types of perception and sense modalities was one of his students, Gustav Fechner, who studied anatomy under Weber at the University of Leipzig. Fechner is credited with mathematically formalizing Weber's ideas as a lawlike relationship between stimulus and perception. Fechner then tested that law in his own studies of the perception of distance, brightness (even going temporarily blind after constantly staring at the sun), and lifted weights. He proposed a modified Fechner-Weber law around 1860 in his book *Elemente der Psychophysik.*

The Fechner-Weber law states that the j.n.d. increases logarithmically with the magnitude of the stimulus. That is, Fechner proposed that the j.n.d. grows to an increasingly greater degree with each linear increment in intensity—not by some constant fraction, as proposed by Weber, but by a common log (i.e., log-base 10) of the fraction. According to the Fechner-Weber law, the j.n.d. would increase as a positively accelerating function of increased exercise intensity.

Hence, according to the Fechner-Weber law, the perception of exertion during exercise would increase in a negatively accelerating fashion. Peak perceptions of exertion would approach a plateau as exercise intensity increases toward maximal effort. However, the Fechner-Weber law is also inconsistent with the increase in perceived exertion that humans experience during increasing exercise intensity.

Modern Psychophysics

In the 1950s, Harvard psychophysicist S.S. Stevens proposed a power law as a replacement for the Fechner-Weber law (Stevens 1957). Whereas Fechner argued that *equal relative increments of stimuli are proportional to equal increments of sensation*, Stevens' power law postulated that *equal stimulus ratios yield equal response ratios.* Computationally, Stevens' law states that the perception or response (R) is proportional to a constant (k) multiplied by the stimulus (S) raised to a power exponent, n.

The exponent n in Stevens power law is determined by first graphically plotting the log10-transformed stimulus values on the x axis and the log10-transformed perception values on the y axis. Then, the best-fitting straight line is drawn (or estimated from statistical software) through all the points on the log–log plot. The slope of this straight line is the exponent n in Stevens' power law. If the exponent is 1.0, the function describing the relationship between the stimulus and the perception is linear. If the exponent is less than 1.0, the function is negatively accelerating; if the exponent is greater than 1.0, the function is positively accelerating. Figure 16.2 illustrates these power functions.

Logarithm or Power Function?

Understanding how logarithms and power functions have been applied to psychophysical relationships is fundamentally important in understanding perceived exertion. The scaling of the human perception of sound provides a good example. The perception of sound is measured on a decibel (dB) scale such that each 10 dB increase represents a doubling of the perceived magnitude of the sound. On the decibel scale, a barely audible sound is given the value of 0 dB. The loudest sound that can be tolerated without pain is about 120 dB. The decibel scale was developed by Bell Laboratories in the early 1900s such that each increment on the scale would represent a doubling of the previous level on the scale. However, while testing the new scale, researchers determined that the human perception of sound did not follow a constant fraction of the sound stimulus as initially proposed by Weber. Rather, it more closely approximated a logarithm of the j.n.d. in sound.

Later, Stevens argued that the growth of sound perception only appeared to describe a logarithm of the j.n.d. because the scientists had used the classical psychophysical methods of limits, adjustment, and constant stimuli, which only indirectly estimated the real growth in perceived loudness. Stevens used more direct scaling methods, such as asking people to judge when a sound was some ratio (e.g., double or half) of a standard sound. He determined that the perception

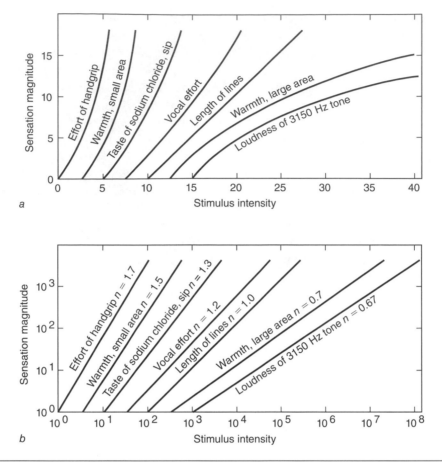

Figure 16.2 Linear *(a)* and log–log *(b)* plots of Stevens' power functions.

Reprinted from S.S. Stevens, 1957, "On the psychophysical law," *The Psychological Review* 64(3): 153-181.

of loudness did not grow as a logarithm of the j.n.d. in the stimulus as proposed by Fechner, but as a power exponent of the stimulus. The function describing the increasing loudness of a 3-kilohertz tone was determined by raising the increments in sound pressure level by an exponent of 0.67. Hence, perceived loudness grew as a negatively accelerating function.

Stevens' power law had a large impact on the field of psychophysics, because it was able to explain the relation among many types of sensation and perception, such as brightness, loudness, the pain of electric shock, the length of lines, and the effort of handgrip contractions, showing that perceptions increase exponentially, accelerating positively or negatively with increases in stimulus intensity.

Methods of Scaling Perception

Measurement of a psychophysical judgment is accomplished by scaling, which is the assignment of categories or numbers to describe or differentiate perceptual events. Four types of scales are used to assess perception: nominal, ordinal, interval, and ratio. Nominal scales simply name the object or event and thus yield the least amount of information. Ordinal scales not only name the object or event but also rank

> **S**tevens' power law explains the relation among many types of sensation and perception, showing that perceptions increase exponentially, accelerating positively or negatively with increases in stimulus intensity.

it, providing a crude index of quantity without specifying how much the ranks differ. Interval scales indicate the magnitude of differences in addition to naming and ranking the object or event. A Fahrenheit thermometer uses an interval scale. It indicates that the difference between 20 °F and 10 °F is the same as the difference between 10 °F and 0 °F. But, 0 °F on the Fahrenheit scale is not absolute zero (i.e., absence of temperature), so 20 °F is not twice as warm as 10 °F. Ratio scales are the most informative, because they have an absolute zero that permits a measure of proportion in addition to naming, ranking, and quantifying distances. A good example is the Kelvin scale of temperature developed in 1848 by British physicist Sir William Thompson, the Baron Kelvin of Largs, Scotland. This scale has an absolute zero. Thus, a temperature of 300 °K is twice as high as a temperature of 150 °K.

The two most commonly used ratio scaling methods in psychophysics are magnitude estimation and magnitude production. **Magnitude estimation** involves presenting a standard stimulus (called a modulus), such as a 10-kilogram weight, and asking the person to label his or her perception of heaviness, or force, with any number. Next, differing weights are presented in a random order, and the person making the ratings is asked to assign a numerical value to each weight in reference to the rating assigned to the modulus. This approach is also called free magnitude estimation, because the person is free to choose any number to label the modulus. In some instances the numerical value for the modulus is chosen by the experimenter; people are then free to choose any number to rate their perception of force.

Magnitude production involves a similar procedure, but the person making the judgments is asked to produce a response that he or she judges to be proportional to a given magnitude of the stimulus. Both estimation and production tasks involve a process called ratio setting. For example, someone might be asked to estimate when a stimulus is half or double the preceding stimulus, or some other percentage of that stimulus.

> **C**ommon rating methods in psychophysics require people to estimate or produce a response that is some ratio of the magnitude of a stimulus.

Power Law and Exercise

Studies using ratio-setting methods during hand-gripping and leg cycling exercise have shown that the growth of perceived exertion during increasing exercise intensities is more consistent with Stevens' power law than with the Fechner-Weber law. Under most circumstances, the exponent describing the relation between exercise intensity and RPE from magnitude estimation ranges between 1.5 and 1.7. This means that as exercise intensity increases, the perception of exertion increases in a positively accelerating fashion; or said another way, at low exercise intensities the perceived exertion should increase more slowly, but at higher exercise intensities the perceived exertion should increase more rapidly.

Types of Measurement Scales

Scale	Purpose	Example
Nominal	Classify or group	Social security number
Ordinal	Rank	Order of finish (first, second, third)
Interval	Indicate distance	Fahrenheit thermometer (10 °F vs. 20 °F)
Ratio	Indicate proportion	Kelvin temperature scale (150 °K vs. 300 °K)

COMPARING PEOPLE

The goal of classical psychophysics was to compare perceptions of various stimuli, not to compare one person's perception of a stimulus with someone else's perception. Indeed, differences among people were considered to be error or noise in the perceptual system. Borg modified Stevens' power law for perceived exertion by including two other terms, as shown in figure 16.3: perceptual noise *(a)* and stimulus threshold *(b)*. Those terms provide the starting point for a graph of the stimulus–response curve for perceived exertion, as shown in figure 16.3. Perceptual noise is a person's perception of exertion at rest, and the stimulus threshold is the work rate that is just noticeable above rest. Adding those terms allows an adjustment for variables that affect a person's level of perceived exertion at rest (e.g., muscle soreness or metal fatigue).

Borg's Range Principle

Ratio scaling methods best yield the true growth function of most perceptions. However, their limitation is that no common standard is used

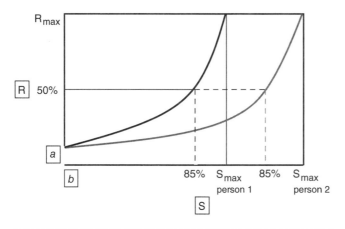

Figure 16.3 This graph illustrates Borg's range principle. The intensity of the response (R), in this case perceived muscular force, is plotted as a function of the intensity of the stimulus (S) (weight lifted) for two people who differ in maximal strength (S_{max}). R_{max} is assumed to be the same for both people according to the range principle. Coefficient *a* represents perceptual noise (i.e., R in the absence of S). Coefficient *b* represents the stimulus threshold. The horizontal dotted line shows the 50% R_{max}. Note that 50% R_{max} is the same for both people, occurring at 85% of S_{max} despite the higher S_{max} of person 2 (as indicated by the vertical dotted lines).

Borg's Modification of Stevens' Power Law

$$R = a + c\,(S - b)^n$$

that permits a comparison of two people's level of perception. Ratio scaling methods can determine whether the rate of growth in the perceived magnitude of a stimulus is twice as great compared to another, but they do not permit a judgment about the absolute level of a perceived magnitude. Ratio scaling of a perception permits each person to choose his or her own starting point for later comparisons. Because people's starting points are based on personal perceptions, which will surely differ, there is no way to compare the level or absolute magnitude of two people's perceptions. For example, the numbers that one person chooses to represent his or her perceptions (e.g., from 1 to 10) may be different from the numbers another person chooses to represent his or her perceptions (e.g., from 100 to 1,000). It is not possible to know that the initial perception rated as 10 was one-tenth the level of another person's initial perception rated as 100.

Borg recognized this limitation of ratio scaling and developed a category rating scale, which performs much like an interval scale, to permit standardized comparisons of perceived exertion. The RPE scales can be used to compare responses across individuals or groups of individuals based on a key assumption known as Borg's range principle (Borg 1961).

Borg's range principle assumes that most people have had similar experiences with physical exertion, retaining memories of past physical exertion levels so that perceptions of "no exertion" and "maximal exertion" have a shared meaning among people. According to the range principle, a judgment of 50% the intensity of maximal exertion would have the same perceptual meaning for two people even if it represented a different absolute exercise intensity for each person. In the example shown in figure 16.3, the exercise intensity (S) perceived

Borg's Range Principle

People who have had similar experiences with physical exertion will have the same perceptual range for feelings of exertion despite the fact that their physiological ranges for tolerating the strain of exercise (e.g., as evidenced by a lower or higher physical working capacity, strength, or maximal aerobic capacity) will differ widely. People's perception of maximal exertion provides a common point of reference, permitting comparisons among people at intensities that represent the same proportion of the perceptual range.

as 50% of R_{max} intersects the same position on the R function curve for person 1 and person 2, about 85% of each person's S_{max} (as indicated by the extrapolated dotted lines). Despite the higher S_{max} of person 2, R_{max} is the same for the two people.

Quantitative Semantics

Another assumption of Borg's approach to rating scales is that the adjectives people use to describe various levels of exertion convey a meaning of quantity that is commonly understood by most people. That assumption has been verified by a method called quantitative semantics, which measures the approximate numerical intervals that separate words according to the quantities they connote to people, on average. So, according to Borg's research, when perceived exertion is rated on an interval scale, the difference between the adjectives *light* and *hard* (or *heavy*) has the same perceptual quantity as does the difference in quantity indicated between the numbers 11 and 15. Hence, the selection and placement of verbal descriptors, or anchors, were intended to help people understand the perceptual meaning of the rating scale.

According to Borg's range principle, RPE during exercise should change in direct proportion to oxygen consumption, expressed not as absolute uptake in liter per minute, but as a

percentage of maximal oxygen uptake capacity. One way to test the validity of Borg's assumptions would be to compare RPE with a measure of relative metabolic strain during physical exertion. Indeed, a consistent finding about perceived exertion is that in many circumstances, RPE is linearly correlated with exercise intensity expressed as the percentage of $\dot{V}O_2max$ (%$\dot{V}O_2max$).

Figure 16.4 shows that RPEs between about 10 and 16 approximate exercise intensities between 45% and 85% of aerobic capacity. That linear relationship between RPE and percentage of $\dot{V}O_2max$ appears inconsistent with Stevens' power law stating that equal stimulus ratios yield equal response ratios, which predicts that the power exponent of exercise intensity will exceed 1. If so, how can RPE be linearly related to an increasing percentage of $\dot{V}O_2max$, maximal power output, or maximal force, when each one is a ratio of the stimulus? One possible explanation, which we address later, is that the power law does not accurately describe the growth of perceived exertion in all circumstances. That

During aerobic exercise, perceived exertion is directly related to relative exercise intensity expressed as %$\dot{V}O_2max$.

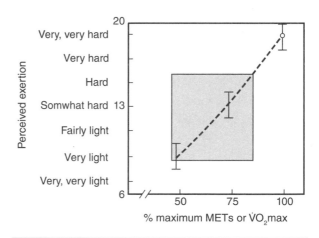

Figure 16.4 Category ratings of perceived exertion are related to the percentage of maximal oxygen consumption or the percentage of maximal METs during exercise.

Based on Borg 1998.

could be the case because perceived exertion is a complex integration of several senses, not a single sense.

Another explanation is that Borg's 15-graded, 6-20 RPE scale, as well as other category scales such as the University of Pittsburgh's 0-10 OMNI pictorial scales of perceived exertion during weightlifting (Robertson et al. 2005) and ratings of fatigue during cycling (Robertson et al. 2000) and running (Robertson et al. 2006; Utter et al. 2002) developed for children, permits comparisons among people on levels of perceived exertion but gives a distorted picture of the true growth of perceived exertion. For example, the OMNI scales link numbers that increase linearly with adjectives that connote growths in sensation using pictures that show a linearly increasing grade of effort (i.e., bigger and bigger dumbbells or running or riding a bicycle up a steep grade). Thus, children can easily guess that they are expected to give higher numbers as exercise progresses because that's what the pictures show.

The 15-graded Borg RPE scale is numbered 6 through 20. Because this scale is a category scale, it does not have an absolute zero point; it has an artificial floor and may not be sensitive to j.n.d.'s at lower exercise intensities. Also, there is a limit, or ceiling, of 20 to the maximal rating that can be made with the 15-graded RPE scale. Thus, if someone's RPE judgments increase as exercise intensity increases (as is common during most graded exercise tests), then it is possible that the ceiling of the scale is reached before the person's actual maximum. From that point on, the person is forced to provide the maximal rating of 20, even though the intensity of exercise, and the perception of exertion, would likely continue to increase beyond the first rating of 20 given. This effect, common to most category scales, is appropriately termed the ceiling effect.

Borg used the principles of ratio setting and quantitative semantics to construct another rating scale with ratio properties, the category–ratio 10-item (CR-10) scale. It is not influenced by the ceiling effect because it does not have a ceiling. The scale is numbered 0 through 10 and includes a maximal point that each person uses to rate perceived exertion in relation to a near-maximal rating of 10. For example, if a muscular contraction felt 20% greater than the value judged as 10,

the person would respond with a rating of 12; if it felt half again as forceful as that perceived at a rating of 10, the person would give a rating of 15. The decision to use the 6-20 or the CR-10 scale depends on the research or practical purpose of measuring RPE, which is addressed in subsequent sections on physiological correlates and exercise testing and prescription. Proper instructions for administrating the scales are very important and can be found elsewhere (Borg 1998, 104).

> **B**org's CR-10 RPE has ratio properties and estimates perceived exertion at low and high exercise intensities better than the original 6-20 category-interval scale does.

Ratings of perceived exertion can be made with both scales for the overall body (sometimes known as global RPE), or ratings can be differentiated to specific body parts (Pandolf 1982). Local or differentiated RPEs are ratings obtained for a specific body part or region, such as chest, leg, or arm effort. The decision to assess global or local ratings, or both, may depend on several factors, including the type of exercise, the clinical health of the person, or a particular research question. For example, during cycling exercise, it might be important to obtain perceived exertion about the legs, as well as the overall RPE. When testing a patient with chronic obstructive pulmonary disease, it might be especially important to know about breathing problems that affect RPE, so one would ask for local ratings of chest or breathing effort during exercise.

SIGNALS TO PERCEIVED EXERTION

In 1830, Charles Bell proposed "muscular sense" as a sixth sense, existing on a par with sight, sound, smell, taste, and touch. He postulated the existence of special peripheral afferent nerves that are activated by changes in posture and locomotion. His view was not widely accepted, and the prevailing view—held by a number of people including Wilhelm Wundt, the father of psychology—was that of a "sensation of innervation," whereby outgoing (efferent) impulses are sent from motor nerve cells to muscle, accounting for the muscular sense without a need to consider peripheral sense organs. That view persisted until late in the 19th century and has resurfaced in debates during the past few years about the biological basis for effort sense (Amann and Dempsey 2011; Marcora 2009a, 2009b, 2011; Meeusen et al. 2009).

A person's feelings of exertion and the ability to judge the quantity of those feelings depend on central commands sent to somatosensory regions of the brain and the perceptual integration of several sensations arising from various signals from all over the body. Unlike the 5 to 10 traditional senses, the sense of exertion does not have a specific sense organ. Rather, feelings of exertion represent an integration, or gestalt, of many signals with different origins. All of these signals are physiological in origin in that they all result in an excitatory or inhibitory postsynaptic electrical potential, consistent with the definition of a prothetic sense by Stevens and Galanter (1957). Nonetheless, it has become common to categorize signals that originate outside of the central nervous system as physiological mediators of exertion. Signals that originate within the central nervous system, such as those that activate brain regions regulating such concepts as personality, attention, and past experience (or

memory), are termed psychological mediators of perceived exertion.

SENSORY NERVOUS SYSTEM

How physiological responses provide signals to sensations during exercise and how those sensations are filtered and integrated into perceived exertion ultimately depend on how those responses are processed by the sensory nervous system. Nerve fibers are named according to whether they are myelinated (classes A and B) or unmyelinated (class C). Class A fibers are further placed into α, β, γ, and δ groups based on their conduction velocity. Class A fibers innervate skeletal muscles (extrafusal and intrafusal fibers). Class A (δ) sensory fibers relay touch, pressure, pain, and temperature; class B motor fibers innervate organs of the autonomic nervous system; and class C sensory fibers also relay pain and temperature. Sensory nerves are also named according to their function as type Ia, Ib, II, III, and IV afferent nerve fibers, which is the nomenclature used in this chapter.

The sensory nerves carry information from peripheral receptors to the spinal cord, where they synapse with sensory neurons that send ascending tracts to the brain that ultimately terminate at the tertiary, primary, or secondary (Brodmann's areas 3, 1, and 2) somatosensory cortexes (see figure 16.5). Signals of muscle fiber position and contraction velocity are transmitted by type I afferent nerve fibers. Sensations of force and stretch in skeletal and respiratory muscles, tendon stretch, and joint position and pressure are transmitted by type II afferent neurons carried through the dorsal column–medial lemniscal system of the spinal cord, which may also transmit signals related to metabolism. Sensations of pain and temperature are carried by a different bundle of afferent fibers, called the anterolateral system, in the spinal cord. Sensory signals sent by noxious chemical stimulation, such as lactate or hydrogen ions (or both), are transmitted by type III and IV afferent fibers via the anterolateral system. Figure 16.6 illustrates the medial lemniscus and anterolateral sensory nervous tracts in the spinal cord.

Muscular Sense

Sir Charles Scott Sherrington, the 19th-century British neuroscientist who coined the term *synapse,* argued that both central and peripheral views about muscle sensations were needed to explain the fact that sensations arise from both passive and active movements. He defined "the muscular sense" as "all reactions on sense arising in motor organs and their accessories" (Sherringto 1900, p. 1002).

Gray Matter

The butterfly-shaped gray matter is composed of cell bodies or nuclei and surrounds the central cerebrospinal canal (see figure 16.7). The dorsal horn (i.e., the posterior spine) contains the sensory neurons that process neural inflow from somatosensory organs, including skeletal muscle. The surrounding white matter consists of the axons from the sensory cells that ascend from the dorsal horn to transmit sensory information to the brain. The intermediate column and the lateral horn consist of autonomic neurons that innervate organs in the gut and pelvis. The ventral horn (i.e., the anterior spine) consists of motor neurons that innervate skeletal muscle.

Spinal neurons are grouped according to the organization of laminae and nuclei. Laminae, or layers, of gray matter in the spinal cord are defined according to their cellular sizes and shapes (i.e., cytoarchitecture) and function based on work in the 1950s by Swedish neuroscientist Bror Rexed. Laminae I to IV process exteroceptive sensation and comprise the dorsal horn. Laminae V and VI mainly process proprioceptive sensations relayed to the midbrain and the cerebellum. Laminae IV to VII also relay pain, temperature, and light or fine touch. Lamina VII is a relay between the muscle spindle to the midbrain and cerebellum. Visceral motor neurons are located in lamina VII and innervate neurons in autonomic ganglia. Laminae VIII and IX in the

Classes of Nerves

A (α), largest and fastest, motor and sensory
A (β), next largest, motor and sensory
A (γ), next largest, only motor
A (δ), next largest, only sensory
B, smaller than A fibers, only motor
C, smallest, motor and sensory

Classes		Sensory Types
A (α)	=	Ia
A (α)	=	Ib
A (β)	=	II
A (δ)	=	III
C	=	IV

ventral horn are composed of α, β, and γ motor neurons and provide the final pathway for the initiation and modulation of motor innervation of skeletal muscle. Lamina X surrounds the central canal and contains neuroglia and the gray commissure that spans the midline of the spinal cord posterior to the central canal. The main nuclear groups of cell columns within the spinal cord are the marginal zone, substantia gelatinosa, nucleus proprius, dorsal nucleus

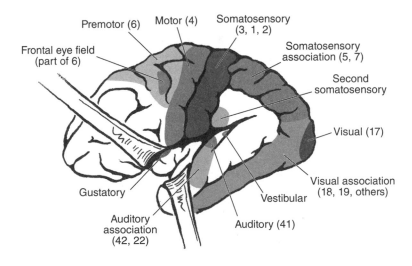

Figure 16.5 Brodmann's areas in the human brain.

Reprinted by permission from *The human brain: An introduction to its functional anatomy*, 4th ed., J. Nolte, pg. 232, copyright 1999, with permission from Elsevier.

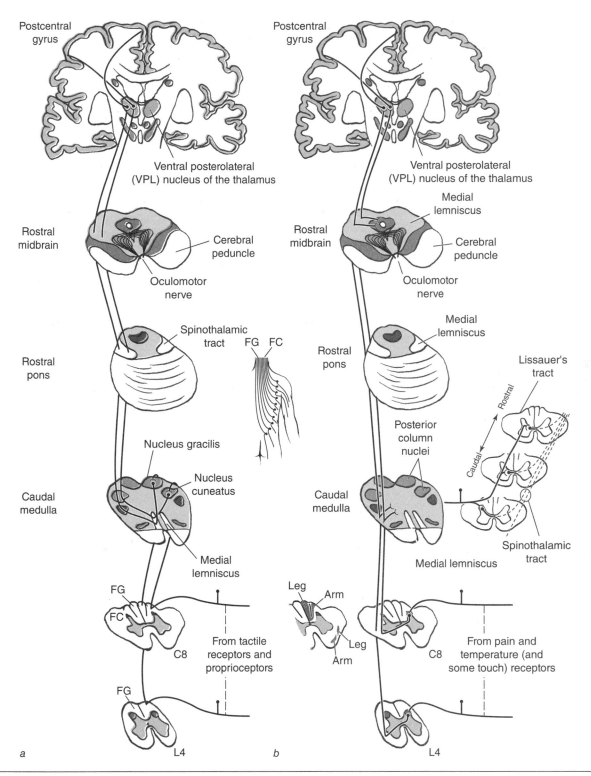

Figure 16.6 Sensory nervous medial lemniscus tracts *(a)* and anterolateral tracts *(b)*.

Reprinted by permission from *The human brain: An introduction to its functional anatomy,* 4th ed., J. Nolte, pg. 236, copyright 1999, with permission of Elsevier.

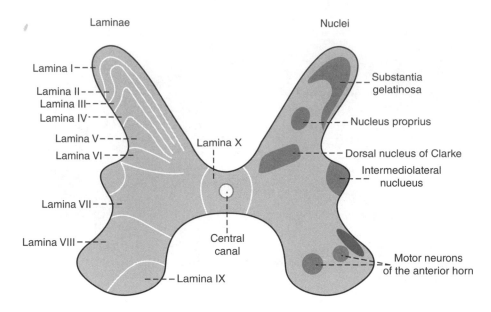

Figure 16.7 Spinal cord nuclei and laminae.

of Clarke, intermediolateral nucleus, and lower motor neuron nuclei.

The *marginal zone nucleus* is a thin layer of column cells at the tip of the dorsal horn. Its axons feed the lateral spinothalamic tract, which relays pain and temperature signals to the diencephalon region of brain.

The *substantia gelatinosa* is found at the head of the dorsal horn. It is composed mostly of intersegmental column cells that synapse at laminae IV to VII to relay pain, temperature, and light touch signals to the brain via the anterior and lateral spinothalamic tracts.

The *nucleus proprius* is the main sensory nucleus of the dorsal horn and is located adjacent to and below the substantia gelatinosa. Together with the dorsal nucleus of Clarke, the nucleus proprius is involved in sensing fine touch and proprioception. It consists of laminae III, IV, and V and receives input from the dorsal root ganglia. Its axons transmit sensations of light touch, proprioception, pain, and temperature to the thalamus and hypothalamus through the spinothalamic tract, and proprioception to the cerebellum through the ventral spinocerebellar tract.

The *dorsal nucleus of Clarke* is a cell column located in the midportion of the base form of the dorsal horn, mainly in the lower thoracic and upper lumbar spine. The axons from these cells pass uncrossed to the lateral funiculus and form the dorsal (posterior) spinocerebellar tract that transmits unconscious proprioception from muscle spindles and Golgi tendon organs to the cerebellum.

The *intermediolateral nucleus* is in the intermediate zone between the dorsal and the ventral horns in the spinal cord levels. In the thoracic to midlumbar spine, it receives sensory information from visceral organs and contains preganglionic sympathetic neurons. It also extends axons into the ventral spinal roots that provide preganglionic sympathetic fibers. Midsacral cell columns contain preganglionic parasympathetic neurons.

The *lower motor neuron nuclei* are located in the ventral horn of the spinal cord. They contain predominantly motor nuclei consisting of α motor neurons to extrafusal contractile skeletal muscle and β and γ motor neurons to intrafusal muscle spindles.

White Matter

The white matter that surrounds the gray matter contains myelinated and unmyelinated nerve fibers that carry neural signals up (ascending) or down (descending) the spinal cord (see figure 16.8). Axon fibers in the white matter are bundled together in four main ways according to either structure (funiculus and fasciculus) or function (tract and pathway). A funiculus is a large group of fibers found in an area of the spinal cord (e.g., posterior funiculus). Within a funiculus, smaller bundles that have different origins but common features constitute a fasciculus (e.g., fasciculus proprius). A tract is a group of nerve fibers that usually have the same origin, destination, and course and also similar functions (e.g., a corticospinal tract originates in the brain cortex and ends in the spinal cord, and a spinothalamic tract originates in the spinal cord and ends in the thalamus).

A pathway includes the nuclei and tracts in a functional neural circuit (e.g., cell bodies in the dorsal root ganglia, their axons as they project through the dorsal roots, synapses in the spinal cord, and projections of higher-level neurons across the white commissure, which ascend to the thalamus in the spinothalamic tracts). The white commissure is the bundle of nerve fibers that cross over the midline of the spinal cord anterior to the gray commissure (lamina X). A (δ) fibers and C fibers carrying pain sensation in the spinothalamic tract contribute to this commissure, as do fibers of the anterior corticospinal tract, which carry motor signals from the primary motor cortex.

Information from the skin, joints, and skeletal muscle is relayed to the spinal cord by sensory cells located in the dorsal root ganglia and then to the brain via the cuneate fasciculus (upper body) or gracile fasciculus (lower body) in the dorsal column of the medial lemniscus system. These fibers carry information related to tactile, two-point discrimination of simultaneously applied pressure, vibration, position, movement sense, and conscious proprioception (see figure 16.9). In the anterolateral column (or lateral funiculus), the lateral spinothalamic tract carries pain, temperature, and crude touch information from somatic and visceral receptors. More laterally, the dorsal and ventral spinocerebellar tracts carry unconscious proprioception information from muscles and joints of the lower extremity to the cerebellum (see figure 16.9). In the ventral column there are four prominent tracts: (1) the anterior spinothalamic tract, which carries pain, temperature, and touch sensations to the brain stem and diencephalon; (2) the spinoolivary tract, which carries information from Golgi tendon organs to the cerebellum; (3) the spinoreticular tract; and (4) the spinotectal tract (see figure 16.10).

The ascending dorsal column medial lemniscal and anterolateral systems carry sensory nerve traffic into several brain regions located beneath the cortex. Afferent fibers also travel to the basal ganglia and the cerebellum, areas involved in the initiation and termination of movement patterns (such as walking) and fine motor control. At the same time, signals are being sent farther up into the thalamus and then finally to the primary sensory cortex. Figure 16.11 uses a homunculus ("little man") to illustrate the relatively small

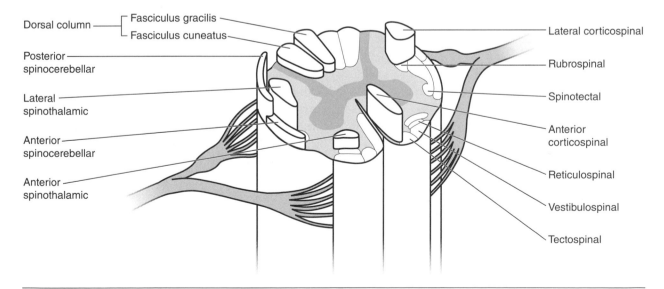

Figure 16.8 Dorsal ascending sensory columns.

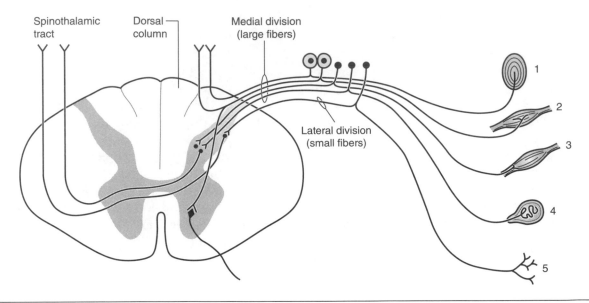

Figure 16.9 Dorsal root ganglia nerves from skin, joints, and skeletal muscle: (1) Pacinian corpuscle (mechano-receptor for changes in skin pressure and vibration); (2) muscle spindle (muscle length); (3) Golgi tendon organ (force); (4) encapsulated nerve ending (e.g., Meissner and Merkel mechanoreceptors for fine touch); and (5) free nerve ending (temperature, pain, and touch).

Adapted, by permission, from S. Waxman, 2009, *Clinical neuroanatomy*, 26th ed. (New York: McGraw-Hill), 47. © The McGraw-Hill Companies.

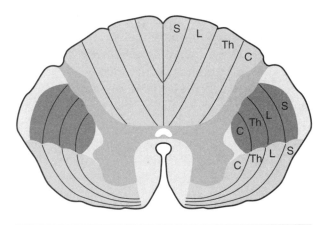

Figure 16.10 Sensory tracts of the dorsal, lateral, and ventral columns. S is sacral; L is lumbar; Th is thoracic; and C is cervical.

Heart rate (HR) increases as exercise intensity increases, but it is not perceived by most people during exercise, as sensations of heavy breathing and muscular force are. Thus, HR provides an index of strain but not a signal or sensation that is perceived as exertion.

representation of the skeletal muscles on the brain cortex compared with the large representation of the head, hands, and feet. The normal integration of all of these sensory signals regulates the homeostasis of physiological systems during the stress of increased metabolism in exercise and also provides the physiological basis for perceived exertion and subjective fatigue.

Because RPE increases as workload or work rate increases, any physiological response that increases with work could be related to RPE. Thus, it is important to distinguish physiological responses providing or modifying a signal that can be sensed during exercise, and therefore mediate RPE, from indexes of the physiological strain of exercise that are merely correlated with perceived exertion. An example of the latter is heart rate (HR), which increases linearly with work rate but is not perceived by most people during exercise. Hence, heart rate (HR) provides an index of strain but not a signal or sensation that is perceived as exertion. The following questions can help distinguish a physiological response as a mediator of RPE.

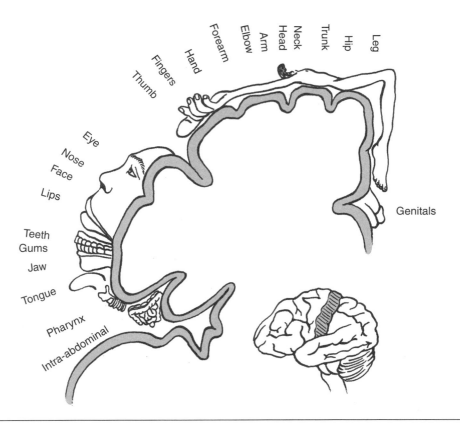

Figure 16.11 Homunculus of the sensory nervous system. A homunculus (little man) is used to show that most of the body can be mapped onto the sensory cortex of the brain using electrical stimulation. The distortions illustrate that the portion of the cortex dedicated to each body part is proportional to the amount of precision needed to control it, not its size.

From *The Brain: A Scientific American Book* by Scientific American © 1979 by Scientific American. Used with the permission of W.H. Freeman and Company.

- Is the factor a biologically plausible cause for altering the perception of effort?

- Does the relationship between the factor and perceived exertion hold under all conditions?

- Can the factor be directly sensed by the individual?

PHYSIOLOGICAL MEDIATORS

Physiological mediators of perceived exertion have been categorized as either respiratory–metabolic or peripheral in origin. Respiratory–metabolic signals are a group of physiological responses that influence the rate and depth of breathing (known as $\dot{V}E$ or minute ventilation) and the relative metabolic strain (i.e., percentage of $\dot{V}O_2$peak) during exercise.

Peripheral signals include sensations of force from the working muscles, sensations of pressure or force from joints and tendons, as well as sensations resulting from noxious chemicals that appear in the blood (such as hydrogen ions) during very intense exercise (e.g., above 50% of $\dot{V}O_2$peak) and repeated lifts of heavy weights.

Rating of perceived exertion is dominated during low-intensity exercise by local factors such as muscle force; but as exercise intensity increases, central factors, including sensations associated with increasing blood lactate and hyperventilation, play a more significant role (see table 16.1). The RPE typically corresponds with the percentage of $\dot{V}O_2$peak at all intensities regardless of the type of exercise mode. However, experimental manipulations of minute ventilation, blood lactate, blood pH, and blood glucose at unchanged levels of power output or

Table 16.1 Physiological Correlates of Rating of Perceived Exertion

Level	Symptoms	Metabolic intensity (% $\dot{V}O_2$peak)	$\dot{V}_E$	RELATIVE CONTRIBUTION	
				Respiratory–metabolic (% $\dot{V}O_2$peak)	Peripheral
I	Movement awareness	<50	Limited	Proportional	Dominant
II	Discomfort tolerance	50-70	Moderate	Proportional	Dominant
III	Noxious pain avoidance	>70	Significant	Proportional	Dominant

Model of the potentiating relationship between respiratory–metabolic and peripheral signals of exertion at low (level I), moderate (level II), and high (level III) metabolic rates.

Based on Robertson 1982.

percentage of $\dot{V}O_2$peak can perturb the association of the percentage of $\dot{V}O_2$peak with RPE.

Respiratory–Metabolic Correlates and Mediators of Perceived Exertion

Heart rate, blood pressure, oxygen uptake, and ventilation are respiratory–metabolic responses to increases in exercise intensity that change along with perceptions of exertion. Only ventilation, however, meets the criteria for a sensory mediator of perceived exertion.

Heart Rate and Blood Pressure

Because HR usually increases linearly with increasing exercise intensity, as does RPE, it is not surprising that HR and RPE are correlated with each other during incremental exercise. This happens not because HR is causing RPE to increase, but rather because HR increases to circulate more blood to meet the increasing energy needs of the active muscles. The relationship with HR was used as early evidence that RPE was a valid estimate of exertion. Borg presumably numbered his 15-graded scale from 6 to 20 to correspond with the typical range of HR from rest to maximal exertion, such that multiplying the RPE by 10 would provide a rough estimate of HR (Borg 1970, 1982). However, that relationship holds only under circumstances in which the environment is strictly controlled

and exercise intensity is incremented in periods of just a few minutes. In many other circumstances of prolonged exercise, HR and RPE can uncouple. A constant of 20 to 30 beats per minute must be added to the calculation of HR, such that

$$HR = RPE \times 10 \; (+ \; 20 \; to \; 30).$$

Blood pressure (BP) during exercise is not highly related to perceived exertion. Systolic blood pressure (SBP) increases with increases in intensity, though not linearly, and diastolic blood pressure remains stable or decreases slightly during dynamic exercise. The result of those responses is a moderate increase in mean arterial pressure (MAP). Because MAP does not change appreciably during exercise, it should not be viewed as a mediator of perceived exertion. However, the rate–pressure product (i.e., SBP × HR) is a good estimate of the oxygen demand of the heart during exercise, which is not related to RPE but can be related to ischemia of the heart and ratings of chest pain in people with heart disease.

It is unlikely that HR and blood pressure (BP) serve as mediators of perceived exertion. Under certain conditions such as thermal stress or the administration of cardiac drugs that alter HR (e.g., propanolol, which blocks β-adrenoreceptors on the heart), perceived exertion is uncoupled from HR. Also, HR can be affected by emotional states; and both humans and monkeys can be taught, using biofeedback of HR, to lower HR during exercise at low intensities. Furthermore, RPE during prolonged exercise at a constant intensity rises with the passage of time despite the fact that HR and BP remain essentially unchanged (Jackson et al. 1981). And it is unlikely that most people can accurately sense changes in HR or BP during exercise.

Oxygen Uptake ($\dot{V}O_2$)

The increase in oxygen consumption during exercise, particularly when expressed as relative exercise intensity (i.e., percentage of $\dot{V}O_2$peak), is strongly related to perceived exertion under many circumstances. As with HR, though, the association between RPE and %$\dot{V}O_2$peak can be altered during exercise. Manipulating other factors (e.g., environmental temperature or blood levels of lactic acid) while keeping the relative exercise intensity constant alters RPE. Also, RPE at a given percentage of $\dot{V}O_2$peak becomes lower after exercise training, so other physiological or psychological factors must also be important influences on perceived exertion. It is also unlikely that a person can directly sense $\dot{V}O_2$. Because the relationship between RPE and $\dot{V}O_2$ can be perturbed, and because it seems unlikely that people can actually sense oxygen consumption, %$\dot{V}O_2$peak is probably an index of perceived exertion rather than a signal to sensations underlying perceived exertion.

Ventilation

At low exercise intensities, signals associated with breathing do not appear to influence perceived exertion. But people can sense increases in the rate and effort of breathing as exercise becomes more effortful, and those sensations become an increasingly important influence on perceived exertion as the intensity of exercise increases (Killian 1987). In patients with asthma or other chronic obstructive lung diseases, ratings of breathlessness are the most important contributor to overall RPE (Yorio et al. 1992). Feelings of force or stretch from the inspiratory muscles also contribute to feelings of exertion, as does the overall breathing rate.

When ventilation is manipulated by changing the content of the oxygen or carbon dioxide in the air, RPE corresponds with the increases and decreases in ventilation, even though the actual intensity of the exercise has not changed. It seems very unlikely that humans can directly perceive the amount of oxygen being consumed or the amount of carbon dioxide being expired. However, the ventilatory equivalent for oxygen ($\dot{V}OE/\dot{V}O_2$) and the percentage of maximal oxygen uptake (%$\dot{V}O_2$max) during exercise provide very good indexes of the relative metabolic strain being experienced.

Rating of perceived exertion at the ventilatory threshold, the point at which the exponential growth of ventilation during heavy exercise is most pronounced, typically ranges between 12 and 14, which approximates *somewhat hard* on Borg's 6-20 category scale (Hill et al. 1987). Some evidence suggests that when the brain recruits more skeletal muscle fibers to generate more force during heavy exercise, it also stimulates heavier breathing to match the increasing metabolic demand of the exercise. In addition, increases in lactic acid during heavy exercise can contribute to increased ventilation.

Peripheral Correlates and Mediators of Perceived Exertion

Peripheral responses to increases in exercise intensity contribute more to perceptions of exertion than do cardiovascular–metabolic responses. There is evidence that RPE during incremental exercise is mediated by the concomitant accumulation of blood lactic acid (via influences on pain and ventilation), the increase in muscle recruitment and contraction, and increase in skin temperature. Although the release of catecholamines and stress hormones is also associated with increases in exercise intensity, the relationship between changes in these substances and RPE is likely not causal. Figure 16.12 presents an illustration of the relationship between perceived exertion and HR and lactic acid responses to increases in power output.

Blood Lactic Acid

At high exercise intensities, concentrations of lactic acid increase in skeletal muscles and the blood when the muscles' need for oxygen exceeds the ability of their oxidative enzymes to

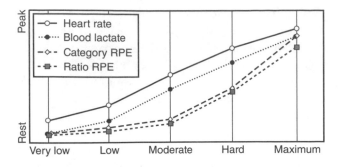

Figure 16.12 Linear and curvilinear relations between perceived exertion and physiological responses during incremental exercise.

use the oxygen being supplied. The major by-product of this increased anaerobic metabolism is the excess production of lactic acid. Borg appears to have been the first to recognize that the blood level of lactic acid during exercise has the same exponential rise as perceived exertion measured by ratio-setting methods (Borg 1962). Later study confirmed that the lactic acid increases in muscle and in blood during heavy incremental exercise correspond closely with RPE measured by an early version of Borg's 0-10 category–ratio scale (Noble et al. 1983). During incremental exercise, RPE measured by Borg's 6-20 category scale will not correspond well with lactic acid accumulation, because RPE increases linearly, whereas lactic acid increases curvilinearly.

The accumulation of lactic acid is accompanied by increased hydrogen ions that decrease the pH level of the blood. Although lactic acid is probably not a signal for perceived exertion, it influences at least two physiological changes that contribute to sensations that can contribute to perceived exertion. The first is pain and the second is ventilation.

Nociceptive nerves (nerves that carry pain signals) are sensitive to increased hydrogen ion concentrations, so lactic acid formation can be sensed as painful and the sense of pain could increase perceived exertion (Kostka and Cafarelli 1982; Robertson et al. 1986). However, the exact role of lactic acid in exercise-induced pain is not known, because other noxious chemicals (e.g., substance P or prostaglandins) that may contribute to perceptions of pain, as well as analgesic chemicals (e.g., β-endorphin), can be elevated in the blood at exercise intensities above 50% of $\dot{V}O_2$peak. The blockade of type III and IV

sensory fibers by the opioid antagonist fentanyl reduces limb discomfort by 13% at a high cycling intensity (325 watts), well above blood lactate threshold, but not at low (≤150-watt) intensities (Amann et al. 2010). Ratings of forearm muscle exertion during incremental maximal handgripping are not affected by the opioid antagonist naltrexone or by the analgesic codeine, an opiate precursor (Cook, O'Connor, and Ray 2000).

The acidosis caused by lactic acid is buffered during light to moderately intense exercise by bicarbonates in the blood. The carbonic acid that is formed is dissociated in the lungs to water and carbon dioxide, which is exhaled and adds to the volume of breathing in proportion to the carbon dioxide formed. At very heavy intensities, the excess carbon dioxide stimulates breathing centers in the brain to further increase ventilation. Because the onset of blood lactate accumulation, or the lactate threshold (the point at which the exponential growth of blood lactate levels during exercise is most pronounced), is closely coupled in time with ventilatory threshold and occurs at the same percentage of $\dot{V}O_2$peak, it is not surprising that RPEs of 12 to 14 on Borg's 6-20 category scale also are usually observed at the lactate threshold during graded incremented exercise (e.g., DeMello et al. 1987), although lower ratings occur when lactate threshold is induced using speed-incremented exercise in fit people (e.g., Boutcher et al. 1989).

Temperature Regulation

Core body temperature (Tc) increases as energy expenditure increases during exercise in proportion to the percentage of maximal working capacity. Thus, like HR, Tc is an index of relative metabolic strain. During prolonged (e.g., 30 min or longer) exercise under conditions in which the body's heat dissipation is burdened by high air temperature and high humidity, Tc increases more because the radiation gradient from the body to air and the evaporation of sweat are lowered. Under these hostile conditions, RPE increases. However, experiments that have manipulated Tc during constant exercise intensity, under conditions of room temperature and humidity, have failed to show that Tc is an independent signal for RPE (see Robertson and Noble 1997).

Skin temperature, on the other hand, can be perceived as a distinct sensation (compared to Tc) and may contribute to feelings of exertion during very hot and humid conditions. Although people can sense changes in skin temperature, the evaporation of sweat during exercise maintains, or can lower, skin temperature when air temperature remains constant because of the heat used to vaporize water on the skin surface and the heat transferred to passing air via convection. However, the dilation of capillaries near the skin surface may lead to sensations of subcutaneous heat that are independent of skin surface temperature.

Catecholamines and Stress Hormones

Epinephrine and norepinephrine (see chapter 3) are catecholamines released from the adrenal medulla by the sympathetic nervous system in response to the stress of heavy exercise. They act as neurotransmitters or as hormones to stimulate the contraction of muscle cells in the heart and to constrict or relax blood vessels that supply skeletal muscles. Similar to what occurs with lactic acid, catecholamines increase exponentially as exercise intensity increases; the rise in epinephrine occurs later and at higher intensities than the rise in norepinephrine and lactic acid. Also as with lactic acid, the increases in the blood levels of catecholamines during heavy incremental exercise correspond to RPE measured by Borg's 0-10 category–ratio scale of RPE (Skrinar, Ingram, and Pandolf 1983).

Much of the increased norepinephrine comes also from nerves that innervate the heart and those that innervate the blood vessels supplying skeletal muscles during exercise, pointing to the role of norepinephrine in increasing circulation

and BP to support increased metabolism. The secretion of epinephrine is more closely related to energy metabolism and to the emotional stress of heavy exercise. The roles of catecholamines in the maintenance of blood glucose levels, the regulation of muscle glycogen, and the control of emotional responses are potential mechanisms by which catecholamines could influence perceived exertion. However, like blood lactic acid, catecholamines may better represent an index of metabolic strain than a signal for RPE.

During exercise at intensities above about 60% of $\dot{V}O_2$peak, the anterior pituitary gland secretes adrenocorticotropin (ACTH) and β-endorphin into the bloodstream. The amount secreted is linear with increasing relative intensity. The role of ACTH is to stimulate the release of cortisol from the adrenal cortex to aid glucose metabolism during stress. The role of β-endorphin is mainly to assist the catecholamines in the regulation of circulation, breathing, and temperature control during increased metabolism, and in some circumstances analgesia (i.e., pain reduction). Anesthesia that blocks type III and IV sensory nerve traffic from the legs during cycling exercise abolishes the secretion of ACTH and β-endorphin without impairing the ability to generate power and without lowering catecholamine levels or RPE (Kjaer et al. 1989). Thus, it is unlikely that ACTH and β-endorphin directly influence perceived exertion. Rather, it is more likely that their increases during exercise result from the stress associated with high perceived exertion.

Muscle Recruitment and Contraction

Neurophysiological signals resulting from muscular contraction during exercise are processed through a feedforward–feedback mechanism (see figure 16.13). A feedforward mechanism occurs when motor (efferent) commands are simultaneously transmitted to the working muscle and the sensory cortex in the brain. A feedback mechanism operates when sensory (afferent) information regarding tension, velocity, position, and pain from peripheral receptors in the muscle (muscle spindles, Golgi tendon organs, mechanoreceptors, and nociceptors) is transmitted to the sensory cortex. The integration of these pathways permits the complex processing of the physiological signals underlying perceived

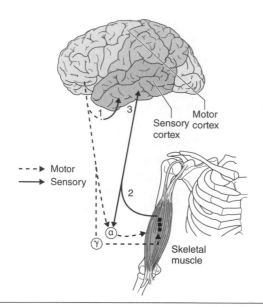

Figure 16.13 The feedforward–feedback mechanism.
Based on Cafarelli, 1982.

force and exertion (Cafarelli and Bigland-Ritchie 1979).

Muscle fiber type may also mediate perceived exertion. The exact differences between the signals sent by slow- and fast-twitch fibers are not fully understood. Lactate production during exercise is positively related to the percentage of fast-twitch fibers, suggesting that people with more fast- than slow-twitch fibers will experience a greater degree of metabolic acidosis, which might act on acid-sensing ion channels in unmyelinated fibers. And, as mentioned previously, some evidence suggests that the brain feeds forward motor commands to breathing centers to increase ventilation at the same time motor commands are sent to skeletal muscles to increase force.

Experiments using curare (a drug that blocks the chemical signals of acetylcholine at the neuromuscular synapse) to partially paralyze muscles indicate that RPE is increased proportionately to the increase in the central motor command from the brain to recruit more muscle fibers (Gandevia 1982). Other studies used the mechanical vibration of the patellar tendon in the thigh (Cafarelli and Kostka 1981) or the flexor tendon in the arm (Jones and Hunter 1985) to test the influence of feedback from muscle on the sense of force. When people tried to produce a force with the vibrated limb that felt the same as the force they were at the same time produc-

ing with the opposite, nonvibrated limb, the force of the vibrated limb was markedly lower. Thus, they experienced the vibrated muscle as producing more force than it actually was. One interpretation of those results is that increased sensations from the muscle, specifically from the muscle spindle (Cafarelli and Kostka 1981) or Golgi tendon organ (Jones and Hunter 1985), led to increased perceived force, presumably because there was no increase in central command during vibration as indexed by EMG. Similarly, submaximal force production during leg extension without patellar tendon vibration is lower when it is matched to perceived exertion with tendon vibration (Ogoh et al. 2002). Brain imaging of increased cerebral blood flow in the motor sensory cortex during handgrip exercise was not influenced by tendon vibration or ischemia in the exercising arm. Hence, it did not depend on neural inflow from muscle spindles or metabolically sensitive nerve fibers (Williamson et al. 1996). However, the involvement of type Ib or III mechanoreceptors was not ruled out.

Central Command

The idea of central command cannot solely explain how people are able to judge an unexpected change in exercise intensity when it is imposed on them, a defining feature of perceived exertion (Borg 1962; Morgan 1981; Skinner et al. 1973). Nonetheless, experiments using anesthetic drugs during exercise seem to show that people can be aware of increased effort during voluntary muscle contractions without needing to rely solely on the peripheral sensations of limb movement. Also, clinical cases of patients with abnormal perception and control of movement (Frith, Blakemore, and Wolpert 2000) are consistent with the idea of a sensorimotor memory of central motor command.

In an early study, perceived exertion during prolonged, constant-load cycling was higher (i.e., rated as *hard* rather than *somewhat hard*) after the blockade of unmyelinated type III and IV sensory fibers with the drug bupivacaine, even though ventilation wasn't affected and blood levels of the stress hormones ACTH and β-endorphin were abolished (Kjaer et al. 1989). Muscular strength in the thigh was reduced by 20% and blood lactate levels were twice as high

(4 mmol vs.2 mmol) during anesthesia, so the results seem to support that the higher perceived exertion paralleled an increase in motor command to recruit more glycolytic muscle fibers. However, proprioception was not affected by bupivacaine, so the study did not rule out that a sense of increased muscle force contributed to higher perceived exertion.

Patients who have Brown-Séquard syndrome have an injury or lesion to one side of the spinal cord, resulting in paralysis and the loss of proprioception on the side of the lesion and the loss of pain and temperature sensation on the opposite side. This type of division, or hemisection, of the spinal cord can result in a lesion on each of the three main neural systems: (1) the principal upper motor neuron pathway of the corticospinal tract, leading to lost motor function; (2) either or both of the medial lemniscus–dorsal columns (fasciculus gracilis and fasciculus cuneatus), leading to the loss of vibration and position sense and the sensation of fine touch; and (3) the anterolateral spinothalamic tract, leading to the loss of pain and temperature sensation.

Because Brown-Séquard patients typically have one side of the body with diminished sensation of pain and temperature but normal motor function, and the other side with diminished motor function (including loss of proprioception) but normal pain and temperature sensation, they provide a clinical model to test the relative contributions of central command and peripheral sensory signals to perceived exertion. In one study, patients used the leg with intact motor function but diminished sensation to produce 2 minutes of voluntary, static contraction, which resulted in an average RPE of 15 on Borg's 6-20 rating scale. When the same muscle force they had produced voluntarily was produced with electrical stimulation of the muscle, perceived exertion ratings were much lower (<10) even in the leg with intact sensory function. Also, when they tried to produce an equal absolute force for 2 minutes with the leg with the motor deficit, perceived exertion ratings were higher (mean RPE of 17) even though the average force produced was one-third less (Winchester, Williamson, and Mitchell 2000). The results seem to support the primacy of central command in the origin of perceived exertion. However, the clinical presentation of Brown-Séquard syndrome is based on the loss of pain and temperature sensations, so this study doesn't rule out that patients in the study had retained some sense of muscle tension during exercise performed with the sensory impaired leg, which could have contributed to their sense of effort.

At other extremes, people with some medical conditions are not aware of movement or have a false memory of muscle sense. Patients who show the anarchic or alien hand sign say they have no control of an arm and hand that writes or grasps without their will, as if the limb has a mind of its own (Marchetti and Della Salla 1998). However, the anarchic hand sign is associated with contralateral damage to the supplementary motor cortex (Goldberg et al. 1981), which, unlike the primary motor cortex, is activated during the planning of movement rather than during muscle force production.

Amputees who experience a phantom limb commonly say they still feel the missing limb, and some claim to be able to "move" the phantom. If the limb was paralyzed before amputation, patients say the phantom limb remains paralyzed and can't be moved despite their efforts (Ramachandran and Hirstein 1998). The phenomenon of the phantom limb is consistent with memories in somatosensory regions of the brain that are also associated with a corollary efference copy of a motor command. Patients who lose peripheral sensations but still have an intact motor output system may be unable to sustain a constant level of muscle contraction or make automatic, reflexive corrections to movements without visual feedback (Rothwell et al. 1982). Similar problems can occur when brain damage in somatosensory areas (e.g., the infra-parietal lobe) leaves patients without a sense of the limb opposite the brain lesion (Jeannerod, Michel, and Prablanc 1986). Overall, patients with peripheral sensory deficits have an impaired sense of muscular effort and the consequences of active movement. Their impaired ability to judge lifted weights indicates that their abnormal effort sense depends at least in part on the loss of large-fiber (i.e., types I and II) sensations during muscle contractions (Sanes and Shadmehr 1995).

The relative importance of sensations and motor commands to perceived exertion can differ according to the type, intensity, and duration of physical exertion. For example, the production of a force requires motor-unit recruitment, which depends on the memory of a central command. However, the effort exerted to sustain that force, in the absence of external knowledge of the actual force produced, depends on the person's perception of strain. When people try to sustain a constant force (e.g., during hand-gripping) without external knowledge (e.g., vision) of the force they are producing, force production gradually declines because of fatigue in tendons or muscles (e.g., the impairment of muscle contraction by the chemical by-products of metabolism). However, the person's perception of the force stays the same. The force was determined by the motor command, and the perception of force was matched to the efference copy of the motor command. There was no way for the person to detect the discrepancy between the expected and actual force. In contrast, with external knowledge of declining force production, the motor drive needed to maintain constant force production increases and is accompanied by an increase in perceived exertion.

Several lines of evidence show that the sense of effort that accompanies central motor command can operate independently of somatosensory inflow to the CNS. Without a change in workload or afferent feedback from muscle sensory receptors, perceived exertion is higher during a drug-induced (curare) partial paralysis that requires a person to try harder to perform the exercise. People can be deceived by hypnotic suggestion to perceive increased exertion when the actual workload has not changed. During normal circumstances of steady, dynamic exercise (e.g., prolonged cycling), perceived exertion can creep higher with the passage of time even when the workload doesn't change.

Clearly, if people had to rely only on sensory feedback for the control of movements, everyday life could not be as we know it to be. Each step or grasp would be hesitant, delayed by waiting for sensory feedback and perception before faulty movement commands could be corrected. An adaptive motor system is needed to overcome this dilemma by sending forward a copy of the motor command to sensory regions of the brain, and possibly the spinal cord, so there are

expected sensory consequences of movements (Christensen et al. 2007; Frith, Blakemore, and Wolpert 2000). In the past few years, brain imaging in humans has supported this long-accepted view. When healthy sensory nerves are experimentally blocked by ischemia (i.e., made numb using a blood pressure cuff), fMRI imaging shows that there is still activation of the primary somatosensory cortex (along with the premotor cortex, the insular cortex, and the intraparietal cortex) when people willfully move an ankle (Christensen et al. 2007). This finding supports the contention that the perception of movements does not depend only on the sensation of movement, but at least partly on predictions of the sensory consequences of voluntary movements by a sensory–motor feedforward network.

Paradoxical to the view that perceived exertion depends solely on central command, exhaustion during maximal muscular effort, when perceived exertion is highest, results in part from a lowered activation of spinal motor neurons. This occurs as a result of reduced central motor drive in response to neural inflow to somatosensory brain regions from muscle spindle, tendon, organ, and type III and IV afferents from fatiguing muscle (Butler, Taylor, and Gandevia 2003; Gandevia 2001). The use of lidocaine anesthesia in the spine during exercise supports the notion that the inhibition of somatosensory feedback from muscles during exercise can influence the conscious or subconscious components (or both) of central motor drive during high-intensity endurance exercise (Amann et al. 2008).

Corollaries of motor command or effort exist at several levels in the CNS to sustain motor, sensory, cardiovascular, respiratory, hormonal, metabolic, and thermoregulatory functions during physical activity. This neural outflow from the CNS to organ systems that support locomotion for a particular type of exercise changes with time as the musculoskeletal system adapts to changes in the amounts or types of physical activity (Duchateau and Enoka 2002). Thus, a change in perceived exertion in response to repeated physical activity that increases physical fitness will necessarily result from the altered central drive to execute the same external task, either directly because of altered corollary outflow operating at a preconscious level or indirectly because of altered sensations from physiological responses to the central driver.

PSYCHOLOGICAL AND SOCIOCULTURAL INFLUENCES

Although perceived exertion is influenced to a large degree by central command and physiological responses that provide or influence the signals underlying sensation, psychological and sociocultural factors also can mediate perceived exertion by (1) filtering sensations at the level of the central nervous system; (2) influencing how sensations, or an integrated perception, are evaluated; and (3) influencing rating behavior (i.e., the act of reporting perceived exertion to another person). Relatively few studies have clearly explained how psychological and sociocultural factors influence RPE. Nonetheless, some results seem plausible, given our current understanding of psychological theory and perception.

> **P**sychological and sociocultural factors can alter perceived exertion by influencing how sensations are processed by the nervous system, how perceptions are evaluated, and how RPE is reported to another person.

Augmentation–Reduction

Classical psychophysicists were interested in scaling sensations—that is, comparing the growth functions of perceptions of various physical stimuli. They considered differences among people in their judgments about the same stimulus to be error or "perceptual noise," probably because these scientists' backgrounds were in mathematics, physics, and physiology. In contrast, psychologists who study the ways people differ from each other (i.e., study personality) consider variations in psychophysical judgments among people to be indicative of real differences that can be explained by psychological variables. Indeed, most of the major theories of personality

include a factor describing how people modulate the intensity of a stimulus.

In the 1960s, Harvard medical psychologist Asenath Petrie had people judge changes in the width of a wooden dowel held between the thumb and forefinger so that she could measure what she termed kinesthetic figural aftereffect. Her research showed that some people consistently overestimated psychophysical stimuli when making judgments about size, whereas others underestimated. She dubbed them **augmenters** and **reducers**, respectively, and proposed that the lower tolerance for pain that she observed among augmenters could be explained by their naturally overstimulated nervous system. In contrast, reducers were believed to be naturally understimulated, so they could tolerate more sensations related to pain.

Petrie's findings were consistent with the earlier research of the famous Russian psychologist Pavlov and the British psychologist Hans Eysenck. Pavlov proposed a temperament trait called strength of excitement (SE) that referred to the ability to perform efficiently under levels of high stimulation without showing emotional disturbance. Eysenck later developed two temperament traits, extroversion–introversion and emotional stability–neuroticism, which linked the nervous system with behavior in much the same way Pavlov's single trait of SE did. An extroverted, stable person would be predicted to judge the intensity of a stimulus as lower than would an introverted, neurotic person. A logical extension of those lines of research is that people characterized as perceptual reducers or as extroverted and emotionally stable would be expected to perceive less exertion when compared with augmenters or introverted neurotics during exercise of the same intensity. Research in the 1970s by Bob Robertson at the University of Pittsburgh on perceptual reducers (Robertson et al. 1977) and by William P. Morgan at the University of Wisconsin on personality and mood (Morgan 1973) suggested that this indeed occurs.

Personality and Mood

Morgan found that people who scored high on self-ratings of anxiety, neuroticism, or depression (or a combination of these) made more errors in rating perceived exertion than did people who scored low on those tests. Also, people with a higher degree of somatic perception (i.e., the awareness of bodily sensations during stressful situations) reported higher RPEs than those who were less aware of such sensations. Compared to introverts, extroverts perceive a given exercise intensity as less effortful, and people with higher extroversion scores may prefer to exercise at higher workloads. Other psychological variables that have been shown to influence perceived exertion in some people are attentional style (whether someone focuses on body perceptions or dissociates from them during exercise), locus of control (whether people feel they have control over themselves and the environment), and self-efficacy (high confidence in personal abilities about physical exertion; Morgan 1981).

Hypnotic Suggestion

Morgan and colleagues also showed that imagined changes in work rate influence RPE even when the actual work rate is not changed (Morgan et al. 1973). After hypnotic suggestions that the exercise was harder, young men reported higher RPE even though they actually were cycling at a constant power output of 100 watts for several minutes. They did not seem to be faking the ratings, because HR and ventilation also increased. The imagined intensity apparently evoked a central command from the brain to the autonomic nervous system to increase heart and breathing rates as though a real increase in the metabolic rate of the exercise were occurring.

Comfort, Fatigue, and Perceived Exertion

The focus of most studies of perceived exertion has been on increasing or decreasing the intensity of exercise across a wide range of intensities with each level lasting a fairly short period of time (e.g., 1 to 5 min). That is a good approach for studying how people judge intensity, but it does not fully simulate exercise experiences, during which people often spend 20 to 60 minutes at an intensity that does not fluctuate very much. Common experience informs us that per-

ceived exertion tends to increase over time even when the actual intensity of the exercise does not change. When someone is asked to maintain a constant force, or workload, perceived exertion increases with time. In contrast, if a person is asked to maintain a constant effort, the amount of force or work the person produces decreases because the work feels harder as the duration of the task increases. Yale researchers observed that the exponent of the power function for perceived effort during cycling exercise doubled when the duration of each increase in power output ranging from 100 to 200 watts increased in duration from 15 seconds to 5 minutes (Cafarelli, Cain, and Stevens 1977). Feelings of fatigue may thus be another factor affecting perceived exertion.

> **P**erceived exertion tends to increase over time, even when the actual intensity of the exercise does not change. Thus, feelings of fatigue may affect perceived exertion.

In the 1970s, Michigan State University psychologist S. Howard Bartley, who studied perception and had an interest in the subjective aspects of fatigue, made an important distinction between the homeostatic perceptual system (composed of internal receptors responsible for regulating the balance or harmony of physiological systems to maintain cellular function) and the comfort perceptual system (consisting of the awareness of senses of pain, temperature, movement and position, and touch, including some of the homeostatic signals). Partly on the basis of Bartley's ideas, military physiologists (Weiser, Kinsman, and Stamper 1973) asked young men to ride a cycle ergometer at about 60% of aerobic capacity until they felt too uncomfortable to continue. The average time was about 36 minutes. Subjective ratings by the men described three main types of related responses: (1) general fatigue (e.g., worn out, tired, weary); (2) leg fatigue (e.g., weak legs, leg cramps), which had a subcomponent of cardiopulmonary symptoms (e.g., shortness of breath, heart pounding); and

(3) task aversion (e.g., sweating, uncomfortable, would rather quit) (see figure 16.14). Those findings were the first to suggest that perceived exertion during prolonged exercise could have both comfort and homeostatic dimensions that might affect perceived exertion as well as preferred exertion, the level of exertion that someone is motivated to endure (Borg 1962).

These important issues of comfort and motivation during exercise have been mainly ignored since the early research by Phil Weiser and his colleagues over 40 years ago. Recent efforts

> **S**ubjective fatigue appears to be composed of both homeostatic, or general, cardiopulmonary and local muscular sensations, and comfort components.

to measure subjective responses to varying intensities of exercise (Ekkekakis et al. 2011; Marcora 2009b) have not used the methods of psychophysics to build on that early research, so the growth and determinants of feelings of discomfort, pleasantness, and task aversion during

incremental or prolonged exercise and their relations with perceived exertion remain unknown.

Type A Behavior

When the type A behavior pattern (TABP) was elaborated in the 1970s as a possible risk factor for developing heart disease, evidence suggested that type A men were so motivated to accomplish more and more in less and less time that they suppressed perceptions of pain and fatigue. They might ignore chest pains or delay seeking medical treatment. There also was concern that type A men would overexert during exercise and underrate perceived exertion. That view has persisted today, without good evidence to support it. Studies showing an association between TABP and RPE or a self-rating of fatigue did a poor job of measuring TABP or exercise intensity. The studies did not control for relative oxygen consumption or training history to ensure that type A and type B subjects had similar fitness levels, or did not use a valid measure of perceived exertion, or used a self-report measure of TABP rather than the structured interview, which is the gold standard measure of TABP (Dishman et al. 1991). More recent research using better methods has shown no difference in RPE during

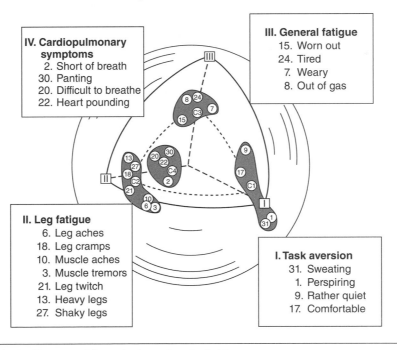

Figure 16.14 Spherical analysis diagram of four clusters at end of ride.

Adapted, by permission, from P.C. Weiser, R.A. Kinsman, and D.A. Stamper, 1973, "Task-specific symptomatology changes resulting from prolonged submaximal bicycle riding," *Medicine and Science in Sports and Exercise* 5(2): 83.

standard exercise testing between men classified as type A and type B by the structured interview (Dishman, Graham, et al. 2001). It is still possible that people who show type A behaviors might overexert or suppress perceived exertion during physical activities that foster competition, but this has not been shown in a scientific study.

Context and Perceived Exertion

Social, cultural, and contextual factors also can influence perceived exertion, but such influences are poorly understood (Acevedo et al. 1999; Boutcher, Fleischer-Curtian, and Gines 1988; Hardy, Hall, and Presholdt 1986; Rejeski 1981). The attitudes people have toward physical activity are shaped by their culture, and these attitudes might affect how a person rates effort during exercise, especially when exercising for prolonged periods at a fairly constant intensity. A person who has learned that exercise is enjoyable may have a different perception of exertion than a person who has learned to expect exercise to be painful or boring. The setting in which exercise occurs can also influence ratings. For example, the RPE of an exerciser could be influenced by characteristics of the scale administrator, such as sex, demeanor, or attractiveness. The preference of an individual for a particular mode of exercise is another potential influence on perceived exertion. A person who views a particular activity as distasteful (task aversion) might rate that activity as more effortful than another activity of equal intensity. The influence of psychological factors may be on a conscious or subconscious level, and people may or may not be aware of the effect of these factors on RPE. Therefore, it is important that scale administrators be aware of the potential psychological and sociocultural influences on perceived exertion and attempt to create a neutral environment to promote accurate responding. In addition, they must stress that honest responses are desired and that there are no right or wrong answers.

Although psychological and sociocultural factors likely influence perceived exertion and RPE, they haven't been adequately studied. The early line of research on the influence of personality traits and mood on RPE has not been pursued and verified. Also, such studies have relied mainly on correlational, not experimental, evidence based on absolute work rate without controlling for various levels of physiological strain among people having different levels of fitness or training. Hence, despite their seeming importance, the relative contributions of psychological and sociocultural influences on perceived exertion remain unknown.

PERCEIVED EXERTION: THE FINAL COMMON PATHWAY

How are central motor command and the sensations during physical activity filtered and evaluated to yield an RPE? The hierarchical model for understanding fatigue (or RPE) illustrated in figure 16.15 proposes four levels of sensory processing of the physiological responses (physiological substrata) in bicycling exercise. The level of discrete symptoms refers to the specific sensations that originate from the physiological responses. At the subordinate level, discrete symptoms are organized into clusters representing differentiated symptoms that are specific to the type (i.e., mode) of exercise. At the ordinate level, these clusters are combined to produce a primary symptom that is specific to the type of exercise (e.g., bicycling fatigue). Task aversion and motivation clusters also emerge at this level. The final level is the superordinate level, which represents an integration of symptoms to produce a global rating of fatigue.

Figure 16.16 presents a similar model for understanding RPE in which the perception of the exercise stimulus is influenced by individual differences that affect central motor command and the person's physiological responses to exercise. For example, a person with a high level of fitness and acquired motor skills will have a different response to a physical task than someone who is untrained and unskilled in the activity. Level 1 responses refer to the activation of efferent (i.e., motor) and afferent (i.e., sensory) pathways specific to the exercise stimulus. At level 2, discrete physiological responses (increased $\dot{V}O_2$, increased hydrogen ions) are processed in the sensory cortex and then fil-

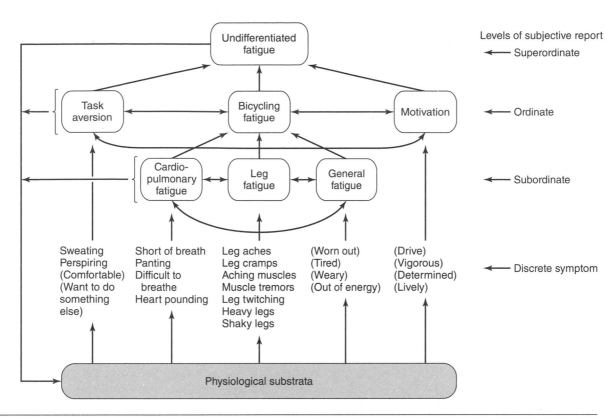

Figure 16.15 Pyramidal schema for subjective symptomatology during exercise.

Reprinted, by permission, from P.C. Weiser and D.A. Stamper, 1977, Psychophysiological interactions leading to increased effort, leg fatigue, and re-spiratory distress during prolonged strenuous bicycle riding. In *Physical work and effort,* edited by G.A. Borg (New York: Pergamon Press), 401-416. Adapted from Pandolf, K.B., R.L. Burse, and R.F. Goldman. 1975. Differentiated ratings of perceived exertion during physical conditioning of older individuals using leg-weight loading. *Perceptual and Motor Skills* 40, 563-574.

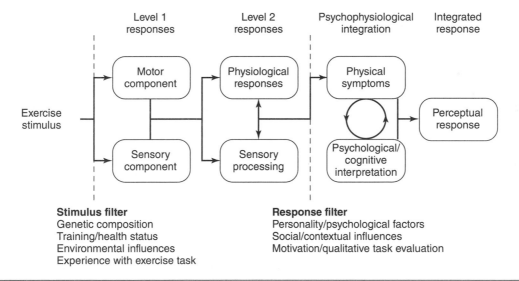

Figure 16.16 An integrated model of perceived exertion.

Provided by Dr. Heather O'Neal, the Exercise Psychology Laboratory, Department of Exercise Science, and Department of Psychology, the University of Georgia.

tered at a subconscious level to yield physical symptoms that are recognized by the person (expected effort, changes in breathing, sweating, etc.). An overall perceptual response results from the conscious interpretation of expected effort and physical symptoms according to the person's unique psychological and cognitive characteristics.

PRACTICAL USE OF RATINGS OF PERCEIVED EXERTION

Ratings of perceived exertion using Borg's RPE scales serve practical purposes in exercise testing, prescription, and monitoring people's progress during training in preventive and rehabilitative medicine and in sport. The concept of perceived exertion is easily understood by most people over the age of 10 (Bar-Or 2001), and about 9 of 10 adults are able to give accurate RPE during most types of exercise (American College of Sports Medicine 2000). Assessments of RPE are time efficient, inexpensive, and easy to administer. However, it is important that the person receive proper instructions. Some people might tend to focus on a single physiological, psychological, or environmental cue instead of rating their overall subjective feelings of exertion. Therefore, people must understand the scale instructions before rating perceived exertion, especially what the beginning and ending points on the scales mean concerning effort. The recent experience of a maximal effort is the best, but most people can remember or imagine what a maximal effort feels like based on past experiences.

Exercise Testing

Ratings of perceived exertion can be used to estimate perceived muscular force during resistance exercise, but RPE is most frequently obtained during a graded exercise test (GXT) in clinical and research settings. A GXT uses progressive increments in exercise intensity to determine a person's maximal exercise capacity (usually not submaximal endurance) and usually lasts 8 to 20 minutes. The most technical GXTs involve 12-lead electrocardiograms, blood sampling, and continuous sampling of oxygen consumption while the person walks or runs on a treadmill at increasing inclines, speeds, or both, or pedals a cycle ergometer while power output is increased. Results from a GXT can be estimated from simple field tests, such as time to complete a standard walking, running, or swimming distance. Graded exercise tests are used to estimate the maximal level of oxygen consumption per unit of time ($\dot{V}O_2$peak), which is the most commonly used criterion measure of cardiorespiratory fitness, or more commonly, how many minutes a person can endure the GXT before quitting.

The way perceived exertion is used during a GXT depends on the test protocol, the group of people being tested, and the exercise setting. In a clinical setting, a GXT is often used to aid in the diagnosis of pathology and to monitor improvement with treatment. Although a GXT is used mainly to assess exercise tolerance and general functional capacity in patients with conditions that limit physical capacity, a GXT may be used to assess patients' ability to perform everyday tasks or for building patients' confidence in their ability to exercise safely. In a research setting, the primary uses of a GXT are to determine the $\dot{V}O_2$peak, evaluate the effect of an intervention, and assess physiological responses to exercise. A GXT is generally used in a sport setting to screen for participation, assess training progress, and predict performance capacity.

The use of RPE during exercise testing has several specific purposes. First, it provides an index of subjective strain, so it can aid the tester in making judgments about a person's progress during the GXT while giving signs when a person is nearing the end of the test. In older adults and patients, it is recommended that preparations to end a maximal GXT begin when the person reports an RPE of 15 to 17 on the 6-20 scale. The use of RPE for monitoring is especially important in people who may not have a normal physiological response to exercise (e.g., patients with heart or lung diseases). Perceived exertion is not sensitive to heart ischemia, so heart rate and rhythm, blood pressure, and chest pain are still key signs of strain during exercise in heart patients. The close relationship between RPE and the percentage of maximal heart rate (%HRmax) reserve still holds in patients taking drugs that blunt HR (e.g., β-blockers), as long as HRreserve is computed from the resting and maximal exercise HRs obtained from a GXT while the patient is medicated at the therapeutic dose.

A second use of RPE during exercise testing is as a subjective indicator of peak exercise intensity. An RPE near the top of the scale is a good indicator that the person exerted a maximal effort. Third, a predetermined RPE can be used to monitor changes in power output after exercise training. For example, the percentage of $\dot{V}O_2$peak at an RPE of 15 after training can be compared with %$\dot{V}O_2$peak obtained before training. After training, most people will be able to exercise at a higher relative intensity without perceiving the exercise as harder. Fourth, the use of RPE during exercise testing can aid in the monitoring of people with health conditions that might lower their tolerance for exercise or put them at risk for circulation problems during a test. Finally, RPE can be used to detect a risk of staleness from overtraining among athletes who must train heavily to be competitive in their sports.

In older adults and heart or lung patients, an RPE between 15 and 17 on Borg's 6-20 scale is a good sign for the tester to be ready to stop a GXT. Perceived exertion is not sensitive to heart ischemia, so heart rate and heart rhythm, blood pressure, and chest pain are still key signs of strain during exercise in heart patients.

Administrators of exercise tests should keep in mind a few factors that may influence the perceptual response. With the activation of smaller muscle mass, RPE at an absolute workload is higher than with the activation of larger muscle mass. For example, RPE at a given workload or MET level should be lower during treadmill running than during leg cycling, although RPE should be similar at a given percentage of $\dot{V}O_2$peak. Although RPE is higher during arm cranking than during leg cycling when exercise intensity is expressed relative to %$\dot{V}O_2$peak of maximal leg cycling, it will be perceived similarly when intensity is expressed relative to %$\dot{V}O_2$peak of maximal arm cranking (Ekblom and Goldbarg 1971). Additionally, small but possibly important differences have been reported between sexes, in aging populations, and during pregnancy and various phases of the menstrual cycle. Hostile environmental conditions (e.g., temperature and humidity extremes) may also influence RPE.

Exercise Prescription and Monitoring

Exercise prescription falls into four areas: type (mode), intensity, duration (time), and frequency (number of bouts per week). Intensity is most directly related to RPE, but duration also affects it. An exercise program is prescribed at an intensity based on the results of the GXT. The American College of Sports Medicine and the American Heart Association guidelines for exercise prescription recommend that healthy people exercise 3 days per week for 20 minutes at a vigorous intensity (60% to 85% of $\dot{V}O_2$peak) or 5 days a week for 30 minutes at a moderate intensity (3 to 6 METs; 40% to 59% of $\dot{V}O_2$peak) (Haskell et al. 2007; see tables 16.2 and 16.3). Because the direct measurement of $\dot{V}O_2$ is time consuming, expensive, and cumbersome, exercise intensity is typically prescribed using one of the following methods to estimate the percentage of $\dot{V}O_2$peak: HR, metabolic equivalents (METs), and/or RPE (see table 16.3).

Heart Rate

Because HR and $\dot{V}O_2$ have a linear relationship, exercise intensity has traditionally been prescribed using a percentage of HRmax or a percentage of HRreserve. For that purpose, it is usually assumed that 60% to 90% of HRmax is equal to 50% to 85% of $\dot{V}O_2$max or HRreserve.

However, a large study of male and female employees at NASA's Johnson Space Center in Houston, Texas, showed that a prescription based on HRreserve underestimated %$\dot{V}O_2$peak by about 5% to 10% at intensities between 50% and 60% of HRreserve, but overestimated %$\dot{V}O_2$peak by about 4% to 8% at intensities between 80% and 85% of HRreserve (Weir and Jackson 1992). Thus, %HRreserve represents an inaccurate index of relative exercise intensity at low and high exercise intensities for many people. Adjusting %$\dot{V}O_2$peak for resting $\dot{V}O_2$ (i.e., $\dot{V}O_2$peak reserve), just as with %HRreserve, corrects this mismatch and yields a linear relationship between %$\dot{V}O_2$peak reserve and %HRpeak reserve. But making this adjustment is not practical in many exercise settings, and most exercise prescriptions are still made without it.

Table 16.2 Recommended Use of Rating of Perceived Exertion and Heart Rate Guidelines Found Successful in the Prescription of Exercise for Healthy Adults

MEASURE OF EXERCISE INTENSITY FOLLOWING EXERCISE		
Heart rate	**RPE**	**Exercise prescription**
<70% of HRmax	11	Increase intensity, duration, or both.
70-80% of HRmax	12-14	Okay. Increase intensity once monthly, usually in 5 s increments for each 1/4 mile. Increase duration once weekly, usually one extra 1/4 mile lap for each increase.
85-90% of HRmax	15	Beware. Check heart rate. Make sure that subject is running at the assigned velocity.
>90% of HRmax	>15	Decrease intensity, duration, or both. Make sure that subject is running at the new (slower) rate.

RPE = rating of perceived exertion; HRmax = maximal heart rate.

Reprinted from E.J. Burke and M.L. Collins, 1984, Using perceived exertion for the prescription of exercise in healthy adults. In *Clinical sports medicine*, edited by Robert Cantu (Lexington, MA: Callamore Press), 10. By permission from Robert Cantu.

Heart Rate Reserve

Heart rate reserve can be calculated by subtracting resting HR from HRmax, and this value can be used to calculate a target training HR range using the Karvonen formula:

[(HRmax − resting HR) × .60] + resting HR = training HR at 60%.

There are other problems with the use of HR for prescribing and monitoring exercise intensity. Often, HRmax is estimated based on a person's age rather than measured. Even when influences on HR due to age, training status, and type of exercise are accounted for, the standard deviation of true HRmax is about 11 beats per minute (bpm). Hence, errors of 11 bpm above or below a true maximum can be expected in about 30% of the adult population when HRmax is estimated but not measured. It is therefore not surprising that some people given age-predicted HR ranges complain that the exercise intensity is too easy or too hard. So, RPE can be used along with HR to provide a more appropriate range of exercise intensity.

METs

The ACSM guidelines for exercise prescription recommend that a person's total weekly energy expenditure from exercise approximate at least 1,000 kilocalories, with an optimal energy expenditure of 2,000 kilocalories per week. The energy cost of a given activity can be calculated using the following formula:

$$\text{kcal/min} = \text{METs} \times 3.5 \times \text{body weight (in kg)} / 200$$

The energy cost in METs has been determined for various physical activities, and most exercise physiology textbooks include tables listing the metabolic costs of various types of physical activity. The prescription of exercise intensity based on the energy cost of the activity is also susceptible to error due to individual differences. A person's training status and skill level can influence the metabolic cost of the activity. For example, an unskilled swimmer expends more energy than an experienced, more economical swimmer who is swimming the same distance. Also, the intensity of the activity may vary within a given exercise session. Hence, the use of RPE during exercise prescribed according to energy cost can help people maintain the appropriate exercise intensity.

Table 16.3 Classification of Physical Activity Intensity Based on Physical Activity Lasting up to 60 Minutes

| | ENDURANCE-TYPE ACTIVITY | | | | | | | RESISTANCE-TYPE EXERCISE |
| | RELATIVE INTENSITY | | | ABSOLUTE INTENSITY (METS) IN HEALTHY ADULTS (AGE IN YEARS) | | | | RELATIVE INTENSITY* |
Intensity	$\dot{V}O_2R$ (%) heart rate reserve (%)	Maximal heart rate (%)	RPE†	Young (29-39 years)	Middle aged (41-64 years)	Old (65-79 years)	Very old (80+ years)	Maximal voluntary contraction (%)
Very light	<20	<35	<10	<2.4	<2.0	<1.6	≤1.0	<30
Light	20-39	35-54	10-11	2.4-4.7	2.0-3.9	1.6-3.1	1.1-1.9	30-49
Moderate	40-59	55-69	12-13	4.8-7.1	4.0-5.9	3.2-4.7	2.0-2.9	50-69
Hard	60-84	70-89	14-16	7.2-10.1	6.0-8.4	4.8-6.7	3.0-4.25	70-84
Very hard	85	90	17-19	10.2	8.5	6.8	4.25	85
Maximal*	100	100	20	12.0	10.0	8.0	5.0	100

*Based on 8-12 repetitions for persons under age 50 years and 10-15 repetitions for persons aged 50 years and older.

†Borg Rating of Perceived Exertion 6-20 scale (Borg 1982).

*Maximal values are mean values achieved during maximal exercise by healthy adults. Absolute intensity (MET) values are approximate mean values for men. Mean values for women are approximately 1-2 METs lower than those for men; $\dot{V}o_dO_2R$ = oxygen uptake reserve.

Reprinted, by permission, from M.L. Pollock et al., 1998, "The recommended quantity and quality of exercise for developing and maintaining cardiorespiratory and muscular fitness, and flexibility in healthy adults," *Medicine and Science in Sports and Exercise* 30: 978. Copyright American College of Sports Medicine; Adapted from U.S. Department of Health and Human Services: Physical activity and health: A report of the Surgeon General, 1996.

Rating of Perceived Exertion as an Adjuvant to Heart Rate

On the basis of Borg's early studies, exercise physiologists thought a model in which RPE × 10 = HR could be effective, but clinical observations suggested that a correction factor of 20 to 30 bpm had to be added (i.e., RPE × 10 + 20 to 30 bpm = HR) for RPE of 11 to 16 and HRs within typical training ranges of 130 to 160 bpm.

Accuracy of Ratings of Perceived Exertion

Ratings of perceived exertion between 12 and 16 usually correspond with recommended exercise intensities between 40% and 85% of maximal METs (multiples of resting metabolic rate), or 40% to 85% of HRreserve during level walking or jogging. Nonetheless, RPE falls outside that range in as many as one-third of adults during their first GXT (Whaley et al. 1997). Normally, exercise intensity is prescribed based on the results of the GXT. During the GXT the participant estimates RPE throughout the test. These estimates are then matched to a percentage of maximum. If RPE is used in an exercise setting, the participant is asked to produce that rating. A problem with this estimation–production method is that the RPE in a GXT is commonly associated with a steady state achieved only briefly (e.g., 2 min). Then the participant moves on to another stage in the GXT, which itself is brief (e.g., 8 to 20 min). Normally, exercise is maintained at about the same intensity for a much longer period. This makes matching the exercise intensity from the GXT with an exercise intensity during training difficult with the use of RPEs. Errors between desired training ranges and actual training ranges are increased, so it is important to administer a production–production protocol when possible.

In a production–production protocol, the participant is asked to produce an RPE associated with a desired intensity (e.g., metabolic rate) for training during the GXT. As the exercise session progresses, the test administrator monitors the metabolic rate at the RPE; if the rate is not in the desired range, the participant is asked to produce a new, appropriate RPE. This process continues until the desired metabolic rate matches well with the RPE. Three practice trials performed on separated days are generally sufficient to reduce errors in the production of exercise intensity using RPE (Dishman et al. 1987).

It is also expected that the reproduction of an intensity will be more accurate if the estimation task is intramodal (i.e., the same activity mode is used for estimation and production, such as cycling) rather than intermodal (i.e., the estimation task is a different mode of activity than the production task, such as cycling and running). Studies have shown acceptable errors of HR, oxygen uptake, and ventilation when intramodal production of intensity has followed RPE estimation during grade-incremented treadmill testing. Errors of production from cycling or treadmill RPE estimation approximate 10% to 15% for HR. Group mean errors for power output approximate 10 to 50 watts and for $\dot{V}O_2$ are less than 5%, although the errors for a single person may be as high as 20% (Dunbar et al. 1992). The just noticeable differences for grade-incremented treadmill or load-incremented cycling have not been clearly established, but reports suggest that they are about 25 watts. The production of exercise intensity during field jogging or running from treadmill RPE yields equivalent HR, lactic acid, and velocity at an RPE that is about 2 units lower in the field setting.

Training Status Effects on Rating of Perceived Exertion

Perceived exertion is influenced by a person's level of physical training. A common indicator that a person has increased in fitness is the ability to perform at a faster pace (i.e., a higher absolute $\dot{V}O_2$) while exercising at the same percentage of maximal capacity as before the increased training. Ventilatory and lactate thresholds, which are physiological predictors of fitness, occur at lower relative work rates (50% to 60% of $\dot{V}O_2$peak) in untrained people and higher relative work rates (65% to 80% of $\dot{V}O_2$peak) in trained people. After increased training, RPE at the ventilatory and lactate thresholds stays around 12 to 15, corresponding with subjective categories of *somewhat hard* to *hard* on Borg's 6-20 category scale, despite the fact that those thresholds are occurring at a higher percentage of $\dot{V}O_2$peak and at a higher absolute level of work (Demello et al. 1987; Hill et al. 1987). Thus, RPE is an accurate indicator of exercise training status (Boutcher et al. 1989; Seip et al. 1991).

The Power Law and Borg's Rating of Perceived Exertion Scales

A potential problem of using category RPE (i.e., Borg's 6-20 RPE scale) to prescribe exercise is the curvilinear growth of perceived exertion when it is measured with ratio-setting methods, such as magnitude estimation or Borg's CR-10 scale. This can especially be a problem when Borg's RPE scale is used because of its linear relationship with increasing exercise intensity. However, within the training range of 40% to 85% of $\dot{V}O_2$ recommended by the ACSM, the relationship of RPE to %$\dot{V}O_2$peak or power output is virtually linear (see figure 16.17). The exception occurs during high-intensity walking, which has a power exponent of about 3. Thus, in most instances in which an exercise program is initiated at moderate intensities (i.e., 40% to 85% of $\dot{V}O_2$peak), the person should be able to use the 6-20 category RPE in a way that is generally linear with increasing exercise intensity. That is, a person who can perceive the increase from 12 to 13 should be able to perceive the increase from 15 to 16 similarly; this would permit the production of a linear increase in relative exercise intensity. However, if there is a shift from walking to running as a mode of exercise, a new learning experience using a production–production approach should probably be conducted for the new mode of exercise. Other shifts in the training mode (e.g., from running to cycling) should not require new learning because the power exponents of those modes of exercise are similar enough for the practical uses of the RPE scale.

Clinical Production of Perceived Force

It is a common practice in physical rehabilitation medicine to ask patients to produce muscular

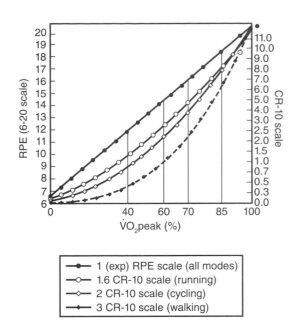

Figure 16.17 Category ratings of perceived exertion as they relate to physiological responses to various intensities and types of exercise.

Provided by J.B. Crabbe, the Exercise Psychology Laboratory, the University of Georgia.

forces relative to a perceived maximal effort. Clinical judgments about treatment and outcome are based on the forces produced by the patient. Studies from psychophysics indicate that people should be able to perform such forces accurately. In the first modern-day study of perceived force, magnitude estimation and production tasks were used to establish that perceived force during handgrip contractions grew exponentially, with power exponents ranging from 1.7 to 2.0 (Stevens and Mack 1959). Since that early research there have been few psychophysical studies of force production, but these have confirmed that perceived force grows according to a power function with the exponent ranging from about 1.4 to 1.7 during thumb opposition, handgrip, and leg or arm cranking on a cycle ergometer (see Borg 1982). These studies indicate that the perception of increments in muscular force grows exponentially, which is consistent with Stevens' power law.

Borg's range principle, which states that perceptual intensities of force for different people are set approximately equal at a subjective maximum, can be extended to predict that people who have had common experiences with resistance forces should be able to produce forces that represent equal proportions of their imagined maximal force. Studies have shown that the growth of the percentage of perceived effort versus the percentage of the maximal force of voluntary opposition of the thumb, static and dynamic extension of the knee, and horizontal adduction of the shoulders during bench pressing exercise is linear, with an exponent approximating 1.0 for the log–log plot of perceived versus actual relative force. Thus, the perceived percentage of force production during horizontal shoulder adduction is directly proportional across ranges of 25% to 75% and 10% to 90% of voluntary maximal force (Jackson and Dishman 2000; Jackson, Dishman, and Martin 2002; Jackson et al. 2006). Although people can produce actual forces that are linearly related to the desired forces, some people make large errors. This means that most patients asked to produce submaximal forces perform at an acceptable level, but some do not. Those who overshoot the desired effort may increase their chance for a rehabilitation setback. Those who undershoot the desired effort may have their recovery rate decreased and recovery time increased.

Preferred Exertion

Prescribing exercise according to preferred exertion is a concept that may have important implications for increasing physical activity in the general public (Borg 1962). **Preferred exertion** is the level of exertion that is desirable to a person during exercise. Preferred exertion refers to the level of exercise a person chooses when allowed to "set the pace." Only a few studies of preferred exertion have been done, but reports on men indicate that they prefer to leg cycle at an intensity around 60% of $\dot{V}O_2$peak, which corresponds to a category RPE of 13 ± 2, or *somewhat hard*. Trained runners prefer a higher intensity of about 75% of $\dot{V}O_2$peak and an RPE of 9 to 12 (see Dishman 1994 for a review). So, it appears that most people prefer to exercise at an intensity around the thresholds for the rapid onset of blood lactic acid and hyperventilation. For most people, this preferred intensity is adequate for improving cardiorespiratory fitness.

If people are allowed to exercise at an intensity they prefer rather than at an intensity that is too easy or too hard, they may be more likely to continue to participate in exercise. A high level of strain during exercise may increase the risks for musculoskeletal and orthopedic injuries that can lead to inactivity. If inactive people select, or are prescribed, an intensity that is perceived as very effortful, relative to their physiological responses, they may be less attracted to continued participation. Conversely, some people may prefer to exercise harder than recommended according to HR (King et al. 1991). Letting people exercise at their own pace could enhance their comfort and enjoyment during exercise. However, it is not known what percentage of the population would prefer to exercise at an intensity that is too low for fitness (e.g., <40% of capacity) or how many people who are at cardiovascular risk might prefer to exercise at dangerously high intensities.

Exertional Symptoms

Compared with the evidence supporting the accuracy of RPE for estimating and producing exercise intensity, little is known about the usefulness of other subjective responses to exercise for prescribing and monitoring exercise intensity (Bayles et al. 1990; Ekkekakis et al. 2011). Although the ACSM recommends the use of self-report scales for angina pectoris, claudication pain, and dyspnea, in addition to RPE (2009), and such scales are common in exercise stress testing, the study and measurement of pain during and after exercise are an emerging area in exercise psychology (Borg 1998; Cook and Koltyn 2000; O'Connor and Cook 1999).

SUMMARY

Gunnar Borg was the first to use a category rating scale that was valid for making interindividual comparisons of RPE. This was based on the assumption of Borg's range principle, that all healthy people have the same perceptual range from which to make judgments of perceived exertion. Perceptions of exertion, when assessed using ratio scaling methods, follow a positively accelerating function as exercise intensity increases. Perceptions of exertion represent a gestalt, which is an integration of central motor commands with sensory signals from working muscles and noxious chemical stimulation plus respiratory and metabolic signals related to respiratory work and the relative metabolic strain of the exercise. In addition, psychological factors, such as memories and focus of attention, interact with these physiological signals, along with information from the external environment. It is only after the brain has integrated these signals that perception of the exercise occurs and a cognitive label can be provided to represent an overall feeling of exertion. The RPE scales can be used during exercise testing and prescription as a valid adjuvant to monitoring exercise intensity.

WEBSITES

http://psychclassics.yorku.ca/Fechner

http://psychclassics.yorku.ca/Fechner/wozniak.htm

www.psych.yorku.ca/classics/Fechner

www.semiophysics.com/SemioPhysics_Articles_mental_10.html

www.sosmath.com/algebra/logs/log4/log4.html#exponential

www.sosmath.com/algebra/logs/log1/log1.html

Glossary

5-HIAA—5-hydroxyindoleacetic acid; a major metabolic breakdown product (metabolite) of serotonin (5-HT).

absolute intensity—Level of work expressed as a value that is the same for all people (e.g., running at 6 mph).

accelerometer—A mechanical device that measures movement through the use of transducers to record the acceleration of the body in one or more planes.

acetylcholine—A neurotransmitter substance at cholinergic synapses that causes cardiac inhibition, vasodilation, gastrointestinal peristalsis, and other parasympathetic effects; also acts in an excitatory manner between motor neurons and skeletal muscles.

actigraphy—The measurement of movement, acceleration, and deceleration in one plane.

active coping—Responses to perceived controllable stress that influence an outcome through mental or physical effort.

acute exercise—A single session of exercise; typically short, but can last for four hours or more (e.g., a marathon).

acute pain—Pain lasting less than three months.

adenosine—A purine nucleoside that has important roles in the reactions and regulation of metabolism and in the regulation of sleep in addition to inhibiting noradrenaline release from sympathetic nerve terminals and reducing adipose tissue sensitivity to noradrenaline.

adherence—Faithfully following a standard of behavior that has been established as part of a negotiated agreement; a person's continuation in an exercise program.

adrenal cortex—The outer covering of the adrenal gland, which is located adjacent to the kidney; secretes glucocorticoid, mineralocorticoid, and sex hormones.

adrenal medulla—The inner core of the adrenal gland; secretes epinephrine, norepinephrine, and enkephalins.

adrenaline—See *epinephrine*.

adrenergic—Relating to cells or fibers of the autonomic or central nervous system that use epinephrine as their neurotransmitter.

adrenocorticotropic hormone (ACTH)—A hormone released by the anterior lobe of the hypophysis (anterior pituitary); controls the production and release of hormones of the adrenal cortex.

aerobic fitness—The ability of the cardiorespiratory system to take up and use oxygen; the capacity to carry out activities that use large-muscle groups at moderate intensities, which permit the body to use oxygen for the production of energy and can be sustained for more than a few minutes.

affect—The conscious expression of a value given to a feeling state; a general category including feelings, emotions, and mood as distinct from cognitions and behavior.

afferent—Referring to a neural axon that carries nerve impulses away from a sensory organ to the central nervous system.

algesics—Endogenous substances that activate nociceptors and can cause pain.

allodynia—Pain resulting from a stimulus that normally doesn't cause pain (e.g., pain when water hits your shoulder during a shower after getting a sunburn).

allostasis—The ability to achieve stability through change; that is, the adaptation to disruptions to homeostasis.

allostatic load—The long-term effects of the physiological response to stress, which include the activation of the autonomic nervous system; the hypothalamic-pituitary-adrenal (HPA) axis; and the metabolic, cardiovascular, and immune systems.

alpha wave—Brain wave activity in the 8- to 12-hertz range; commonly described as relaxed wakefulness.

amygdala—A group of nuclei located in the limbic system; involved in the control of appropriate behavior in social situations, emotional memory, and the generation of anger and fear.

analgesia—A reduction in pain to the point that it is no longer present (see *hypoalgesia*).

analogue model—A set of properties that represents the actual set of properties of an idea or event using transformation rules, such as in maps and graphs; for example, the study of normal behavior or psychological function as a proxy for the study of abnormal behavior or mental disorder.

angina—A pathological heart condition involving severe chest pain.

antecedents—Events, whether internal (i.e., thoughts and affect) or external, that precede a target behavior; can be temporally close to or during the behavior (proximal) or occur a long time before the behavior (distal).

anterior cingulate cortex—A brain structure that monitors and detects behavioral errors and is involved in conflict detection processes.

anxiety—An emotional response to a perceived threat. Consists of feelings of tension, apprehension, and nervousness; unpleasant thoughts or worries; and physiological changes.

anxiety disorder—A mental illness characterized by apprehension or worry that is accompanied by restlessness, muscular tension, elevated heart rate, and breathlessness. Anxiety disorders include phobias, panic disorders, obsessive-compulsive disorder, and generalized anxiety disorder.

anxiolytic—Having the effect of decreasing anxiety.

arousal—A unidimensional state of physiological activation that runs on a continuum from sleep to extreme activation.

attitude—An evaluation of and reaction to an object, person, event, or idea; includes cognitive, affective, and behavioral components.

augmenters—People who consistently overestimate psychophysical stimuli while making judgments about size.

autonomic nervous system—The part of the peripheral nervous system that innervates smooth muscle, cardiac muscle, and glands; composed of the sympathetic, parasympathetic, and enteric divisions.

basal ganglia—The part of the telencephalon that consists of the corpus striatum and cell groups associated with the corpus striatum, such as the subthalamic nucleus and substantia nigra.

behavioral intention—What one aims to do or accomplish; intention is thought of in degrees (e.g., 90% likely that I will do something) rather than dichotomously (i.e., I will or I won't do something).

behavioral management—An intervention approach that targets changes in behavior through stimulus control, reinforcement control, contracting, and other strategies based on behaviorism and cognitive behaviorism.

behavioral neuroscience and comparative psychology—Subdisciplines of psychology that involve the study of perception and learning, neuroscience, cognitive psychology, and comparative psychology; the application of neural events to the study of the brain and behavior.

behaviorism—A subdiscipline of psychology that developed out of learning theory to describe the associations among observable stimuli, responses, and outcomes as the basis for understanding behavior, with no role for personality or mental states in predicting and describing behavior.

beliefs—Expectations, convictions, or opinions.

β-endorphin—An endogenous opioid peptide secreted by the anterior pituitary along with adrenocorticotropic hormone in response to stress.

bias—The systematic departure of results from the correct values as a consequence of errors in design or investigational technique; the effects of any factor that the researcher did not expect to influence the outcome (dependent variable); In respect to perception, bias or response criteria is a decision rule based on factors such as past experiences, instructions, and the expected cost and benefits.

biological psychology—A subdiscipline of psychology in which methods of natural science, such as those in physiology, endocrinology, pharmacology, and molecular biology, are applied to the study of the brain and behavior.

biopsychosocial model of disease—A model of disease introduced by George Engel in 1977 that proposes multicausal factors in health and disease, emphasizing the interaction of biological, psychological, and social factors.

bipolar scale—A measurement tool that conceptualizes two polar opposites, such as energy and fatigue, on a single continuum (see also *multidimensional scale* and *unipolar scale*).

brain-derived neurotrophic factor (BDNF)—A neurotrophin that supports the survival of existing neurons and promotes the growth and differentiation of new neurons and synapses.

brain plasticity/resources—Interchangeable terms often used to describe how people learn to adapt to environmental conditions and challenges.

brain stem—The continuous extension of the spinal cord upward into the cranial cavity; consists of the medulla, pons, and cerebellum (rhombencephalon) and midbrain (mesencephalon).

Cannon-Bard theory—A theory of emotion that describes a common physiological response, regardless of the type of emotion, involving sympathetic activation to prepare the body for flight or fight. When confronted with a stimulus, the brain decides the appropriate response, and the corresponding emotional response and the physiological activation occur simultaneously.

case-control design—A retrospective design in which healthy controls are matched with sick people ("cases"), often from the same setting, on age, sex, and race. Comparisons are made between the groups on past exposure to potential risk factors for a disease.

catecholamines—A class of synaptic transmitters that contain a single amine group (monoamines), including dopamine, norepinephrine, and epinephrine.

cerebellum—The portion of the brain that coordinates voluntary movement and adjusts the speed, force, and other factors involved during a period of muscular activity; organizes motor impulses before they are transferred to the muscles.

chronic exercise—Bouts of exercise that are repeated on a fairly regular basis over a period of time; exercise training or regular exercise that is defined by the type of activity, intensity, duration, frequency per week, and time period (e.g., weeks, months).

chronic fatigue syndrome—A debilitating and complex medical condition of unknown cause characterized by profound fatigue that is not improved by bed rest and that may be worsened by physical or mental activity.

chronic pain—Pain lasting three or more months.

classical conditioning—A form of behavior modification in which the stimulus for a reflexive response (unconditioned stimulus) is paired repeatedly with a neutral stimulus until the neutral stimulus (now the conditioned stimulus) elicits the response in the absence of the unconditioned stimulus.

claudication—From the Latin word for limping, it refers to pain in the lower leg during walking.

cognition—A general term for any process that reflects a person's knowledge or awareness; includes perceiving, remembering, judging, and reasoning.

cognitive behavioral modification—The use of principles from learning theory to modify the cognitions and activities related to a behavior that is to be changed.

cognitive behaviorism—A theory of human behavior based on interactive dualism in that behavior is seen as an outcome of cognition, and changes in cognition are seen as determinants of behavior.

cognitive restructuring—A behavior change strategy based on cognitive behaviorism in which negative or faulty thoughts are modified or replaced with positive thoughts or thoughts that enable or enhance the behavior change process.

compliance—Following a prescribed standard of behavior, usually related to immediate and short-term health advice to alleviate symptoms, such as taking a specific regimen of medications; a sense of coercive obedience.

computerized axial tomogram (CAT scan, CT scan)—A method that uses X-ray absorption to examine brain structure in humans.

conditioned stimulus—A previously neutral stimulus that has been paired repeatedly with an unconditioned stimulus and now elicits the target conditioned response in the absence of the unconditioned stimulus.

confounder—An extraneous factor that is not a consequence of exposure or an experimental manipulation. A confounding variable exerts an effect on the outcome such that there is a distortion in a study's effects. Confounders are determinants or correlates of the outcome under study and are unequally distributed among the exposed and unexposed individuals, making it difficult or impossible to interpret the relations among the other variables.

consequence—An abstract or concrete event that follows a target behavior; can be temporally close (proximal) to or far (distal) from the behavior; can be reinforcing and thus increase the frequency of the target behavior, or punishing and thus decrease the frequency of the target behavior.

construct—An abstract idea that was developed (constructed) to describe the relationships among phenomena or for other research purposes; exists theoretically but is not directly observable.

contingency contract—A behavior change strategy in which a person forms a contract with another person detailing rewards and punishments that are contingent (depend) on the performance or nonperformance of a target behavior.

control group—In experimental research, the group that does not experience, for the sake of comparison, the treatment the researcher is interested in studying.

convergent validity—Validity as indicated by the overlap between tests or instruments that are presumed to measure the same variable; related to concurrent validity, which is indicated by the correlation between one instrument and another instrument that measures the same construct and is assumed to be valid.

corpus striatum—Part of the basal ganglia that consists of the globus pallidus and the striatum, which is further divided into the caudate nucleus and the putamen.

correlates—Variables for which there are established reproducible associations or predictive relationships.

corticotropin-releasing hormone (CRH)—A hormone released by the parvocellular area of the paraventricular nucleus of the anterior hypothalamus; controls the diurnal rhythms of adrenocorticotropic hormone release.

cortisol—A steroid hormone that is the major glucocorticoid secreted by the adrenal cortex; plays a primary role in the stress response and central nervous dysregulation associated with mood disorders; also involved in the stimulation of formation and storage of glycogen and the maintenance of blood glucose.

cosmology—The study of the physical universe considered as a totality of phenomena in time and space.

cranial nerves—Twelve pairs of sensory and motor nerves that are connected directly to the brain.

cross-sectional design—A research plan in which data from a single point in time are collected and participants are classified on predictor (independent) and outcome (dependent) variables.

cross-stressor adaptation hypothesis—The proposal that physiological adaptations to the repeated stress of exercise will result in adaptations to the physiological response to mental stress.

cytokines—Cell-signaling molecules that modulate the responses of the immune system.

decisional balance—One of the three components of the transtheoretical model of behavior change (stages of change model) that are proposed to affect behavior change; the differences between the pros, or perceived benefits, of the target behavior and the cons, or perceived costs.

dependent variable—The variable in a study whose values are predicted by the independent (predictor) variable, or that "depend" on another variable; the outcome variable.

depletion hypothesis—See *monoamine depletion hypothesis.*

diencephalon—The posterior part of the forebrain; major structures are the thalamus and the hypothalamus.

discipline—A branch of knowledge or teaching.

discriminative stimulus—A stimulus that is paired with a reinforcing stimulus during operant conditioning; provides information about the consequences of a response.

distal—Referring to an outcome or event that is temporally distant from the target behavior.

distraction hypothesis—An explanation of the beneficial psychological effects of exercise based on "time-out" from worrisome thoughts and daily stressors during exercise.

diurnal—Referring to a pattern that repeats once every 24 hours.

divergent validity—The validity of a measure indicated by the lack of association with another measure that it should not be related to if it is valid; the mirror image of convergent validity.

dopamine—A biogenic amine and neurotransmitter that is the precursor for norepinephrine and epinephrine.

dorsolateral prefrontal cortex—The region of the frontal lobe that has been linked to goal selection, planning, sequencing, verbal and spatial working memory, self-monitoring, and self-awareness.

down-regulation—The development of a tolerance after repeated administration of a pharmacologically or physiologically active substance, or in response to excessively high levels of a substance; often characterized by an initial decrease in the affinity of receptors for the substance and a subsequent decrease in the number of receptors.

dualism—The philosophical view that the world consists of or is explicable as two fundamental entities, such as mind and matter; the perspective that the mind and body function separately, without interchange.

dysregulation—Disruption in self-regulation.

dysthymia—A mild, chronic form of major depression.

ecological validity—A type of external validity that refers to how well the measurement taken in an experiment generalizes to nonlaboratory conditions, or how well a finding from research with one group generalizes to another group.

effect size—The measure of an association or the strength of a relationship; the difference in the outcome for the average subject who received the treatment from that for the average subject who did not; broadly, any measure of the association or strength of a relationship, often thought of as an indication of practical significance.

effectiveness—The ability of an intervention or method to work in other settings or to be practically applied outside of a laboratory setting; a level of ecological validity.

efferent—Referring to a neural axon that carries nerve impulses from the central nervous system to the muscles and glands.

efficacy—The ability of an intervention or method to do what it was intended to do.

ego orientation—A motivational orientation in which success is determined by comparing one's performance to that of others or to an external standard.

electroencephalography (EEG)—The recording of the gross electrical activity of the brain using large electrodes placed on the scalp in a standardized pattern.

electromyography (EMG)—The recording of the gross electrical activity of muscle contractions.

electrophysiology—A technique to measure neural activity in the brain; electrodes are positioned in the brain cortex or in specific regions of brain neurons to record electrical potentials during behavior or in response to stress.

emotion—An intense mental state that arises subjectively rather than through conscious effort and is accompanied by physiological changes related to autonomic activation; brief responses of negative or positive feelings.

empirical research—Data-based research that can be verified by observation or experience.

endocannabinoids—Endogenous physiological ligands that bind to cannabinoid receptors, which mediate the psychoactive effects of cannabis (i.e., marijuana), including the reduction of anxiety and pain, elevation of mood, and impairment of short-term memory.

endocrine—Referring to glands that secrete hormones and other biochemicals to the interior of the body.

endogenous—Produced within the body.

endorphin—An endogenous opioid peptide that can act as a neurotransmitter, neuromodulator, and hormone.

endorphin hypothesis—The proposition that the mood enhancement associated with exercise is due to actions of endorphins, which are secreted during exercise.

energy symptoms—Subjective feelings of having the capacity to complete mental or physical activities.

enkephalin—One of three kinds of endogenous opioids, which are a class of compounds that exert an effect like that of opium, such as reduced pain sensitivity.

enteric system—The branch of the autonomic nervous system that regulates the intestines.

epidemiology—The study of the distribution and determinants of health-related states and events in a population, and the application of this study to the control of health problems.

epinephrine (Epi)—Also known as adrenaline, a compound that acts as a hormone secreted by the adrenal medulla and as a neurotransmitter; a postganglionic adrenergic mediator acting as a sympathomimetic substance; plays an important role in preparing for responding to stress.

executive function—Mental processes that are central to decision making, goal planning, and attentional control.

exercise—A subset of physical activity that consists of planned, structured, repetitive bodily movements with the purpose of improving or maintaining one or more components of physical fitness or health.

exercise adoption—Behavioral and cognitive components of beginning regular, purposeful, and structured physical activity; includes some degree of psychological commitment.

exercise maintenance—Sustaining a regular exercise program for a specific period of time, usually at least six months.

exercise prescription—A recommendation for a specific exercise mode, intensity, duration, and frequency per week to meet specific goals.

exercise psychology—The interdisciplinary field of study of the psychobiological, behavioral, and social factors at play in exercise and physical activity settings.

experimental design—The art of planning and executing an experiment in which the researcher has some control over the conditions in which the study takes place and the independent variables.

face validity—Logical or conceptual validity; according to experts, the extent to which the measurement instrument seems to make sense.

factor analysis—Statistical analysis used to determine whether the structure of a test seems consistent with the construct it purports to measure; an analysis designed to find patterns in the variations among several variables to see whether large numbers of variables can be grouped into "factors" that are conceptually or statistically related.

fatigue—Subjective feelings of having a reduced capacity to complete mental or physical activities.

feeling—A subjective experience that can be overt or covert.

feeling state—Bodily sensations, cognitive appraisals, actual or potential instrumental responses, or some combination of these responses.

fibromyalgia—A chronic medical condition characterized by widespread musculoskeletal pain, fatigue, and tenderness in localized areas.

field theory—A post-Freudian theory of personality developed by Kurt Lewin that proposes that behavior is determined by the person and the person's environment; takes into account contemporary interrelations and interconnections.

frontal lobe—The part of the brain that receives multiple inputs from cortical and subcortical areas and integrates information in ways that lead to unified, goal-directed behavior.

functional MRI (fMRI)—A method to determine brain activity that applies the magnetic resonance principle for the purpose of finding out which parts of the brain are activated by various types of physical sensations or motor activity.

galanin—An amino acid peptide neurotransmitter that hyperpolarizes noradrenergic neurons and inhibits locus coeruleus firing in vitro.

galvanic skin response—A change in the electrical resistance of the skin, or in its converse, conduction, through autonomic activation; measured by placing two electrodes on the skin and recording the changes in skin conductance or resistance in the tissue path between them.

γ-aminobutyric acid (GABA)—A major inhibitory transmitter in the nervous system.

ganglion (plural: **ganglia**)—An aggregation of nerve cell bodies located in the peripheral nervous system.

general adaptation syndrome (GAS)—Hans Selye's theory that many diseases are "diseases of adaptation" and develop because of insufficient, excessive, or poorly regulated responses to environmental stressors; likewise, the GAS could be beneficially altered by experiences that could enhance the resistance to psychosomatic and neurotic diseases.

generalized anxiety disorder (GAD)—A disorder characterized by excessive or pathological worry about multiple concerns; exaggerated vigilance; and somatic symptoms of stress and anxiety, such as muscular tension.

genotype—The sum of all the genetic information in an organism.

gestalt—A configuration or pattern of elements so unified as a whole that its properties cannot be derived from a simple summation of its parts; the whole is more than the sum of its parts.

glucocorticoid—A class of hormones that affect carbohydrate metabolism and are released by the adrenal cortex (e.g., in response to stress).

glutamate (glutamic acid)—An amino acid that is a small-molecule, rapidly acting neurotransmitter; the major excitatory transmitter in the central nervous system.

goal setting—The process by which specific plans are established to achieve a desired outcome.

halo effect—An effect that occurs when the researcher ascribes certain characteristics to a subject based on other known characteristics, resulting in a bias on the part of the researcher (experimenter expectancy effect).

Hawthorne effect—The tendency for people in a research study to change simply because they are being studied.

health education—Programs and strategies based on a medical model that target behaviors related to the promotion of health; educational programs and mass media campaigns.

health psychology—The subdomain of psychology devoted to understanding the psychological influences on and consequences of health and illness, as well as the impact of health policy and health interventions.

heart rate variability—Variability described by the standard deviation of intervals between successive R waves of the cardiac cycle; provides an index of the modulation of heart rate by the autonomic nervous system.

hemispheric asymmetry—The differences in neural circuits between the left and right hemispheres of the brain.

high-risk situation—Any situation that challenges a person's confidence in the ability to maintain a positive health behavior or to abstain from an unhealthy behavior.

hippocampus—The portion of the limbic system thought to be important in learning and memory.

homeostasis—The ability or tendency of an organism or a cell to maintain internal equilibrium by adjusting its physiological processes; the tendency for an internal environment to remain constant.

homologous model—An animal model of disease that meets the standards of predictive validity and isomorphism and also has the same etiology as that of the human disease.

hypoalgesia—A reduction in pain, but pain is still present (see *analgesia*).

hypothalamic-pituitary-adrenal axis (HPA axis)—The hypothalamus, pituitary, and adrenal cortex.

hypothalamus—Part of the diencephalon; controls vegetative functions, regulates hormone balance, and plays a role in emotional behavior.

iconic model—A two- or three-dimensional model that looks similar to what it represents but is larger or smaller. Examples include pictures, sculptures, holograms, and virtual realities.

idealism—A philosophical theory contending that objective reality is actually perception and that it consists of ideas; the contention that the essential nature of reality lies in consciousness.

immunocytochemistry—The study of cell components by immunological methods, such as the use of fluorescent antibodies.

in situ—Referring to a technique to examine processes inside a cell or organism in its original, natural setting.

in situ hybridization histochemistry—A technique that uses a labeled, complementary single strand of DNA to detect steady-state levels of messenger RNA in a cell that is fixed in its natural position in a tissue.

in vitro—Occurring "in glass"; usually with reference to biological testing done outside the body, as in a laboratory dish.

in vivo—Within a living body, usually with reference to testing done with intact, live subjects.

incidence—The number of new cases of a disease or condition divided by the number of people exposed over a specified period of time.

independent variable—A variable that is manipulated by the researcher with the idea that it will have an effect on another variable (dependent variable); a variable that can be used to explain or predict the values of another variable.

indolamines—A class of biogenic amines that includes serotonin and melatonin.

intensity—The amount of work performed during exercise; expressed as an absolute quantity (e.g., watts), or relative to maximal capacity (e.g., 70% of maximal aerobic capacity), or as a perception of effort (a rating of perceived exertion of 13 on the Borg scale).

intention—See *behavioral intention*.

isomorphic model—An animal model of disease that evokes the same features as the human disease, which abate after the administration of drugs that are clinically useful in humans; the features generated may not have the same etiology or course of development as the human disease.

James-Lange theory—A theory proposing that emotions result from the evaluation of various physiological responses; different emotions have different constellations of physiological responses, and the perception of these responses results in the corresponding emotion—thus, bodily responses during emotion are the source of the emotional response.

just noticeable difference (j.n.d.)—The smallest amount of change in the intensity of a stimulus required for the change to be perceived.

latency—The length of time between the application of a stimulus and the response.

ligand—A molecule that binds to another, usually larger, molecule (e.g., a hormone or neurotransmitter binding to a receptor).

Likert scaling—A questionnaire format in which respondents are given statements and are asked to respond to each statement by indicating how they relate to it by choosing among several qualifiers anchored around a neutral point by two extreme responses (e.g., *strongly agree* and *strongly disagree*); the most widely used type of attitude scale in the social sciences.

limbic system—A heterogeneous array of brain nuclei located near the edge of the medial wall of the cerebral hemisphere that innervate each other; includes the hippocampus, amygdala, and gyrus fornicatus; influences the endocrine systems, as well as emotion and learning.

locus coeruleus (LC)—Located in the pons, the major nucleus for the production of norepinephrine; has a major role in the inhibition of spontaneous firing in areas of the brain to which it projects.

magnetic resonance imaging (MRI)—A method to measure structural details of a living brain using radio waves and a strong magnetic field.

magnetoencephalography (MEG)—a noninvasive method used to measure magnetic fields in the brain that are generated by small intracellular electrical currents flowing tangential to the scalp, corresponding to sulcal activations; provides direct information about the dynamics of evoked and spontaneous neural activity and the location of their sources in the brain.

magnitude estimation—Presenting someone with a standard stimulus (modulus), such as a 10-pound (4.5 kg) weight, and asking that person to label his or her perception of sensation (e.g., heaviness or force) with any number; then asking the person to assign a numerical value to various stimuli (e.g., weights) presented in random order in reference to the rating assigned to the modulus.

magnitude production—Presenting someone with a standard stimulus (modulus) and asking that person to produce a response or choose a stimulus that is proportional to a given magnitude (e.g., twice as heavy) of the stimulus.

major depression—One of two major categories of mood disorders (the other being manic-depressive disorder) characterized by depressed mood or loss of interest or pleasure and other behavioral and psychological symptoms.

manic-depressive disorder—One of two major categories of mood disorders (the other being major depression) characterized by periods of depression alternating with periods of elevated mood and associated behavior.

mastery hypothesis—An explanation of enhanced mood, self-efficacy, and self-esteem based on the positive consequences of the successful completion of an important task, such as exercise.

materialism—The philosophical theory that material objects are the only reality, and that thoughts and feelings can be explained through states of and changes in matter and physical phenomena.

maximal aerobic capacity—The maximal amount of oxygen the body can take up and use.

McArdle's syndrome—A congenital condition that prevents people from using muscle glycogen during exercise and increases muscle pain during exercise.

mediation—Mechanism by which an independent variable affects an outcome; the amount of mediation is measured by the indirect effect, which equals the reduction of the effect of the independent variable on the outcome when the contribution of the mediating variable is removed.

mediator—A variable that transmits the effects of another variable (predictor) on the outcome.

medulla—The part of the brain stem that marks the transition from the spinal cord to the brain stem; contains motor and sensory nerves; the dorsal surface of its upper half forms the floor of the fourth ventricle.

melancholia—A severe form of major depressive episode. Key features are a pervasive loss of pleasure or interest in pleasurable activities, dark mood that is worse in the morning, early morning awakening, psychomotor retardation or agitation, weight loss, and extreme feelings of guilt.

melatonin—A hormone that is released by the pineal gland in a true circadian rhythm; involved in the sleep–wake cycle.

mental chronometry—The use of measures of response time to separate mental processes.

messenger ribonucleic acid (mRNA)—Messenger or template RNA; RNA produced by transcription that reflects the exact nucleoside sequence of the genetically active DNA; carries the code for a particular protein from the nuclear DNA to a ribosome in the cytoplasm where protein is made in amino acid sequences specified by the mRNA.

meta-analysis—A quantitative procedure for summarizing the effects of a number of research studies on a common topic.

metabolic equivalent (MET)—Metabolic equivalent; the ratio of energy expended in kilocalories divided by resting energy expenditure in kilocalories, either measured or estimated from body size; 1 MET is 3.5 ml/kg/min.

metacognition—Higher-order thinking that controls the thought processes required for problem solving.

method of adjustment—A technique in which a stimulus having a standard, objectively measured intensity is presented along with a comparison stimulus that is adjusted until it is perceived to be of the same intensity as the standard stimulus.

method of constant stimuli—The presentation of a standard stimulus and a comparison stimulus; the task is to determine whether the comparison stimulus is perceived and/or whether it is the same as or different from the standard stimulus.

method of limits—A technique used to determine the lower and upper thresholds for perception by recording judgments of the magnitude of stimuli that are presented in a series across a range of intensities in ascending and descending order.

MHPG—3-methoxy-4-hydroxyphenylglycol; the major metabolic breakdown product (metabolite) of norepinephrine that is secreted in the urine.

microdialysis—A method to determine the extracellular levels of a substance through dialysis, which is the separation of molecules of various sizes through the use of an artificial membrane that is permeable to only some molecules.

midbrain—Also known as the mesencephalon; forms the top of the brain stem and includes the reticular formation, substantia nigra, and red nucleus.

model—A generalized, simplified representation of some aspect(s) of living and nonliving systems; models should be considered provisional and subject to change, improvement, and eventual replacement.

moderation—Weakening, amplifying, or reversing a causal effect when a moderator variable is a particular value.

moderator—A variable that influences the relationship between two other variables; influences how an intervention or mediator affects the outcome.

monism—The philosophical view that material and immaterial matter are different manifestations of one underlying phenomenon; the mind exists only by the function of the body.

monoamine depletion hypothesis—The theory that depression is caused by a deficiency of norepinephrine at the central adrenergic receptors or of serotonin (or of both), and that mania results from excessive norepinephrine.

monoamine dysregulation hypothesis—The theory that depression is the result of a disruption in the noradrenergic and serotonergic systems' self-regulating ability and the overstimulation of neural centers such as the prefrontal cortex, amygdala, hippocampus, and periventricular gray; a major proposed site of dysregulation is the locus coeruleus (LC).

mood—A type of affective state that is accompanied by anticipation, either conscious or unconscious, of pleasure or pain; moods can last less than a minute or for days.

motivated response distortion—See *social desirability responding.*

multidimensional scale—A measurement instrument that simultaneously measures several constructs (see also *bipolar scale* and *unipolar scale*).

muscle dysmorphia—A pathological preoccupation with muscularity that occurs in both men and women; can be associated with body dysmorphic disorder.

muscle sense—Sensations arising from muscles and related structures as a result of changes in posture and locomotion.

negative feedback—Output that inhibits the activity of an initial input.

neocortex—The relatively recently evolved portion of the cerebral cortex that is composed of nerve cells arranged in six layers; characterized by the elaborate folding of tissue.

neurobiology—The study of the biological processes of the brain; areas of study include the anatomy, physiology, and pathology of the nervous system.

neurogenic reserve hypothesis—The supposition that exercise leads to a cascade of neurological changes in the brain and an increase in the number of neurons in the dentate gyrus of the hippocampus.

neuroimaging—Methods to measure brain activity using techniques such as X-ray and computer technology (e.g., CAT scan, MRI).

neuropathic—A disturbance of the function of or a pathological change in a nerve.

neuropeptide Y (NPY)—An amino acid peptide that inhibits the locus coeruleus from firing in vitro, providing feedback inhibition to locus coeruleus neurons.

neurotransmitter—Any specific chemical agent that is released by the presynaptic cell, upon excitation, and crosses the synapse to stimulate, inhibit, or modify the postsynaptic cell; serves as the basis of communication between neurons.

nociception—The neural process of encoding noxious stimuli.

nociceptor—The high-threshold sensory receptor of the peripheral somatosensory nervous system that is capable of transducing and encoding noxious stimuli.

noradrenergic—Relating to cells or fibers of the autonomic or central nervous system that use norepinephrine as their neurotransmitter.

norepinephrine (NE)—A neurotransmitter, also known as noradrenaline, that is the postganglionic adrenergic mediator. It is also produced in the adrenal medulla and centrally in the locus coeruleus; principal effects are excitatory.

noxious stimulus—A stimulus that is damaging or threatens damage to normal tissues.

nucleus (plural: **nuclei**)—A collection of neural cell bodies located within the brain.

obsessive-compulsive disorder (OCD)—A recurrent and persistent unwanted idea, thought, or impulse to carry out an unwanted act that the person cannot voluntarily suppress; typified by repetitive acts or rituals to relieve anxiety.

ontology—The branch of philosophy that deals with the nature of being.

operant conditioning—A type of behavior modification in which a reinforcing or punishing event is paired with a voluntary behavior to change the frequency with which the behavior occurs; the goal is to change the rate of responding.

orbitofrontal cortex—The region of the frontal lobe associated with the inhibition of inappropriate responses; is implicated in judging the likelihood of reward and in assessing risk.

orthogonal—Referring to variables that are uncorrelated, or unrelated to each other.

osteoarthritis—A degenerative joint disease that can affect any joint in the body but is especially common in the hips, knees, and spine.

outcome expectation—The anticipated results of an event or of engaging in a specific behavior.

outcome value—The reinforcement or incentive value of an expected outcome; can be something people want to obtain or avoid.

pain—An unpleasant sensory and emotional experience associated with actual or potential tissue damage, or described in terms of such damage.

panic disorder—Repeated episodes of intense fear that strike abruptly and without obvious cause. Predominant symptoms include heart palpitations, breathing distress, tingling sensations, and a fear of dying.

parasympathetic nervous system—One of three divisions of the autonomic nervous system; arises from the cranial nerves and the sacral portions of the spinal cord; primarily involved in energy conservation.

perceived behavioral control—The degree to which people believe they can have an effect on a specific outcome; ranges on a continuum from no control to total control.

perceived exertion—The subjective judgment of strain or effort during physical activity; a perception of the quantity more than of the quality of sensations.

perceptual sensitivity—A person's capacity to discriminate changes in signal strength.

phenomenology—The study of the expression of subjective experience; concerned primarily with the description of experience.

phobia—An obsessive, persistent, and unrealistic fear of an external situation or object that is out of proportion to the actual threat or danger.

physical activity—Any bodily movement produced by skeletal muscles that results in energy expenditure.

physical fitness—The capacity to meet the present and potential physical challenges of life; a set of attributes that people have or achieve that relate to overall health, the ability to perform daily tasks and physical activities; components include cardiorespiratory fitness, body composition, flexibility, agility, muscular strength and endurance, and metabolic variables such as glucose tolerance.

placebo—A treatment given to a control group in experimental research that is meant to have no effect; used in comparison to the treatment, or independent variable, that is being tested.

placebo effect—Changes that cannot be attributed to a treatment; the changes are due instead to subjects' erroneous beliefs that they received an effective treatment.

polysomnography—The simultaneous measurement of multiple physiological indicators of sleep stages, such as brain waves, respiration, and muscle and chin movements, to detect rapid eye movement.

pons—A part of the brain stem that wraps around the base of the cerebellum; contains the locus coeruleus, the major nuclei in the brain that produce norepinephrine.

positron emission tomography (PET)—A method that uses radioactive chemicals to measure the dynamic activity of a living brain by detecting the positrons emitted by radioactive glucose or another metabolic analog.

posttraumatic stress disorder—Anxiety and behavioral disturbances that develop within the first month after exposure to an extreme trauma.

predictive design—A research plan whose goal is to explain the values of a variable (e.g., disease) by using the values of one or more other variables; disease-free subjects are grouped according to their exposure to the variable(s) suspected to influence disease occurrence and are then evaluated over time to determine disease in exposed and unexposed groups.

predictive model—An animal model that includes specific signs or behaviors that can be reliably changed by drugs known to have clinical efficacy in humans.

preferred exertion—The level of exertion that someone is motivated to endure.

prevalence—The number of existing cases of a disease or condition divided by the total population at a point in time. Prevalence is used to measure the burden of the disease and to plan for the implementation of services.

processes of change—One of the three components of the transtheoretical model of behavior change that is said to explain behavior change; consists of 10 covert and overt activities that are used to change thinking, affect, behavior, or relationships.

projection neurons—Neurons with cell bodies in the spinal cord that send their axons to the brain.

proopiomelanocorticotropin (POMC)—A precursor peptide found predominantly in the anterior pituitary from which the endogenous opioid β-endorphin and adrenocorticotropic hormone (ACTH) are derived.

prostaglandin—A physiologically active substance present in many tissues, with effects such as vasodilation, vasoconstriction, stimula-

tion of intestinal or bronchial smooth muscle, uterine stimulation, and antagonism to hormones influencing lipid metabolism.

proximal—Referring to an outcome or event that is temporally close to the target behavior.

psychology—A scientific discipline concerned with the study and application of principles of behavior and mental processes in humans and other animals in their interactions with the environment; areas of study include processes of sense perception, thinking, learning, cognition, emotions and motivations, personality, abnormal behavior, interactions among individuals, and interactions with the environment.

psychometrics—The psychological theory and measurement of psychological variables; includes the design, administration, and interpretation of quantitative tests for the measurement of psychological variables.

psychophysics—The study of psychological judgments (sensations and perceptions) of physical stimuli using standardized methods to manipulate physical stimuli and to measure the perceptual response to the stimuli; the measurement of judgments people make about their physical environment.

punishment—Consequences of a specific behavior that decrease the frequency of the behavior.

randomized controlled trial (RCT)—Research with large populations to test the associations among variables found in epidemiological or small laboratory experiments; includes representative population and treatment and control groups matched with respect to characteristics thought to affect outcome.

raphe nuclei—The major nuclei for the production of serotonin; located in the center line of the brain stem.

rapid eye movement (REM) sleep—The portion of the sleep cycle characterized by dreaming, rapid eye movement, and an alert EEG pattern; predominates during the last one-third of the night's sleep.

receiver operating characteristic (ROC)—A method of assessing the balance between correct decisions (true positives and true negatives) and errors of commission (false positives).

receptor—A structural protein molecule, usually on the cell surface or within the cytoplasm, that combines with a specific factor, such as a hormone or neurotransmitter; the interaction of the factor and the receptor results in a change in cell function.

reciprocal determinism—The central concept of causation for social cognitive theory; describes the bidirectional interacting influence of determinants of behavior; a mutually influencing relationship among two or more variables.

reducers—People who consistently underestimate stimuli while making judgments.

referred appraisal—External standards people apply to themselves that are based on how they believe significant others perceive them.

reinforcement—Consequences of a target behavior that increase the frequency of the behavior.

reinforcement control—A behavior change strategy that manipulates the consequences of the target behavior to increase the frequency of the behavior.

reinforcing stimulus—A stimulus that is capable of eliciting a reflexive response (e.g., the smell of bread baking can be a reinforcing stimulus that elicits salivation).

relapse prevention—A set of strategies to keep people from returning to undesired behavior after successful behavior modification.

relative intensity—The work rate expressed in relation to maximal intensity, aerobic capacity, or workload.

relative risk—The ratio of the rates of occurrence of disease in two groups.

reliability—The characteristic of a measure that includes precision, accuracy, and stability across time; freedom from measurement or random error.

REM sleep—See *rapid eye movement (REM) sleep*.

reticular formation—The network of nerves that extends from the medulla through the thalamus; involved in the sleep–wake cycle and forebrain arousal.

rhabdomyolysis—A rapid breakdown of skeletal muscle due to a muscle injury.

rheumatoid arthritis—An autoimmune disease that causes joint pain, especially in the finger and wrist joints.

RNA—Ribonucleic acid; nucleic acids that are associated with the control of cellular chemical activities.

Rosenthal effect—Also known as the self-fulfilling prophecy or the Pygmalion effect; the tendency of participants to want to meet the expectations that the investigator has communicated about the participant's attributes or abilities.

scaling—The assignment of objects to numbers according to a rule; the development of an instrument to assign objects or statements to a response scale (numbers) according to specific rules; creating a scale by grouping items into a logical sequence.

Schachter's theory of emotion—A theory that proposes that emotions are the result of the interaction between the physiological activation and cognitive interpretation of a nonspecific arousal; the cognitive interpretation (appraisal) of the context and intensity of the autonomic response leads to the subjective experience of a particular emotion.

self-concept—The organized configuration of perceptions about one's attributes and qualities that are within conscious awareness.

self-efficacy—The perception of one's ability to carry out behavior with a known outcome; expectations of personal mastery regarding the initiation and persistence of behavior.

self-enhancement hypothesis—The view that behavioral choices are made based on the evaluation of outcome expectations with respect to the potential for enhanced feelings of competence and self-esteem.

self-esteem—The evaluation of one's self-concept and the feelings associated with that evaluation.

self-monitoring—Actions taken to assess the antecedents, consequences, and characteristics of attempts to engage in or avoid a target behavior.

self-motivation—An internal factor that arouses, directs, and integrates a person's behavior; an energizing condition that causes people to internalize evaluations of their own performance and then to seek to meet these standards; the behavioral tendency to persevere independent of situational reinforcements.

self-reflection—The ability to symbolize that enables people to anticipate and plan for future events and actions.

self-regulation—Ways people modify their own behavior; based on the assumption that behavior is under the direct control of the person and is guided by internalized standards whose achievement will elicit positive self-evaluation.

self-schemata—The cognitive structure of the self and the personal attributes that serve to guide the selection, retrieval, and storage of information about the self.

sensitivity—The ability of a test to detect a disease or attribute; a test with high sensitivity will not miss the disease or condition if it is present.

serotonin—Also known as 5-HT, a synaptic transmitter classified as an indolamine that is produced and secreted by the raphe nuclei; the general suppressor of neural gain.

signal detection theory (SDT)—Proposed that a person's likelihood of reporting a change of signal strength is due to two interacting factors, perceptual sensitivity (i.e., capacity to discriminate changes in signal strength) and bias or response criteria, which is a decision rule based on factors such as past experiences, instructions, and the expected cost and benefits.

slow-wave sleep (SWS)—Sleep stages 3 and 4 combined; characterized by delta waves; the stage at which people are hardest to awaken; occurs during about 20% of a night's sleep and predominates during the first one-third of a night's sleep.

social cognitive theory—The theory of human behavior, evolved from social learning theory, in which behavior is a function of social cognitions; the key concept is triadic reciprocality.

social desirability responding—The tendency for people to respond in ways that they perceive as conforming to the socially desirable images they have of themselves.

social psychology—The subdiscipline of psychology concerned with the effects of various social environments on the individual; includes the study of attitude measurement and change, group dynamics, social learning and personality, social cognition, aggression, and self-perception.

specificity—The ability of a test to discriminate; a test with high specificity will not incorrectly indicate the presence of the disease or condition if it is not present.

spinal cord—The part of the central nervous system containing neural circuits that control reflexive function, bring sensory information from the periphery to the brain, and carry motor signals to the periphery.

spinal nerves—Sensory and motor pathways in 31 pairs that join the spinal cord at regularly spaced intervals. Sensory information is carried from the periphery to the spinal cord, and motor impulses are transmitted from the spinal cord to the muscles.

state anxiety—The immediate response to a conscious or unconscious threat; somatic and cognitive symptoms include elevated heart rate, muscle tension, and visceral motility, as well as transient feelings of lack of control, low confidence, and uncertainty.

stimulus control—Strategies to change the frequency of a target behavior by modifying the antecedents of the behavior.

strain—The deformation, distortion, or tension in an object as a result of stress.

stress—The way load impinges on a physical object; an imbalance in physiological systems that activates physiological and behavioral responses to restore balance, or homeostasis.

stressor—A force that acts on a biological system to cause stress, an imbalance, or a disruption in homeostasis.

striatum—The area of the brain around the lateral ventricle that includes the caudate nucleus and putamen; the striatum and the globus pallidus or pallidum form the corpus striatum.

superior sagittal sinus—One of the six venous channels located in the posterior of the dura mater; drains blood from the anterior cerebral hemispheres into the internal jugular vein.

sympathetic medullary system—The system consisting of the sympathetic nervous system and the adrenal medulla; actions are associated with the stress response.

sympathetic nervous system—One of three divisions of the autonomic nervous system; arises from the thoracic and lumbar portions of the spinal cord; primarily involved in activities that require energy expenditure.

task orientation—A motivational orientation in which success is seen in terms of personal mastery and self-improvement.

telencephalon—Part of the forebrain; major structures are the neocortex, basal ganglia, and limbic system.

temperament—The mainly stable, core component of personality that predisposes people to varying degrees of emotional responsiveness and changing moods.

thalamus—A structure of the brain located in the diencephalon; composed of sensory relay nuclei with bidirectional connections with many areas in the cerebral cortex.

theory—The formulation of underlying principles of certain observed phenomena that have been verified to some degree and are used to explain and predict; a symbolic model used to guide the design, execution, and interpretation of research.

thermogenic hypothesis—A perspective that attributes the enhanced mood associated with exercise to increased body temperature.

thyroid-stimulating hormone—A hormone secreted by the anterior hypothalamus; causes the anterior pituitary to release thyrotropic hormone, which stimulates the thyroid gland to secrete thyroxin.

topiramate—An anti-epilepsy drug used also to treat migraines.

trait—The tendency to respond to an internal or external event with a particular mood state; traits are relatively consistent over time, but changes in traits are also possible.

trait anxiety—Chronically generalized anxiety that predisposes people to appraise events as threatening.

transcription—The transfer of genetic code information from one kind of nucleic acid to another; the process by which mRNA forms bases that are complementary to a strand of DNA.

transient hypofrontality hypothesis—A hypothesis that cerebral blood flow during exercise is down-regulated in brain areas not directly involved in motor control.

translation—The process directed by messenger RNA (mRNA) in which amino acids are linked together to form a protein molecule; the specificity of the synthesis is controlled by the base sequences of the mRNA.

transtheoretical model of behavior change—A dynamic model of intentional behavior change that is based on the stages and processes people go through to bring about long-term behavior.

triadic reciprocality—Key assumption of social cognitive theory that characteristics of the person, environment, and behavior are mutually influencing.

unconditioned stimulus—A stimulus that automatically elicits a response that is typically reflexive.

unipolar scale—A measurement instrument that conceptualizes a psychological construct as a single dimension ranging from the absence of something to a very high degree of the thing being measured (see also *bipolar scale* and *multidimensional scale*).

ventrolateral prefrontal cortex—The region of the frontal lobe associated with the maintenance of information in working memory while blocking distractions.

vigilance—The ability to maintain attention and alertness over a prolonged period of time; also known as sustained attention.

working memory—The temporary storage and manipulation of information necessary for complex tasks such as learning, language comprehension, and reasoning.

Yerkes-Dodson law—A law that describes an inverted-U-shaped relationship between arousal and performance.

Bibliography

Aarts, H., T. Paulussen, and H. Schaalma. 1997. Physical exercise habit: On the conceptualization and formation of habitual health behaviors. *Health Education Research* 12: 363-374.

Abeles, A.M., M.H. Pillinger, B.M. Solitar, and M. Abeles. 2007. Narrative review: The pathophysiology of fibromyalgia. *Annals of Internal Medicine* 146 (10): 726-734.

Abraham, C., and S. Michie. 2008. A taxonomy of behavior change techniques used in interventions. *Health psychology* 27 (3): 379-387.

Abrantes, A.M., D.R. Strong, A. Cohn, et al. 2009. Acute changes in obsessions and compulsions following moderate-intensity aerobic exercise among patients with obsessive-compulsive disorder. *Journal of Anxiety Disorders* 23 (7): 923-927.

Abu-Omar, K., A. Rutten, and V. Lehtinen. 2004. Mental health and physical activity in the European Union. *Sozial- und Praventivmedizin* 49 (5): 301-309.

Achrousos, G.P. 1998. Stressors, stress, and neuroendocrine integration of the adaptive response. The 1997 Hans Selye Memorial Lecture. *Annals of the New York Academy of Sciences* 851 (June 30): 311-335.

Adlard, P.A., and C.W. Cotman. 2004. Voluntary exercise protects against stress-induced decreases in brain-derived neurotrophic factor protein expression. *Neuroscience* 124 (4): 985-992.

Ainsworth, B.E., W.L. Haskell, S.D. Herrmann, N. Meckes, D.R. Bassett, Jr., C. Tudor-Locke, J. L. Greer, J. Vezina, M.C. Whitt-Glover, and A.S. Leon. 2011. 2011 Compendium of physical activities: A second update of codes and MET values. *Medicine and Science in Sports and Exercise.* 43 (8): 1575-81. doi: 10.1249/MSS.0b013e31821ece12.

Ajzen, I. 1988. *Attitudes, personality and behavior.* Chicago, IL: Dorsey Press.

Ajzen, I. and M. Fishbein. 1974. Factors influencing intentions and the intention-behavior relation. *Human Relations* 27 (1): 1-15.

Akil, H., C. Owens, H. Gutstein, L. Taylor, E. Curran, and S. Watson. 1998. Endogenous opioids: Overview and current issues. *Drug and Alcohol Dependence* 51 (1-2): 127-140.

Alder, J., S. Thakker-Varia, D.A. Bangasser, et al. 2003. Brain-derived neurotrophic factor-induced gene expression reveals novel actions of VGF in hippocampal synaptic plasticity. *Journal of Neuroscience* 23 (34):10800-10808.

Alessi, C.A., J.L. Martin, A.P. Webber, E. Cynthia Kim, J.O. Harker, and K.R. Josephson. 2005. Randomized, controlled trial of a nonpharmacological intervention to improve abnormal sleep/wake patterns in nursing home residents. *Journal of the American Geriatrics Society* 53 (5): 803-810.

Alfermann, D. and O. Stoll. 2000. Effects of physical exercise on self-concept and well-being. *International Journal of Sport Psychology* 30: 47-65.

Allen, M.T., and M.D. Crowell. 1989. Patterns of autonomic response during laboratory stressors. *Psychophysiology* 26: 603-614.

Allgulander, C., B. Bandelow, E. Hollander, et al. 2003. WCA recommendations for the long-term treatment of generalized anxiety disorder. *CNS Spectrums* 8 (8 Suppl. 1): 53-61.

Alpert, B., T.M. Field, S. Goldstein, and S. Perry. 1990. Aerobics enhances cardiovascular fitness and agility in preschoolers. *Health Psychology* 9 (1): 48-56.

Amann, M., G.M. Blain, L.T. Proctor, J.J. Sebranek, D.F. Pegelow, and J.A. Dempsey. 2010. Group III and IV muscle afferents contribute to ventilatory and cardiovascular response to rhythmic exercise in humans. *Journal of Applied Physiology* 109 (4): 966-976.

Amann, M., and J.A. Dempsey. 2011. Reply to Marcora. *Journal of Applied Physiology* 110: 1500.

Amann, M., L.T. Proctor, J.J. Sebranek, M.W. Eldridge, D.F. Pegelow, and J.A. Dempsey. 2008. Somatosensory feedback from the limbs exerts inhibitory influences on central neural drive during whole body endurance exercise. *Journal of Applied Physiology* 105 (6): 1714-1724.

Amann, M., L.T. Proctor, J.J. Sebranek, D.F. Pegelow, and J.A. Dempsey. 2009. Opioid-mediated muscle afferents inhibit central motor drive and limit peripheral muscle fatigue development in humans. *Journal of Physiology* 587 (Pt 1): 271-283.

American College Health Association. 2011. American College Health Association—National College Health Assessment II: Reference Group Executive Summary. Fall 2010. Linthicum, MD.

American College of Sports Medicine. 2000. *Guidelines for exercise testing and prescription.* 6th ed. Baltimore: Lippincott Williams & Wilkins.

American College of Sports Medicine. 2009. *Guidelines for exercise testing and prescription.* 8th ed. Philadelphia: Wolters Kluwer; Lippincott Williams & Wilkins.

American Psychiatric Association. 1994. *Diagnostic and statistical manual.* 4th ed. Washington, DC: American Psychiatric Association.

American Psychiatric Association. 2000. Practice guidelines for the treatment of patients with major depressive disorders (revision). *American Journal of Psychiatry* 157 (4 Suppl.): 1-45.

Anderson, B.J., D.P. McCloskey, D.A. Tata, and H.E. Gorby. 2003. Physiological psychology: Biological and behavioral outcomes of exercise. In *Handbook of research methods in experimental psychology*, edited by S.F. Davis. Malden, MA: Blackwell Publishing.

Anderson, B.J., D.N. Rapp, D.H. Baek, D.P. McCloskey, P.S. Coburn-Litvak, and J.K. Robinson. 2000. Exercise influences spatial learning in the radial arm maze. *Physiology & Behavior* 70 (5): 425-429.

Anderson, L.B. 1996. Tracking of risk factors for coronary heart disease from adolescence to young adulthood with special emphasis on physical activity and fitness: A longitudinal study. *Danish Medical Bulletin* 43(5): 407-418.

Anderson, R.J., and S. Brice. 2011. The mood-enhancing benefits of exercise: Memory biases augment the effect. *Psychology of Sport and Exercise* 12 (2): 79-82.

André N., and Dishman R.K. 2012. Evidence for the construct validity of self-motivation as a correlate of exercise adherence in French older adults. *Journal of Aging and Physical Activity* 20 (2): 231-245.

Angevaren, M., G. Aufdemkampe, H.J.J. Verhaar, A. Aleman, and L. Vanhees. 2008. Physical activity and enhanced fitness to improve cognitive function in older people without known cognitive impairment. *Cochrane Database of Systematic Reviews*. Issue 3. Art. No.: CD005381. doi: 10.1002/14651858.CD005381.pub3.

Annesi, J.J., and A.C. Whitaker. 2010. Psychological factors associated with weight loss in obese and severely obese women in a behavioral physical activity intervention. *Health Education & Behavior* 37 (4): 593-606.

Annesi, J.J., J.L. Unruh, C.N. Marti, S. Gorjala, and G. Tennant. 2011. Effects of the Coach Approach intervention on adherence to exercise in obese women: Assessing mediation of social cognitive theory factors. *Research Quarterly for Exercise and Sport*. 82 (1): 99-108.

Anshel, M.H., D. Muller, and V.L. Owens. 1986. Effect of a sports camp experience on the multidimensional self-concepts of boys. *Perceptual & Motor Skills* 63 (2, Pt 1): 363-366.

Anton, S.D., M.G. Perri, J. Riley, et al. 2005. Differential predictors of adherence in exercise programs with moderate versus higher levels of intensity and frequency. *Journal of Sport & Exercise Psychology* 27 (2): 171-187.

Artham, S.M., C.J. Lavie, and R.V. Milani. 2008. Cardiac rehabilitation programs markedly improve high-risk profiles in coronary patients with high psychological distress. *Southern Medical Journal* 101 (3): 262-267. doi: 10.1097/SMJ.0b013e318164dfa8.

Artinian, N.T., G.F. Fletcher, D. Mozaffarian, et al. on behalf of the American Heart Association Prevention Committee of the Council on Cardiovascular Nursing. 2010. Interventions to promote physical activity and dietary lifestyle changes for cardiovascular risk factor reduction in adults: A scientific statement from the American Heart Association. *Circulation* 122 (4): 406-441.

Ashford, S., J. Edmunds, and D.P. French. 2010. What is the best way to change self-efficacy to promote lifestyle and recreational physical activity? A systematic review with meta-analysis. *British Journal of Health Psychology* 15 (2): 265-288.

Atallah, L., J.J. Leong, B. Lo, and G.Z. Yang. 2011. Energy expenditure prediction using a miniaturized ear-worn sensor. *Medicine & Science in Sports & Exercise* 43 (7): 1369-1377.

Auweele, Y.A., R. Rzewnicki, and V. Van Mele. 1997. Reasons for not exercising and exercise intentions: A study of middle-aged sedentary adults. *Journal of Sports Sciences* 15: 151-165.

Averill, J. R., G. L. Clore, J. E. LeDoux, J. Panksepp, D. Watson, L. A. Clark, P. Ekman, and R. J. Davidson. 1994. What influences the subjective experience of emotion? In *The nature of emotions: Fundamental questions*. edited by P. Ekman and R.J. Davidson. New York: Oxford University Press.

Babyak, M., J.A. Blumenthal, S. Herman, et al. 2000. Exercise treatment for major depression: Maintenance of therapeutic benefit at 10 months. *Psychosomatic Medicine* 62 (5): 633-638.

Backmand, H.M., J. Kaprio, U.M. Kujala, and S. Sarna. 2009. Physical activity, mood and the functioning of daily living A longitudinal study among former elite athletes and referents in middle and old age. *Archives of Gerontology and Geriatrics* 48 (1): 1-9.

Baddeley, A.D. 1986. *Working memory*. New York: Oxford.

Baekeland, F. 1970. Exercise deprivation: Sleep and psychological reactions. *Archives of General Psychiatry* 22: 365-369.

Bahrke, M. and W.P. Morgan. 1978. Anxiety reduction following exercise and meditation. *Cognitive Therapy & Research* 2 (4): 323-333.

Baker, L.D., L.L. Frank, K. Foster-Schubert, et al. 2010. Effects of aerobic exercise on mild cognitive impairment. *Archives of Neurology* 67 (1): 71-79.

Baker, P.R.A., D.P. Francis, J. Soares, A.L. Weightman, and C. Foster. 2011. Community wide interventions for increasing physical activity. *Cochrane Database of Systematic Reviews* Issue 4. Art. No.: CD008366. doi: 10.1002/14651858.CD008366.pub2.

Balducci, S., G. Iacobellis, L. Parisi, et al. 2006. Exercise training can modify the natural history of diabetic peripheral neuropathy. *Journal of Diabetes and Its Complications* 20 (4): 216-223.Ball, K., N.W. Burton, and W.J. Brown. 2009. A prospective study of overweight, physical activity, and depressive symptoms in young women. *Obesity* 17 (1): 66-71.

Ballenger, J.C. 2001. Overview of different pharmacotherapies for attaining remission in generalized anxiety disorder. *Journal of Clinical Psychiatry* 62 (Suppl. 19): 11-19.

Baltes, P.B., U. Staudinger, and U. Lindenberger. 1999. Lifespan psychology: Theory and application to intellectual functioning. In *Annual Review of Psychology*, edited by J.T. Spence, J.M. Darley and D.J. Foss. Palo Alto, CA: Annual Reviews.

Bandura, A. 1977. Self-efficacy: Toward a unifying theory of behavioral change. *Psychological Review* 1984: 191-215.

Bandura, A. 1986. *Social foundations of thought and action*. Englewood Cliffs, NJ: Prentice Hall.

Bandura, A. 1997. *Self-efficacy: The exercise of control*. New York: W.H. Freeman and Company.

Bandura, A. 2004. Health promotion by social cognitive means. *Health Education & Behavior* 31 (2): 143-164.

Bantick, S.J., R.G. Wise, A. Ploghaus, S. Clare, S.M. Smith, and I. Tracey. 2002. Imaging how attention modulates pain in humans using functional MRI. *Brain* 125 (2): 310-319.

Bar-Or, O. 2001.Exertional perception in children and adolescents with a disease or disability. *International Journal of Sport and Exercise Psychology* 21 (2): 127-136.

Bar-Sela, A., Hoff, H.E., and Faris, E. (trans.-eds.). 1964 *Moses Maimonides' Two Treatises on the Regimen of Health*, Philadelphia: American Philosophical Society 1-50.

Barak, A., B. Klein, and J.G. Proudfoot. 2009. Defining internet-supported therapeutic interventions. *Annals of Behavioral Medicine:* 38 (1): 4-17.

Baranowski, T., C. Anderson, and C. Carmack. 1998. Mediating variable framework in physical activity interventions: How are we doing? How might we do better? *American Journal of Preventive Medicine* 15: 266-297.

Barger, L.K., K.P. Wright, Jr., R.J. Hughes, and C.A. Czeisler. 2004. Daily exercise facilitates phase delays of circadian melatonin rhythm in very dim light. *American Journal of Physiology* 286 (6): R1077-R1084.

Barkley, R.A. 1998. *Attention-deficit hyperactivity disorder: A handbook for diagnosis and treatment*. 2nd ed. New York: The Guilford Press.

Barnes, R.T., S.A. Coombes, N.B. Armstrong, T.J. Higgins, and C.M. Janelle. 2010. Evaluating attentional and affective changes following an acute exercise bout using a modified dot-probe protocol. *Journal of Sports Sciences* 28 (10): 1065-1076.

Baron, R.M., and D.A. Kenny. 1986. The moderator-mediator variable distinction in social psychological research: Conceptual, strategic, and statistical considerations. *Journal of Personality and Social Psychology* 51: 1173-1182.

Barr-Anderson, D.J., M. AuYoung, M.C. Whitt-Glover, B.A. Glenn, and A.K. Yancey. 2011. Integration of short bouts of physical activity into organizational routine: A systematic review of the literature. *American Journal of Preventive Medicine* 40 (1): 76-93.

Barrett, L.F., and T.D. Wager. 2006. The structure of emotion: Evidence from neuroimaging studies. *Current Directions in Psychological Science* 15: 79-85.

Bartholomew, J.B. 1999. The effect of resistance exercise on manipulated preexercise mood states for male exercisers. *Journal of Sport & Exercise Psychology* (21): 39-51.

Bartholomew, J.B., and D.E. Linder. 1998. State anxiety following resistance exercise: The role of gender and exercise intensity. *Journal of Behavioral Medicine* 21 (2): 205-219.

Bartholomew, J.B., D. Morrison, and J.T. Ciccolo. 2005. Effects of acute exercise on mood and well-being in patients with major depressive disorder. *Medicine & Science in Sports & Exercise* 37 (12): 2032-2037.

Bartlett, M.S., J.C. Hager, P. Ekman, and T.J. Sejnowski, 1999. Measuring facial expressions by computer image analysis. *Psychophysiology* 36: 253-263.

Bartlewski, P.P., J L. Van Raalte, and B.W. Brewer. 1996. Effects of aerobic exercise on the social physique anxiety and body esteem of female college students. *Women in Sport and Physical Activity Journal* 5 (2): 49-61.

Bartlo, P., and P.J. Klein. 2011. Physical activity benefits and needs in adults with intellectual disabilities: Systematic review of the literature. *American Journal on Intellectual and Developmental Disabilities* 116 (3): 220-232.

Basbaum, A.I., and M.C. Bushnell. 2009. *Science of pain*. San Diego: Academic Press.

Bastian, H.C. 1887-1889. The "muscular sense," its nature and cortical localisation. *Brain* 10: 1-137.

Batson, C.D., L.L. Shaw, and K.C. Oleson. 1992. Differentiating affect, mood, and emotion: Toward functionally based conceptual distinctions. In *Emotion*: Review of personality and social psychology, vol. 13, edited by M.S. Clark. Newbury Park, CA: Sage..

Baumeister, R.F. 1993. *Self-esteem: The puzzle of low self-regard*. New York: Plenum Press.

Bayles, C.M., K.F. Metz, R. Robertson, F.L. Gross, J. Cosgrove, and D. McBurney. 1990. Perceptual regulation of prescribed exercise. *Journal of Cardiopulmonary Rehabilitation* 10: 25-31.

Bazargan, M. 1996. Self-reported sleep disturbance among African-American elderly: The effects of depression, health status, exercise, and social support. *International Journal of Aging & Human Development* 42 (2): 143-160.

Beard, J.R., K. Heathcote, R. Brooks, A. Earnest, and B. Kelly. 2007. Predictors of mental disorders and their outcome in a community based cohort. *Social Psychiatry and Psychiatric Epidemiology* 42 (8): 623-630.

Beaupre, L.A, D. Lier, D.M Davies, and D.B.C Johnston. 2004. The effect of a preoperative exercise and education program on functional recovery, health related quality of life, and health service utilization following primary total knee arthroplasty. *Journal of Rheumatology* 31 (6): 1166-1173.

Beecher, H.K. 1956. Relationship of significance of wound to pain experienced. *Journal of the American Medical Association* 161 (17): 1609-1613.

Bélanger-Gravel, A., G. Godin, L.A. Vezina-Im, S. Amireault, and P. Poirier. 2010. The effect of theory-based interventions on physical activity participation among overweight/obese individuals: A systematic review. *Obesity Review*. 12 (6): 430-9. doi: 10.1111/j.1467-789X.2010.00729.x.

Bell, C. 1826. On the nervous circle which connects the voluntary muscles with the brain. *Philosophical Transactions of the Royal Society of London* 116: 163-173.

Bell, C. 1830. *The nervous system of the human body.* London: Longman.

Beltrame, K.F., A.J. Weekes, C. Morgan, R. Tavella, and J.A. Spertus. 2009. The prevalence of weekly angina among patients with chronic stable angina in primary care practices: The Coronary Artery Disease in General Practice (CADENCE) Study. *Archives of Internal Medicine* 169 (16): 1491-1499.

Benington, J.H., S.K. Kodali, and H.C. Heller. 1995. Stimulation of A1 adenosine receptors mimics the electroencephalographic effects of sleep deprivation. *Brain Research* 692 (1-2): 79-85.

Bennett, J.A., K.S. Lyons, K. Winters-Stone, L.M. Nail, and J. Scherer. 2007. Motivational interviewing to increase physical activity in long-term cancer survivors: A randomized controlled trial. *Nursing Research* 56 (1): 18-27.

Bennett, R., J. Jones, D. Turk, I.J. Russell, and L. Matallana. 2007. An internet survey of 2,596 people with fibromyalgia. *BMC Musculoskeletal Disorders* 8 (1): 27.

Berchtold, N.C., G. Chinn, M. Chou, J.P. Kesslak, and C.W. Cotman. 2005. Exercise primes a molecular memory for brain-derived neurotrophic factor protein induction in the rat hippocampus. *Neuroscience* 133 (3): 853-861.

Berger, B.G. and R.W. Motl. 2000. Exercise and mood: A selective review and synthesis of research employing the profile of mood states. *Journal of Applied Sport Psychology* 12: 69-92.

Berger, B.G., D.R. Owen, R.W. Motl, and L. Parks. 1998. Relationship between expectancy of psychological benefits and mood alteration in joggers. *International Journal of Sport Psychology* 29 (1): 1-16.

Berkowitz, J.M., M. Huhman, and M.J. Nolin. 2008. Did augmenting the VERB campaign advertising in select communities have an effect on awareness, attitudes, and physical activity? *American Journal of Preventive Medicine* 34 (6 Suppl.): S257-S266.

Bernard, C.L. 1867. *Rapport sur les progres et la marche de la physiologie generale.* Paris: Bailliere.

Berntson, G.G., J.T. Cacioppo, and K.S. Quigley. 1991. Autonomic determinism: The modes of autonomic control, the doctrine of autonomic space, and the laws of autonomic constraint. *Psychological Review* 98 (Oct): 459-487.

Berntson, G.G., J.T. Cacioppo, and K.S. Quigley. 1993. Cardiac psychophysiology and autonomic space in humans: Empirical perspectives and conceptual implications. *Psychological Bulletin* 114 (2): 296-322.

Berridge, K.C., and T.E. Robinson. 1998. What is the role of dopamine in reward: Hedonic impact, reward learning, or incentive salience? *Brain Research. Brain Research Reviews* 28 (3): 309-369.

Best, J.R. 2010. Effects of physical activity on children's executive function: Contributions of experimental research on aerobic exercise. *Developmental Review* 30 (4): 331-351.

Best, J.R., P.H. Miller, and L.L. Jones. 2009. Executive function after age 5: Changes and correlates. *Developmental Review* 29: 180-200.

Beunen, G., and M. Thomis. 1999. Genetic determinants of sports participation and daily physical activity. *International Journal of Obesity and Related Metabolic Disorders* 23 (Suppl. 3): S55-S63.

Biddle, S., D. Akande, N. Armstrong, M. Ashcroft, R. Brooke, and M. Goudas. 1996. The self-motivation inventory modified for children: Evidence on psychometric properties and its use in physical exercise. *International Journal of Sport Psychology*. 27 (3): 237-250.

Biddle, S.J.H. 1997. Cognitive theories of motivation and the physical self. In *The physical self: From motivation to well-being*, edited by K.R. Fox. Champaign, IL: Human Kinetics.

Biddle, S.J.H., and R. Fuchs. 2009. Exercise psychology: A view from Europe. *Psychology of Sport and Exercise* 10 (4): 410-419.

Biddle, S J., T. Gorely, and S.J. Marshall. 2009. Is television viewing a suitable marker of sedentary behavior in young people? *Annals of Behavioral Medicine* 38 (2): 147-153.

Biddle, S.J.H., and C.R. Nigg. 2000. Theories of exercise behavior. *International Journal of Sport Psychology* 31 (2): 290-304.

Binder, D.K., and H.E. Scharfman. 2004. Brain-derived neurotrophic factor. *Growth factors* 22 (3): 123-131.

Bircan, C., S. Karasel, B. Akgün, O. El, and S. Alper. 2008. Effects of muscle strengthening versus aerobic exercise program in fibromyalgia. *Rheumatology International* 28 (6): 527-532.

Birdsong, W.T., L. Fierro, F.G. Williams, et al. 2010. Sensing muscle ischemia: Coincident detection of acid and ATP via interplay of two ion channels. *Neuron* 68 (4): 739-749.

Bixby, W.R., and M.R. Lochbaum. 2006. Affect responses to acute bouts of aerobic exercise in fit and unfit participants: An examination of opponent-process theory. *Journal of Sport Behavior* 29 (2): 111.

Black, C.D., M.P. Herring, D.J. Hurley, and P.J. O'Connor. 2010. Ginger (Zingiber officinale) reduces muscle pain caused by eccentric exercise. *Journal of Pain* 11 (9): 894-903.

Black, C.D., and P.J. O'Connor. 2008. Acute effects of dietary ginger on quadriceps muscle pain during moderate-intensity cycling exercise. *International Journal of Sport Nutrition & Exercise Metabolism* 18 (6): 653-664.

Blair, S.N., M. Booth, I. Gyarfas, et al. 1996. Development of public policy and physical activity initiatives internationally. *Sports Medicine* 21 (3): 157-163.

Blamey, A., N. Mutrie, and T. Aitchison. 1995. Health promotion by encouraged use of stairs. *British Medical Journal* 311: 289-290.

Blanchard, C., M. Fortier, S. Sweet, et al. 2007. Explaining physical activity levels from a self-efficacy perspective: The physical activity counseling trial. *Annals of Behavioral Medicine* 34 (3): 323-328.

Blascovich, J., and J. Tomaka. 1991. Measures of self-esteem. In *Measures of personality and social psychological attitudes*, edited by J.P. Robinson, P.R. Shaver, and L.S. Wrightsman. San Diego, CA: Academic Press.

Blissmer, B., and E. McAuley. 2002. Testing the requirements of stages of physical activity among adults: The comparative effectiveness of stage-matched, mismatched, standard care, and control interventions. *Annals of Behavioral Medicine* 24 (3): 181-189.

Blumberg, S.J., and J.V. Luke. 2011. *Wireless substitution: Early release of estimates from the National Health Interview Survey, January-June 2010.* National Center for Health Statistics, December 21, 2010 [cited September 2, 2011]. www.cdc.gov/nchs/nhis.htm.

Blumenthal, J.A., M.A. Babyak, K.A. Moore, et al. 1999. Effects of exercise training on older patients with major depression. *Archives of Internal Medicine* 159 (Oct 25): 2349-2356.

Blumenthal, J.A., S. Herman, P. Khatri, et al. 2000. Exercise treatment for major depression: Maintenance of therapeutic benefit at 10 months. *Psychosomatic Medicine* 62 (5): 633-638.

Blumenthal, J.A., S. Rose, and J.L. Chang. 1985. Anorexia nervosa and exercise. Implications from recent findings. *Sports Medicine* 2 (Jul-Aug): 237-247.

Bock, B.C., B.H. Marcus, T.K. King, B. Borrelli, and M.R. Roberts. 1999. Exercise effects on withdrawal and mood among women attempting smoking cessation. *Addictive Behaviors* 24 (3): 399-410.

Boecker, H., T. Sprenger, M.E. Spilker, et al. 2008. The runner's high: Opioidergic mechanisms in the human brain. *Cerebral Cortex* 18 (11): 2523-2531.

Boecker, H., A. Othman, S. Mueckter, L. Scheef, M. Pensel, M. Daamen, J. Jankowski, H.H. Schild, T.R. Tölle, and M. Schreckenberger. 2010. Advocating Neuroimaging Studies of Transmitter Release in Human Physical Exercise Challenges Studies. *Open Access Journal of Sports Medicine* 1: 167-175.

Bol, Y., A.A. Druits, R.M. Hupperts, J.W. Valaeyen, and F.R. Verhey. 2009. The psychology of fatigue in patients with multiple sclerosis: A review. *Journal of Psychosomatic Research* 66 (1): 3-11.

Bollen, K.A. 1989. *Structural equations with latent variables.* New York: Wiley.

Bollen, K.A., P.J. Curran, and J. Wiley. 2006. *Latent curve models: A structural equation perspective.* Hoboken, NJ: Wiley-Interscience.

Bolognesi, M., C.R. Nigg, M. Massarini, and S. Lippke. 2006. Reducing obesity indicators through brief physical activity counseling (PACE) in Italian primary care settings. *Annals of Behavioral Medicine* 31 (2): 179-185.

Bonnet, M., M.M. Bradley, P.J. Lang, and J. Requin. 1995. Modulation of spinal reflexes: Arousal, pleasure, action. *Psychophysiology* 32 (4): 367-372.

Booth, M.L., N. Owen, A. Bauman, O. Clavisi, and E. Leslie. 2000. Social-cognitive and perceived environmental influences associated with physical activity in older Australians. *Preventive Medicine* 31: 15-22.

Bopp, M., S. Wilcox, M. Laken, K. Butler, R.E. Carter, L. McClorin, and A. Yancey. 2006. Factors associated with physical activity among African-American men and women. *American Journal of Preventive Medicine* 30 (4): 340-346.

Borg, G.A. 1961. Interindividual scaling and perception of muscular force. *Kungliga Fysiografiska Sällskapets I Lund Förhandlinger* 12 (31): 117-125.

Borg, G.A. 1962. *Physical performance and perceived exertion.* Vol. XI, *Studia Psychologica et Paedagogica. Seris altera.* Lund, Sweden: Gleerup.

Borg, G.A. 1970. Perceived exertion as an indicator of somatic stress. *Scandinavian Journal of Rehabilitative Medicine* 23: 92-98.

Borg, G.A. 1972. The basic "noise constant" in the psychophysical function of perceived exertion. *Reports from the Institute of Applied Psychology, U.Stockholm* (33).

Borg, G.A. 1982. Psychophysical bases of perceived exertion. *Medicine & Science in Sports & Exercise* 14: 377-381.

Borg, G.A. 1998. *Borg's perceived exertion and pain scales.* Champaign, IL: Human Kinetics.

Borg, P., K. Kukkonen-Harjula, M. Fogelholm, and M. Pasanen. 2002. Effects of walking or resistance training on weight loss maintenance in obese, middle-aged men: A randomized trial. *International Journal of Obesity* 26 (5): 676-683.

Borges, G., M.K. Nock, J.M. Haro Abad, et al. 2010. Twelve-month prevalence of and risk factors for suicide attempts in the World Health Organization World Mental Health Surveys. *Journal of Clinical Psychiatry* 71 (12): 1617-1628.

Borkowski, J.H., M. Carr, and M. Pressely. 1987. "Spontaneous" strategy use: Perspectives from metacognitive theory. *Intelligence* 11: 61-75.

Bouchard, C. 2011. Overcoming barriers to progress in exercise genomics. *Exercise and Sport Sciences Reviews*. 39(4) :212-217. doi: 10.1097/JES.0b013e31822643f6.

Bouchard, C., and T. Rankinen. 2001. Individual differences in response to regular physical activity. *Medicine & Science in Sports & Exercise* 33 (6 Suppl.): S446-S451; discussion S452-S453.

Bouchard, C., M.A. Sarzynski, T.K. Rice, et al. 2011. Genomic predictors of the maximal O uptake response to standardized exercise training programs. *Journal of Applied Physiology* 110 (5): 1160-1170.

Bouchard, C., R. Shephard, and T. Stephens. 1994. *Physical activity, fitness, and health: International proceedings and consensus statement.* Champaign, IL: Human Kinetics.

Boutcher, S.H., L.A. Fleischer-Curtian, and S.D. Gines. 1988. The effects of self-presentation on perceived exertion. *Journal of Sport & Exercise Psychology* 10 (3): 270-280.

Boutcher, S.H., F.W. Nugent, P.F. McLaren, and A.L. Weltman. 1998. Heart period variability of trained and untrained men at rest and during mental challenge. *Psychophysiology* 35 (Jan): 16-22.

Boutcher, S.H., R.L. Seip, R.K. Hetzler, E.F. Pierce, D. Snead, and A. Weltman. 1989. The effects of specificity of training on rating of perceived exertion at the lactate threshold. *European Journal of Applied Physiology* 59: 365-369.

Boyd, K.R., and D.W. Hrycaiko. 1997. The effect of a physical activity intervention package on the self-esteem of pre-adolescent and adolescent females. *Adolescence* 32 (Fall): 693-708.

Bozdagi, O., E. Rich, S. Tronel, et al. 2008. The neurotrophin-inducible gene Vgf regulates hippocampal function and behavior through a brain-derived neurotrophic factor-dependent mechanism. *Journal of Neuroscience* 28 (39): 9857-9869.

Bozoian, S., W.J. Rejeski, and E. McAuley. 1994. Self-efficacy influences feeling states associated with acute exercise. *Journal of Sport & Exercise Psychology* 16 (3): 326-333.

Bradley, M.M., and P.J. Lang. 1994. Measuring emotion: The Self-Assessment Manikin and the semantic differential. *Journal of Behavior Therapy and Experimental Psychiatry.* 25 (1): 49-59.

Bray, M.S., J.M. Hagberg, L. Perusse, et al. 2009. The human gene map for performance and health-related fitness phenotypes: The 2006-2007 update. *Medicine & Science in Sports & Exercise* 41 (1): 35-73.

Breivik, H., B. Collett, V. Ventafridda, R. Cohen, and D. Gallacher. 2006. Survey of chronic pain in Europe: Prevalence, impact on daily life, and treatment. *European Journal of Pain* 10 (4): 287-333.

Breslau, J., S. Aguilar-Gaxiola, K.S. Kendler, M. Su, D. Williams, and R.C. Kessler. 2006. Specifying race-ethnic differences in risk for psychiatric disorder in a USA national sample. *Psychological Medicine* 36 (1): 57-68.

Breus, M.J. and P.J. O'Connor. 1998. Exercise-induced anxiolysis: A test of the "time out" hypothesis in high anxious females. *Medicine & Science in Sports & Exercise* 30 (7): 1107-1112.

Breus, M.J., P.J. O'Connor, and S.T. Ragan. 2000. Muscle pain induced by novel eccentric exercise does not disturb the sleep of normal young men. *Journal of Pain* 1 (1): 67-76.

Briones, T.L. 2006. Environment, physical activity, and neurogenesis: Implications for prevention and treatment of Alzheimer's Disease. *Current Alzheimer Research* 3: 49-54.

Brisswalter, J.B., M. Collardeau, and R Arcelin. 2002. Effects of acute physical exercise on cognitive performance. *Sports Medicine* 32: 555-566.

Brodie, D.A., and A. Inoue. 2005. Motivational interviewing to promote physical activity for people with chronic heart failure. *Journal of Advanced Nursing* 50 (5): 518-527.

Bronfenbrenner, U. 1979. *The Ecology of Human Development.* Cambridge, MA: Harvard University Press.

Broocks, A., B. Bandelow, G. Pekrun, et al. 1998. Comparison of aerobic exercise, clomipramine, and placebo in the treatment of panic disorder [see comments]. *American Journal of Psychiatry* 155 (May): 603-609.

Broocks, A., T.F. Meyer, B. Bandelow, et al. 1997. Exercise avoidance and impaired endurance capacity in patients with panic disorder. *Neuropsychobiology* 36: 182-187.

Brown, R.D., and J.M. Harrison. 1986. The effects of a strength training program on the strength and self-concept of two female age groups. *Research Quarterly for Exercise and Sport* 57: 315-320.

Brown, G.G., J.E. Perthen, T.T. Liu, and R.B. Buxton. 2007. A primer on functional magnetic resonance imaging. *Neuropsychology Review.* 17 (2): 107-25. doi: 10.1007/s11065-007-9028-8.

Brown, S G., and R.E. Rhodes. 2006. Relationships among dog ownership and leisure-time walking in Western Canadian adults. *American Journal of Preventive Medicine* 30 (2): 131-136.

Brown, W.J., J.H. Ford, N.W. Burton, A.L. Marshall, and A.J. Dobson. 2005. Prospective study of physical activity and depressive symptoms in middle-aged women. *American Journal of Preventive Medicine* 29 (4): 265-272.

Brown, W.J., G. Mishra, C. Lee, and A. Bauman. 2000. Leisure time physical activity in Australian women: Relationship with well being and symptoms. *Research Quarterly for Exercise and Sport* 71 (3): 206-216.

Brownell, K., A.J. Stunkard, and J. Albaum. 1980. Evaluation and modification of exercise patterns in the natural environment. *American Journal of Psychiatry* 136: 1540-1545.

Brownson, R.C., E.A. Baker, R.A. Housemann, L.K. Brennan, and S.J. Bacak. 2001. Environmental and policy determinants of physical activity in the United States. *American Journal of Public Health* 91 (12): 1995-2003.

Brownson, R.C., C.M. Hoehner, K. Day, A. Forsyth, and J.F. Sallis. 2009. Measuring the built environment for physical activity: State of the science. *American Journal of Preventive Medicine* 36 (4): S99-S123; E12.

Bryne, A. and D.G. Bryne. 1993. The effect of exercise on depression, anxiety and other mood states: a review. *Journal of Psychosomatic Research* 17: 565-574.

Bryan, R.J. 1990. Cerebral blood flow and energy metabolism during stress. *American Journal of Physiology* 259 (Aug): H269-H280.

Brynteson, P., and T.M.I. Adams. 1993. The effects of conceptually based physical education programs on attitudes and exercise habits of college alumni after 2 to 11 years of follow-up. *Research Quarterly for Exercise & Sport* 64: 208-212.

Buckworth, J. 2000. Exercise determinants and interventions. *International Journal of Sport Psychology* 31 (2): 305-320.

Buckworth, J. 2001. Exercise adherence in college students: Issues and preliminary results. *Quest* 53 (3): 335-345.

Buckworth, J., R.K. Dishman, and K.J. Cureton. 1994. Effects of aerobic fitness on cardiovascular reactivity and the carotid baroreflex in women with parental hypertension. *Medicine & Science in Sports & Exercise* 26 (Suppl. 5): S198.

Buckworth, J., R.E. Lee, G. Regan, L.K. Schneider, and C.C. DiClemente. 2007. Decomposing intrinsic and extrinsic motivation for exercise: Application to stages of motivational readiness. *Psychology of Sport and Exercise* 8 (4): 441-461.

Bulbulian, R., and B.L. Darabos. 1986. Motor neuron excitability: The Hoffmann reflex following exercise of low and high intensity. *Medicine & Science in Sports & Exercise* 18 (Dec): 697-702.

Bull, F.C., K. Jamrozik, and B.A. Blanksby. 1998. Tailoring advice on exercise: Does it make a difference? *American Journal of Preventive Medicine* 16 (3): 230-239.

Bullitt, E., F.N. Rahman, J.K. Smith, et al. 2009. The effect of exercise on the cerebral vasculature of healthy aged subjects as visualized by MR angiography. *American Journal of Neuroradiology* 30 (10): 1857-1863.

Buman, M.P., E.B. Hekler, D.L. Bliwise, and A.C. King. 2011a. Exercise effects on night-to-night fluctuations in self-rated sleep among older adults with sleep complaints. *Journal of Sleep Research* 20 (1 Pt 1): 28-37.

Buman, M.P., E.B. Hekler, D.L. Bliwise, and A.C. King. 2011b. Moderators and mediators of exercise-induced objective sleep improvements in midlife and older adults with sleep complaints. *Health Psychology* 30 (5): 579-587.

Burgess, M.L., J.M. Davis, T.K. Borg, and J. Buggy. 1991. Intracranial self-stimulation motivates treadmill running in rats. *Journal of Applied Physiology* 71 (Oct): 1593-1597.

Burghardt, P.R., L.J. Fulk, G.A. Hand, and M.A. Wilson. 2004. The effects of chronic treadmill and wheel running on behavior in rats. *Brain Research* 1019 (1-2): 84-96.

Burke, E.J. and M.L. Collins. 1984. Using perceived exertion for the prescription of exercise in healthy adults. In *Clinical sports medicine*, Lexington, MA: Callamore Press.

Burton, R. 1632. *The anatomy of melancholy*. Oxford: Printed by Ion Lichfield for Henry Cripps.

Busch, V., and C. Gaul. 2008. Exercise in migraine therapy: Is there any evidence for efficacy? A critical review. *Headache: The Journal of Head and Face Pain* 48 (6): 890-899.

Butler, J.E., J.L. Taylor, and S.C. Gandevia. 2003. Responses of human motoneurons to corticospinal stimulation during maximal voluntary contractions and ischemia. *Journal of Neuroscience* 23 (32): 10224-10230.

Buxton, O.M., C.W. Lee, M. L'Hermite-Baleriaux, F.W. Turek, and E. Van Cauter. 2003. Exercise elicits phase shifts and acute alterations of melatonin that vary with circadian phase. *American Journal of Physiology* 284 (3): R714-R724.

Buxton, R.B. 2009. *Introduction to functional magnetic resonance imaging: Principles and techniques*. Cambridge, UK: Cambridge University Press.

Buxton, R.B., L.R. Frank, E.C. Wong, B. Siewert, S. Warach, and R.R. Edelman. 1998. A general kinetic model for quantitative perfusion imaging with arterial spin labeling. *Magnetic Resonance in Medicine* 40 (3): 383-396.

Cacioppo, J.T., G.G. Berntson, J.T. Larsen, K.M. Poehlmann, and T.A. Ito. 2000. The psychophysiology of emotion. In *Handbook of emotions*, edited by M. Lewis, J.M. Haviland-Jones, and L.F. Barrett. New York: Guilford Press.

Cacioppo, J.T., D.J. Klein, G.G. Bernsten, and E. Hatfield. 1993. The psychophysiology of emotion. In *Handbook of emotions*, edited by M. Lewis and J.M. Haviland. New York: Guilford Press.

Cacioppo, J.T., R.E. Petty, M.E. Losch, and H.S. Kim. 1986. Electromyographic activity over facial muscle regions can differentiate the valence and intensity of affective reactions. *Journal of Personality and Social Psychology* 50: 260-268.

Cafarelli, E., and B. Bigland-Ritchie. 1979. Sensation of static force in muscles of different length. *Experimental Neurology* 65: 511-525.

Cafarelli, E., W.S. Cain, and J.C. Stevens. 1977. Effort of dynamic exercise: Influence of load, duration, and task. *Ergonomics* 20 (2): 147-158.

Cafarelli, E., and C.E. Kostka. 1981. Effect of vibration on static force sensation in man. *Experimental Neurology* 74 (2): 331-340.

Cain, W.S., and J.C. Stevens. 1971. Effort in sustained and phasic handgrip contractions. *American Journal of Psychology* 84: 51-65.

Cain, W.S., and J.C. Stevens. 1973. Constant-effort contractions related to the electromyogram. *Medicine and Science in Sports* 5 (2): 121-127.

Calfas, K.J., B.J. Long, J.F. Sallis, W. Wooten, M. Pratt, and K. Patrick. 1996. A controlled trial of physician counseling to promote the adoption of physical activity. *Preventive Medicine* 25 (3): 225-233.

Calfas, K.J., J.F. Sallis, B. Oldenburg, and M. French. 1997. Mediators of change in physical activity following an intervention in primary care: PACE. *Preventive Medicine* 26: 297-304.

Calhoun, L.G. 1999. Gender and ethnic differences in the relationship between body esteem and self-esteem. *Journal of Psychology* 133 (4): 357-368.

California Department of Education. 2005. *A study of the relationship between physical fitness and academic achievement in California using 2004 test results.* Sacramento: California Department of Education.

Callaghan, P., E. Khalil, and I. Morres. 2009. Pragmatic randomised controlled trial of a preferred intensity exercise programme to improve wellbeing outcomes of women living with depression. University of Nottingham. Nottingham, UK.

Camacho, T.C., R.E. Roberts, N.B. Lazarus, G.A. Kaplan, and R.D. Cohen. 1991. Physical activity and depression: Evidence from the Alameda County Study. *American Journal of Epidemiology* 134: 220-231.

Camacho-Minano, M.J., N.M. Lavoi, and D.J. Barr-Anderson. 2011. Interventions to promote physical activity among young and adolescent girls: A systematic review. *Health Education Research*. 26 (6): 1025-1049. doi: 10.1093/her/cyr040.

Campbell, A., and H.A. Hausenblas. 2009. Effects of exercise interventions on body image: A meta-analysis. *Journal of Health Psychology* 14 (6): 780-793.

Campbell, D.D., and J.E. Davis. 1939-1940. Report of research and experimentation in exercise and recreational therapy. *American Journal of Psychiatry* 96: 915-933.

Campbell, D.T., and D.W. Fiske. 1959. Convergent and discriminant validation by the multitrait-multimethod matrix. *Psychological Bulletin* 56: 81-105.

Cannon, W.B. 1929. Organization for physiological homeostasis. *Physiological Review* 9: 399-431.

Carlson, J.M., D. Foti, L.R. Mujica-Parodi, E. Harmon-Jones, and G. Hajcak. 2011. Ventral striatal and medial prefrontal BOLD activation is correlated with reward-related electrocortical activity: A combined ERP and fMRI study. *NeuroImage* 57 (4): 1608-1616.

Carlson, N. R. 1998. *Physiology of behavior.* 6th ed. Needham Heights, MA: Allyn and Bacon.

Carlson, N.R. 2010. *Physiology of behavior.* 10th ed. Needham Heights, MA: Allyn and Bacon.

Carlson, S.A., J.E. Fulton, S.M. Lee, et al. 2008. Physical education and academic achievement in elementary school: Data from the Early Childhood Longitudinal study. *American Journal of Public Health* 98 (4): 721-727.

Carroll, J.B. 1993. *Human cognitive abilities.* Cambridge: Cambridge University Press.

Carron, A.V., H.A. Hausenblas, and D. Mack. 1996. Social influence and exercise: A meta-analysis. *Journal of Sport & Exercise Psychology* 18: 1-16.

Carskadon, M.A., and W.C. Dement. 1989. Normal human sleep: An overview. In *Principles and practice of sleep medicine*, edited by M.H. Kryger, T. Roth, and W.C. Dement. Philadelphia: Saunders.

Caruso, C.M., and D.L. Gill. 1992. Strengthening physical self-perceptions through exercise. *Journal of Sports Medicine and Physical Fitness* 32: 416-427.

Carver, C.S. 2004. Negative affects deriving from the behavioral approach system. *Emotion* 4 (1): 3-22.

Carver, C.S., and J. Connor-Smith. 2010. Personality and coping. *Annual Review of Psychology* 61: 679-704.

Carver, C.S., and E. Harmon-Jones. 2009a. Anger is an approach-related affect: Evidence and implications. *Psychological Bulletin* 135 (2): 183-204.

Carver, C.S., and E. Harmon-Jones. 2009b. Anger and approach: Reply to Watson (2009) and to Tomarken and Zald (2009). *Psychological Bulletin* 135 (2): 215-217.

Carver, C.S., H.J. Scheier, C.J. Miller, and D. Fulford. 2009. Optimism. In *Oxford handbook of positive psychology*, edited by C.R. Snyder and S.J. Lopez. New York: Oxford University Press.

Carver, C.S., and T.L. White. 1994. Behavioral inhibition, behavioral activation, and affective responses to impending reward and punishment: The BIS/BAS Scales. *Journal of Personality and Social Psychology* 67 (2): 319-333.

Casey, B.J., A. Galvan, and T.A. Hare. 2005. Changes in cerebral functional organization during cognitive development. *Current Opinion in Neurobiology* 15 (2): 239-244.

Cash, T.F. 2000. *Multidimensional Body-Self Relations Questionnaire: MBSRQ user's manual.* Norfolk, VA: Old Dominion University.

Casper, R.C. 1993. Exercise and Mood. *World Review of Nutrition and Dietetics* (71): 115-143.

Caspersen, C.J. 1989. Physical activity epidemiology: concepts, methods, and applications to exercise science. *Exercise and Sport Sciences Reviews* 17: 423-473.

Caspersen, C.J., M.A. Pereira, and K.M. Curran. 2000. Changes in Physical Activity Patterns in the United States, by Sex and Cross-Sectional Age. *Medicine and Science in Sports and Exercise* 32, 9: 1601-1609.

Caspersen, C.J., K.E. Powell, and G.M. Christenson. 1985. Physical activity, exercise, and physical fitness: Definitions and distinctions for health-related research. *Public Health Reports* 100: 126-131.

Castro, C., J.F. Sallis, S.A. Hickmann, R.E. Lee, and A.H. Chen. 1999. A prospective study of psychosocial correlates of physical activity for ethnic minority women. *Psychology & Health* 14 (2): 277-293.

Centers for Disease Control and Prevention. 2001. Increasing physical activity: A report on recommendations of the Task Force on Community Preventive Services. *Morbidity and Mortality Weekly Reports* 50(No. RR-18); 7-12.

Centers for Disease Control and Prevention (CDC). 2001a. Physical activity trend—United States, 1990-1998. *Morbidity and Mortality Weekly Reports* 50: 166-169.

Centers for Disease Control and Prevention (CDC). 2001b. Prevalence of disabilities and associated health conditions among adults—United States, 1999. *Journal of the American Medical Association* 285 (12): 1571.

Centers for Disease Control and Prevention (CDC). 2005. Public health strategies for preventing and controlling overweight and obesity in school and worksite settings: A report on recommendations of the task force on community preventative services. *CDC Recommendations and Reports,* October 7, 2005/54(RR10). www.cdc.gov/mmwR/preview/mmwrhtml/rr5410a1.htm.

Centers for Disease Control and Prevention (CDC). 2010a. Web-based Injury Statistics Query and Reporting System (WISQARS) [Online]. National Center for Injury Prevention and Control, CDC (producer). www.cdc.gov/injury/wisqars/index.html.

Centers for Disease Control and Prevention (CDC). 2012. Youth Risk Behavior Surveillance—United States, 2011. Surveillance Summaries, June 8. *Morbidity and Mortality Weekly Report* 61 (No. SS-4).

Chaddock, L., M.B. Pontifex, C.H. Hillman, and A.F. Kramer. 2011. A review of the relation of aerobic fitness and physical activity to brain structure and function in children. *Journal of the International Neuropsychological Society* 7 (6): 975-85. doi: 10.1017/S1355617711000567.

Challenges and a call for action. *Psychology of Sport and Exercise* 12: 1-6.

Chaouloff, F. 1997. Effects of acute physical exercise on central serotonergic systems. *Medicine & Science in Sports & Exercise* 29 (Jan): 58-62.

Charney, D.S., S.W. Woods, W.K. Goodman, and G.R. Heninger. 1987. Serotonin function in anxiety. II. Effects of the serotonin agonist MCPP in panic disorder patients and healthy subjects. *Psychopharmacology* 92: 14-24.

Charney, D.S., S.W. Woods, J.H. Krystal, L.M. Nagy, and G.R. Heninger. 1992. Noradrenergic neuronal dysregulation in panic disorder: The effects of intravenous yohimbine and clonidine in panic disorder patients. *Acta Psychiatrica Scandinavica* 86 (Oct): 273-282.

Chida, Y., and A. Steptoe. 2009. The association of anger and hostility with future coronary heart disease: A meta-analytic review of prospective evidence. *Journal of the American College of Cardiology* 53 (11): 936-946.

Chilcott, L.A., and C.M. Shapiro. 1996. The socioeconomic impact of insomnia. An overview. *Pharmaco-Economics* 10 (Suppl. 1): 1-14.

Chodzko-Zajko, W.J., and K.A. Moore. 1994. Physical fitness and cognitive functioning in aging. In *Exercise and sport science reviews*, edited by J.O. Holloszy. Baltimore, PA: Williams & Wilkins.

Chodzko-Zajko, W.J., D.N. Proctor, M.A.F. Singh, C.T. Minson, C.R. Nigg, G.J. Salem, and J.S. Skinner. Exercise and Physical Activity for Older Adults. *Medicine & Science in Sports & Exercise* 41, 7 (2009): 1510-30 doi: 10.249/MSS.0b013e3181a0c95c.

Chomitz, V.R., M.M. Slinning, R.J. McGowan, S.E. Mitchell, G.F. Dawson, and K.A. Hacker. 2009. Is there a relationship between physical fitness and academic achievement? Positive results from public school children in the Northeastern United States. *Journal of School Health* 79 (1): 30-37.

Chou, R., and L. Hoyt Huffman. 2007. Nonpharmacologic therapies for acute and chronic low back pain: A review of the evidence for an American Pain Society/American College of Physicians clinical practice guideline. *Annals of Internal Medicine* 147 (7): 492-504.

Chouinard, G. 2004. Issues in the clinical use of benzodiazepines: Potency, withdrawal, and rebound. *Journal of Clinical Psychiatry* 65 (Suppl. 5): 7-12.

Christensen, M.S., J. Lundbye-Jensen, S.S. Geertsen, T.H. Petersen, O.B. Paulson, and J.B. Nielsen. 2007. Premotor cortex modulates somatosensory cortex during voluntary movements without proprioceptive feedback. *Nature Neuroscience* 10 (4): 417-419.

Chronicle of Higher Education. 2000. Information bank. Available from www.chronicle.com.

Chrousos, G.P., and P.W. Gold. 1998. A healthy body in a healthy mind—and vice versa—the damaging power of"uncontrollable"stress[editorial;comment].*Journal of Clinical Endocrinology and Metabolism* 83 (June): 1842-1845.

Chung, S., M.E. Domino, S.C. Stearns, and B.M. Popkin. 2009. Retirement and physical activity: Analyses by occupation and wealth. *American Journal of Preventive Medicine* 36 (5): 422-428.

Churchill, J.D., R. Galvez, S. Colcombe, R.A. Swain, A.F. Kramer, and W.T. Greenough. 2002. Exercise, experience and the aging brain. *Neurobiology of Aging* 23 (5): 941-955.

Ciubotariu, A., L. Arendt-Nielsen, and T. Graven-Nielsen. 2007. Localized muscle pain causes prolonged recovery after fatiguing isometric contractions. *Experimental Brain Research* 181 (1): 147-158.

Clarac, F. 2008. Some historical reflections on the neural control of locomotion. *Brain Research Reviews* 57 (1): 13-21.

Clark, P.J., T.K. Bhattacharya, D.S. Miller, and J.S. Rhodes. 2011. Induction of c-Fos, Zif268, and Arc from acute bouts of voluntary wheel running in new and pre-existing adult mouse hippocampal granule neurons. *Neuroscience* 184: 16-27.

Clausen, J.P., and J. Trap-Jensen. 1976. Heart rate and arterial blood pressure during exercise in patients with angina pectoris. Effects of training and of nitroglycerin. *Circulation* 53 (3): 436-442.

Clausen, R.P., K.B. Hansen, P. Cali, et al. 2004. The respective N-hydroxypyrazole analogues of the classical glutamate receptor ligands ibotenic acid and (RS)-2-amino-2-(3-hydroxy-5-methyl-4-isoxazolyl) acetic acid. *European Journal of Pharmacology* 499 (1-2): 35-44.

Cleland, V., D. Crawford, L.A. Baur, C. Hume, A. Timperio, and J. Salmon. 2008. A prospective examination of children's time spent outdoors, objectively measured physical activity and overweight. *International Journal of Obesity* 32 (11): 1685-1693.

Cloninger, C.R. 2005. Character strengths and virtues: A handbook and classification. *American Journal of Psychiatry* 162 (4): 820-821.

Clore, G.L., N. Schwarz, and M. Conway. 1994. Affective causes and consequences of social information processing. In *Handbook of social cognition, Vol.1: Basic processes; Vol.2: Applications*, edited by R.S. Wyer, Jr., and T.K. Srull. 2nd ed. Hillsdale, NJ: Lawrence Erlbaum.

Clutter, W., D. Bier, S. Shah, and P.E. Cryer. 1980. Epinephrine: Plasma metabolic clearance rates and physiologic thresholds for metabolic and hemodynamic actions in man. *Journal of Clinical Investigation* 66: 94-101.

Coats, A.J.S. 1992. Heart rate variability and physical training. In *Blood pressure and heart rate variability*, edited by M. Di Rienzo. Amsterdam, Netherlands: IOS Press.

Cockerill, I.M., and M.E. Riddington. 1996. Exercise dependence and associated disorders: A review. *Counseling Psychology Quarterly* 9 (2): 119-129.

Coghill, R.C., C.N. Sang, J.M. Maisog, and M.J. Iadarola. 1999. Pain intensity processing within the human brain: A bilateral, distributed mechanism. *Journal of Neurophysiology* 82 (4): 1934-1943.

Cohen, M.S., and S.Y. Bookheimer. 1994. Localization of brain function using magnetic resonance imaging. *Trends in Neurosciences* 17 (Jul): 268-277.

Colabianchi, N., M. Dowda, K.A. Pfeiffer, D.E. Porter, M.J. Almeida, and R.R. Pate. 2007. Towards an understanding of salient neighborhood boundaries: Adolescent reports of an easy walking distance and convenient driving distance. *International Journal of Behavioral Nutrition and Physical Activity* 4: 66.

Colcombe, S.J., K.I. Erickson, P. Scalf, et al. 2006. Aerobic exercise training increases brain volume in aging humans. *Journal of Gerontology: Medical Sciences* 61A (11): 1166-1170.

Colcombe, S.J., and A. F Kramer. 2003. Fitness effects on the cognitive function of older adults: A meta-analytic study. *Psychological Science* 14: 125-130.

Colcombe, S.J., A.F. Kramer, K.I. Erickson, et al. 2004. Cardiovascular fitness, cortical plasticity, and aging. *Proceedings of the National Academy of Science* 101 (9): 3316-3321.

Cole, D.A., S.E. Maxwell, J.M. Martin, et al. 2001. The development of multiple domains of child and adolescent self-concept: A cohort sequential longitudinal design. *Child Development* 72 (6): 1723-1746.

Cole, R.J., D.F. Kripke, J. Wisbey, et al. 1995. Seasonal variation in human illumination exposure at two different latitudes. *Journal of Biological Rhythms* 10 (4): 324-334.

Colombe, S.J., A. F Kramer, K.I. Erickson, et al. 2004. Cardiovascular fitness, cortical plasticity, and aging. *Proceedings of the National Academy of Science.* 101: 3316-3321.

Conn, V.S., A.R. Hafdahl, and L.M. Brown. 2009. Meta-analysis of quality-of-life outcomes from physical activity interventions. *Nursing Research* 58 (3): 175-183.

Conn, V.S., A.R. Hafdahl, P.S. Cooper, L.M. Brown, and S.L. Lusk. 2009. Meta-analysis of workplace physical activity interventions. *American Journal of Preventive Medicine* 37 (4): 330-339.

Conn, V.S., A.R. Hafdahl, and D.R. Mehr. 2011. Interventions to increase physical activity among healthy adults: A meta-analysis of outcomes. *American Journal of Public Health* 101 (4): 751-758.

Connor-Smith, J.K., and C. Flachsbart. 2007. Relations between personality and coping: A meta-analysis. *Journal of Personality and Social Psychology* 93 (6): 1080-1107.

Cook, D.B., E.M. Jackson, P.J. O'Connor, and R.K. Dishman. 2004. Muscle pain during exercise in normotensive African American women: Effect of parental hypertension history. *Journal of Pain* 5 (2): 111-118.

Cook, D.B., and K.F. Koltyn. 2000. Pain and exercise. *International Journal of Sport Psychology* 31 (2): 256-277.

Cook, D.B., P.R. Nagelkirk, A. Poluri, J. Mores, and B.H. Natelson. 2006. The influence of aerobic fitness and fibromyalgia on cardiorespiratory and perceptual responses to exercise in patients with chronic fatigue syndrome. *Arthritis and Rheumatism* 54 (10): 3351-3362.

Cook, D.B., P.J. O'Connor, S.A. Eubanks, J.C. Smith, and M. Lee. 1997. Naturally occurring muscle pain during exercise: Assessment and experimental evidence. *Medicine & Science in Sports & Exercise* 29 (8): 999-1012.

Cook, D.B., P.J. O'Connor, G. Lange, and J. Steffener. 2007. Functional neuroimaging correlates of mental fatigue induced by cognition among chronic fatigue syndrome patients and controls. *NeuroImage* 36 (1): 108-122.

Cook, D.B., P.J. O'Connor, S.E. Oliver, and Y. Lee. 1998. Sex differences in naturally occurring leg muscle pain and exertion during maximal cycle ergometry. *International Journal of Neuroscience* 95 (3-4): 183-202.

Cook, D.B., P.J. O'Connor, and C.A. Ray. 2000. Muscle pain perception and sympathetic nerve activity to exercise during opioid modulation. *American Journal of Physiology.* 279 (5): R1565-R1573.

Cook, D.B., A.J. Stegner, and L.D. Ellingson. 2010. Exercise alters pain sensitivity in Gulf War veterans with chronic musculoskeletal pain. *Journal of Pain* 11 (8): 764-772.

Coopersmith, S. 1967. *The antecedents of self-esteem.* San Francisco: Freeman.

Coopersmith, S. 1975. *Coopersmith Self-Esteem Inventory, technical manual.* Palo Alto, CA: Consulting Psychologists Press.

Costa, P.T., and R.R. McCrae. 1985. *The NEO Personality Inventory: Manual, Form S and Form R.* Odessa, FL: Psychological Assessment Resources.

Cotman, C.W., N.C. Berchtold, and L.A. Christie. 2007. Exercise builds brain health: Key roles of growth factor cascades and inflammation. *Trends in Neurosciences* 30 (9): 464-472.

Courneya, K.S. 2010. Efficacy, effectiveness, and behavior change trials in exercise research. *International Journal of Behavioral Nutrition and Physical Activity* 7: 81.

Courneya, K.S., and C.M. Friedenreich. 1999. Physical exercise and quality of life following cancer diagnosis: A literature review. *Annals of Behavioral Medicine* 21 (Spring): 171-179.

Courneya, K.S., and L.M. Hellsten. 1998. Personality correlates of exercise behavior, motives, barriers, and preferences: An application of the five-factor model. *Personality and Individual Differences* 24 (5): 625-633.

Courneya, K.S., and E. McAuley. 1995. Cognitive mediators of the social influence-exercise adherence relationship: A test of the Theory of Planned Behavior. *Journal of Behavioral Medicine* 18 (5): 499-515.

Cox, J.J., F. Reimann, A.K. Nicholas, et al. 2006. An SCN9A channelopathy causes congenital inability to experience pain. *Nature* 444 (7121): 894-898.

Cox, K.L., V. Burke, L.J. Beilin, and I.B. Puddey. 2010. A comparison of the effects of swimming and walking on body weight, fat distribution, lipids, glucose, and insulin in older women : The Sedentary Women Exercise Adherence Trial 2 (Report). *Metabolism* 59 (11): 1562-1573.

Crabbe, J.B., and R.K. Dishman. 2001. Exercise and brain electrocortical activity: A quantitative synthesis. *Medicine and Science in Sports and Exercise.* 32 (suppl. 5): S43, S38.

Crabbe, J.B., and R.K. Dishman. 2004. Brain electrocortical activity during and after exercise: A quantitative synthesis. *Psychophysiology* 41 (4): 563-574.

Crabbe, J.B., J.C. Smith, and R.K. Dishman. 2007. Emotional & electroencephalographic responses during affective picture viewing after exercise. *Physiology & Behavior* 90 (2-3): 394-404.

Craft, L.L., and D.M. Landers. 1998. The effect of exercise on clinical depression and depression resulting from mental illness: A meta-analysis. *Journal of Sport and Exercise Psychology* 20: 339-357.

Crapse, T.B., and M.A. Sommer. 2008. Corollary discharge across the animal kingdom. *Nature reviews. Neuroscience* 9 (8): 587-600.

Crespo, C.J., E. Smit, R.E. Andersen, O. Carter-Pokras, and B.E. Ainsworth. 2000. Race/ethnicity, social class and their relation to physical inactivity during leisure time: Results from the third National Health and Nutrition Examination Survey, 1988-1994. *American Journal of Preventive Medicine* 18 (1): 46-53.

Crews, D.J., and D.M. Landers. 1987. A meta-analytic review of aerobic fitness and reactivity to psychosocial stressors. *Medicine & Science in Sports & Exercise* 19 (Suppl. 5): S114-S120.

Crocker, P.R.E. 1997. A confirmatory factor analysis of the Positive Affect Negative Affect Schedule (PANAS) with a youth sport sample. *Journal of Sport & Exercise Psychology* 19 (1): 91-97.

Cronbach, L.J., and P.E. Meehl. 1955. Construct validity in psychological tests. *Psychological Bulletin* 52: 281-302.

Cuijpers, P., A. van Straten, P. van Oppen, and G. Andersson. 2008a. Are psychological and pharmacologic interventions equally effective in the treatment of adult depressive disorders? A meta-analysis of comparative studies. *Journal of Clinical Psychiatry* 69 (11): 1675-1685; quiz 1839-1841.

Cuijpers, P., A. Van Straten, L. Warmerdam, and N. Smits. 2008b. Characteristics of effective psychological treatments of depression: A metaregression analysis. *Psychotherapy Research* 18 (2): 225-236.

Cuthbert, B.N., M.M. Bradley, and P.J. Lang. 1996. Probing picture perception: Activation and emotion. *Psychophysiology* 33 (2): 103-111.

Cuthbert, B.N., H.T. Schupp, M. Bradley, M. McManis, and P.J. Lang. 1998. Probing affective pictures: Attended startle and tone probes. *Psychophysiology* 35 (May): 344-347.

Cutt, H., B. Giles-Corti, M. Knuiman, and V. Burke. 2007. Dog ownership, health and physical activity: A critical review of the literature. *Health & Place* 13 (1): 261-272.

Dalgas, U., E. Stenager, J. Jakobsen, et al. 2010. Fatigue, mood and quality of life improve in MS patients after progressive resistance training. *Multiple Sclerosis* 16 (4): 480-490.

Dallenbach, K.M. 1939. Pain: History and present status. *American Journal of Psychology* 52 (3): 331-347.

Daly, J., A.P. Sindone, D.R. Thompson, K. Hancock, E. Chang, and P. Davidson. 2002. Barriers to participation in and adherence to cardiac rehabilitation programs: A critical literature review. *Progress in Cardiovascular Nursing* 17 (1): 8-17.

Damasio, H., T. Grabowski, R. Frank, A.M. Galaburda, and A.R. Damasio. 1994. The return of Phineas Gage: Clues about the brain from the skull of a famous patient [published erratum appears in Science 1994 Aug 26; 265 (5176): 1159]. *Science* 264 (May 20): 1102-1105.

Danaher, B.G., and J.R. Seeley. 2009. Methodological issues in research on web-based behavioral interventions. *Annals of Behavioral Medicine* 38 (1): 28-39.

Darwin, C. 1872. *The expression of the emotions in man and animals*. London: Murray.

Davidson, R.J. 1992. Anterior cerebral asymmetry and the nature of emotion. *Brain and Cognition* 20: 125-151.

Davidson, R.J. 1998a. Affective style and affective disorders: Perspectives from affective neuroscience. *Cognition & Emotion* 12 (3): 307-330.

Davidson, R.J. 1998b. Anterior electrophysiological asymmetries, emotion, and depression: Conceptual and methodological conundrums. *Psychophysiology* 35 (5): 607-614.

Davidson, R.J. 2000. Cognitive neuroscience needs affective neuroscience (and vice versa). *Brain and Cognition*. 42 (1): 89-92. doi: 10.1006/brcg.1999.1170.

Davidson, R.J., P. Ekman, C.D. Saron, J.A. Senulius, and W.V. Friesen. 1990. Approach-withdrawal and cerebral asymmetry: Emotional expression and brain physiology I. *Journal of Personality and Social Psychology* 58: 330-341.

Davidson, R.J., and W. Irwin. 1999. The functional neuroanatomy of emotion and affective style. *Trends in Cognitive Sciences* 3 (1): 11-21.

Davis, C. 1997. Body image, exercise, and eating disorders. In *The physical self: From motivation to wellbeing*, edited by K.R. Fox. Champaign, IL: Human Kinetics.

Davis, C. 2000. Exercise abuse. *International Journal of Sport Psychology* 31: 278-289.

Davis, C., and K.R. Fox. 1993. Excessive exercise and weight preoccupation in women. *Addictive Behaviors* 18: 201-211.

Davis, C.L., P.D. Tomporowski, J.E. McDowell, et al. 2011. Exercise improves executive function and achievement and alters brain activation in overweight children: A randomized, controlled trial. *Health Psychology* 30 (1): 91-98.

Davis, H.P., M.R. Rosenzweig, L.A. Becker, and K.J. Sather. 1988. Biological psychology's relationships to psychology and neuroscience. *American Psychologist* 43: 359-371.

Davis, M. 1997. The neurophysiological basis of acoustic startle modulation: Research on fear motivation and sensory gating. In *Attention and orienting: Sensory and motivational processes*, edited by P.J. Lang, R.F. Simons, and M. Balaban. Mahwah, NJ: Erlbaum.

Davis, M., W.A. Falls, S. Campeau, and M. Kim. 1993. Fear-potentiated startle: A neural and pharmacological analysis. *Behavioural Brain Research* 58 (1-2): 175-198.

Dawson, D., Y.I. Noy, M. Harma, T. Akerstedt, and G. Belenky. 2011. Modelling fatigue and the use of fatigue models in work settings. *Accident: Analysis and Prevention* 43 (2): 549-564.

Day, H.E., B.N. Greenwood, S.E. Hammack, et al. 2004. Differential expression of 5HT-1A, alpha 1b adrenergic, CRF-R1, and CRF-R2 receptor mRNA in serotonergic, gamma-aminobutyric acidergic, and catecholaminergic cells of the rat dorsal raphe nucleus. *Journal of Comparative Neurology* 474 (3): 364-378.

De Bruijn, G.-J. 2011. Exercise habit strength, planning and the theory of planned behaviour: An action control approach. *Psychology of Sport and Exercise* 12 (2): 106-114.

de Jong, J., K.A. Lemmink, A.C. King, M. Huisman, and M. Stevens. 2006. Twelve-month effects of the Groningen active living model (GALM) on physical activity, health and fitness outcomes in sedentary and underactive older adults aged 55-65. *Patient Education and Counseling* 66 (2): 167-176.

De Moor, M.H., A.L. Beem, J.H. Stubbe, D.I. Boomsma, and E.J. De Geus. 2006. Regular exercise, anxiety, depression and personality: A population-based study. *Preventive Medicine* 42 (4): 273-279.

De Moor, M.H., D.I. Boomsma, J.H. Stubbe, G. Willemsen, and E.J. de Geus. 2008. Testing causality in the association between regular exercise and symptoms of anxiety and depression. *Archives of General Psychiatry* 65 (8): 897-905.

De Moor, M.H., Y.J. Liu, D.I. Boomsma, et al. 2009. Genome-wide association study of exercise behavior in Dutch and American adults. *Medicine & Science in Sports & Exercise* 41 (10): 1887-1895.

De Moor, M.H., G. Willemsen, I. Rebollo-Mesa, J.H. Stubbe, E.J. De Geus, and D.I. Boomsma. 2011. Exercise participation in adolescents and their parents: Evidence for genetic and generation specific environmental effects. *Behavior Genetics* 41 (2): 211-222.

de Morree, H.M., and S.M. Marcora. 2010. The face of effort: Frowning muscle activity reflects effort during a physical task. *Biological Psychology* 85 (3): 377-382.

de Morree, H.M., and S.M. Marcora. 2012. Frowning muscle activity and perception of effort during constant-workload cycling. *European Journal of Applied Physiology* 112(5), 1967-1972.

Deci, E.L., and R.M. Ryan. 1980. The empirical exploration of intrinsic motivational processes. In L. Berkowitz (Ed.), *Advances in experimental social psychology* (pp. 39-80). New York: Academic Press.

Deci, E.L., and R.M. Ryan. 1983. The basis of self-determination: Intrinsic motivation and integrated internalizations. *Academic Psychology Bulletin* 5 (1): 21-29.

Deci, E.L., and R.M. Ryan. 1985. The general causality orientations scale: Self-determination in personality. *Journal of Research in Personality* 19 (2): 109-134.

Deci, E.L., and R.M. Ryan. (1991). A motivational approach to self: Integration in personality. In R. Dienstbier (Ed.), *Nebraska symposium on motivation: Perspectives on motivation, 38* (pp. 237-288). Lincoln, NE: University Of Nebraska Press.

Deci, E.L., and R.M. Ryan. 1994. Promoting self-determined education. *Scandinavian Journal of Educational Research* 38 (1): 3-14.

Deci, E.L., and N.D. Ryan. 2008. Self-determination theory: A macrotheory of human motivation, development and health. *Canadian Psychology* 49 (3): 182-185.

Deeny, S.P., D. Poeppel, J.B. Zimmerman, et al. 2008a. Exercise, APOE, and working memory: MEG and behavioral evidence for benefit of exercise in epsilon4 carriers. *Biological Psychology* 78 (2): 179-187.

DeLuca, J. 2005. *Fatigue as a window to the brain.* Cambridge, MA: The MIT Press.

Demeersman, R.E. 1993. Heart rate variability and aerobic fitness. *American Heart Journal* 125: 726-731.

Demello, J.J., K.J. Cureton, R.E. Boineau, and M.M. Singh. 1987. Ratings of perceived exertion at the lactate threshold in trained and untrained men and women. *Medicine & Science in Sports & Exercise* 19 (Aug): 354-362.

Demyttenaere, K., J. De Fruyt, and S.M. Stahl. 2005. The many faces of fatigue in major depressive disorder. *International Journal of Neuropsychopharmacology* 8 (1): 93-105.

Derbyshire, S.W.G., M.G. Whalley, and D.A. Oakley. 2009. Fibromyalgia pain and its modulation by hypnotic and non-hypnotic suggestion: An fMRI analysis. *European Journal of Pain* 13 (5): 542-550.

Derbyshire, S.W.G., M.G. Whalley, V.A. Stenger, and D.A. Oakley. 2004. Cerebral activation during hypnotically induced and imagined pain. *NeuroImage* 23 (1): 392-401.

Desharnais, R., J. Jobin, C. Cote, L. Levesque, and G. Godin. 1993. Aerobic exercise and the placebo effect: A controlled study. *Psychosomatic Medicine* 55: 149-154.

Deslandes, A., H. Moraes, C. Ferreira, et al. 2009. Exercise and mental health: Many reasons to move. *Neuropsychobiology* 59: 191-198.

Detry, J.-M.R., A. Robert, R.J. Luwaert, et al. 1985. Diagnostic value of computerized exercise testing in men without previous myocardial infarction. A multivariate, compartmental and probabilistic approach. *European Heart Journal* 6 (3): 227-238.

Detterman, D.K. 1986. Human intelligence is a complex system of separate processes. In *What is intelligence? Contemporary viewpoints on its nature and definition*, edited by R.J. Sternberg and D.K. Detterman. Norwood, NJ: Ablex.

deVries, H.A., and G.M. Adams. 1972. Electromyographic comparisons of single doses of exercise and meprobamate as to effects on muscular relaxation. *American Journal of Physical Medicine* 51: 130-141.

deVries, H.A., C.P. Simard, R.A. Wiswell, E. Heckathorne, and V. Carabetta. 1982. Fusimotor system involvement in the tranquilizer effect of exercise. *American Journal of Physical Medicine* 61 (Jun): 111-122.

deVries, H.A., R.A. Wiswell, R. Bulbulian, and T. Moritani. 1981. Tranquilizer effect of exercise. Acute effects of moderate aerobic exercise on spinal reflex activation level. *American Journal of Physical Medicine* 60 (Apr): 57-66.

Diamond, A. 1991. Guidelines for the study of brain-behavior relationships during development. In *Frontal lobe function and dysfunction*, edited by H.M.E.H. S. Levin, and A.L. Benton. New York: Oxford University Press.

Diamond. A. 2006. Bootstrapping conceptual deduction using physical connection: Rethinking frontal cortex. *Trends in Cognitive Sciences* 10 (5): 212-218.

Diamond, A., and K. Lee. 2011. Interventions shown to aid executive function development in children 4 to 12 years old. *Science* 333 (6045): 959-964.

Dick, B.D., and S. Rashiq. 2007. Disruption of attention and working memory traces in individuals with chronic pain. *Anesthesia & Analgesia* 104 (5): 1223-1229.

Diehm, C., A. Schuster, J.R. Allenberg, et al. 2004. High prevalence of peripheral arterial disease and comorbidity in 6880 primary care patients: Cross-sectional study. *Atherosclerosis* 172 (1): 95-105.

Dietrich, A. 2003. Functional neuroanatomy of altered states of consciousness: The transient hypofrontality hypothesis. *Consciousness and Cognition* 12 (2): 231-256.

Dietrich, A. 2006. Transient hypofrontality as a mechanism for the psychological effects of exercise. *Psychiatry Research* 145 (1): 79-83.

Dietrich, A., and M. Audiffren. 2011. The reticular-activating hypofrontality (RAH) model of acute exercise. *Neuroscience and Biobehavioral Reviews* 35 (6): 1305-1325.

Dietrich, A., and W.F. McDaniel. 2004. Endocannabinoids and exercise. *British Journal of Sports Medicine* 38 (5): 536-541.

Dietz, W.H. 1996. The role of lifestyle in health: The epidemiology and consequences of inactivity. *Proceedings of the Nutrition Society* 55: 829-840.

Digman, J.M. 1990. Personality structure: Emergence of the five-factor model. *Annual Review of Psychology* 41 (1): 417-440.

DiLorenzo, T.M., E.P. Bargman, R. Stucky-Ropp, G.S. Brassington, P.A. Frensch, and T. LaFontaine. 1999. Long-term effects of aerobic exercise on psychological outcomes. *Preventive Medicine: An International Devoted to Practice & Theory* 28 (1): 75-85.

Dishman, R.K. 1982. Compliance/adherence in health-related exercise. *Health Psychology* 1 (3): 237-267.

Dishman, R.K. 1985. Medical Psychology in Exercise and Sport. *Medical Clinics of North America* 69, 1: 123-43.

Dishman, R.K. 1986. Exercise compliance: A new view for public health. *Physician and Sportsmedicine* 14 (5): 127-145.

Dishman, R.K. 1992. Physiological and psychological effects of overtraining. edited by K. Brownell, J. Rodin, and J. Wilmore. *Eating, body weight, and performance in athletes: Disorders of modern society.* Philadelphia: Lea & Febiger.

Dishman, R.K. 1994. Prescribing exercise intensity for healthy adults using perceived exertion. *Medicine & Science in Sports & Exercise* 26 (9): 1087-1094.

Dishman, R.K. 1997. Brain monoamines, exercise, and behavioral stress: Animal models. *Medicine & Science in Sports & Exercise* 29 (Jan): 63-74.

Dishman, R.K. 1998. Physical activity and mental health. In *Encyclopedia of mental health*, edited by H.S. Friedman. Vol. 3. San Diego: Academic Press.

Dishman, R.K. 2000. Introduction. *International Journal of Sports Medicine* 31: 103-109.

Dishman, R.K. 2008. Gene-physical activity interactions in the etiology of obesity: Behavioral considerations. *Obesity* 16 (Suppl. 3): S60-S65.

Dishman, R.K., H.R. Berthoud, F.W. Booth, et al. 2006. Neurobiology of exercise. *Obesity* 14 (3): 345-356.

Dishman, R.K., K. Brownell, and J. Rodin. 1992. Physiological and psychological effects of overtraining. In *Eating, body weight, and performance in athletes: Disorders of modern society.* Philadelphia: Lea & Febiger.

Dishman, R.K., and J. Buckworth. 1996a. Adherence to physical activity. In *Physical activity and mental health*, edited by W.P. Morgan. Washington, DC: Taylor & Francis.

Dishman, R.K., and J. Buckworth 1996b. Increasing physical activity: A quantitative synthesis. *Medicine & Science in Sports & Exercise* 28 (6): 706-719.

Dishman, R.K., D.M. DeJoy, M.G. Wilson, and R.J. Vandenberg. 2009. Move to Improve: a randomized workplace trial to increase physical activity. *American Journal of Preventive Medicine* 36 (2): 133-141.

Dishman, R.K., A.L. Dunn, S.D. Youngstedt, et al. 1996. Increased open field locomotion and decreased striatal GABAa binding after activity wheel running. *Physiology and Behavior* 60 (3): 699-705.

Dishman, R.K., R.P. Farquhar, and K.J. Cureton. 1994. Responses to preferred intensities of exertion in men differing in activity levels. *Medicine & Science in Sports & Exercise* 26 (Jun): 783-790.

Dishman, R.K., R.E. Graham, J. Buckworth, and J.E. White-Welkley. 2001. *Perceived exertion during incremental cycling is not influenced by the Type A Behavior Pattern.* I *International Journal of Sports Medicine.* 22 (Apr): 209-214.

Dishman, R.K., R.E. Graham, R.G. Holly, and J.G. Tieman. 1991. Estimates of Type A behavior do not predict perceived exertion during graded exercise. *Medicine & Science in Sports & Exercise* 23 (11): 1276-1282.

Dishman, R.K., D.P. Hales, M.J. Almeida, K.A. Pfeiffer, M. Dowda, and R.R. Pate. 2006. Factorial validity and invariance of the Physical Self-Description Questionnaire among black and white adolescent girls. *Ethnicity & Disease* 16 (2): 551-558.

Dishman, R.K., D.P. Hales, K.A. Pfeiffer, et al. 2006. Physical self-concept and self-esteem mediate cross-sectional relations of physical activity and sport participation with depression symptoms among adolescent girls. *Health Psychology* 25 (3): 396-407.

Dishman, R.K., and P.V. Holmes. 2012. Exercise and opioids: Animal models. In *Functional neuroimaging in exercise and sport sciences*, edited by H. Boecker, C.H. Hillman, L. Scheef, and H. Strüder. New York: Springer.

Dishman, R.K., S. Hong, J. Soares, et al. 2000. Activity-wheel running blunts suppression of splenic natural killer cell cytotoxicity after sympathectomy and footshock. *Physiology & Behavior* 71 (3-4): 297-304.

Dishman, R.K., and E.M. Jackson. 2000. Exercise, fitness, and stress. *International Journal of Sport Psychology* 31 (2): 175-203.

Dishman, R.K., E.M. Jackson, and Y. Nakamura. 2002. Influence of fitness and gender on blood pressure responses during active or passive stress. *Psychophysiology* 39 (5): 568-576.

Dishman, R.K., R.W. Motl, R. Saunders, et al. 2002. Factorial invariance and latent mean structure of questionnaires measuring social-cognitive determinants of physical activity among black and white adolescent girls. *Preventive Medicine.* 34 (1): 100-108.

Dishman, R.K., R.W. Motl, R. Saunders, et al. 2004. Self-efficacy partially mediates the effect of a school-based physical-activity intervention among adolescent girls. *Preventive Medicine* 38: 628-636.

Dishman, R.K., Y. Nakamura, M.E. Garcia, R.W. Thompson, A.L. Dunn, and S.N. Blair. 2000. Heart rate variability, trait anxiety, and perceived stress among physically fit men and women. *International Journal of Psychophysiology* 37 (Aug): 121-133.

Dishman, R.K., Y. Nakamura, E.M. Jackson, and C.A. Ray. 2003. Blood pressure and muscle sympathetic nerve activity during cold pressor stress: Fitness and gender. *Psychophysiology* 40 (3): 370-380.

Dishman, R.K., and P.J. O'Connor. 2009. Lessons in exercise neurobiology: The case of endorphins. *Mental Health and Physical Activity* 2 (1): 4-9.

Dishman, R.K., B. Oldenburg, H. O'Neal, and R. Shephard. 1998. Worksite physical activity interventions. *American Journal of Preventive Medicine* 15 (4): 344-361.

Dishman, R.K., R.W. Patton, J. Smith, R. Weinberg, and A. Jackson. 1987. Using perceived exertion to prescribe and monitor exercise training heart rate. *International Journal of Sports Medicine* 8 (June): 208-213.

Dishman, R.K., K.J. Renner, J.E. White-Welkley, K.A. Burke, and B.N. Bunnell. 2000. Treadmill exercise training augments brain norepinephrine response to familiar and novel stress. *Brain Research Bulletin.* 52 (5) : 337-42.

Dishman, R.K., K.J. Renner, S.D. Youngstedt, et al. 1997. Activity wheel running reduces escape latency and alters brain monoamine levels after footshock. *Brain Research Bulletin* 42: 399-406.

Dishman, R.K., J.F. Sallis, and D.R. Orenstein, 1985, The determinants of physical activity and exercise. *Public Health Reports* 100 (2): 161.

Dishman, R.K., X. Sui, T.S. Church, G.A. Hand, M.H. Trivedi, and S.N. Blair. 2012. Decline in cardiorespiratory fitness and odds of incident depression. *American Journal of Preventive Medicine.* October issue (number 10).

Dishman, R.K., X. Sui, T.S. Church, S.D. Youngstedt, and S.N. Blair. 2013. *Decline in cardiorespiratory fitness and increased incidence of sleep complaints.* Athens, GA: University of Georgia.

Dishman, R.K., N.J. Thom, T.W. Puetz, P.J. O'Connor, and B.A. Clementz. 2010. Effects of cycling exercise on vigor, fatigue, and electroencephalographic Activity among young adults who report persistent fatigue. *Psychophysiology* 47 (6): 1066-1074.

Dishman, R.K., N.J. Thom, C.R. Rooks, R.W. Motl, C. Horwath, and C.R. Nigg. 2009. Failure of post-action stages of the transtheoretical model to predict change in regular physical activity: A multiethnic cohort study. *Annals of Behavioral Medicine* 37 (3): 280-293.

Dishman, R.K., R.J. Vandenberg, R.W. Motl, and C.R. Nigg. 2010. Using constructs of the transtheoretical model to predict classes of change in regular physical activity: A multi-ethnic longitudinal cohort study. *Annals of Behavioral Medicine* 40 (2): 150-163.

Dishman, R.K., J.M. Warren, S. Hong, et al. 2000. Treadmill exercise training blunts suppression of splenic natural killer cell cytolysis after footshock. *Journal of Applied Physiology* 88 (6): 2176-2182.

Dishman, R.K., J.M. Warren, S.D. Youngstedt, et al. 1995. Activity-wheel running attenuates suppression of natural killer cell activity after footshock. *Journal of Applied Physiology* 78 (Apr): 1547-1554.

Dishman, R.K., R.A. Washburn, and D.A. Schoeller. 2001. Measurement of physical activity. *Quest* 53: 295-309.

Dittrich, S.M., V. Günther, G. Franz, M. Burtscher, B. Holzner, and M. Kopp. 2008. Aerobic exercise with relaxation: Influence on pain and psychological well-being in female migraine patients. *Clinical Journal of Sport Medicine* 18 (4): 363-365. doi: 10.1097/JSM.0b013e31817efac9.

Division of Labor Force Statistics. 2011. *College enrollment and work activity of 2010 high school graduates* [News release]. U.S. Department of Labor Statistics, April 08, 2011 [cited September 1, 2011]. www.bls.gov/news.release/hsgec.nr0.htm.

Donnelly, J.E., and K. Lambourne. 2011. Classroom-based physical activity, cognition, and academic achievement. *Preventive Medicine* 52: S36-S42.

Donta, S.T., D.J. Clauw, C.C. Engel, et al. and for the VA Cooperative Study #470 Study Group. 2003. Cognitive behavioral therapy and aerobic exercise for Gulf War veterans' illnesses. *Journal of the American Medical Association* 289 (11): 1396-1404.

Doyne, E.J., D.J. Ossip-Klein, E.D. Bowman, K.M. Osborn, I.B. McDougall-Wilson, and R.A. Neimeyer. 1987. Running versus weight lifting in the treatment of depression. *Journal of Consulting and Clinical Psychology* 555: 748-754.

Drevets, W.C. 1998. Functional neuroimaging studies of depression: The anatomy of melancholia. *Annual Review of Medicine* 49: 341-361.

Driver, S., and A. Ede. 2009. Impact of physical activity on mood after TBI. *Brain Injury* 23 (3): 203-212.

Driver, H.S., and S.R. Taylor. 2000. Exercise and sleep. *Sleep Medicine Reviews* 4: 387-402.

Dubreucq, S., M. Koehl, D.N. Abrous, G. Marsicano, and F. Chaouloff. 2010. CB1 receptor deficiency decreases wheel-running activity: Consequences on emotional behaviours and hippocampal neurogenesis. *Experimental Neurology* 224 (1): 106-113.

Duchateau, J., and R.M. Enoka. 2002. Neural adaptations with chronic activity patterns in able-bodied humans. *American Journal of Physical Medicine & Rehabilitation* 81 (11 Suppl.): S17-S27.

Duchenne, G.B. 1867. *Physiologie des mouvements démontrée à l'aide de l'expérimentation électrique et de l'observation clinique et applicable à l'étude des paralysies et des déformations [Physiology of movements demonstrated with electrical experimentation and with clinical observation and applied to the study of paralysis and deformations].* Paris: Baillère.

Duda, J.L., and J.G. Nicholls. 1992. Dimensions of achievement motivation in schoolwork and sport. *Journal of Educational Psychology* 84 (3): 290.

Dunbar, C.C., R.J. Robertson, R. Baun, et al. 1992. The validity of regulating exercise intensity by ratings of perceived exertion. *Medicine & Science in Sports & Exercise* 24 (Jan): 94-99.

Duncan, M., and K. Mummery. 2005. Psychosocial and environmental factors associated with physical activity among city dwellers in regional Queensland. *Preventive Medicine* 40 (4): 363-372.

Duncan, S.C., T.E. Duncan, L.A. Strycker, and N.R. Chaumeton. 2004. A multilevel approach to youth physical activity research. *Exercise and Sport Sciences Reviews* 32 (3): 95-99.

Duncan, T.E., S.C. Duncan, and E. McAuley. 1993. The role of domain and gender-specific provisions of social relations in adherence to a prescribed exercise regimen. *Journal of Sport and Exercise Psychology* 15 (2): 220-231.

Dunn, A.L. 2009. The effectiveness of lifestyle physical activity interventions to reduce cardiovascular disease. *American Journal of Lifestyle Medicine* 3 (1): 11S-18S.

Dunn, A.L., R.E. Andersen, and J.M. Jakicic. 1998. Lifestyle physical activity interventions. History, short- and long-term effects, and recommendations. *American Journal of Preventive Medicine* 15 (4): 398-412.

Dunn, A. L. and R. K. Dishman. 1991. Exercise and the neurobiology of depression. *Exercise and Sport Sciences Reviews* 19: 41-98.

Dunn, A.L., and J.S. Jewell. 2010. The effect of exercise on mental health. *Current Sports Medicine Reports* 9 (4): 202-207.

Dunn, A.L., B.H. Marcus, J.B. Kampert, M.E. Garcia, H.W. Kohl, and S.N. Blair. 1997. Reduction in cardiovascular disease risk factors: Six-month results from Project Active. *Preventive Medicine* 26 (6): 883-892.

Dunn, A.L., B.H. Marcus, J.B. Kampert, M.E. Garcia, H.W. Kohl, and S.N. Blair. 1999. Comparison of lifestyle and structured interventions to increase physical activity and cardiorespiratory fitness: A randomized trial. *Journal of the American Medical Association* 281 (4): 327-334.

Dunn, A.L., T.G. Reigle, S.D. Youngstedt, R.B. Armstrong, and R.K. Dishman. 1996. Brain norepinephrine and metabolites after treadmill training and wheel running in rats. *Medicine and Science in Sports and Exercise.* 28 (2): 204-209.

Dunn, A.L., M.H. Trivedi, J.B. Kampert, C.G. Clark, and H.O. Chambliss. 2005. Exercise treatment for depression: Efficacy and dose response. *American Journal of Preventive Medicine* 28 (1): 1-8.

Dupont, R.L., D.P. Rice, L.S. Miller, S.S. Shiraki, C.R. Rowland, and H.J. Harwood. 1996. Economic cost of anxiety disorders. *Anxiety* 2: 167-172.

Durante, R., and B.E. Ainsworth. 1996. The recall of physical activity: Using a cognitive model of the question-answering process. *Medicine & Science in Sports & Exercise* 28 (10): 1282-1291.

Dustman, R.E., R. Emmerson, and D. Shearer. 1994. Physical activity, age, and cognitive-neuropsychological function. *Journal of Aging and Physical Activity* 2: 143-181.

Dworkin, R.H., M. Backonja, M.C. Rowbotham, et al. 2003. Advances in neuropathic pain: Diagnosis, mechanisms, and treatment recommendations. *Archives of Neurology* 60 (11): 1524-1534.

Dykens, E.M., and D.J. Cohen. Effects of Special Olympics International on Social Competence in Persons with Mental Retardation. *Journal of the American Academy of Child and Adolescent Psychiatry* 35, 2 (Feb 1996): 223-229.

Dzewaltowski, D.A. 1994. Physical activity determinants: A social cognitive approach. *Medicine and Science in Sports and Exercise.* 26 (11): 1395-1399.

Eakin, E.G., S.P. Lawler, C. Vandelanotte, and N. Owen. 2007. Telephone interventions for physical activity and dietary behavior change: A systematic review. *American Journal of Preventive Medicine* 32 (5): 419-434.

Edmunds, J., N. Ntoumanis, and J.L. Duda. 2006. Examining exercise dependence symptomatology from a self-determination perspective. *Journal of Health Psychology* 11 (6): 887-903.

Eggermont, L., D. Swaab, P. Luiten, and E. Scherder. 2006. Exercise, cognition and Alzheimer's disease: More is not necessarily better. *Neuroscience and Biobehavioral Reviews* 30: 562-575.

Einerson, J., A. Ward, and P. Hanson. 1988. Exercise responses in females with anorexia nervosa. *International Journal of Eating Disorders* 7: 253-260.

Ekblom, B., and A.N. Goldbarg. 1971. The influence of physical training and other factors on the subjective rating of perceived exertion. *Acta Physiologica Scandinavica* 83: 399-406.

Ekeland, E., F. Heian, K.B. Hagen, J. Abbott, and L. Nordheim. 2004. Exercise to improve self-esteem in children and young people. *Cochrane Database of Systematic Reviews.* 1: CD003683.

Ekkekakis, P., E.E. Hall, and S.J. Petruzzello. 2008. The relationship between exercise intensity and affective responses demystified: To crack the 40-year-old nut, replace the 40-year-old nutcracker! *Annals of Behavioral Medicine* 35 (2): 136-149.

Ekkekakis, P., G. Parfitt, and S.J. Petruzzello. 2011. The pleasure and displeasure people feel when they exercise at different intensities: Decennial update and progress towards a tripartite rationale for exercise intensity prescription. *Sports Medicine* 41 (8): 641-671.

Ekkekakis, P., and S.J. Petruzzello. 1999. Acute aerobic exercise and affect: Current status, problems and prospects regarding dose-response. *Sports Medicine* 28 (Nov): 337-374.

Ekkekakis, P., and S.J. Petruzzello. 2000. Analysis of the affect measurement conundrum in exercise psychology. *Psychology of Sport and Exercise* 1: 71-88.

Ekkekakis, P., and S.J. Petruzzello. 2001a. Analysis of the affect measurement conundrum in exercise psychology: II. A conceptual and methodological critique of the Exercise-induced Feeling Inventory. *Psychology of Sport and Exercise* 2 (1): 1-26.

Ekkekakis, P., and S.J. Petruzzello. 2001b. Analysis of the affect measurement conundrum in exercise psychology. III. A conceptual and methodological critique of the Subjective Exercise Experiences Scale. *Psychology of Sport and Exercise* 2 (4): 205-232.

Ekkekakis, P., and S.J. Petruzzello. 2002. Analysis of the affect measurement conundrum in exercise psychology: IV. A conceptual case for the affect circumplex. *Psychology of Sport and Exercise* 3 (1): 35-63.

Ekman, P. 1989. The argument and evidence about universals in facial expressions of emotions. In *Handbook of psychophysiology: The biological psychology of emotions and social processes*, edited by H. Wagner and A. Manstead. London: Wiley.

Ekman, P. 1992. Are there basic emotions? *Psychological Review.* 99 (3): 550-3.

Ekman, P. 1994. Moods, emotions, and traits. In *The nature of emotion: Fundamental questions,* edited by P. Ekman and R.J. Davidson. New York: Oxford University Press.

Ekman, P., R.J. Davidson, and W.V. Friesen. 1990. The Duchenne smile: Emotional expression and brain physiology II. *Journal of Personality and Social Psychology* 582: 342-353.

Ekman, P., and W.V. Friesen. 1971. Constants across cultures in the face and emotion. *Journal of Personality & Social Psychology* 17: 124-129.

Ekman, P., and W.V. Friesen. 1976. Measuring facial movement. *Journal of Environmental Psychology and Nonverbal Behavior* 11: 56-75.

Ekman, P., W.V. Friesen, and P. Ellsworth. 1972 *Emotion in the human face: Guidelines for research and an integration of findings.* New York: Pergamon Press.

Elavsky, S. 2010. Longitudinal examination of the exercise and self-esteem model in middle-aged women. *Journal of Sport & Exercise Psychology* 32: 862-880.

Elavsky, S., and E. McAuley. 2007. Lack of perceived sleep improvement after 4-month structured exercise programs. *Menopause* 14 (3 Pt 1): 535-540.

Elias, M.F., and A.L. Goodell. 2010. Diet and exercise: Blood pressure and cognition. *Hypertension* 55 (6): 1296-1298.

Ellis, A. 1957. Rational psychotherapy and individual psychology. *Journal of Individual Psychology* 13: 38-44.

Ellis, A. 2003. Early theories and practices of rational emotive behavior therapy and how they have been augmented and revised during the last three decades. *Journal of Rational-Emotive & Cognitive-Behavior Therapy* 21 (3): 219-243.

Ellis, A. 2003. Early theories and practices of rational emotive behavior therapy and how they have been augmented and revised during the last three decades. *Journal of Rational-Emotive & Cognitive-Behavior Therapy,* 21(3-4) , page 236-237

Emery, C.F. 1994. Effects of age on physiological and psychological functioning among COPD patients in an exercise program. *Journal of Aging and Health* 6: 3-16.

Emery, C.F. 2008. Exercise, chronic obstructive pulmonary disease and cognition. In *Exercise and its mediating effects on cognition*, edited by W.W. Spirduso, L.W. Poon, and W.J. Chodzko-Kajko. Champaign, IL: Human Kinetics.

Emery, C.F., V.J. Honn, D.J. Frid, K.R. Lebowitz, and P.T. Diaz. 2001. Acute effects of exercise on cognition in patients with chronic obstructive pulmonary disease. *American Journal of Respiratory and Critical Care Medicine* 164: 1624-1627.

Emery, C.F., N.E. Leatherman, E.J. Burker, and N.R. MacIntyre. 1991. Psychological outcomes of a pulmonary rehabilitation program. *Chest* 100: 613-617.

Emery, C.F., R.L. Schein, E.R. Hauck, and N.R. MacIntyre. 1998. Psychological and cognitive outcomes of a randomized trial of exercise among patients with chronic obstructive pulmonary disease. *Health Psychology* 17 (3): 232-240.

Emery, C.F., R.L. Shermer, E.R. Hauck, E.T. Hsiao, and N.R. MacIntyre. 2003. Cognitive and psychological outcomes of exercise in a 1-year follow-up study of patients with chronic obstructive pulmonary disease. *Health Psychology* 22 (6): 598-604.

Engel, G.L. 1977. The need for a new medical model: A challenge for biomedicine. *Science* 196 (4286): 129-136.

Englund, C.E., D.H. Ryman, P. Naitoh, and J.A. Hodgdon. 1985. Cognitive performance during successive sustained physical work episodes. *Behavior Research Methods, Instruments, & Computers* 17: 75-85.

Epping, J.N. 2011. Dog ownership and dog walking to promote physical activity and health in patients. *Current Sports Medicine Reports* 10 (4): 224.

Epstein, L.H. 1998. Integrating theoretical approaches to promote physical activity. *American Journal of Preventive Medicine* 15 (4): 257-265.

Epstein, L.H., B.E. Saelens, M.D. Myers, and D. Vito. 1997. Effects of decreasing sedentary behaviors on activity choice in obese children. *Health Psychology* 16: 107-113.

Epstein, L.J., and P.S. Valentine. 2010. Starting a sleep center. *Chest* 137 (5): 1217-1224.

Erickson, K.I., S.J. Colcombe, S. Elavsky, et al. 2007. Interactive effects of fitness and hormone treatment on brain health in postmenopausal women. *Neurobiology of Aging* 28 (2): 179-185.

Erickson, K.I., and A.F. Kramer. 2009. Aerobic exercise effects on cognitive and neural plasticity in older adults. *British Journal of Sports Medicine* 43 (1): 22-24.

Ernst, E., J.I. Rand, and C. Stevinson. 1998. Complementary therapies for depression: an overview. *Archives Of General Psychiatry* 55 (Nov): 1026-1032.

Espiritu, R.C., D.F. Kripke, S. Ancoli-Israel, et al. 1994. Low illumination by San Diego adults: Association with atypical depressive symptoms. *Biological Psychiatry* 35: 403-407.

Estabrooks, P.A. 2000. Sustaining exercise participation through group cohesion. *Exercise and Sport Sciences Reviews* 28 (Apr): 63-67.

Etnier, J.L., and M. Berry. 2001. Fluid intelligence in an older COPD sample after short- or long-term exercise. *Medicine & Science in Sport and Exercise* 33: 1620-1628.

Etnier, J.L., R. Johnston, D. Dagenbach, R.J. Pollard, W.J. Rejeski, and M. Berry. 1999. The relationships among pulmonary function, aerobic fitness, and cognitive functioning in older COPD patients. *Chest* 116: 953-960.

Etnier, J.L., K.S. Matt, D.M. Landers, and S.M. Arent. 2005. Dose-response and mechanistic issues in the resistance training and affect relationship. *Journal of Sport and Exercise Psychology* 27 (1): 92-110.

Etnier, J.L., P.M. Nowell, D.M. Landers, and B.A. Sibley. 2006. A meta-regression to examine the relationship between aerobic fitness and cognitive performance. *Brain Research Reviews* 52: 119-130.

Etnier, J.L., W. Salazar, D.M. Landers, S.J. Petruzzello, M. Han, and P. Nowell. 1997. The influence of physical fitness and exercise upon cognitive functioning: A meta-analysis. *Journal of Sport and Exercise Psychology* 19: 249-277.

Evans, C.J. 1988. The opioid peptides. In *The opiate receptors*, edited by G.W. Pasternak. New York: Humana Press.

Eyler, A.A., R.C. Brownson, S.J. Bacak, and R.A. Housemann. 2003. The epidemiology of walking for physical activity in the United States. *Medicine & Science in Sports & Exercise* 35 (9): 1529-1536.

Eysenck, H.J. 1990. Biological dimensions of personality. In *Handbook of personality: Theory and research*, edited by L.A. Pervin. New York: Guilford Press.

Faigenbaum, A., L.D. Zaichkowsky, W.L. Wescott, et al. 1997. Psychological effects of strength training on children. *Journal of Sport Behavior* 20 (2): 164-175.

Farmer, M.E., B.Z. Locke, E.K. Moscicki, A.L. Dannenberg, D.B. Larson, and L.S. Radloff 1988. Physical activity and depressive symptoms: The NHANES I epidemiologic follow-up study. *American Journal of Epidemiology* 128: 1340-1351.

Faulkner, G.E.J., and A.H. Taylor. 2005. *Exercise, health and mental health: Emerging relationships.* New York: Routledge.

Fechner, G. 1966. *Elements of psychophysics* (Trans. Helmut Adler). New York: Holt, Rinehart & Winston. (Original work published 1860).

Felson, D.T., J. Niu, M. Clancy, B. Sack, P. Aliabadi, and Y. Zhang. 2007. Effect of recreational physical activities on the development of knee osteoarthritis in older adults of different weights: The Framingham Study. *Arthritis Care & Research* 57 (1): 6-12.

Fernandez de Molina, A. and R.W. Hunsperger 1962. Organization of the subcortical system governing defense and flight reactions in the cat. *Journal of Physiology*, 160(2): 200-213.

Ferrari, M., L. Mottola, and V. Quaresima. 2004. Principles, techniques, and limitations of near infrared spectroscopy. *Canadian Journal of Applied Physiology [Revue Canadienne de Physiologie Appliquee]* 29 (4): 463-487.

Ferreira, I., K. van der Horst, W. Wendel-Vos, S. Kremers, F.J. van Lenthe, and J. Brug. 2007. Environmental correlates of physical activity in youth: A review and update. *Obesity Reviews* 8 (2): 129-154.

Ferrier, S., C.M. Blanchard, M. Vallis, and N. Giacomantonio. 2011. Behavioural interventions to increase the physical activity of cardiac patients: A review. *European Journal of Cardiovascular Prevention and Rehabilitation* 18 (1): 15-32.

Fichna, J., A. Janecka, J. Costentin, and J.C. Do Rego. 2007. The endomorphin system and its evolving neurophysiological role. *Pharmacological Reviews* 59 (1): 88-123.

Fillingim, R.B., D.L. Roth, and E.W. Cook. 1992. The effects of aerobic exercise on cardiovascular, facial EMG, and self-report responses to emotional imagery. *Psychosomatic Medicine* 54 (1): 109-120.

Finch, C., and E. Cassell. 2006. The public health impact of injury during sport and active recreation. *Journal of Science and Medicine in Sport* 9 (6): 490-497.

Finucane, M. M., Stevens, G. A., Cowan, M. J., Danaei, G., Lin, J. K., Paciorek, C. J., et al. (2011). National, regional, and global trends in body-mass index since 1980: Systematic analysis of health examination surveys and epidemiological studies with 960 country-years and 9.1 million participants. *The Lancet.* doi: 10.1016/S0140-6736(10)62037-5.

Fishbein, M. 2008. A reasoned action approach to health promotion. *Medical Decision Making* 28 (6): 834-844.

Fitts, W.H. 1965. *Tennessee Self-Concept Scale: Manual*. Los Angeles: Western Psychological Services.

Flagel, S.B., J.J. Clark, T.E. Robinson, et al. 2011. A selective role for dopamine in stimulus-reward learning. *Nature* 469 (7328): 53-57.

Flavell, J.H. 1979. Metacognition and cognitive monitoring: A new area of cognitive-developmental inquiry. *American Psychologist* 34: 906-911.

Fleming, J.S., and B.E. Courtney. 1984. The dimensionality of self-esteem: II. Hierarchical facet model for revised measurement scales. *Journal of Personality & Social Psychology* 46 (2): 404-421.

Fleming, J.S., and W.A. Watts. 1980. The dimensionality of self-esteem: Some results of a college sample. *Journal of Personality & Social Psychology* 39 (5): 921-929.

Flemons, W.W., N.J. Douglas, S.T. Kuna, D.O. Rodenstein, and J. Wheatley. 2004. Access to diagnosis and treatment of patients with suspected sleep apnea. *American Journal of Respiratory and Critical Care Medicine* 169 (6): 668-672.

Fleury, J., and S.M. Lee. 2006. The social ecological model and physical activity in African American women. *American Journal of Community Psychology* 37 (1-2): 129-140.

Flor, H., D.C. Turk, and B.O. Scholz. 1987. Impact of chronic pain on the spouse: Marital, emotional and physical consequences. *Journal of Psychosomatic Research* 31 (1): 63-71.

Flora, J.A., E.W. Maibach, and N. Maccoby. 1989. The role of media across four levels of health promotion intervention. *Annual Review of Public Health* 10: 181-201.

Focht, B.C., and K.F. Koltyn. 1999. Influences of resistance exercise of different intensities on state anxiety and blood pressure. *Medicine & Science in Sports & Exercise* 31 (3): 456-463.

Folkins, C.H., and W.E. Sime. 1981. Physical fitness training and mental health. *American Psychologist*. 36 (4): 373-389.

Foley, T.E., B.N. Greenwood, H.E. Day, L.G. Koch, S.L. Britton, and M. Fleshner. 2006. Elevated central monoamine receptor mRNA in rats bred for high endurance capacity: Implications for central fatigue. *Behavioural Brain Research* 174 (1): 132-142.

Folkman, S., and R.S. Lazarus. 1988. *Manual for the ways of coping questionnaire*. Palo Alto, CA: Consulting Psychologists Press.

Folkman, S., and J.T. Moskowitz. 2004. Coping: Pitfalls and promise. *Annual Review of Psychology* 55: 745-774.

Forcier, K., L.R. Stroud, G.D. Papandonatos, et al. 2006. Links between physical fitness and cardiovascular reactivity and recovery to psychological stressors: A meta-analysis. *Health Psychology* 25 (6): 723-739.

Ford, D.H., and H.B. Urban. 1998. *Contemporary models of psychotherapy: A comparative analysis*. New York: Wiley.

Fordyce, D.E., and R.P. Farrar. 1991a. Enhancement of spatial learning in F344 rats by physical activity and related learning-associated alterations in hippocampal and cortical cholinergic functioning. *Behavioural Brain Research* 46 (2): 123-133.

Fordyce, D.E., and R.P. Farrar. 1991b. Physical activity effects on hippocampal and parietal cortical cholinergic function and spatial learning in F344 rats. *Behavioural Brain Research* 43 (2): 115-123.

Fordyce, D.E., and J.M. Wehner. 1993. Physical activity enhances spatial learning performance with an associated alteration in hippocampal protein kinase C activity in C57BL/6 and DBA/2 mice. *Brain Research*. 619(1-2): 111-119.

Fox, J.H., S.E. Hammack, and W.A. Falls. 2008. Exercise is associated with reduction in the anxiogenic effect of mCPP on acoustic startle. *Behavioral Neuroscience* 122 (4): 943-948.

Fox, K.R. 1990. *The Physical Self Perception Profile manual*. DeKalb, IL: Office for Health Promotion, Northern Illinois University.

Fox, K.R. 1997. The physical self and processes in self-esteem development. In *The physical self: From motivation to well-being*, edited by K.R. Fox. Champaign, IL: Human Kinetics.

Fox, K.R. 1997. *The physical self: From motivation to well-being*. Champaign, IL: Human Kinetics.

Fox, K.R. 1998. Advances in the measurement of the physical self. In *Advances in sport and exercise psychology measurement*, edited by J.L. Duda. Morgantown, WV: Fitness Information Technology.

Fox, K.R. 2000. Self-esteem, self-perceptions and exercise. *International Journal of Sport Psychology* 31 (2): 228-240.

Fox, K.R., and C.B. Corbin. 1989. The Physical Self-Perception Profile: Development and preliminary validation. *Journal of Sport & Exercise Psychology* 11 (4): 408-430.

Frankenhaeuser, M. 1971. Behavior and circulating catecholamines. *Brain Research* 31 (Aug 20): 241-262.

Franklin, B.A. 1988. Program factors that influence exercise adherence: Practical adherence skills for the clinical staff. In *Exercise adherence*, edited by R.K. Dishman. Champaign, IL: Human Kinetics.

Fransen, M., S. McConnell, and M. Bell. 2002. Therapeutic exercise for people with osteoarthritis of the hip or knee. A systematic review. *Journal of Rheumatology* 29 (8): 1737-1745.

Fransen, M., S. McConnell, G. Hernandez-Molina, and S. Reichenbach. 2010. Does land-based exercise reduce pain and disability associated with hip osteoarthritis? A meta-analysis of randomized controlled trials. *Osteoarthritis and Cartilage* 18 (5): 613-620.

Franz, S.I., and G.V. Hamilton. 1905. The effects of exercise upon the retardation in conditions of depression. *American Journal of Insanity* 62: 239-256.

Franzoi, S.L., and S.A. Shields. 1984. The Body Esteem Scale: Multidimensional structure and sex differences in a college population. *Journal of Personality Assessment* 48 (2): 173-178.

Freburger, J.K., G.M. Holmes, R.P. Agans, et al. 2009. The rising prevalence of chronic low back pain. *Archives of Internal Medicine* 169 (3): 251-258.

Frederick, C.M., and R.M. Ryan. 1995. Self-determination in sport: A review using cognitive evaluation theory. *International Journal of Sport Psychology* 26: 5-23.

Freedson, P., H.R. Bowles, R. Troiano, and W. Haskell. 2012. Assessment of physical activity using wearable monitors: Recommendations for monitor calibration and use in the field. *Medicine & Science in Sports & Exercise* 44 (1 Suppl. 1):S1-S4. doi: 10.1249/MSS.0b013e3182399b7e.

Freeman, M.P., M. Fava, J. Lake, M.H. Trivedi, K.L. Wisner, and D. Mischoulon. 2010. Complementary and alternative medicine in major depressive disorder: The American Psychiatric Association Task Force report. *Journal of Clinical Psychiatry* 71 (6): 669-681.

Fremont, J., and L.W. Craighead. 1987. Aerobic exercise and cognitive therapy in the treatment of dysphoric moods. *Cognitive Therapy and Research* 112: 241-251.

Freud, S. 1959. *The justification from neurasthenia of a particular syndrome: The anxiety neurosis.* Vol. 1, *Collected Papers.* New York: Basic Books.

Fridlund, A.J., and J.T. Cacioppo. 1986. Guidelines for human electromyographic research. *Psychophysiology* 23: 567-589.

Friedman, H.S., and S. Booth-Kewley. 1987. The "disease-prone personality". A meta-analytic view of the construct. *American Psychologist.* 42 (6): 539-55.

Frijda, N.H. 1986. *The emotions.* New York: Cambridge University Press.

Frith, C.D., S.J. Blakemore, and D.M. Wolpert. 2000. Abnormalities in the awareness and control of action. *Philosophical Transactions of the Royal Society of London. Series B, Biological Sciences* 355 (1404): 1771-1788.

Frost, H., S.E. Lamb, and S. Robertson. 2002. A randomized controlled trial of exercise to improve mobility and function after elective knee arthroplasty. Feasibility, results and methodological difficulties. *Clinical Rehabilitation* 16 (2): 200-209.

Frost, S.S., R.T. Goins, R.H. Hunter, et al. 2010. Effects of the built environment on physical activity of adults living in rural settings. *American Journal of Health Promotion* 24 (4): 267-283.

Fullerton, G.S., and J.M. Cattell. 1892. *On the perception of small differences.* Philadelphia: University of Pennsylvania Press.

Fuss, J., and P. Gass. 2010. Endocannabinoids and voluntary activity in mice: Runner's high and long-term consequences in emotional behaviors. *Experimental neurology* 224 (1): 103-105.

Galea, M.N., and S.R. Bray. 2007. Determinants of walking exercise among individuals with intermittent claudication: Does pain play a role? *Journal of Cardiopulmonary Rehabilitation and Prevention* 27 (2):107-113. doi: 10.1097/01.HCR.0000265045.36725.97.

Gandevia, S.C. 1982. The perception of motor commands on effort during muscular paralysis. *Brain* 105: 151-159.

Gandevia, S.C. 1996. Kinesthesia: Roles for afferent signals and motor commands In *Handbook of physiology: Sec. 12. Exercise: Regulation and integration of multiple systems,* edited by L.B. Rowell and J.T. Shepherd. New York: Oxford University Press.

Gandevia S.C. 2001. Spinal and supraspinal factors in human muscle fatigue. *Physiological Reviews.* 81(4): 1725-1789.

Gandevia, S.C., K. Killian, D.K. McKenzie, et al. 1993. Respiratory sensations, cardiovascular control, kinaesthesia and transcranial stimulation during paralysis in humans. *Journal of Physiology* 470: 85-107.

Ganio, M.S., L.E. Armstrong, E.C. Johnson, et al. 2010. Effect of quercetin supplementation on maximal oxygen uptake in men and women. *Journal of Sports Sciences* 28 (2): 201-208.

Garavan, H., J.C. Pendergrass, T.J. Ross, E.A. Stein, and R.C. Risinger. 2001. Amygdala response to both positively and negatively valenced stimuli. *Neuroreport* 12 (12): 2779-2783.

Garcia, A.W., and A.C. King. 1991. Predicting long-term adherence to aerobic exercise: A comparison of two models. *Journal of Sport and Exercise Psychology* 13: 394-410.

Gardner, A.W., P.S. Montgomery, R.M. Ritti-dias, and U. Thadani. 2011. Exercise performance, physical activity, and health-related quality of life in participants with stable angina. *Angiology* 62 (6): 461-466.

Garland, T., S.A. Kelly, J.L. Malisch, et al. 2011. How to run far: Multiple solutions and sex-specific responses to selective breeding for high voluntary activity levels. *Proceedings of the Royal Society B: Biological Sciences* 278 (1705): 574-581.

Garvin, A.W., K.F. Koltyn, and W.P. Morgan. 1997. Influence of acute physical activity and relaxation on state anxiety and blood lactate in untrained college males. *International Journal of Sports Medicine* 18 (Aug): 470-476.

Gary, R., and S.Y. Lee. 2007. Physical function and quality of life in older women with diastolic heart failure: Effects of a progressive walking program on sleep patterns. *Progress in Cardiovascular Nursing* 22 (2): 72-80.

Gatchel, R.J., and A. Okifuji. 2006. Evidence-based scientific data documenting the treatment and cost-effectiveness of comprehensive pain programs for chronic nonmalignant pain. *Journal of Pain* 7 (11): 779-793.

Gauvin, L. and W.J. Rejeski. 1993. The exercise-induced feeling inventory: Development and initial validation. *Journal of Sport & Exercise Psychology* 15 (4): 403-423.

Gauvin, L., W.J. Rejeski, and B.A. Reboussin. 2000. Contributions of acute bouts of vigorous physical activity to explaining diurnal variations in feeling states in active, middle-aged women. *Health Psychology* 19 (4): 365-375.

Gauvin, L., and J.C. Spence. 1998. Measurement of exercise-induced changes in feeling states, affect, mood, and emotions. In *Advances in sport and exercise psychology measurement*, edited by J.L. Duda. Morgantown, WV: Fitness Information Technology.

Gaynes, B.N., D. Warden, M.H. Trivedi, S.R. Wisniewski, M. Fava, and A.J. Rush. 2009. What did STAR*D teach us? Results from a large-scale, practical, clinical trial for patients with depression. *Psychiatric Services* 60 (11): 1439-1445.

Geisser, M.E., W. Wang, M. Smuck, L.G. Koch, S.L. Britton, and R. Lydic. 2008. Nociception before and after exercise in rats bred for high and low aerobic capacity. *Neuroscience Letters* 443 (1): 37-40.

Gelenberg, A.J., M.P. Freeman, J.C. Markowitz, et al. 2010. *Practice guidelines for the treatment of patients with major depressive disorder.* 3rd edition. American Psychiatric Association, 1-152, doi: 10.1176/appi.books.9780890423387.654001.

Genova, H.M., G.R. Wylie, and J. DeLuca. 2011. Neuroimaging of fatigue. In *Brain imaging in behavioral medicine and clinical neuroscience*, edited by R.A. Cohen and L.H. Sweet. New York: Springer.

Georges, F., and G. Aston-Jones. 2001. Potent regulation of midbrain dopamine neurons by the bed nucleus of the stria terminalis. *Journal of Neuroscience* 21 (16): RC160.

Gerhard, T., B. Chavez, M. Olfson, and S. Crystal. 2009. National patterns in the outpatient pharmacological management of children and adolescents with autism spectrum disorder. *Journal of Clinical Psychopharmacology* 29 (3): 307-310.

Gibbons, R.J., K. Chatterjee, J. Daley et al. 1999. ACC/AHA/ACP-ASIM guidelines for the management of patients with chronic stable angina: A report of the American College of Cardiology/American Heart Association Task Force on Practice Guidelines (Committee on Management of Patients With Chronic Stable Angina). *Journal of the American College of Cardiology* 33 (7): 2092-2197.

Gillison, F.B., S.M. Skevington, A. Sato, M. Standage, and S. Evangelidou. 2009. The effects of exercise interventions on quality of life in clinical and healthy populations: A meta-analysis. *Social Science & Medicine* 68 (9): 1700-1710.

Ginsberg, H.N., and S.C. Woods. 2009. The endocannabinoid system: Potential for reducing cardiometabolic risk. *Obesity* 17 (10): 1821-1829.

Godbey, G.C., L.L. Caldwell, M. Floyd, and L.L. Payne. 2005. Contributions of leisure studies and recreation and park management research to the active living agenda. *American Journal of Preventive Medicine* 28 (2 Suppl. 2): 150-158.

Goddard, A.W., and D.S. Charney. 1997. Toward an integrated neurobiology of panic disorder. *Journal of Clinical Psychiatry* 58 (Suppl. 2): 4-11.

Goddard, A.W., and D.S. Charney. 1998. SSRIs in the treatment of panic disorder. *Depression and Anxiety* 8 (Suppl. 1): 114-120.

Godin, G. 1994. Social-cognitive models. In *Advances in exercise adherence*, edited by R.K. Dishman. 2nd ed. Champaign, IL: Human Kinetics.

Gold, P.W., and G.P. Chrousos. 1999. The endocrinology of melancholic and atypical depression: Relation to neurocircuitry and somatic consequences. *Proceedings of the Association of American Physicians* 111 (1): 22-34.

Goldberg, G., N.H. Mayer, and J.U. Toglia. 1981. Medial frontal cortex infarction and the alien hand sign. *Archives of Neurology* 38 (11): 683-686.

Goldberg, L.R. 1981. Language and individual differences: The search for universals in personality lexicons. In *Review of personality and social psychology*, edited by L. Wheeler. Beverly Hills, CA: Sage.

Golden, R.N., B.N. Gaynes, R.D. Ekstrom, et al. 2005. The efficacy of light therapy in the treatment of mood disorders: A review and meta-analysis of the evidence. *American Journal of Psychiatry* 162 (4): 656-662.

Goldfarb, A.H., and A.Z. Jamurtas. 1997. Beta-endorphin response to exercise. An update. *Sports Medicine* 24: 8-16.

Goldfield, G.S., R. Mallory, T. Parker, et al. 2007. Effects of modifying physical activity and sedentary behavior on psychosocial adjustment in overweight/obese children. *Journal of Pediatric Psychology* 32 (7): 783-793.

Gomez, L.F., J.C. Mateus, and G. Cabrera. 2004. Leisure-time physical activity among women in a neighbourhood in Bogota, Colombia: Prevalence and socio-demographic correlates. *Cadernos de Saude Publica/Ministerio da Saude, Fundacao Oswaldo Cruz, Escola Nacional de Saude Publica* 20 (4): 1103-1109.

Gomez-Pinilla, F., S. Vaynman, and Z. Ying. 2008. Brain-derived neurotrophic factor functions as a metabotrophin to mediate the effects of exercise on cognition. *European Journal of Neuroscience* 28 (11): 2278-2287.

Gomez-Pinilla, F., Z. Ying, P. Opazo, R.R. Roy, and V.R. Edgerton. 2001. Differential regulation by exercise of BDNF and NT-3 in rat spinal cord and skeletal muscle. *European Journal of Neuroscience* 13 (6): 1078-1084.

Goode, K.T., and D.L. Roth. 1993. Factor analysis of cognitions during running: Association with mood change. *Journal of Sport & Exercise Psychology* 15 (4): 375-389.

Goodwin, R.D. 2003. Association between physical activity and mental disorders among adults in the United States. *Preventive Medicine* 36 (6): 698-703.

Gorman, J.M., and L.K. Gorman. 1987. Drug treatment of social phobia. *Journal of Affective Disorders* 13 (Sep-Oct): 183-192.

Goudas, L.C., R. Bloch, M. Gialeli-Goudas, J. Lau, and D.B. Carr. 2005. The epidemiology of cancer pain. *Cancer Investigation* 23 (2): 182-190.

Graham, R.E., A. Zeichner, L.J. Peacock, and R.K. Dishman. 1996. Bradycardia during baroreflex stimulation and active or passive stressor tasks: Cardiorespiratory fitness and hostility. *Psychophysiology* 33: 566-575.

Graven-Nielsen, T., L. Arendt-Nielsen, and S. Mense. 2008. *Fundamentals of musculoskeletal pain*. Seattle: IASP Press.

Gray, H., and W.H. Lewis. 1918. *Anatomy of the Human Body* (*20th Edition*) Philadelphia: Lea & Febiger. New York: Bartleby.com 2000

Gray, J.A. 1973. The structure of the emotions and the limbic system. In *Physiology, emotion and psychosomatic illness*, edited by J. Willis. Amsterdam: Elsevier.

Gray, J.A. 1987. *The neuropsychology of anxiety: An enquiry into the functions of the septo-hippocampal system*. Oxford, UK: Clarendon Press.

Gray, J.A. 1994a. Personality dimensions and emotion systems. In *The nature of emotion: Fundamental questions*, edited by P. Ekman and R.J. Davidson. New York: Oxford University Press.

Gray, J.A. 1994b. Three fundamental emotion systems. In *The nature of emotion: Fundamental questions*, edited by P. Ekman and R.J. Davidson. New York: Oxford University Press.

Green, D.M., and J.A. Swets. 1974. *Signal detection theory and psychophysics*. Huntington, NY: Krieger.

Greenberg, P.E., R.C. Kessler, H.G. Birnbaum, et al. 2003. The economic burden of depression in the United States: How did it change between 1990 and 2000? *The Journal of Clinical Psychiatry*. 64 (12): 1465-75.

Greenberg, P.E., T. Sisitsky, R.C. Kessler, et al. 1999. The economic burden of anxiety disorders in the 1990s. *Journal of Clinical Psychiatry* 60 (Jul): 427-435.

Greenberg, P.E., L.E. Stiglin, S.N. Finkelstein, and E.R. Berndt. 1993. Depression: A neglected major illness. *The Journal of Clinical Psychiatry*. 54 (11): 419-24.

Greenwald, M.K., E.W. Cook, III, and P.J. Lang. 1989. Affective judgment and psychophysiological response: Dimensional covariation in the evaluation of pictorial stimuli. *Journal of Psychophysiology* 3: 51-64.

Greenwood, B.N., P.V. Strong, T.E. Foley, and M. Fleshner. 2009. A behavioral analysis of the impact of voluntary physical activity on hippocampus-dependent contextual conditioning. *Hippocampus*. 19 (10): 988-1001. doi: 10.1002/hipo.20534.

Greenwood, B.N., and M. Fleshner. 2011. Exercise, stress resistance, and central serotonergic systems. *Exercise and Sport Sciences Reviews* 39 (3): 140-149.

Greenwood, B.N., T.E. Foley, H.E. Day, et al. 2003. Freewheel running prevents learned helplessness/behavioral depression: Role of dorsal raphe serotonergic neurons. *Journal of Neuroscience* 23 (7): 2889-2898.

Greenwood, B.N., T.E. Foley, H.E.W. Day, et al. 2005. Wheel running alters serotonin (5-HT) transporter, 5-HT1A, 5-HT1B, and alpha1b-adrenergic receptor mRNA in the rat raphe nuclei. *Biological Psychiatry* 57 (5): 559-568.

Greenwood, B.N., T.E. Foley, T.V. Le, et al. 2011. Long-term voluntary wheel running is rewarding and produces plasticity in the mesolimbic reward pathway. *Behavioural Brain Research* 217 (2): 354-362.

Greenwood, B.N., P.V. Strong, L. Brooks, and M. Fleshner. 2008. Anxiety-like behaviors produced by acute fluoxetine administration in male Fischer 344 rats are prevented by prior exercise. *Psychopharmacology* 199 (2): 209-222.

Greer, T.L., and M.H. Trivedi. 2009. Exercise in the treatment of depression. *Current Psychiatry Reports* 11 (6): 466-472.

Grego, F., J.-M. Vallier, M. Collardeau, et al. 2004. Effects of long duration exercise on cognitive function, blood glucose, and counterregulatory hormones in male cyclists. *Neuroscience Letters* 362: 76-80.

Greist, J.H., M.H. Klein, R.R. Eischens, J. Faris, A.S. Gurman, and W.P. Morgan. 1978. Running through your mind. *Journal of Psychosomatic Research* 22: 259-294.

Greist, J.H., M.H. Klein, R.R. Eischens, J. Faris, A.S. Gurman, and W.P. Morgan. 1979. Running as treatment for depression. *Comprehensive Psychiatry* 20 (Jan-Feb): 41-54.

Gross, P.M., M.L. Marcus, and D.D. Heistad. 1980. Regional distribution of cerebral blood flow during exercise in dogs. *Journal of Applied Physiology* 48 (Feb): 213-217.

Grosz, H.J., and B.B. Farmer. 1972. Pitts' and McClure's lactate-anxiety study revisited. *British Journal of Psychiatry* 120: 415-418.

Gruber, A.J., and H.J. Pope. 2000. Psychiatric and medical effects of anabolic-androgenic steroid use in women. *Psychotherapy and Psychosomatics* 69: 19-26.

Gruber, J.J. 1986. Physical activity and self-esteem development in children: A meta-analysis. In *Effects of physical activity on children*. edited by G.A Stull and E.M. Eckert. *The Academy Papers* 19: 330-348.

Guardiola-Lemaitre, B. 1997. Toxicology of melatonin. *Journal of Biological Rhythms* 12: 697-706.

Guilleminault, C., A. Clerk, J. Black, M. Labanowski, R. Pelayo, and D. Claman. 1995. Nondrug treatment trials in psychophysiologic insomnia. *Annals of Internal Medicine* 155: 838-844.

Gunstad, J., J.T. Kearney, M.B. Spitznagel, et al. 2009. Blood pressure and cognitive function in older adults with cardiovascular disease. *International Journal of Neuroscience* 119: 2228-2242.

Guttman, L. 1950. The basis for scalogram analysis. In *Measurement and prediction*, edited by S.A. Stouffer. Princeton, NJ: Princeton University Press.

Guy, P. 2008. The role of physical activity in rheumatoid arthritis. *Physiology & Behavior* 94 (2): 270-275.

Haeckel, Ernst Heinrich Philipp. August 2011. 2008 [cited August 23, 2011]. www.encyclopedia.com/doc/1G2-2830901809.html.

Hahm, S., T.M. Mizuno, T.J. Wu, et al. 1999. Targeted deletion of the Vgf gene indicates that the encoded secretory peptide precursor plays a novel role in the regulation of energy balance. *Neuron* 23 (3): 537-548.

Hall, E.E., P. Ekkekakis, and S.J. Petruzzello. 2002. The affective beneficence of vigorous exercise revisited. *British Journal of Health Psychology* 7 (Pt 1): 47-66.

Hamaoka, T., K.K. McCully, V. Quaresima, K. Yamamoto, and B. Chance. 2007. Near-infrared spectroscopy/imaging for monitoring muscle oxygenation and oxidative metabolism in healthy and diseased humans. *Journal of Biomedical Optics*. 12 (6): 062105. doi: 10.1117/1.2805437.

Hambrecht, R., C. Walther, S. Möbius-Winkler, et al. 2004. Percutaneous coronary angioplasty compared with exercise training in patients with stable coronary artery disease. *Circulation* 109 (11): 1371-1378.

Hamer, M., and Y. Chida. 2009. Physical activity and risk of neurodegenerative disease: A systematic review of prospective evidence. *Psychological Medicine* 39: 3-11.

Hamer, M., A. Taylor, and A. Steptoe. 2006. The effect of acute aerobic exercise on stress related blood pressure responses: A systematic review and meta-analysis. *Biological Psychology* 71 (2): 183-190.

Hankey, G.J., P.E. Norman, and J.W. Eikelboom. 2006. Medical treatment of peripheral arterial disease. *Journal of the American Medical Association* 295 (5): 547-553.

Hansen, C.J., L.C. Stevens, and J.R. Coast. 2001. Exercise duration and mood state: How much is enough to feel better? *Health Psychology* 20 (4): 267-275.

Hardy, C.J., E.G. Hall, and P.H. Presholdt. 1986. The mediational role of social influence in the perception of exertion. *Journal of Sport and Exercise Psychology* 8: 88-104.

Hardy, C.J., and W.J. Rejeski. 1989. Not what, but how one feels: The measurement of affect during exercise. *Journal of Sport & Exercise Psychology* 11 (3): 304-317.

Harlow, H.F., and J.A. Bromer. 1938. A test apparatus for monkeys. *The Psychological Record* 2: 434-436.

Harlow, J.M. 1868. Recovery from the passage of an iron bar through the head. *Publication of the .Massachusetts Medical Society.* 2: 327-347.

Harmon-Jones, E., P.A. Gable, and C.K. Peterson. 2010. The role of asymmetric frontal cortical activity in emotion-related phenomena: A review and update. *Biological Psychology* 84 (3): 451-462.

Harmon-Jones, E., C. Harmon-Jones, L. Abramson, and C.K. Peterson. 2009. PANAS positive activation is associated with anger. *Emotion* 9 (2): 183-196.

Harris, A.H., R. Cronkite, and R. Moos. 2006. Physical activity, exercise coping, and depression in a 10-year cohort study of depressed patients. *Journal of Affective Disorders* 93 (1-3): 79-85.

Harris, S.S., C.J. Caspersen, G.H. DeFriese, and E.J. Estes. 1989. Physical activity counseling for healthy adults as a primary preventive intervention in the clinical setting. Report for the U.S. Preventive Services Task Force [published erratum appears in *Journal of the American Medical Association,* 1989 Oct 20; 262 (15): 2094] [see comments]. *Journal of the American Medical Association* 261 (June 23-30): 3588-3598.

Harter, S. 1982. The Perceived Competence Scale for Children. *Child Development* 53 (1): 87-97.

Harter, S. 1985. Competence as a dimension of self-evaluation: Toward a comprehensive model of self-worth. In *The development of the self*, edited by R.H. Leahy. New York: Academic Press.

Harter, S. 1986. Cognitive-developmental processes in the integration of concepts about emotions and the self. *Social Cognition* 4 (2): 119-151.

Harter, S. 1996. Historical roots of contemporary issues involving self-concept. In *Handbook of self-concept: Developmental, social, and clinical considerations*, edited by B.A. Bracken, 1-37. New York: Wiley.

Hartman, F.A., K.A. Brownell, and J.E. Lockwood. 1932. Cortin as a general tissue hormone. *American Journal of Physiology* 101: 50.

Haskell, W.L. 2012. Physical activity by self-report: A brief history and future issues. *Journal of Physical Activity & Health* 9 (Suppl. 1): S5-10.

Haskell, W.L., I.M. Lee, R.R. Pate, et al. 2007. Physical activity and public health: Updated recommendation for adults from the American College of Sports Medicine and the American Heart Association. *Circulation* 116:1081-1093.

Hatfield, B.D., A.H. Goldfarb, G.A. Sforzo, and M.G. Flynn. 1987. Serum beta-endorphin and affective responses to graded exercise in young and elderly men. *Journals of Gerontology*. 42 (4): 429-31.

Heart Association. *Medicine & Science in Sports & Exercise*, 39 (8), 1423-1434. doi: 10.1249/mss.0b013e3180616b27.

Hausenblas, H.A., A.V. Carron, and D.E. Mack. 1997. Application of the theories of reasoned action and planned behavior to exercise behavior: A meta-analysis. *Journal of Sport & Exercise Psychology*. 19 (1): 36-51.

Hauser, W. 2010. Efficacy of different types of aerobic exercise in fibromyalgia syndrome: A systematic review and meta-analysis of randomised controlled trials. *Arthritis Research & Therapy* 12:R79. doi: 10.1186/ar3002.

Häuser, W., K. Thieme, and D.C. Turk. 2010. Guidelines on the management of fibromyalgia syndrome: A systematic review. *European Journal of Pain* 14 (1): 5-10.

Hayden, J.A., M.W. van Tulder, and G. Tomlinson. 2005. Systematic review: Strategies for using exercise therapy to improve outcomes in chronic low back pain. *Annals of Internal Medicine* 142 (9): 776-785.

Heaney, J.L., A.T. Ginty, D. Carroll, and A.C. Phillips. 2011. Preliminary evidence that exercise dependence is associated with blunted cardiac and cortisol reactions to acute psychological stress. *International Journal of Psychophysiology* 79 (2): 323-329.

Heesch, K.C., N.W. Burton, and W.J. Brown. 2011. Concurrent and prospective associations between physical activity, walking and mental health in older women. *Journal of Epidemiology and Community Health* 65 (9): 807-813.

Heimer, L., D.S. Zahm, L. Churchill, P.W. Kalivas, and C. Wohltmann. 1991. Specificity in the projection patterns of accumbal core and shell in the rat. *Neuroscience* 41 (1): 89-125.

Heisler, L.K., L. Zhou, P. Bajwa, J. Hsu, and L.H. Tecott. 2007. Serotonin 5-HT(2C) receptors regulate anxiety-like behavior. *Genes, Brain, and Behavior* 6 (5): 491-496.

Hemingway, H., C. Langenberg, J Damant, et al. 2008. Prevalence of angina in women versus men. *Circulation* 117 (12): 1526-1536.

Hensley, L.D. 2000. State of required physical education in colleges and universities. *Research Quarterly for Exercise & Sport* 71: A71-A72.

Hergenhahn, B.R. 1992. *An introduction to the history of psychology*. 2nd ed. Belmont, CA: Wadsworth.

Hernández-Molina, G., S. Reichenbach, B. Zhang, M. Lavalley, and D.T. Felson. 2008. Effect of therapeutic exercise for hip osteoarthritis pain: Results of a meta-analysis. *Arthritis Care & Research* 59 (9): 1221-1228.

Herring, M.P., and P.J. O'Connor. 2009. The effect of acute resistance exercise on feelings of energy and fatigue. *Journal of Sports Sciences* 27 (7): 701-709.

Herring, M.P., P.J. O'Connor, and R.K. Dishman. 2010. The effect of exercise training on anxiety symptoms among patients: A systematic review. *Archives of Internal Medicine* 170 (4): 321-331.

Herring, M.P., T.W. Puetz, J. O'Connor P, and R.K. Dishman. 2012. Effect of exercise training on depressive symptoms among patients with a chronic illness: A systematic review and meta-analysis of randomized controlled trials. *Arch Intern Med.* 172 (2): 101-11. doi: 10.1001/archinternmed.2011.696.

Herring, M.P., M.L. Jacob, C. Suveg, R.K. Dishman, and P.J. O'Connor. 2012. Feasibility of exercise training for the short-term treatment of generalized anxiety disorder: A randomized controlled trial. *Psychotherapy and Psychosomatics* 81 (1): 21-28.

Herrmann, L.L., G.M. Goodwin, and K.P. Ebmeier. 2007. The cognitive neuropsychology of depression in the elderly. *Psychological Medicine* 37: 1693-1702.

Hertzog, C., A.F. Kramer, R.S. Wilson, and U. Lindenberger. 2009. Enrichment effects on adult cognitive development. *Psychological Science in the Public Interest* 9 (1): 1-65.

Herva, A., J. Laitinen, J. Miettunen, et al. 2005. Obesity and depression: Results from the longitudinal Northern Finland 1966 Birth Cohort Study. *International Journal of Obesity* 30 (3): 520-527.

Hetta, J., M. Almqvist, H. Agren, G. Hambert, B. Liljenberg, and B.A. Roos. 1985. Prevalence of sleep disturbances and related symptoms in a middle-aged Swedish population. In *Sleep '84*, edited by W.P. Koella, E. Ruther, and H. Schulz. Stuttgart, New York: Gustav Fischer Verlag.

Heyn, P., B.C. Abreu, and K.J. Ottenbacher. 2004. The effects of exercise training on elderly persons with cognitive impairment and dementia: A meta-analysis. *Archives of Physical Medicine and Rehabilitation* 85: 1694-1704.

Hilgard, E.R. 1989. *Psychology in America: A historical survey*. New York: Harcourt Brace Jovanovich.

Hill, D.W., K.J. Cureton, S.C. Grisham, and M.A. Collins. 1987. Effect of training on the rating of perceived exertion at the ventilatory threshold. *European Journal of Applied Physiology and Occupational Physiology* 56: 206-211.

Hill, M.N., and B.S. McEwen. 2010. Involvement of the endocannabinoid system in the neurobehavioural effects of stress and glucocorticoids. *Progress in Neuro-Psychopharmacology & Biological Psychiatry* 34 (5): 791-797.

Hillman, C.H., S.M. Buck, J.R. Themanson, M.B. Pontifex, and D. Castelli. 2009. Aerobic fitness and cognitive development: Event-related brain potential and task performance indices of executive control in preadolescent children. *Developmental Psychology* 45 (1): 114-129.

Hillman, C.H., K.I. Erickson, and A. F Kramer. 2008. Be smart, exercise your heart: Exercise effects on brain and cognition. *Nature Reviews Neuroscience* 9 (1): 58-65.

Hillman, C.H., M.B. Pontifex, L.B. Raine, D. Castelli, E.E. Hall, and A.F. Kramer. 2009. The effect of acute treadmill walking on cognitive control and academic achievement in preadolescent children. *Neuroscience* 159: 1044-1054.

Hillman, C.H., E.M. Snook, and G. Jerome, J. 2003. Acute cardiovascular exercise and executive control function. *International Journal of Psychophysiology* 48: 307-314.

Hillsdon, M., C. Foster, and M. Thorogood. 2005. Interventions for promoting physical activity. *Cochrane Database of Systematic Reviews* [Online] (1): CD003180.

Hirsch, B. and D.T. Lykken. 1993. Age and the self-perception of ability: A twin study analysis. *Psychology & Aging* 8 (1): 72-80.

Hockey, G.R.J. 1997. Compensatory control in the regulation of human performance under stress and high workload: A cognitive-energetical framework. *Biological Psychology* 45: 73-93.

Hoehner, C.M., J. Soares, D. Parra Perez, et al. 2008. Physical activity interventions in Latin America: A systematic review. *American Journal of Preventive Medicine* 34 (3): 224-233.

Hoffman, B.M., J.A. Blumenthal, M.A. Babyak, et al. 2008. Exercise fails to improve neurocognition in depressed middle-aged and older adults. *Medicine & Science in Sports & Exercise* 40 (7): 1344-1352.

Hoffman, M.D., and D.R. Hoffman. 2008. Exercisers achieve greater acute exercise-induced mood enhancement than nonexercisers. *Archives of Physical Medicine and Rehabilitation* 89 (2): 358-363.

Holets, V.R., T. Hokfelt, A. Rokaeus, L. Terenius, and M. Goldstein. 1988. Locus coeruleus neurons in the rat containing neuropeptide Y, tyrosine hydroxylase or galanin and their efferent projections to the spinal cord, cerebral cortex and hypothalamus. *Neuroscience* 24 (Mar): 893-906.

Hollmann, W., H.G. Fischer, M.K. de, H. Herzog, K. Herzog, and L.E. Feinendegen. 1994. The brain—regional cerebral blood flow, metabolism, and psyche during ergometer exercise. In *Physical activity, fitness and health: International proceedings and consensus statement*, edited by C. Bouchard, R. Shephard, and T. Stephens. Champaign, IL: Human Kinetics.

Holmes, P.V. 2003. Rodent models of depression: Re-examining validity without anthropomorphic inference. *Critical Reviews in Neurobiology* 15 (2): 143-174.

Hootman, J.M., Dick, R., and Agel, J. 2007. Epidemiology of collegiate injuries for 15 sports: Summary and recommendations for injury prevention initiatives. *Journal of Athletic Training* 42 (2): 311-319.

Hormes, J.M., L.A. Lytle, C.R. Gross, R.L. Ahmed, A.B. Troxel, and K.H. Schmitz. 2008. The body image and relationships scale: Development and validation of a measure of body image in female breast cancer survivors. *Journal of Clinical Oncology* 26 (8): 1269.

Horne, J.A., and V.J. Moore. 1985. Sleep EEG effects of exercise with and without additional body cooling. *Electroencephalography and Clinical Neurophysiology* 60: 33-38.

Horne, J.A., and L.H.E. Staff. 1983. Exercise and sleep: Body heating effects. *Sleep* 6: 36-46.

Horowitz, A.L. 1995. *MRI physics for radiologists: A visual approach*. 3rd ed. New York: Springer-Verlag.

Hsiao, E.T., and R.E. Thayer. 1998. Exercising for mood regulation: The importance of experience. *Personality & Individual Differences* 24 (6): 829-836.

Hughes, C.F., C. Uhlmann, and J.W. Pennebaker. 1994. The body's response to processing emotional trauma: Linking verbal text with autonomic activity. *Journal of Personality* 62 (Dec): 565-585.

Huhman, M., L.D. Potter, F.L. Wong, S.W. Banspach, J.C. Duke, and C.D. Heitzler. 2005. Effects of a mass media campaign to increase physical activity among children: Year-1 results of the VERB campaign. *Pediatrics* 116 (2): e277-284.

Hung, J.-W., C.-W. Liou, P.-W. Wang, et al. 2009. Effect of 12-week tai chi chuan exercise on peripheral nerve modulation in patients with type 2 diabetes mellitus. *Journal of Rehabilitation Medicine* 41 (11): 924-929.

Hunsberger, J.G., S.S. Newton, A.H. Bennett, et al. 2007. Antidepressant actions of the exercise-regulated gene VGF. *Nature Medicine* 13 (12): 1476-1482.

Huotari, P., H. Nupponen, L. Mikkelsson, L. Laakso, and U. Kujala. 2011. Adolescent physical fitness and activity as predictors of adulthood activity. *Journal of Sports Sciences* 29 (11): 1135-1141.

Huppert, T.J., R.D. Hoge, S.G. Diamond, M.A. Franceschini, and D.A. Boas. 2006. A temporal comparison of BOLD, ASL, and NIRS hemodynamic responses to motor stimuli in adult humans. *NeuroImage* 29 (2): 368-382.

IASP Task Force on Taxonomy. 1994. Part III: Pain terms—A current list with definitions and notes on usage. In *Classification of chronic pain*, edited by B. Merskey and N. Bogduk. Seattle: IASP Press.

Institute of Medicine. 2011. *Relieving pain in America: A blueprint for transforming prevention, care, education and research*. Washington, DC: The National Academies Press.

International Human Genome Sequencing Consortium. 2004. Finishing the euchromatic sequence of the human genome. *Nature* 431 (7011): 931-945.

Intille, S.S., C. Kukla, R. Farzanfar, and W. Bakr. 2003. Just-in-time technology to encourage incremental, dietary behavior change. *Annual Symposium proceedings/AMIA Symposium*: 874.

Irwin, W., R.J. Davidson, M.J. Lowe, B.J. Mock, J.A. Sorenson, and P.A. Turski. 1996. Human amygdala activation detected with echo-planar functional magnetic resonance imaging. *Neuroreport* 711: 1765-1769.

Ismail, A.H. 1967. The effects of a well-organized physical education programme on intellectual performance. *Research in Physical Education* 1: 31-38.

Jackson, A.S., X. Sui, J.R. Hebert, T.S. Church, and S.N. Blair. 2009. Role of lifestyle and aging on the longitudinal change in cardiorespiratory fitness. *Archive of Internal Medicine*. 169 (19): 1781-7. doi: 10.1001/archinternmed.2009.312.

Jackson, A.W., and R.K. Dishman. 2000. Perceived submaximal force production in young men and women. *Medicine & Science in Sports & Exercise* 32: 448-451.

Jackson, A.W., R.K. Dishman, and S.B. Martin. 2002. Perceived leg extension and flexion forces of young adult men and women: Comparison to previous findings. *Research Quarterly for Exercise and Sport* 73 (2): 225-228.

Jackson, A., R.K. Dishman, C.S. La, R. Patton, and R. Weinberg. 1981. The heart rate, perceived exertion, and pace of the 1.5 mile run. *Medicine & Science in Sports & Exercise* 13: 224-228.

Jackson, A.W., A.W. Ludtke, S.B. Martin, L.P. Koziris, and R.K. Dishman. 2006. Perceived submaximal force production in young adults. *Research Quarterly for Exercise and Sport* 77 (1): 50-57.

Jackson, E.M., and R.K. Dishman. 2002. Hemodynamic responses to stress among black women: Fitness and parental hypertension. *Medicine & Science in Sports & Exercise* 34 (7): 1097-1104; discussion 1105.

Jackson, E.M., and R.K. Dishman 2006. Cardiorespiratory fitness and laboratory stress: A meta-regression analysis. *Psychophysiology* 43 (1): 57-72.

Jakicic, J.M., C. Winters, W. Lang, and R.R. Wing. 1999. Effects of intermittent exercise and use of home exercise equipment on adherence, weight loss, and fitness in overweight women. *Journal of the American Medical Association* 282: 1554-1560.

Janis, I.L., and L. Mann. 1977. *Decision making: a psychological analysis of conflict, choice, and commitment.* New York, NY: The Free Press.

James, W. 1884. What is an emotion? *Mind* 9: 188-205.

James, W. 1890. *The principles of psychology.* Vol. 2. New York: Holt.

James, W. 1899. *Talks to teachers on psychology: And to students on some of life's ideals.* New York: Holt.

James, W. 1899. Physical training in the educational curriculum. *American Physical Education Review.* Boston: American Association for the Advancement of Physical Education.

Jamison, R.N. 2010. Unraveling the secrets to chronic pain and disability: More than meets the eye. *Journal of Pain* 11 (5): 405-407.

Janis, I.L., and P.B. Field. 1959. Sex differences and factors related to personality. In *Personality and persuasibility.* edited by C.I. Hovland and I.L. Janis. New Haven, CT: Yale University Press.

Janson, C., T. Gislason, W. De Backer, et al. 1995. Insomnia and sleep: Prevalence of sleep disturbances among young adults in three European countries. *Sleep* 18: 589-597.

Jeannerod, M., F. Michel, and C. Prablanc. 1986. The control of hand movements in case of hemianaesthesia following a parietal lesion. *Brain* 107: 899-920.

Jensen, M.C., M.N. Brant-Zawadzki, N. Obuchowski, M.T. Modic, D. Malkasian, and J.S. Ross. 1994. Magnetic resonance imaging of the lumbar spine in people without back pain. *New England Journal of Medicine* 331 (2): 69-73.

Jensen, M.P., M.J. Chodroff, and R.H. Dworkin. 2007. The impact of neuropathic pain on health-related quality of life. *Neurology* 68 (15): 1178-1182.

Jerstad, S.J., K.N. Boutelle, K.K. Ness, and E. Stice. 2010. Prospective reciprocal relations between physical activity and depression in female adolescents. *Journal of Consulting and Clinical Psychology* 78 (2): 268-272.

Johannes, C.B., T. Kim Le, X. Zhou, J.A. Johnston, and R.H. Dworkin. 2010. The prevalence of chronic pain in United States adults: Results of an Internet-based survey. *Journal of Pain* 11 (11): 1230-1239.

John, P.J., N. Sharma, C.M. Sharma, and A. Kankane. 2007. Effectiveness of yoga therapy in the treatment of migraine without aura: A randomized controlled trial. *Headache: Journal of Head and Face Pain* 47 (5): 654-661.

Johnson, M., and M. Martinson. 2007. Efficacy of electrical nerve stimulation for chronic musculoskeletal pain: A meta-analysis of randomized controlled trials. *Pain* 130 (1): 157-165.

Jonas, B.S., P. Franks, and D.D. Ingram. 1997. Are symptoms of anxiety and depression risk factors for hypertension? Longitudinal evidence from the National Health and Nutrition Examination Survey I Epidemiologic Follow-up Study. *Archives of Family Medicine* 6 (Jan-Feb): 43-49.

Jónás, I., K.A. Schubert, A.C. Reijne, et al. 2010. Behavioral traits are affected by selective breeding for increased wheel-running behavior in mice. *Behavior Genetics* 40 (4): 542-550.

Jones, J., D.N. Rutledge, K. Dupree Jones, L. Matallana, and D.S. Rooks. 2008. Self-assessed physical function levels of women with fibromyalgia: A national survey. *Women's Health Issues* 18 (5): 406-412.

Jones, K.D., C.S. Burckhardt, and J.A. Bennett. 2004. Motivational interviewing may encourage exercise in persons with fibromyalgia by enhancing self efficacy. *Arthritis Care & Research* 51 (5): 864-867.

Jones, K.D., C.S Burckhardt, S.R Clark, R.M Bennett, and K.M Potempa. 2002. A randomized controlled trial of muscle strengthening versus flexibility training in fibromyalgia. *Journal of Rheumatology* 29 (5): 1041-1048.

Jones, L.A., and I.W. Hunter. 1985. Effect of muscle tendon vibration on the perception of force. *Experimental Neurology* 87 (1): 35-45.

Jonsdottir, I.H. 2000. Special feature for the Olympics: Effects of exercise on the immune system: Neuropeptides and their interaction with exercise and immune function. *Immunology and Cell Biology* 78 (5): 562-570.

Jonsdottir, I.H., L. Rodjer, E. Hadzibajramovic, M. Borjesson, and G. Ahlborg, Jr. 2010. A prospective study of leisure-time physical activity and mental health in Swedish health care workers and social insurance officers. *Preventive Medicine* 51 (5): 373-377.

Kahn, E.B., L.T. Ramsey, R.C. Brownson, et al. 2002. The effectiveness of interventions to increase physical activity: A systematic review. *American Journal of Preventive Medicine* 22 (May): 73-107.

Kahneman, D. 1973. *Attention and effort.* Englewood Cliffs, NJ: Prentice Hall.

Kamijo, K. 2009. Effects of acute exercise on event-related brain potentials. In *Enhancing cognitive functioning and brain plasticity,* edited by W.J. Chodzko-Kajko, A.F. Kramer, and L.W. Poon. Champaign, IL: Human Kinetics.

Kandel, E.R. 1998. A new intellectual framework for psychiatry. *American Journal of Psychiatry.* 155: 457-469.

Kankaanp, M., S. Taimela, O. Airaksinen, and O. Hänninen. 1999. The efficacy of active rehabilitation in chronic low back pain: Effect on pain intensity, self-experienced disability, and lumbar fatigability. *Spine* 24 (10): 1034.

Kann, L. et al. 1998. CDC surveillance summaries: Youth Risk Behavior Survey—United States, 1997. *Morbidity and Mortality Weekly Reports* 47 (3): 1-89.

Kaplan, G.A., W.J. Strawbridge, R.D. Cohen, and L.R. Hungerford. 1996. Natural history of leisure-time physical activity and its correlates: Associations with mortality from all causes and cardiovascular disease over 28 years. *American Journal of Epidemiology* 144 (8): 793-797.

Kardel, K.R., B. Johansen, N. Voldner, P. Ole Iversen, and T. Henriksen. 2009. Association between aerobic fitness in late pregnancy and duration of labor in nulliparous women. *Acta Obstetricia et Gynecologica Scandinavica* 88 (8): 948-952.

Kaski, J.C. 2004. Pathophysiology and management of patients with chest pain and normal coronary arteriograms (cardiac syndrome X). *Circulation* 109 (5): 568-572.

Kelley, G.A., K.S. Kelley, J.M. Hootman, and D.L. Jones. 2011. Effects of community-deliverable exercise on pain and physical function in adults with arthritis and other rheumatic diseases: A meta-analysis. *Arthritis Care & Research* 63 (1): 79-93.

Kelley, G.A, K.S. Kelley, and D.L. Jones. 2011. Efficacy and effectiveness of exercise on tender points in adults with fibromyalgia: A meta-analysis of randomized controlled trials. *Arthritis Care & Research.* 63 (1): 79-93. doi: 10.1002/acr.20347.

Kempermann, G. 2008. The neurogenic reserve hypothesis: What is adult hippocampal neurogenesis good for? *Trends in Neuroscience* 31 (4): 163-169.

Kemppainen, P., A. Pertovaara, T. Huopaniemi, G. Johansson, and S.-L. Karonen. 1985. Modification of dental pain and cutaneous thermal sensitivity by physical exercise in man. *Brain Research* 360 (1-2): 33-40.

Kendall, A.R., M. Mahue-Giangreco, C.L. Carpenter, P.A. Ganz, and L. Bernstein. 2005. Influence of exercise activity on quality of life in long-term breast cancer survivors. *Quality of Life Research* 14 (2): 361-371.

Kendzierski, D. 1994. Schema theory: An information processing focus. in *Advances in Exercise Adherence.* edited by R.K. Dishman, Champaign, IL: Human Kinetics.

Kerlinger, F.N. 1973. *Foundations of behavioral research.* 2nd ed. New York: Holt, Rinehart, & Winston.

Kessler, R.C., P. Berglund, O. Demler, R. Jin, K.R. Merikangas, and E.E. Walters. 2005a. Lifetime prevalence and age-of-onset distributions of DSM-IV disorders in the National Comorbidity Survey Replication. *Archives of General Psychiatry* 62 (6): 593-602.

Kessler, R.C., P. Berglund, O. Demler, et al. 2003. The epidemiology of major depressive disorder: Results from the National Comorbidity Survey Replication (NCS-R). *Journal of the American Medical Association* 289 (23): 3095-3105.

Kessler, R.C., W.T. Chiu, O. Demler, K.R. Merikangas, and E.E. Walters. 2005b. Prevalence, severity, and comorbidity of 12-month DSM-IV disorders in the National Comorbidity Survey Replication. *Archives of General Psychiatry* 62 (6): 617-627.

Kessler, R.C., O. Demler, R.G. Frank, et al. 2005c. Prevalence and treatment of mental disorders, 1990 to 2003. *New England Journal of Medicine* 352 (24): 2515-2523.

Kessler, R.C., K.A. McGonagle, S. Zhao, et al. 1994. Lifetime and 12-month prevalence of DSM-III-R psychiatric disorders in the United States: Results from the National Comorbidity Survey. *Archives of General Psychiatry* 51: 8-19.

Khanna, S., and J.G. Sinclair. 1989. Noxious stimuli produce prolonged changes in the CA1 region of the rat hippocampus. *Pain* 39 (3): 337-343.

Khatri, P., J.A. Blumenthal, M.A. Babyak, et al. 2001. Effects of exercise training on cognitive functioning among depressed older men and women. *Journal of Aging and Physical Activity* 9: 43-57.

Killian, K.J. 1987. Limitations of exercise by dyspnea. *Canadian Journal of Sport Science* 12 (Suppl. 1): 53S-60S.

Kimiecik, J. 1992. Predicting vigorous physical activity of corporate employees: Comparing the theories of reasoned action and planned behavior. *Journal of Sport & Exercise Psychology.* 14 (2): 192-206.

King, A.C., K. Baumann, P. O'Sullivan, S. Wilcox, and C. Castro. 2002. Effects of moderate-intensity exercise on physiological, behavioral, and emotional responses to family caregiving: A randomized controlled trial. *Journals of Gerontology. Series A, Biological Sciences and Medical Sciences* 57 (1): M26-M36.

King, A.C., C. Castro, S. Wilcox, A.A. Eyler, J.F. Sallis, and R.C. Brownson. 2000. Personal and environmental factors associated with physical inactivity among different racial-ethnic groups of U.S. middle-aged and older-aged women. *Health Psychology* 19 (4): 354-364.

King, A.C., W.L. Haskell, C.B. Taylor, H.C. Kraemer, and R.F. DeBusk. 1991. Group-vs home-based exercise training in healthy older men and women. *Journal of the American Medical Association.* 266: 1535-1542.

King, A.C., and J.E. Martin. 1993. Exercise adherence and maintenance. In *Resource manual for guidelines for exercise testing and prescription*, edited by J.L. Durstine, A.C. King, P.L. Painter, J.L. Roitman, and L.D. Zwiren. Philadelphia: Lea & Febiger.

King, A.C., R.F. Oman, G.S. Brassington, D.L. Bliwise, and W.L. Haskell. 1997. Moderate-intensity exercise and self-rated quality of sleep in older adults: A randomized controlled trial. *Journal of the American Medical Association* 277 (1): 32-37.

King, A.C., L.A. Pruitt, S. Woo, et al. 2008. Effects of moderate-intensity exercise on polysomnographic and subjective sleep quality in older adults with mild to moderate sleep complaints. *Journals of Gerontology: Series A: Biological Sciences & Medical Sciences* 63 (9): 997-1004.

King, A.C, D. Stokols, E. Talen, G.S. Brassington, and R. Killingsworth. 2002. Theoretical approaches to the promotion of physical activity: Forging a transdisciplinary paradigm. *American Journal of Preventive Medicine* 23 (Aug): 15-25.

King, A.C., C.B. Taylor, and W.L. Haskell. 1993. Effects of differing intensities and formats of 12 months of exercise training on psychological outcomes in older adults. *Health Psychology* 124: 292-300.

King, N., N. Byrne, A. Hunt, and A. Hills. 2010. Comparing exercise prescribed with exercise completed: Effects of gender and mode of exercise. *Journal of Sports Sciences* 28 (6): 633-640.

Kingsley, J.D., L.B. Panton, T. Toole, P. Sirithienthad, R. Mathis, and V. McMillan. 2005. The effects of a 12-week strength-training program on strength and functionality in women with fibromyalgia. *Archives of Physical Medicine and Rehabilitation* 86 (9): 1713-1721.

Kirk, A., J. Barnett, G. Leese, and N. Mutrie. 2009. A randomized trial investigating the 12-month changes in physical activity and health outcomes following a physical activity consultation delivered by a person or in written form in type 2 diabetes: Time2Act. *Diabetic Medicine* 26 (3): 293-301.

Kirkcaldy, B.D., and R.J. Shephard. 1990. Therapeutic implications of exercise. *International Journal of Sport Psychology* 21 (2): 165-184.

Kjaer, M., N.H. Secher, F.W. Bach, S. Sheikh, and H. Galbo. 1989. Hormonal and metabolic responses to exercise in humans: Effect of sensory nervous blockade. *American Journal of Physiology* 257 (1 Pt 1): E95-E101.

Klink, M., and S.F. Quan. 1987. Prevalence of reported sleep disturbances in a general adult population and their relationship to obstructive airways diseases. *Chest* 91: 540-546.

Knab, A.M., R.S. Bowen, A.T. Hamilton, A.A. Gulledge, and J.T. Lightfoot. 2009. Altered dopaminergic profiles: Implications for the regulation of voluntary physical activity. *Behavioural Brain Research* 204 (1): 147-152.

Knab, A.M., and J.T. Lightfoot. 2010. Does the difference between physically active and couch potato lie in the dopamine system? *International Journal of Biological Sciences* 6 (2): 133-150.

Knapp, D.N. 1988. Behavioral management techniques and exercise promotion. In *Exercise adherence*, edited by R.K. Dishman. Champaign, IL: Human Kinetics.

Knight, J.A., S. Thompson, J.M. Raboud, and B.R. Hoffman. 2005. Light and exercise and melatonin production in women. *American Journal of Epidemiology* 162 (11): 1114-1122.

Knox, S., A. Barnes, C. Kiefe, et al. 2006. History of depression, race, and cardiovascular risk in CARDIA. *International Journal of Behavioral Medicine* 13 (1): 44-50.

Kobasa, S.C., S.R. Maddi, and S. Kahn. 1982. Hardiness and health: A prospective study. *Journal of Personality and Social Psychology* 42 (1): 168-177.

Koch, L.G., and S.L. Britton. 2001. Artificial selection for intrinsic aerobic endurance running capacity in rats. *Physiological Genomics* 5 (1): 45-52.

Koch, L.G., and S.L. Britton. 2008. Development of animal models to test the fundamental basis of gene-environment interactions. *Obesity* 16 (Suppl. 3): S28-S32.

Kohl, H.W., and W. Hobbs. 1998. Development of physical activity behavior among children and adolescents. *Pediatrics* 101 (Suppl. 5): 549-554.

Kollesch, J. 1989. Knidos as the center of early scientific medicine in ancient Greece. *Gesnerus* 46 (1-2): 11-28.

Koltyn, K.F. 1997. The thermogenic hypothesis. In *Physical activity and mental health*, edited by W.P. Morgan. Washington, DC: Taylor & Francis.

Koltyn, K.F. 2002. Exercise-induced hypoalgesia and intensity of exercise. *Sports Medicine* 32 (8): 477-487.

Koltyn, K.F., N.A. Lynch, and D.W. Hill. 1998. Psychological responses to brief exhaustive cycling exercise in the morning and evening. *International Journal of Sport Psychology* 29: 145-156.

Koltyn, K.F., and W.P. Morgan. 1992. Influence of underwater exercise on anxiety and body temperature. *Scandinavian Journal of Medicine and Science in Sports* 2: 249-253.

Koltyn, K.F., and W.P. Morgan. 1997. Influence of wet suit wear on anxiety responses to underwater exercise. *Undersea & Hyperbaric Medicine* 24 (1): 23-28.

Koltyn, K.F., H.I. Robins, C.L. Schmitt, J.D. Cohen, and W.P. Morgan. 1992. Changes in mood state following whole-body hyperthermia. *International Journal of Hyperthermia* 8 (3): 305-307.

Kong, J., N.S. White, K.K. Kwong, et al. 2006. Using fMRI to dissociate sensory encoding from cognitive evaluation of heat pain intensity. *Human Brain Mapping* 27 (9): 715-721.

Konorski, J. 1967. *Integrative activity of the brain: An interdisciplinary approach*. Chicago: University of Chicago Press.

Koob, G.F., and M. Le Moal. 1997. Drug abuse: Hedonic homeostatic dysregulation. *Science* 278 (5335): 52-58.

Kopp, M., M. Steinlechner, G. Ruedl, L. Ledochowski, G. Rumpold, and A.H. Taylor. 2012. Acute effects of brisk walking on affect and psychological well-being in individuals with type 2 diabetes. *Diabetes Research and Clinical Practice*. 25(1): 25-29. doi: 10.1016/j.diabres.2011.09.017.

Kosek, E., J. Ekholm, and P. Hansson. 1996. Modulation of pressure pain thresholds during and following isometric contraction in patients with fibromyalgia and in healthy controls. *Pain* 64 (3): 415-423.

Kostka, C.E., and E. Cafarelli. 1982. Effect of pH on sensation and vastus lateralis electromyogram during cycling exercise. *Journal of Applied Physiology* S2: 1181-1185.

Kovacs, K.J. 1998. C-Fos as a transcription factor: A stressful (re)view from a functional map. *Neurochemistry International* 33 (Oct): 287-297.

Kramer, A.F., S. Hahn, E. McAuley, N.J. Cohen, M.T. Banich, and C Harrison, R. 2002. Exercise, aging, and cognition: Healthy body, healthy mind? In *Human factors interventions for the health care of older adults*, edited by W.A. Rogers and A.D. Fisk. Mahwah, NJ: Erlbaum.

Kremers, S.P.J., and J. Brug. 2008. Habit strength of physical activity and sedentary behavior among children and adolescents. *Pediatric Exercise Science* 20 (1): 5-17.

Kriemler, S., U. Meyer, E. Martin, E.M. van Sluijs, L.B. Andersen, and B.W. Martin. 2011. Effect of school-based interventions on physical activity and fitness in children and adolescents: A review of reviews and systematic update. *British Journal of Sports Medicine* 45 (11): 923-930.

Kripke, D.F. 2000. Chronic hypnotic use: Deadly risks, doubtful benefit. *Sleep Medicine Reviews*. 4 (1): 5-20.

Kripke, D.F., M.R. Klauber, D.L. Wingard, R.L. Fell, J.D. Assmus, and L. Garfinkel. 1998. Mortality hazard associated with prescription hypnotics. *Biological Psychiatry*. 43 (9): 687-93.

Kriska, A.M., and C. Caspersen. 1997. Introduction to a collection of physical activity questionnaires. *Medicine & Science in Sports & Exercise* 29 (S6): S5-S9.

Krogh, J., M. Nordentoft, J.A. Sterne, and D.A. Lawlor. 2011. The effect of exercise in clinically depressed adults: Systematic review and meta-analysis of randomized controlled trials. *Journal of Clinical Psychiatry* 72 (4): 529-538.

Krogh, J., B. Saltin, C. Gluud, and M. Nordentoft. 2009. The DEMO trial: A randomized, parallel-group, observer-blinded clinical trial of strength versus aerobic versus relaxation training for patients with mild to moderate depression. *Journal of Clinical Psychiatry* 70 (6): 790-800.

Ku, P.W., K.R. Fox, and L.J. Chen. 2009. Physical activity and depressive symptoms in Taiwanese older adults: A seven-year follow-up study. *Preventive Medicine* 48 (3): 250-255.

Kubitz, K.A., D.M. Landers, S.J. Petruzzello, and M. Han. 1996. The effects of acute and chronic exercise on sleep. A meta-analytic review. *Sports Medicine* 21 (4): 277-291.

Kubitz, K.A., and A.A. Mott. 1996. EEG power spectral densities during and after cycle ergometer exercise. *Research Quarterly for Exercise & Sport* 67: 91-96.

Kugler, J., H. Seelbach, and G.M. Kruskemper. 1994. Effects of rehabilitation exercise programmes on anxiety and depression in coronary patients: A meta-analysis. *British Journal of Clinical Psychology* 33 (Pt 3) (Sept): 401-410.

Kujala, U.M., S. Orava, J. Parkkari, J. Kaprio, and S. Sarna. 2003. Sports career–related musculoskeletal injuries: Long-term health effects on former athletes. *Sports Medicine* 33 (12): 869-875.

Kujala, U.M., S. Taimela, and T .Viljanen. 1999. Leisure physical activity and various pain symptoms among adolescents. *British Journal of Sports Medicine* 33 (5): 325-328.

Kulinna, P.H., W.W. Warfield, S. Jonaitis, M. Dean, and C. Corbin. 2009. The progression and characteristics of conceptually based fitness/wellness courses at American universities and colleges. *Journal of American College Health* 58 (2): 127-131.

Kunst-Wilson, W.R., and R.B. Zajonc. 1980. Affective discrimination of stimuli that cannot be recognized. *Science* 207 (4430): 557-558.

Kuphal, K.E., E.E. Fibuch, and B.K. Taylor. 2007. Extended swimming exercise reduces inflammatory and peripheral neuropathic pain in rodents. *Journal of Pain* 8 (12): 989-997.

Kyllo, L.B., and D.M. Landers. 1995. Goal setting in sport and exercise: A research synthesis to resolve the controversy. *Journal of Sport and Exercise Psychology* 17: 117-137.

LaBar, K.S., J.C. Gatenby, J.C. Gore, J.E. Ledoux, and E.A. Phelps. 1998. Human amygdala activation during conditioned fear acquisition and extinction: A mixed-trial fMRI study. *Neuron* 205: 937-945.

Lamb, K.L., and R.G. Eston. 1997. Effort perception in children. *Sports Medicine* 23 (3): 139-148.

Lambourne, K., and P.D. Tomporowski. 2010. The effect of acute exercise on cognitive task performance: A meta-regression analysis. *Brain Research Reviews* 1341: 12-24.

Land, B.B., M.R. Bruchas, S. Schattauer, et al. 2009. Activation of the kappa opioid receptor in the dorsal raphe nucleus mediates the aversive effects of stress and reinstates drug seeking. *Proceedings of the National Academy of Sciences of the United States of America* 106 (45): 19168-19173.

Landers, D.M., and S.J. Petruzzello. 1994. Physical activity, fitness, and anxiety. In *Physical activity, fitness, and health: International proceedings and consensus statement*, edited by C. Bouchard, R. Shephard, and J.C. Stevens. Champaign, Il: Human Kinetics.

Landolt, H.P., V. Meier, H.J. Burgess, L. Finelli, F. Cattelin, and A.A. Borbely. 1998. SR 46349B, a selective 5-HT2 receptor antagonist, enhances delta activity and reduces sigma activity in nonREM sleep in humans. *Sleep* 21S: 85.

Lang, P.J. 1995. The emotion probe: Studies of motivation and attention. *American Psychologist* 50 (5): 372-385.

Lang, P.J. 2000. Emotion and motivation: Attention, perception, and action. *Journal of Sport & Exercise Psychology* 20: S122-S140.

Lang, P.J., M.M. Bradley, and B.N. Cuthbert. 1998. Emotion, motivation, and anxiety: Brain mechanisms and psychophysiology. *Biological Psychiatry* 44 (Dec 15): 1248-1263.

LaPorte, R.E., H.J. Montoye, and C.J. Caspersen. 1985. Assessment of physical activity in epidemiologic research: Problems and prospects. *Public Health Reports* 100 (Mar-Apr): 131-146.

Larun, L., L.V. Nordheim, E. Ekeland, K.B. Hagen, and F. Heian. 2006. Exercise in prevention and treatment of anxiety and depression among children and young people. *Cochrane Database of Systematic Reviews* 3: CD004691.

Latimer, A.E., L.R. Brawley, and R.L. Bassett. 2010. A systematic review of three approaches for constructing physical activity messages: What messages work and what improvements are needed? *International Journal of Behavioral Nutrition and Physical Activity* 7: 36.

Lautenschlager, N.T., K.L. Cox, L. Flicker, et al. 2008. Effect of physical activity on cognitive function in older adults at risk for Alzheimer Disease. *Journal of the American Medical Association* 300 (9): 1027-1037.

Lawlor, D.A., and S.W. Hopker. 2001. The effectiveness of exercise as an intervention in the management of depression: systematic review and meta-regression analysis of randomised controlled trials. *British Medical Journal.* 322 (7289): 763-767.

Lawrence, R.C., D.T. Felson, C.G. Helmick, et al. 2008. Estimates of the prevalence of arthritis and other rheumatic conditions in the United States: Part II. *Arthritis & Rheumatism* 58 (1): 26-35.

Layman, E.M. 1960. Contributions of exercise and sports to mental health and social adjustment. In *Science and medicine of exercise and sports*, edited by W.R. Johnson. New York: Harper.

Lazarus, A.A. 2000. Will reason prevail? From classical psychoanalysis to New Age therapy. *American Journal of Psychotherapy* 54 (2): 152-155.

Lazarus, R.S. 1966. *Psychological stress and the coping process.* New York: McGraw-Hill.

Lazarus, R.S. 1991. Emotion theory and psychotherapy. in *Emotion, Psychotherapy, and Change*: edited by J.D. Safran and L.S. Greenberg. New York: Guilford Press.

Lazarus, R.S. 1993. From psychological stress to the emotions: A history of changing outlooks. *Annual Review of Psychology* 44: 1-21.

Lazarus, R. S. 2003a. Does the positive psychology movement have legs? *Psychological Inquiry*, 14: 93-109.

Lazarus, R.S. 2003b. The Lazarus manifesto for positive psychology and psychology in general. *Psychological Inquiry*, 14: 173-189.

Lazarus, R.S. 2006. Emotions and interpersonal relationships: Toward a person-centered conceptualization of emotions and coping. *Journal of Personality* 74 (1): 9-46.

Lazarus, R.S., and S. Folkman. 1984. *Stress, appraisal, and coping.* New York: Springer.

Le Bihan, D. Moderator. 1995. NIH conference: Functional magnetic resonance imaging of the brain.

Leary, T.F. 1957. *Interpersonal diagnosis of personality*: New York: Ronald Press.

LeClerc, D. 1723. *Histoire de la medicine.* Amsterdam: Aux Dépens De La Compagnie.

LeDoux, J.E. 1994. Emotion, memory, and the brain. *Scientific American* (June): 50-57.

LeDuc, P.A., J.A. Caldwell, and P.S. Ruyak. 2000. The effects of exercise as a countermeasure for fatigue in sleep-deprived aviators. *Military Psychology* 12 (4): 249-266.

Lee, S.M., C.R. Burgeson, J.E. Fulton, and C.G. Spain. 2007. Physical education and physical activity: Results from the School Health Policies and Programs Study 2006. *Journal of School Health* 77 (8):435-463.

Lee, Y., D.E. Lopez, E.G. Meloni, and M. Davis. 1996. A primary acoustic startle pathway: Obligatory role of cochlear root neurons and the nucleus reticularis pontis caudalis. *Journal of Neuroscience* 16 (Jun 1): 3775-3789.

Leggio, M.G., L. Mandolesi, F. Federico, et al. 2005. Environmental enrichment promotes improved spatial abilities and enhanced dendritic growth in the rat. *Behavioural Brain Research* 163 (1): 78-90.

Lehtinen, V., and M. Joukamaa. 1994. Epidemiology of depression: Prevalence, risk factors and treatment situation. *Acta Psychiatrica Scandinavica* (Suppl.) 377: 7-10.

Leibenluft, E. 1998. Why are so many women depressed? *Scientific American Presents* 9 (2): 52-60.

Leng, G.C., B. Fowler, and E. Ernst. 2000. Exercise for intermittent claudication. *Cochrane Database of Systematic Reviews* (2): CD000990.

Leonard, F.E. 1919. Pioneers of modern physical training. New York: Association Press.

Letourneau, C. 1878. *Physiologie des passions*. Paris: C. Reinwald et Cie.

LeUnes, A., and J. Burger. 1998. Bibliography on the Profile of Mood States in sport and exercise psychology research, 1971-1998. *Journal of Sport Behavior* 21 (1): 53-70.

Levi, A., J.D. Eldridge, and B.M. Paterson. 1985. Molecular cloning of a gene sequence regulated by nerve growth factor. *Science* 229 (4711): 393-395.

Levi, A., G.L. Ferri, E. Watson, R. Possenti, and S.R. Salton. 2004. Processing, distribution, and function of VGF, a neuronal and endocrine peptide precursor. *Cellular and Molecular Neurobiology* 24 (4): 517-533.

Lewin, K. 1935. *A dynamic theory of personality*. New York: McGraw-Hill.

Lewis, S.J. G., A. Dove, T.W. Robbins, R.A. Barker, and A.M. Owen. 2003. Cognitive impairments in early Parkinson's disease are accompanied by reductions in activity in frontostriatal neural circuitry. *Journal of Neuroscience* 23 (15): 6351-6356.

Lezak, M.D., D.B. Howieson, and D.W. Loring. 2004. *Neuropsychological assessment*. 4th ed. New York: Oxford University Press.

Li, F., K.J. Fisher, P. Harmer, D. Irbe, R.G. Tearse, and B.S. Weimer. 2004. Tai Chi and self-rated quality of sleep and daytime sleepiness in older adults: A randomized controlled trial. *Journal of the American Geriatrics Society* 58: 892-900.

Liddle, S.D., G.D. Baxter, and J.H. Gracey. 2004. Exercise and chronic low back pain: What works? *Pain* 107 (1-2): 176-190.

Lieberman, H.R., C.M. Falco, and S.S. Slade. 2002. Carbohydrate administration during a day of sustained aerobic activity improves vigilance, as assessed by a novel ambulatory monitoring device, and mood. *American Journal of Clinical Nutrition* 76 (1): 120-127.

Lief, A. Ed. 1948. *The commonsense psychiatry of Dr. Adolf Meyer*. New York: McGraw-Hill.

Lightfoot, J.T. 2011. Current understanding of the genetic basis for physical activity. *Journal of Nutrition* 141 (3): 526.

Likert, R. 1932. The method of constructing an attitude scale. *Archives of Psychology* 140: 44-53.

Lim, J., and D.F. Dinges. 2010. A meta-analysis of the impact of short-term sleep deprivation on cognitive variables. *Psychological Bulletin* 136 (3): 375-389.

Lindsley, D.B. 1952. Psychological phenomena and the electroencephalogram. *Electroencephalography and Clinical Neurophysiology* 4: 443-456.

Lindwall, M., H. Asci, and M.S. Hagger. 2011. Factorial validity and measurement invariance of the Revised Physical Self-Perception Profile (PSPP-R) in three countries. *Psychology, Health & Medicine* 16 (1): 115-128.

Lindwall, M., M. Rennemark, and T. Berggren. 2008. Movement in mind: The relationship of exercise with cognitive status for older adults in the Swedish National Study on Aging and Care (SNAC). *Aging & Mental Health* 12 (2): 212-220.

Linenger, J.M., C.V. Chesson, II, and D.S. Nice. 1991. Physical fitness gains following simple environmental change. *American Journal of Preventive Medicine* 7 (5): 298-310.

Lippke, S., R. Schwarzer, J.P. Ziegelmann, U. Scholz, and B. Schuz. 2010. Testing stage-specific effects of a stage-matched intervention: A randomized controlled trial targeting physical exercise and its predictors. *Health Education & Behavior* 37 (4): 533-546.

Lirgg, C.D. 1991. Gender differences in self-confidence in physical activity: A meta-analysis of recent studies. *Journal of Sport & Exercise Psychology* 13 (3): 294-310.

Littre, E. 1839-1861. *Oeuvres completes d'Hippocrate*. Paris: Brillière.

Liu, W.T., C.H. Wang, H.C. Lin, et al. 2008. Efficacy of a cell phone-based exercise programme for COPD. *European Respiratory Journal* 32 (3): 651-659.

Lloyd-Jones, D., R. Adams, M. Carnethon, et al. 2009. Heart disease and stroke statistics—2009 Update. *Circulation* 119 (3): e21-e181.

Long, B.C., and R. van Stavel. 1995. Effects of exercise training on anxiety: A meta-analysis. *Journal of Applied Sport Psychology* 7: 167-189.

Long, M.A. 1995. A study of dental anxiety in a Belfast population. *Journal of the Irish Dental Association* 41 (1): 2-5.

Lopez, A.D., C.D. Mathers, M. Ezzati, D.T. Jamison, and C.J. Murray. 2006. Global and regional burden of disease and risk factors, 2001: Systematic analysis of population health data. *Lancet* 367 (9524): 1747-1757.

Lox, C.L., E. McAuley, and R.S. Tucker. 1995. Exercise as an intervention for enhancing subjective well-being in an HIV-1 population. *Journal of Sport & Exercise Psychology; Journal of Sport & Exercise Psychology.* 17 (4): 345-362.

Lowry, R., S.M. Lee, J.E. Fulton, and L. Kann. 2009. Healthy People 2010 objectives for physical activity, physical education, and television viewing among adolescents: National trends from the Youth Risk Behavior Surveillance System, 1999-2007. *Journal of Physical Activity & Health* 6 (Suppl. 1): S36-S45.

Lubans, D.R., C. Foster, and S.J.H. Biddle. 2008. A review of mediators of behavior in interventions to promote physical activity among children and adolescents. *Preventive Medicine* 47 (5): 463-470.

Luck, S.J. 2005. *An introduction to the event-related potential technique.* Boston: MIT Press.

Luepker, R.V., D.M. Murray, D.R. Jacobs, et al. 1994. Community education for cardiovascular disease prevention: Risk factor changes in the Minnesota Heart Health Program. *American Journal of Public Health* 84: 1383-1393.

Luepker, R.V., C.L. Perry, S.M. McKinlay, et al. 1996. Outcomes of a field trial to improve children's dietary patterns and physical activity. The Child and Adolescent Trial for Cardiovascular Health. CATCH collaborative group. *Journal of the American Medical Association* 275 (Mar 13): 768-776.

Lundahl, B.W., C. Kunz, C. Brownell, D. Tollefson, and B.L. Burke. 2010. A meta-analysis of motivational interviewing: Twenty-five years of empirical studies. *Research on Social Work Practice* 20 (2): 137-160.

Luppino, F.S., L.M. de Wit, P.F. Bouvy, et al. 2010. Overweight, obesity, and depression: A systematic review and meta-analysis of longitudinal studies. *Archives of General Psychiatry* 67 (3): 220.

Lutter, M., and E.J. Nestler. 2009. Homeostatic and hedonic signals interact in the regulation of food intake. *Journal of Nutrition* 139 (3): 629-632.

Maas, J.W. 1979. Biochemistry of the affective disorders. *Hospital Practice* 14 (May): 113-120.

MacDonald, J.R. 2002. Potential causes, mechanisms, and implications of post exercise hypotension. *Journal of Human Hypertension* 16 (4): 225-236.

Macedo, L.G, C.G Maher, J. Latimer, and J.H McAuley. 2009. Motor control exercise for persistent, nonspecific low back pain: A systematic review. *Physical Therapy* 89 (1): 9-25.

Macera, C.A., K.L. Jackson, G.W. Hagenmaier, J.J. Kronenfeld, H.W. Kohl, and S.N. Blair. 1989. Age, physical activity, physical fitness, body composition, and incidence of orthopedic problems. *Research Quarterly for Exercise & Sport* 60 (3): 225-233.

Macmillan, M.B. 2000. Restoring Phineas Gage. *Journal of the History of Neurosciences* 9: 42-62.

Madden, D.J., J. Spaniol, M.C. Costello, et al. 2009. Cerebral white matter integrity mediates adult age differences in cognitive performance. *Journal of Cognitive Neuroscience* 21 (2): 289-302.

Maddock, R.J., C.S. Carter, and D.W. Gietzen. 1991. Elevated serum lactate associated with panic attacks induced by hyperventilation. *Psychiatry Research* 38 (Sept): 301-311.

Maddocks, M., S. Mockett, and A. Wilcock. 2009. Is exercise an acceptable and practical therapy for people with or cured of cancer? A systematic review. *Cancer Treatment Reviews* 35 (4): v383-390.

Maimonides, M. 1199. *Treatise on a hygiene.*

Manchikanti, L., V. Singh, S. Datta, S.P. Cohen, and J.A. Hirsch. 2009. Comprehensive review of epidemiology, scope and impact of spinal pain. *Pain Physician* 12: E35-E70.

Mancuso, C.A., M. Rincon, W. Sayles, and S.A. Paget. 2007. Comparison of energy expenditure from lifestyle physical activities between patients with rheumatoid arthritis and healthy controls. *Arthritis Care & Research* 57 (4): 672-678.

Mansour, A., C.A. Fox, H. Akil, and S.J. Watson. 1995. Opioid-receptor mRNA expression in the rat CNS: Anatomical and functional implications. *Trends in Neurosciences* 18 (1): 22-29.

Marchetti, C., and S. Della Sala. 1998. Disentangling the alien and anarchic hand. *Cognitive Neuropsychiatry* 3 (3): 191-207.

Marcora, S. 2009a. Last word on viewpoint: Perception of effort during exercise is independent of afferent feedback from skeletal muscles, heart, and lungs. *Journal of Applied Physiology* 106 (6): 2067.

Marcora, S. 2009b. Perception of effort during exercise is independent of afferent feedback from skeletal muscles, heart, and lungs. *Journal of Applied Physiology* 106 (6): 2060-2062.

Marcora, S.M. 2011. Role of feedback from Group III and IV muscle afferents in perception of effort, muscle pain, and discomfort. *Journal of Applied Physiology* 110 (5): 1499; author reply 1500.

Marcus, B.H., J.T. Ciccolo, and C.N. Sciamanna. 2009. Using electronic/computer interventions to promote physical activity. *British Journal of Sports Medicine* 43 (2): 102-105.

Marcus, B.H., C.A. Eaton, J.S. Rossi, et al. 1994. Self-efficacy, decision-making and the stages of change: An integrative model of physical exercise. *Journal of Applied Social Psychology* 24: 489-508.

Mason, J.W., J.T. Maher, L.H. Hartley, E. Mougey, M.J. Perlow, and L.G. Jones. 1976. Selectivity of corticosteroid and catecholamine responses to various natural stimuli. In *Psychopathology of human adaptation*, edited by G. Serban, 147-171. New York: Plenum.

Marcus, B.H., V.C. Selby, R.S. Niaura, and J.S. Rossi. 1992. Self-efficacy and the stages of exercise behavior change. *Research Quarterly for Exercise and Sport* 63 (1): 60-66.

Marcus, B.H., and L.R. Simkin. 1993. The stages of exercise behavior. *Journal of Sports Medicine and Physical Fitness* 33: 83-88.

Marcus, B.H., and A.L. Stanton. 1993. Evaluation of relapse prevention and reinforcement interventions to promote exercise adherence in sedentary females. *Research Quarterly for Exercise and Sport* 64: 447-452.

Marcus, B.H., D.M. Williams, P.M. Dubbert, et al. 2006. Physical activity intervention studies: What we know and what we need to know: A scientific statement from the American Heart Association Council on Nutrition, Physical Activity, and Metabolism (Subcommittee on Physical Activity); Council on Cardiovascular Disease in the Young; and the Interdisciplinary Working Group on Quality of Care and Outcomes Research. *Circulation* 114 (24): 2739-2752.

Markland, D., and L. Hardy. 1993. The exercise motivation inventory: Preliminary development and validity of a measure of individuals' reasons for participation in regular physical exercise. *Personality and Individual Differences* 15 (3): 289-296.

Marks, B.L., D.J. Madden, B. Bucur, et al. 2007. Role of aerobic fitness and aging on cerebral white matter integrity. *Annals of the New York Academy of Sciences* 1097: 171-174.

Marlatt, G.A., and J.R. Gordon. 1985. *Relapse prevention: Maintenance strategies in addictive behavior change.* New York: Guilford Press.

Maroulakis, E., and Y. Zervas. 1993. Effects of aerobic exercise on mood of adult women. *Perceptual and Motor Skills* 76 (3): 795-801.

Marsh, H.W. 1990. The structure of academic self-concept: The Marsh/Shavelson model. *Journal of Educational Psychology* 82 (4): 623-636.

Marsh, H.W. 1993. Physical fitness self-concept: Relations of physical fitness to field and technical indicators for boys and girls aged 9-25. *Journal of Sport & Exercise Psychology* 15 (2): 184-206.

Marsh, H.W. 1997. The measurement of physical self-concept: A construct validation approach. In *The physical self: From motivation to well-being.* edited by K.R. Fox. Champaign, IL: Human Kinetics.

Marsh, H.W. 1998. Age and gender effects in physical self-concepts for adolescent elite athletes and non-athletes: A multicohort-multioccasion design. *Journal of Sport & Exercise Psychology* 20 (3): 237-259.

Marsh, H.W. 1999. Cognitive discrepancy models: Actual, ideal, potential, and future self-perspectives of body image. *Social Cognition* 17 (1): 46-75.

Marsh, H.W., J. Hey, L.A. Roche, and C. Perry. 1997. Structure of physical self-concept: Elite athletes and physical education students. *Journal of Educational Psychology* 89 (2): 369-380.

Marsh, H.W., A.J. Martin, and S. Jackson. 2010. Introducing a short version of the physical self description questionnaire: New strategies, short-form evaluative criteria, and applications of factor analyses. *Journal of Sport & Exercise Psychology* 32 (4): 438-482.

Marsh, H.W., and R. O'Neill. 1984. Self Description Questionnaire III: The construct validity of multidimensional self-concept ratings by late adolescents. *Journal of Educational Measurement* 21 (2): 153-174.

Marsh, H.W., J. Parker, and J. Barnes. 1985. Multidimensional adolescent self-concepts: Their relationship to age, sex, and academic measures. *American Educational Research Journal* 22 (3): 422-444.

Marsh, H.W., G.E. Richards, S. Johnson, and L. Roche. 1994. Physical Self-Description Questionnaire: Psychometric properties and a multitrait-multimethod analysis of relations to existing instruments. *Journal of Sport & Exercise Psychology* 16 (3): 270-305.

Marsh, H.W., I.D. Smith, and J. Barnes. 1983. Multitrait-multimethod analyses of the Self-Description Questionnaire: Student-teacher agreement on multidimensional ratings of student self-concept. *American Educational Research Journal* 20 (3): 333-357.

Marsh, H.W., and A.S. Yeung. 1998. Top-down, bottom-up, and horizontal models: The direction of causality in multidimensional, hierarchical self-concept models. *Journal of Personality and Social Psychology* 75 (2): 5509-5527.

Martin, C.K., T.S. Church, A.M. Thompson, C.P. Earnest, and S.N. Blair. 2009. Exercise dose and quality of life: A randomized controlled trial. *Archives of Internal Medicine* 169 (3): 269-278.

Martin, J.L., M.R. Marler, J.O. Harker, K.R. Josephson, and C.A. Alessi. 2007. A multicomponent nonpharmacological intervention improves activity rhythms among nursing home residents with disrupted sleep/wake patterns. *Journals of Gerontology. Series A, Biological Sciences and Medical Sciences* 62 (1): 67-72.

Martin, P., A. Bishop, L. Poon, and M.A. Johnson. 2006. Influence of personality and health behaviors on fatigue in late and very late life. *Journals of Gerontology. Series B, Psychological Sciences and Social Sciences* 61 (3): P161-P166.

Martin Ginis, K.A., S.M. Burke, and Lise Gauvin. 2007. Exercising with others exacerbates the negative effects of mirrored environments on sedentary women's feeling states. *Psychology & Health* 22 (8): 945-962.

Martin Ginis, K.A., and A.E. Latimer. 2007. The effects of single bouts of body-weight supported treadmill training on the feeling states of people with spinal cord injury. *Spinal Cord* 45 (1): 11112-11115.

Martinsen, E.W. 1990. Physical fitness, anxiety and depression. *British Journal of Hospital Medicine* 43 (3): 194, 196, 199.

Martinsen, E.W. 1993. Therapeutic implications of exercise for clinically anxious and depressed patients. *International Journal of Sport Psychology.* 24 (2): 185-199.

Martinsen, E.W. 2008. Physical activity and depression: Clinical experience. *Acta Psychiatrica Scandinavica* (Suppl.) 377: 23-27.

Martinsen, E.W. 2008. Physical activity in the prevention and treatment of anxiety and depression. *Nordic Journal of Psychiatry* 62 (Suppl. 47): 25-29.

Martinsen, E.W., A. Hoffart, and O. Solberg. 1989. Comparing aerobic with nonaerobic forms of exercise in the treatment of clinical depression: A randomized trial. *Comprehensive Psychiatry* 30 (Jul-Aug): 324-331.

Martinsen, E.W., A. Medhus, and L. Sandvik. 1985. Effects of aerobic exercise on depression: A controlled study. *British Medical Journal (Clinical Research Ed.)* 291 (July 13): 109.

Martinsen, E.W., T. Olsen, E. Tonset, K.E. Nyland, and T.F. Aarre. 1998B. Cognitive-behavioral group therapy for panic disorder in the general clinical setting: A naturalistic study with 1-year follow-up. *Journal of Clinical Psychiatry* 59 (8): 437-442; quiz 443.

Martinsen, E.W., J.S. Raglin, A. Hoffart, and S. Friis. 1998. Tolerance to intensive exercise and high levels of lactate in panic disorder. *Journal of Anxiety Disorders* 12 (4): 333-342.

Martinsen, E.W., L. Sandvik, and O.B. Kolbjornsrud. 1989. Aerobic exercise in the treatment of nonpsychotic mental disorders: An exploratory study. *Nordisk Psykiatrisk Tidsskrift* 43 (6): 521-529.

Martinsen, E.W., J. Strand, G. Paulsson, and J. Kaggestad. 1989. Physical fitness level in patients with anxiety and depressive disorders. *International Journal of Sports Medicine* 10 (Feb): 58-61.

Masley, S., R. Roetzheim, and T. Gualtieri. 2009. Aerobic exercise enhances cognitive flexibility. *Journal of Clinical Psychology in Medical Settings* 16 (2): 186-193.

Masse, L.C., C. Nigg, K. Basen-Engquist, and A.A. Atienza. 2011. Understanding the mechanism of physical activity behavior change:

Mathers, C.D., and D. Loncar. 2006. Projections of global mortality and burden of disease from 2002 to 2030. *PloS Medicine* 3 (11): e442.

Mathes, W.F., D.L. Nehrenberg, R. Gordon, K. Hua, T. Garland, Jr., and D. Pomp. 2010. Dopaminergic dysregulation in mice selectively bred for excessive exercise or obesity. *Behavioural Brain Research* 210 (2): 155-163.

Matthews, C.E., K.Y. Chen, P.S. Freedson, et al. 2008. Amount of time spent in sedentary behaviors in the United States, 2003-2004. *American Journal of Epidemiology* 167 (7): 875-881.

Matthews, V.B., M.B. Astrom, M.H. Chan, et al. 2009. Brain-derived neurotrophic factor is produced by skeletal muscle cells in response to contraction and enhances fat oxidation via activation of AMP-activated protein kinase. *Diabetologia* 52 (7): 1409-1418.

Mauger, A.R., A.M. Jones, and C.A. Williams. 2010. Influence of acetaminophen on performance during time trial cycling. *Journal of Applied Physiology* 108 (1): 98-104.

Mausner, J.S., and S. Kramer. 1985. *Epidemiology: An introductory text.* 2nd ed. Philadelphia: Saunders.

McAuley, E. 1994. Physical activity and psychosocial outcomes. In *Physical activity, fitness, and health: International proceedings and consensus statement,* edited by Bouchard, C. and R.J. Shephard Champaign, IL: Human Kinetics.

McAuley, E., S.M. Bane, D.L. Rudolph, and C.L. Lox. 1995. Physique anxiety and exercise in middle-aged adults. *Journals of Gerontology: Series B: Psychological Sciences and Social Sciences* 50 (5): 229-235.

McAuley, E., and B. Blissmer. 2000. Self-efficacy determinants and consequences of physical activity. *Exercise and Sport Sciences Reviews* 28: 85-88.

McAuley, E., and K.S. Courneya. 1994. The Subjective Exercise Experiences Scale (SEES): Development and preliminary validation. *Journal of Sport & Exercise Psychology* 16 (2): 163-177.

McAuley, E., K.S. Courneya, D.L. Rudolph, and C.L. Lox. 1994. Enhancing exercise adherence in middle-aged males and females. *Preventive Medicine.* 23: 498-506.

McAuley, E., S. Elavsky, R.W. Motl, J.F. Konopack, L. Hu, and D.X. Marquez. 2005. Physical activity, self-efficacy, and self-esteem: Longitudinal relationships in older adults. *Journals of Gerontology. Series B, Psychological Sciences and Social Sciences* 60 (5): P268-P275.

McAuley, E., C.L. Lox, and S.C. Duncan. 1993. Long-term maintenance of exercise, self-efficacy, and physiological change in older adults. *Journal of Gerontology* 48 (4): 218-224.

McAuley, E., S.L. Mihalko, and S.M. Bane. 1997. Exercise and self-esteem in middle-aged adults: Multidimensional relationships and physical fitness and self-efficacy influences. *Journal of Behavioral Medicine* 20 (1): 67-83.

McCabe, P.M., J.F. Sheridan, J.M. Weiss, J.P. Kaplan, B.H. Natelson, and W.P. Pare. 2000. Animal models of disease. *Physiology and Behavior* 68 (Feb): 501-507.

McCloskey, D.I. 1978. Kinesthetic sensibility. *Physiological reviews* 58 (4): 763-820.

McCrae, R.R., and P.T. Costa. 2003. *Personality in adulthood: A five-factor theory perspective.* New York: Guilford Press.

McCrae, R.R., P.T. Costa, Jr., F. Ostendorf, et al. 2000. Nature over nurture: Temperament, personality, and life span development. *Journal of Personality and Social Psychology* 78 (1): 173-186.

McCrae, R.R., and O.P. John. 1992. An introduction to the five-factor model and its applications. *Journal of Personality* 60 (2): 175-215.

McCulloch, T.L., and J.S. Bruner. 1939. The effect of electric shock upon subsequent learning in the rat. *Journal of Psychology* 7: 333-336.

McDermott, L.M., and K.P. Ebmeir. 2009. A meta-analysis of depression severity and cognitive function. *Journal of Affective Disorders* 119: 1-8.

McDonald, D.G., and J.A. Hodgdon. 1991. *The psychological effects of aerobic fitness training: Research and theory.* New York: Springer-Verlag.

McEwen, B.S. 1998. Protective and damaging effects of stress mediators. *New England Journal of Medicine* 338: 171-179.

McFarland, M.B., and P.L. Kaminski. 2009. Men, muscles, and mood: The relationship between self-concept, dysphoria, and body image disturbances. *Eating Behaviors* 10 (1): 68-70.

McGinty, D., and R. Szymusiak. 1990. Keeping cool: A hypothesis about the mechanisms and functions of slow wave sleep. *Trends in Neurosciences* 13: 480-487.

McGrae McDermott, M., S. Mehta, and P. Greenland. 1999. Exertional leg symptoms other than intermittent claudication are common in peripheral arterial disease. *Archives of Internal Medicine* 159 (4): 387-392.

McMahon, S.B., and M. Koltzenburg. 2005. *Wall and Melzack's textbook of pain*. 5th ed. Philadelphia: Churchill Livingstone.

McMorris, T., and J. Graydon. 2000. The effect of incremental exercise on cognitive performance. *International Journal of Sport Psychology* 31: 66-81.

McMorris, T., J. Sproule, A. Turner, and B.J. Hale. 2011. Acute, intermediate intensity exercise, and speed and accuracy in working memory tasks: A meta-analytical comparison of effects. *Physiology & Behavior* 102 (3-4): 421-428.

McMorris, T., P.D. Tomporowski, and M. Audiffren, eds. 2009. *Exercise and cognition*. Chichester, UK: John Wiley & Sons.

McNair, D.M., M. Lorr, and L.F. Droppleman. 1981. *Manual for the Profile of Mood States*. San Diego, CA: Educational and Industrial Testing Service.

McNally, R.J., E.B. Foa, and C.D. Donnell. 1989. Memory bias for anxiety information in patients with panic disorder. *Cognition & Emotion* 3 (1): 27-44.

McNeely, M.L., M.B. Parliament, H. Seikaly, et al. 2008. Effect of exercise on upper extremity pain and dysfunction in head and neck cancer survivors. *Cancer* 113 (1): 214-222.

McNeil, J.K., E.M. LeBlanc, and M. Joyner. 1991. The effect of exercise on depressive symptoms in the moderately depressed elderly. *Psychology & Aging* 6 (3): 487-488.

McNeill, L.H., M.W. Kreuter, and S.V. Subramanian. 2006. Social environment and physical activity: A review of concepts and evidence. *Social Science & Medicine* 63 (4): 1011-1022.

McSherry, J.A. 1984. The diagnostic challenge of anorexia nervosa. *American Family Physician* 29 (Feb): 141-145.

Mead, G.E., W. Morley, P. Campbell, C.A. Greig, M. McMurdo, and D.A. Lawlor. 2009. Exercise for depression. *Cochrane Database of Systematic Reviews* (3): CD004366.

Meeusen, R. 2009. Commentaries on Viewpoint: Perception of effort during exercise is independent of afferent feedback from skeletal muscles, heart, and lungs. *Journal of Applied Physiology* 106 (6): 2063.

Meeusen, R., and K. De Meirleir. 1995. Exercise and brain neurotransmission. *Sports Medicine* 20 (3): 160-188.

Meeusen, R., I. Smolders, S. Sarre, et al. 1997. Endurance training effects on neurotransmitter release in rat striatum: An in vivo microdialysis study. *Acta Psychiatrica Scandinavica* 159 (Apr): 335-341.

Mehrabian, A. 1970. A semantic space for nonverbal behavior. *Journal of Consulting and Clinical Psychology*. 35 (2): 248-257.

Mehrabian, A, and J.A. Russell. 1974. *An approach to environmental psychology*. Cambridge, MA: MIT.

Meichenbaum, D. 1977. *Cognitive-behavior modification: An integrative approach*. New York: Plenum Press.

Meichenbaum, D., and R. Cameron. 1974. The clinical potential of modifying what clients say to themselves. *Psychotherapy: Theory, Research & Practice* 11 (2): 103-117.

Meichenbaum, D.H., and J. Goodman. 1971. Training impulsive children to talk to themselves: A means of developing self-control. *Journal of Abnormal Psychology* 77 (2): 115-126.

Mellinger, G.D., M.B. Balter, and E.H. Uhlenhuth. 1985. Insomnia and its treatment. Prevalence and correlates. *Archives of General Psychiatry* 42: 225-232.

Meloni, E.G., and M. Davis. 1999. Enhancement of the acoustic startle response in rats by the dopamine D-sub-1 receptor agonist SKF 82958. *Psychopharmacology* 144 (4): 373-380.

Menard, J., and D. Treit. 1999. Effects of centrally administered anxiolytic compounds in animal models of anxiety. *Neuroscience and Biobehavioral Reviews* 23 (Mar): 591-613.

Mense, S. 2009. Algesic agents exciting muscle nociceptors. *Experimental Brain Research* 196 (1): 89-100.

Merom, D., A. Bauman, P. Phongsavan, et al. 2009. Can a motivational intervention overcome an unsupportive environment for walking: Findings from the Step-by-Step study. *Annals of Behavioral Medicine* 38 (2): 137-146.

Merom, D., P. Phongsavan, R. Wagner, et al. 2008. Promoting walking as an adjunct intervention to group cognitive behavioral therapy for anxiety disorders: A pilot group randomized trial. *Journal of Anxiety Disorders* 22 (6): 959-968.

Messick, S. 1989. Validity. In *Educational measurement*, edited by R.L. Linn. 3rd ed. New York: Macmillan.

Messier, S.P., R.F. Loeser, G.D. Miller, et al. 2004. Exercise and dietary weight loss in overweight and obese older adults with knee osteoarthritis: The arthritis, diet, and activity promotion trial. *Arthritis & Rheumatism* 50 (5): 1501-1510.

Michael, E.D. 1957. Stress adaptations through exercise. *American Association for Health, Physical Education, and Recreation: Research Quarterly* 28: 50-54.

Michie, S., S. Ashford, F.F. Sniehotta, S.U. Dombrowski, A. Bishop, and D.P. French. 2011. A refined taxonomy of behaviour change techniques to help people change their physical activity and healthy eating behaviours: The CALO-RE taxonomy. *Psychology & Health* 26: 1479-1498.

Michie, S., M. Johnston, J. Francis, W. Hardeman, and M. Eccles. 2008. From theory to intervention: Mapping theoretically derived behavioural determinants to behaviour change techniques. *Applied Psychology* 57 (4): 660-680.

Mikkelsen, S.S., J.S. Tolstrup, E.M. Flachs, E.L. Mortensen, P. Schnohr, and T. Flensborg-Madsen. 2010. A cohort study of leisure time physical activity and depression. *Preventive Medicine* 51 (6): 471-475.

Milani, R.V., and C.J. Lavie. 2007. The role of exercise training in peripheral arterial disease. *Vascular Medicine* 12 (4): 351-358.

Miller, G.A. 1956. The magical number seven, plus or minus two: Some limits on our capacity for processing information. *Psychological Review* 63: 81-97.

Mikkelsen, S.S., J.S. Tolstrup, E.M. Flachs, E.L. Mortensen, P. Schnohr, and T. Flensborg-Madsen. 2010. A cohort study of leisure time physical activity and depression. *Preventive Medicine* 51 (6): 471-475.

Milne, H.M., K.E. Wallman, S. Gordon, and K.S. Courneya. 2008. Effects of a combined aerobic and resistance exercise program in breast cancer survivors: A randomized controlled trial. *Breast Cancer Research and Treatment* 108 (2): 279-288.

Mitchell J.H, and P.B. Raven. 1994. Cardiovascular adaptation to physical activity. In *Physical activity, fitness, and health: International proceedings and consensus statement*, edited by C. Bouchard, R.J. Shephard, and T. Stephens. Champaign, IL: Human Kinetics.

Mittenberg, W., C. Patton, E.M. Canyock, and D.C. Condit. 2002. Base rates of malingering and symptom exaggeration. *Journal of Clinical and Experimental Neuropsychology* 24 (8): 1094-1102.

Miyake, A., N.P. Friedman, M.J. Emerson, A.H. Witzki, A. Howerter, and T.D. Wager. 2000. The unity and diversity of executive functions and their contributions to complex "frontal lobe" tasks: A latent variable analysis. *Cognitive Psychology* 41: 49-100.

Mogenson, G.J. 1987. Limbic-motor integration. *Progress in Psychobiology and Physiological Psychology* 12: 117-170.

Molloy, G.J., D. Dixon, M. Hamer, and F.F. Sniehotta. 2010. Social support and regular physical activity: Does planning mediate this link? *British Journal of Health Psychology* 15: 859-870.

Molteni, R., R.J. Barnard, Z. Ying, K. Roberts, and F. Gomez-Pinilla. 2002. A high-fat, refined sugar diet reduces hippocampal brain-derived neurotrophic factor, neuronal plasticity, and learning. *Neuroscience* 112 (4): 803-814.

Moore, J.B., N.G. Mitchell, W.S. Bibeau, and J.B. Bartholomew. 2011. Effects of a 12-week resistance exercise program on physical self-perceptions in college students. *Research Quarterly for Exercise and Sport* 82, 291-301.

Moos, R.H. 1979. Social-ecological perspectives on health. Edited by G.C. Stone, F. Cohen and N.E. Adler. In *Health psychology: A handbook*. San Francisco: Jossey–Bass.

Monahan, T. 1988. Perceived exertion: An old exercise tool finds new applications. *Physician and Sportsmedicine* 16: 174-179.

Mondin, G.W., W.P. Morgan, P.N. Piering, and A.J. Stegner. 1996. Psychological consequences of exercise deprivation in habitual exercisers. *Medicine & Science in Sports & Exercise* 28 (9): 1199-1203.

Monti, J.M. 2010. Serotonin 5-HT(2A) receptor antagonists in the treatment of insomnia: Present status and future prospects. *Drugs of Today* 46 (3): 183-193.

Morabia, A., and M.C. Costanza. 2011. Physical activity or academic achievement? Both! *Preventive Medicine* 52: S1-S2.

Morey, M.C., D.C. Snyder, R. Sloane, et al. 2009. Effects of home-based diet and exercise on functional outcomes among older, overweight long-term cancer survivors: RENEW: A randomized controlled trial. *Journal of the American Medical Association* 301 (18): 1883-1891.

Morgan, K. 2003. Daytime activity and risk factors for late-life insomnia. *Journal of Sleep Research* 12 (3): 231-238.

Morgan, W.P. 1968. Selected physiological and psychomotor correlates of depression in psychiatric patients. *Research Quarterly* 39 (Dec): 1037-1043.

Morgan, W.P. 1969. A pilot investigation of physical working capacity in depressed and nondepressed psychiatric males. *Research Quarterly* 40 (Dec): 859-861.

Morgan, W.P. 1970. Physical working capacity in depressed and non-depressed psychiatric females: A preliminary study. *American Corrective Therapy Journal* 24 (Jan-Feb): 14-16.

Morgan, W.P. 1973a. Influences of acute physical activity on state anxiety. In *Proceedings, Annual Meeting of the College Physical Education Association for Men*, edited by C.E. Mueller. Minneapolis: University of Minnesota.

Morgan, W.P. 1973b. Psychological factors influencing perceived exertion. *Medicine and Science in Sports* 5 (2): 97-103.

Morgan, W.P. 1977. Involvement in vigorous physical activity with special reference to adherence. In *Proceedings of the National College Physical Education Association*, edited by L.I. Gedvilas and M.W. Kneer. Chicago: University of Illinois–Chicago Publications.

Morgan, W.P. 1979a. Anxiety reduction following acute physical activity. *Psychiatric Annals* 9 (3): 36-45.

Morgan, W.P. 1979b. Negative addiction in runners. *Physician and Sportsmedicine* 7: 57-70.

Morgan, W.P. 1981. Psychophysiology of self-awareness during vigorous physical activity. *Research Quarterly for Exercise and Sport.* 52 (3): 385-427.

Morgan WP. 1985. Affective beneficence of vigorous physical activity. *Medicine and Science in Sports and Exercise.* 17(1), 94-100.

Morgan, W.P. 1986. Presidential message. *American Psychological Association Newsletter, Division 47, Exercise and Sport Psychology* 1 (1): 1-2.

Morgan, W.P. 1994a. 40 years of progress: Sport psychology in exercise science and sports medicine. *40th Anniversary Lecture.* American College of Sports Medicine: 81-92.

Morgan, W.P. 1994b. Physical activity, fitness, and depression. In *Physical activity, fitness, and health: International proceedings and consensus statement,* edited by C. Bouchard, R.J. Shephard, and T. Stephens. Champaign, IL: Human Kinetics.

Morgan, W.P. 1997. Methodological considerations. In *Physical activity and mental health,* edited by W. P. Morgan. From *The series in psychology and behavioral medicine.* Washington, DC: Taylor & Francis.

Morgan, W., D. Brown, J. Raglin, P. O'connor, and K. Ellickson. 1987. Psychological monitoring of overtraining and staleness. *British Journal of Sports Medicine.* 21 (3): 107-114.

Morgan, W.P., D.L. Costill, M.G. Flynn, and J.S. Raglin. 1988. Mood disturbance following increased training in swimmers. *Medicine & Science in Sports & Exercise* 20 (4): 408-414.

Morgan, W.P. and S.E. Goldston. 1987. *Exercise and mental health.* Washington, DC: Hemisphere.

Morgan, W.P., K. Hirota, G.A. Weitz, and B. Balke. 1976. Hypnotic perturbation of perceived exertion: Ventilatory consequences. *American Journal of Clinical Hypnosis* 18 (3): 182-190.

Morgan, W.P., P.B. Raven, B.L. Drinkwater, and S.M. Horvath. 1973. Perceptual and metabolic responsivity to standard bicycle ergometry following various hypnotic suggestions. *International Journal of Clinical & Experimental Hypnosis* (2): 86-101.

Morgan, W. P. and P. J. O'Connor. 1988. Exercise and Mental Health. In *Exercise adherence: Its impact on public health,* edited by R.K. Dishman. Champaign, IL: Human Kinetics.

Morgan, W.P., J.A. Roberts, F.R. Brand, and A.D. Feinerman. 1970. Psychological effect of chronic physical activity. *Medicine & Science in Sports & Exercise* 2 (Winter): 213-217.

Morgan, W.P., J.A. Roberts, and A.D. Feinerman. 1971. Psychologic effect of acute physical activity. *Archives of Physical Medicine and Rehabilitation* 52 (Sep): 422-425.

Morrato, E.H., J.O. Hill, H.R. Wyatt, V. Ghushchyan, and P.W. Sullivan. 2007. Physical activity in U.S. adults with diabetes and at risk for developing diabetes, 2003. *Diabetes Care* 30 (2): 203-209.

Morrow, J.R., Jr., J.A. Krzewinski-Malone, A.W. Jackson, T.J. Bungum, and S.J. FitzGerald. 2004. American adults' knowledge of exercise recommendations. *Research Quarterly for Exercise and Sport* 75 (3): 231-237.

Mosely, L. 2002. Combined physiotherapy and education is efficacious for chronic low back pain. *Australian Journal of Physiotherapy* 48: 297-302.

Motl, R.W., and R.K. Dishman. 2003. Acute leg-cycling exercise attenuates the H-reflex recorded in soleus but not flexor carpi radialis. *Muscle Nerve* 28 (5): 609-614.

Motl, R.W., and R.K. Dishman. 2004. Effects of acute exercise on the soleus H-reflex and self-reported anxiety after caffeine ingestion. *Physiology & Behavior* 80 (4): 577-585.

Motl, R.W., R.K. Dishman, R. Saunders, et al. 2002. Examining social-cognitive determinants of intention and physical activity in adolescent girls using structural equation modeling. *Health Psychology* 21 (5): 459-467.

Motl, R.W., R.K. Dishman, D.S. Ward, et al. 2002. Examining social-cognitive determinants of intention and physical activity among black and white adolescent girls using structural equation modeling. *Health Psychology.* 21 (5): 459-467.

Motl, R.W., D. Dlugonski, T.R. Wojcicki, E. McAuley, and D.C. Mohr. 2011. Internet intervention for increasing physical activity in persons with multiple sclerosis. *Multiple Sclerosis* 17 (1): 116-128.

Motl, R.W., R.C. Gliottoni, and J.A. Scott. 2007. Self-efficacy correlates with leg muscle pain during maximal and submaximal cycling exercise. *Journal of Pain* 8 (7): 583-587.

Motl, R.W., and J.L. Gosney. 2008. Effect of exercise training on quality of life in multiple sclerosis: A meta-analysis. *Multiple Sclerosis* 14 (1): 129-135.

Motl, R.W., B.D. Knowles, and R.K. Dishman. 2003. Acute bouts of active and passive leg cycling attenuate the amplitude of the soleus H-reflex in humans. *Neuroscience Letters* 347 (2): 69-72.

Motl, R.W., J.F. Konopack, E. McAuley, S. Elavsky, G.J. Jerome, and D.X. Marquez. 2005. Depressive symptoms among older adults: Long-term reduction after a physical activity intervention. *Journal of Behavioral Medicine* 28 (4): 385-394.

Motl, R.W., and E. McAuley. 2009a. Pathways between physical activity and quality of life in adults with multiple sclerosis. *Health Psychology* 28 (6): 682-689.

Motl, R.W., and E. McAuley. 2009b. Symptom cluster as a predictor of physical activity in multiple sclerosis: Preliminary evidence. *Journal of Pain and Symptom Management* 38 (2): 270-280.

Motl, R.W., E. McAuley, D. Wynn, Y. Suh, and M. Weikert. 2011. Effects of change in fatigue and depression on physical activity over time in relapsing-remitting multiple sclerosis. *Psychology, Health & Medicine* 16 (1): 1-11.

Motl, R.W., P.J. O'Connor, and R.K. Dishman. 2003. Effect of caffeine on perceptions of leg muscle pain during moderate intensity cycling exercise. *Journal of Pain* 4 (6): 316-321.

Motl, R.W., P.J. O'Connor, and R.K. Dishman. 2004. Effects of cycling exercise on the soleus H-reflex and state anxiety among men with low or high trait anxiety. *Psychophysiology* 41 (1): 96-105.

Motl, R.W., P.J. O'Connor, L. Tubandt, T. Puetz, and M.R. Ely. 2006. Effect of caffeine on leg muscle pain during cycling exercise among females. *Medicine & Science in Sports & Exercise* 38 (3): 598-604. doi: 10.1249/01.mss.0000193558.70995.03.

Motl, R.W., E.M. Snook, and R.T. Schapiro. 2008. Symptoms and physical activity behavior in individuals with multiple sclerosis. *Research in Nursing & Health* 31 (5): 466-475.

Mudry, E., C. Hodgins, N. el-Guebaly, et al. 2011. Conceptualizing excessive behaviour syndromes: A systematic review. *Current Psychiatry Reviews* 7 (2): 138-151.

Müller-Riemenschneider, F., T. Reinhold, M. Nocon, and S.N. Willich. 2008. Long-term effectiveness of interventions promoting physical activity: A systematic review. *Preventive Medicine* 47 (4): 354-368.

Murphy, F.C., I. Nimmo-Smith, and A.D. Lawrence. 2003. Functional neuroanatomy of emotions: A meta-analysis. *Cognitive, Affective & Behavioral Neuroscience* 3 (3): 207-233.

Murray, P.S., J.L. Groves, B.J. Pettett, et al. 2010. Locus coeruleus galanin expression is enhanced after exercise in rats selectively bred for high capacity for aerobic activity. *Peptides* 31 (12): 2264-2268.

Muscio, B. 1921. Is a fatigue test possible? *British Journal of Psychology* 12: 31-46.

Muthén, L.K., and B.O. Muthén. 1998-2010. *Statistical analysis with latent variables, Mplus user's guide.* 4th ed. (edition 6.1). Los Angeles: Muthén & Muthén.

Mutrie, N. 1997. The therapeutic effects of exercise on the self. In *The physical self: From motivation to well-being*, edited by K.R. Fox. Champaign, IL: Human Kinetics.

Mutrie, N., A.M Campbell, F. Whyte, et al. 2007. Benefits of supervised group exercise programme for women being treated for early stage breast cancer: Pragmatic randomised controlled trial. *BMJ* 334 (7592): 517.

Myllymäki, T., H. Kyröläinen, K. Savolainen, et al. 2011. Effects of vigorous late-night exercise on sleep quality and cardiac autonomic activity. *Journal of Sleep Research* 20 (1 Pt 2): 146-153.

Naglieri, J.A., and D. Johnson. 2000. Effectiveness of a cognitive strategy intervention to improve math calculation based on the PASS theory. *Journal of Learning Disabilities* 33: 591-597.

Nakabeppu, Y., and D. Nathans. 1991. A naturally occurring truncated form of FosB that inhibits Fos/Jun transcriptional activity. *Cell* 64 (4): 751-759.

Narayan, K.M.V, J.P. Boyle, L.S. Geiss, J.B. Saaddine, and T.J. Thompson. 2006. Impact of recent increase in incidence on future diabetes burden. *Diabetes Care* 29 (9): 2114-2116.

Narin, S., L. Osün, D. Pinar, V. Erbas, V. Oztürk, and F. Idiman. 2003. The effects of exercise and exercise-related changes in blood nitric oxide level on migraine headache. *Clinical Rehabilitation* 17 (6): 624-630.

National Center for Education Statistics, Integrated Postsecondary Education Data System. 2009. Fall enrollment survey (IPEDS-EF:92–99), and spring 2001 through spring 2007; and enrollment in degree-granting institutions model, 1980–2006. Washington, DC: U.S. Department of Education.

National Center for Health Statistics (NCHS), Centers for Disease Control and Prevention. 2011. *Healthy People 2010 final review*. Accessed April 17, 2012. www.cdc.gov/nchs/healthy_people/hp2010/hp2010_final_review.htm.

National Commission on Sleep Disorders Research. 1993. *Wake up America: A national sleep alert*. Executive summary and executive report. Washington, DC: National Institutes of Health, US Government Printing Office.

National Institutes of Health. 2010. *NIH State-of-the-Science Conference: Manifestations and management of chronic insomnia in adults*. June 13-15, 2005 [cited June 9, 2010]. http://consensus.nih.gov/previous.htm.

Nauta, W.J. H., and M. Feirtag. 1979. *The organization of the brain*. San Francisco: Freeman.

Neeper, S.A., F. Gomez-Pinilla, J. Choi, and C.W. Cotman. 1996. Physical activity increases mRNA for brain-derived neurotrophic factor and nerve growth factor in rat brain. *Brain Research* 726 (1-2): 49-56.

Nelson, M.C., M. Story, N.I. Larson, D. Neumark-Sztainer, and L.A. Lytle. 2008. Emerging adulthood and college-aged youth: An overlooked age for weight-related behavior change. *Obesity* 16 (10): 2205-2211.

Nemeroff, C.B. 1998. The neurobiology of depression. *Scientific American* 278 (6): 42-47.

Nes, L.S., and S.C. Segerstrom. 2006. Dispositional optimism and coping: A meta-analytic review. *Personality and Social Psychology Review* 10 (3): 235-251.

Nestler, E.J., and W.A. Carlezon, Jr. 2006. The mesolimbic dopamine reward circuit in depression. *Biological Psychiatry* 59 (12): 1151-1159.

Nettelbeck, T., and C. Wilson. 1997. Speed of information processing and cognition. In *Ellis' handbook of mental deficiency, psychological theory and research*, edited by W.E. MacLean, Jr. Mahwah, NJ: Erlbaum.

Netz, Y., M.J. Wu, B.J. Becker, and G. Tenenbaum. 2005. Physical activity and psychological well-being in advanced age: A meta-analysis of intervention studies. *Psychology and Aging* 20 (2): 272-284.

Newbold, R.F. 1990. Patterns of anxiety in Sallust, Suetonius and Procopius. *The Ancient History Bulletin* 4 (2): 44-50.

Nigg, C.R., B. Borrelli, J. Maddock, and R.K. Dishman. 2008. A theory of physical activity maintenance. *Applied Psychology* 57 (4): 544-560.

Nigg, C.R., R.W. Motl, C.C. Horwath, K.K. Wertin, and R.K. Dishman. 2011. A research agenda to examine the efficacy and relevance of the transtheoretical model for physical activity behavior. *Psychology of Sport and Exercise* 12 (1): 7-12.

Nigg, C.R., and R.J. Paxton. 2008. Conceptual perspectives. In *Youth physical activity and inactivity: Challenges and solutions*, edited by A.L. Smith and S.J. H. Biddle. Champaign, IL: Human Kinetics.

Noack, H., M. Lovden, F. Schmiedek, and U. Lindenberger. 2009. Cognitive plasticity in adulthood and old age: Gauging the generality of cognitive intervention effects. *Restorative Neurology and Neuroscience* 27: 435-453.

Noble, B.J., G.A. Borg, I. Jacobs, and P. Kaiser. 1983. A category-ratio perceived exertion scale: Relationship to blood and muscle lactates and heart rate. *Medicine & Science in Sports & Exercise* 15: 523-528.

Noble, B.J., and R.J. Robertson. 1996. *Perceived exertion*. Champaign, IL: Human Kinetics.

Nock, M.K., I. Hwang, N.A. Sampson, and R.C. Kessler. 2010. Mental disorders, comorbidity and suicidal behavior: Results from the National Comorbidity Survey Replication. *Molecular Psychiatry* 15 (8): 868-876.

Nock, M.K., I. Hwang, N. Sampson, et al. 2009. Cross-national analysis of the associations among mental disorders and suicidal behavior: Findings from the WHO World Mental Health Surveys. *PloS medicine* 6 (8): e1000123.

North, T.C., P. McCullagh, and Z. Vu Tran. 1990. Effect of exercise on depression. *Exercise and Sport Sciences Reviews* 18: 379-415.

Nunez, P.L., and R. Srinivasan. 2006. *Electric fields of the brain: The neurophysics of EEG*. New York: Oxford University Press.

Nunnally, J.C., and I.H. Bernstein. 1994. *Psychometric theory*. 3rd ed. New York: McGraw-Hill.

Nybo, L., and N.H. Secher. 2004. Cerebral perturbations provoked by prolonged exercise. *Progress in Neurobiology* 72 (4): 223-261.

O'Brien, P.M., and P.J. O'Connor. 2000. Effect of bright light on cycling performance. *Medicine & Science in Sports & Exercise* 32 (2): 439.

O'Connell, A.A., and D.B. McCoach. 2004. Applications of hierarchical linear models for evaluations of health interventions: Demystifying the methods and interpretations of multilevel models. *Evaluation & the Health Professions* 27 (2): 119-151.

O'Connor, P.J., L.E. Aenchbacher, and R.K. Dishman. 1993. Physical activity and depression in the elderly. *Journal of Aging and Physical Activity* 1: 34-58.

O'Connor, P.J., M.J. Breus, and S.D. Youngstedt. 1998. Exercise-induced increase in core temperature does not disrupt a behavioral measure of sleep. *Physiology and Behavio*r 64: 213-217.

O'Connor, P.J., C.X. Bryant, J.P. Veltri, and S.M. Gebhardt. 1993. State anxiety and ambulatory blood pressure following resistance exercise in females. *Medicine & Science in Sports & Exercise* 25 (Apr): 516-521.

O'Connor, P.J., R.D. Carda, and B.K. Graf. 1991. Anxiety and intense running exercise in the presence and absence of interpersonal competition. *International Journal of Sports Medicine* 12: 423-426.

O'Connor, P.J., and D.B. Cook. 1999. Exercise and pain: The neurobiology, measurement, and laboratory study of pain in relation to exercise in humans. *Exercise and Sport Sciences Reviews* 27: 119-166.

O'Connor, P.J., and D.B. Cook. 2001. Moderate-intensity muscle pain can be produced and sustained during cycle ergometry. *Medicine & Science in Sports & Exercise* 33 (6): 1046-1051.

O'Connor, P.J., and J.C. Davis. 1992. Psychobiologic responses to exercise at different times of the day. *Medicine & Science in Sports & Exercise* 24: 714-719.

O'Connor, P.J., M.P. Herring, and A. Caravalho. 2010. Mental health benefits of strength training in adults. *American Journal of Lifestyle Medicine* 45 (5): 377-396.

O'Connor, P.J., R.W. Motl, S.P. Broglio, and M.R. Ely. 2004. Dose-dependent effect of caffeine on reducing leg muscle pain during cycling exercise is unrelated to systolic blood pressure. *Pain* 109 (3): 291-298.

O'Connor, P.J., S.J. Petruzzello, K.A. Kubitz, and T.L. Robinson. 1995. Anxiety responses to maximal exercise testing. *British Journal of Sports Medicine* 29: 97-102.

O'Connor, P.J., J.S. Raglin, and E.W. Martinsen. 2000. Physical activity, anxiety and anxiety disorders. *International Journal of Sport Psychology* 31 (2): 136-155.

O'Connor, P.J., and J.C. Smith. 1999. Physical activity and eating disorders. In *Lifestyle medicine*, edited by J.M. Rippe. Cambridge, MA: Blackwell Science.

O'Connor, P.J., J.C. Smith, and W.P. Morgan. 2000. Physical activity does not provoke panic attacks in patients with panic disorder: A review of the evidence. *Anxiety, Stress & Coping* 13: 333-353.

O'Connor, P.J., and S.D. Youngstedt. 1995. Influence of exercise on human sleep. In *Exercise and sport sciences review*, edited by J.O. Holloszy. Baltimore: Williams and Wilkins.

O'Connor, T.M., R. Jago, and T. Baranowski. 2009. Engaging parents to increase youth physical activity: A systematic review. *American Journal of Preventive Medicine* 37 (2): 141-149.

O'Neal, H.A., A.L. Dunn, and E.W. Martinsen. 2000. Depression and exercise. *International Journal of Sport Psychology* 31 (2): 110-135.

O'Neal, H., J.D. Van Hoomissen, P.V. Holmes, and R.K. Dishman. 2001. *Preprogalanin messenger RNA levels are increased in rat locus coeruleus after exercise training. Neuroscience Letters.* 299 (1-2): 69-72.

O'Reilly, R.A. 2010. The what and how of prefrontal cortical organization. *Trends in Neuroscience* 33: 355-361.

O'Shea, S.D., N.F. Taylor, and J.D. Paratz. 2007. Factors affecting adherence to progressive resistance exercise for persons with COPD. *Journal of Cardiopulmonary Rehabilitation and Prevention* 27 (3): 166-174.

Ogawa, S., T.M. Lee, A.S. Nayak, and P. Glynn. 1990. Oxygenation-sensitive contrast in magnetic resonance image of rodent brain at high magnetic fields. *Magnetic Resonance in Medicine* 14 (1): 68-78.

Ogoh, S., W.L. Wasmund, D.M. Keller, et al. 2002. Role of central command in carotid baroreflex resetting in humans during static exercise. *Journal of Physiology* 543 (1): 349.

Ohayon, M.M., M. Caulet, and C. Guilleminault. 1998. How a general population perceives its sleep and how this relates to the complaint of insomnia. *Sleep* 20: 715-723.

Oken, B.S., S. Kishiyama, D. Zajdel, D. Bourdette, D. Carlsen, and M. Haas. 2004. Randomized controlled trial of yoga and exercise in multiple sclerosis. *Neurology* 62 (11): 2058-2064.

Olds, J. 1956. Pleasure centers in the brain. *Scientific American*: 105-116.

Olds, J., and P. Milner. 1954. Positive reinforcement produced by electrical stimulation of septal area and other regions of rat brain. *Journal of Comparative and Physiological Psychology* 47 (6): 419-427.

Olfson, M., and S.C. Marcus. 2009. National patterns in antidepressant medication treatment. *Archives of General Psychiatry* 66 (8): 848-856.

Olivardia, R., H.J. Pope, and J.I. Hudson. 2000. Muscle dysmorphia in male weightlifters: A case-control study. *American Journal of Psychiatry* 157 (Aug): 1291-1296.

Oman, R.F., and A.C. King. 1998. Predicting the adoption and maintenance of exercise participation using self-efficacy and previous exercise participation rates. *American Journal of Health Promotion.* 12 (3): 154-161.

Opdenacker, J., C. Delecluse, and F. Boen. 2009. The longitudinal effects of a lifestyle physical activity intervention and a structured exercise intervention on physical self-perceptions and self-esteem in older adults. *Journal of Sport & Exercise Psychology* 31 (6): 743-760.

Orth, U., K.H. Trzesniewski, and R.W. Robins. 2010. Self-esteem development from young adulthood to old age: A cohort-sequential longitudinal study. *Journal of Personality and Social Psychology* 98 (4): 645-658.

Orwin, A. 1974. Treatment of a situational phobia: A case for running. *British Journal of Psychiatry* 125: 96-98.

Osborn, J., and S.W.G. Derbyshire. 2010. Pain sensation evoked by observing injury in others. *Pain* 148 (2): 268-274.

Osei-Tutu, K.B., and P.D. Campagna. 2005. The effects of short- vs. long-bout exercise on mood, V\od\ O_2max, and percent body fat. *Preventive Medicine* 40 (1): 92-98.

Osgood, C.E., G.J. Suci, and P.H. Tannenbaum. 1957. *The measurement of meaning.* Urbana: University of Illinois Press.

Ossip-Klein, D.J., E.J. Doyne, E.D. Bowman, K.M. Osborn, and R.A. Neimeyer. 1989. Effects of running or weight lifting on self-concept in clinically depressed women. *Journal of Consulting and Clinical Psychology.* 57 (1): 158.

Ottawa Panel Members, Ottawa Methods Group, L. Brosseau, G.A. Wells, et al. 2004. Ottawa Panel evidence-based clinical practice guidelines for therapeutic exercises in the management of rheumatoid arthritis in adults. *Physical Therapy* 84 (10): 934-972.

Ouslander, J.G., B.R. Connell, D.L. Bliwise, Y. Endeshaw, P. Griffiths, and J.F. Schnelle. 2006. A nonpharmacological intervention to improve sleep in nursing home patients: Results of a controlled clinical trial. *Journal of the American Geriatrics Society* 54 (1): 38-47.

Owen, A.M. 2004. Cognitive dysfunction in Parkinson's disease: The role of frontostriatal circuitry. *Neuroscientist* 10 (6): 525-537.

Owen, C.G., C.M. Nightingale, A.R. Rudnicka, et al. 2010. Family dog ownership and levels of physical activity in childhood: Findings from the Child Heart and Health Study in England. *American Journal of Public Health* 100 (9): 1669-1671.

Owen, N., G.N. Healy, C.E. Matthews, and D.W. Dunstan. 2010. Too much sitting: The population health science of sedentary behavior. *Exercise and Sport Sciences Reviews* 38 (3): 105-113.

Owen, N., E. Leslie, J. Salmon, and M.J. Fotheringham. 2000. Environmental determinants of physical activity and sedentary behavior. *Exercise and Sport Sciences Reviews* 28: 153-158.

Ozminkowski, R.J., S. Wang, and J.K. Walsh. 2007. The direct and indirect costs of untreated insomnia in adults in the United States. *Sleep* 30 (3): 263-273.

Paffenbarger, R.S., I.M. Lee, and R. Leung. 1994. Physical activity and personal characteristics associated with depression and suicide in American college men. *Acta Psychiatrica Scandinavia* (Suppl. 377): 16-22.

Pagliari, R., and L. Peyrin. 1995. Norepinephrine release in the rat frontal cortex under treadmill exercise: A study with microdialysis. *Journal of Applied Physiology* 78 (Jun): 2121-2130.

Palkovitz, M., and M.J. Brownstein. 1988. *Maps and guide to microdissection of the rat brain.* New York: Elsevier.

Palmer, L.K. 1995. Effects of a walking program on attributional style, depression, and self-esteem in women. *Perceptual & Motor Skills* 81 (3, Pt 1): 891-898.

Pan, S., C. Cameron, M. DesMeules, H. Morrison, C. Craig, and X.H. Jiang. 2009. Individual, social, environmental, and physical environmental correlates with physical activity among Canadians: A cross-sectional study. *BMC Public Health* 9 (1): 21.

Pandolf, K.B. 1982. Differentiated ratings of perceived exertion during physical exercise. *Medicine & Science in Sports & Exercise* 14: 397-405.

Pandolf, K.B., R.I. Burse, and R.F. Goldman. 1975. Differentiated ratings of perceived exertion during physical conditioning of older individuals using leg-weight loading. *Perceptual and motor Skills* 40, 563-574.

Panksepp, J. 1998. The sources of fear and anxiety in the brain. In *Affective neuroscience: The foundations of human and animal emotions,* edited by J. Panksepp. New York: Oxford University Press.

Papez, J.W. 1937. A proposed mechanism of emotion. *Archives of neurology and psychiatry.* 38 (4): 725-743.

Partonen, T., J. Leppert, C. Hursch, and J. Lonnqvist. 1999. Randomized trial of physical exercise alone or combined with bright light on mood and health-related quality of life. *Psychological Medicine* 28: 1359-1364.

Passos, G.S., D. Poyares, M.G. Santana, S.A. Garbuio, S. Tufik, and M.T. Mello. 2010. Effect of acute physical exercise on patients with chronic primary insomnia. *Journal of Clinical Sleep Medicine* 6 (3): 270-275.

Pate, R.R., G.W. Heath, M. Dowda, and S.G. Trost. 1996. Associations between physical activity and other health behaviors in a representative sample of U.S. adolescents. *American Journal of Public Health* 86 (11): 1577-1581.

Pate, R.R., M. Pratt, S.N. Blair, et al. 1995. Physical activity and public health: a recommendation from the Centers for Disease Control and Prevention and the American College of Sports Medicine. *Journal of the American Medical Association.* 273 (5): 402-407.

Pate, R.R., R. Saunders, R.K. Dishman, C. Addy, M. Dowda, and D.S. Ward. 2007. Long-term effects of a physical activity intervention in high school girls. *American Journal of Preventive Medicine* 33 (4): 276-280.

Paterson, D.H., and D.E. R. Warburton. 2010. Physical activity and functional limitations in older adults: A systematic review related to Canada's Physical Activity Guidelines. *International Journal of Behavioral Nutrition and Physical Activity* 7: 38. www.ijbnpa. org/content/7/1/38.

Paterson, D.J., J.S. Friedland, D.A. Bascom, et al. 1990. Changes in arterial K+ and ventilation during exercise in normal subjects and subjects with McArdle's syndrome. *Journal of Physiology* 429: 339-348.

Patten, S.B., J.V. Williams, D.H. Lavorato, and M. Eliasziw. 2009. A longitudinal community study of major depression and physical activity. *General Hospital Psychiatry* 31 (6): 571-575.

Paulhus, D.L. 1984. Two-component models of socially desirable responding. *Journal of Personality & Social Psychology* 46 (3): 598-609.

Pearman, S.N., R.F. Valois, R.G. Sargent, R.P. Saunders, J.W. Drane, and C.A. Macera. 1997. The impact of a required college health and physical education course on the health status of alumni. *Journal of American College Health* 4: 77-85.

Penttinen, J., and R. Erkkola. 1997. Pregnancy in endurance athletes. *Scandinavian Journal of Medicine & Science in Sports* 7 (4): 226-228.

Peppard, P.E., and T. Young. 2004. Exercise and sleep-disordered breathing: An association independent of body habitus. *Sleep* 27 (3): 480-484.

Pereira, A.C., D.E. Huddleston, A.M. Brickman, et al. 2007. An in vivo correlate of exercise-induced neurogenesis in adult dentate gyrus. *Proceedings of the National Academy of Science* 104 (13): 5638-5643.

Perrey, S. 2008. Non-invasive NIR spectroscopy of human brain function during exercise. *Methods* 45 (4): 289-299.

Perri, M.G., S.D. Anton, P.E. Durning, et al. 2002. Adherence to exercise prescriptions: Effects of prescribing moderate versus higher levels of intensity and frequency. *Health Psychology* 21 (5): 452-458.

Perrin, E.M., J. Boone-Heinonen, A.E. Field, T. Coyne-Beasley, and P. Gordon-Larsen. 2010. Perception of overweight and self-esteem during adolescence. *International Journal of Eating Disorders* 43 (5): 447-454.

Perrine, S.A., I.S. Sheikh, C.A. Nwaneshiudu, J.A. Schroeder, and E.M. Unterwald. 2008. Withdrawal from chronic administration of cocaine decreases delta opioid receptor signaling and increases anxiety- and depression-like behaviors in the rat. *Neuropharmacology* 54 (2): 355-364.

Peterson, C., and M.E.P. Seligman. 2004. *Character strengths and virtues: A handbook and classification.* New York: Oxford University Press.

Petronis, K.R., J.F. Samuels, E.K. Moscicki, and J.C. Anthony. 1990. An epidemiologic investigation of potential risk factors for suicide attempts. *Social Psychiatry and Psychiatric Epidemiology* 25 (July): 193-199.

Petruzzello, S.J., E.E. Hall, and P. Ekkekakis. 2001. Regional brain activation as a biological marker of affective responsivity to acute exercise: Influence of fitness. *Psychophysiology* 38 (1): 99-106.

Petruzzello, S.J., and D.M. Landers. 1994. State anxiety reduction and exercise: Does hemispheric activation reflect such changes? *Medicine & Science in Sports & Exercise* 26 (8): 1028-1035.

Petruzzello, S. J., D.M. Landers, B.D. Hatfield, K.A. Kubitz, and W. Salazar. 1991. A meta-analysis on the anxiety-reducing effects of acute and chronic exercise. Outcomes and mechanisms. *Sports Medicine* 11 (Mar):143-182.

Petruzzello, S.J., and A.K. Tate. 1997. Brain activation, affect, and aerobic exercise: An examination of both state-independent and state-dependent relationships. *Psychophysiology* 34 (5): 527-533.

Petruzzello, S. J., E. E. Hall, and P. Ekkekakis. 2001. Regional brain activation as a biological marker of affective responsivity to acute exercise: influence of fitness. *Psychophysiology* 38 (1):99-106.

Pew Internet and American Life Project. 2011a. *Home broadband adoption, 2000-2010.* Pew Internet & American Life Project 2010 [cited May 13, 2011]. www.pewinternet.org/Static-Pages/Trend-Data/Home-Broadband-Adoption.aspx.

Pew Internet and American Life Project. 2011b. *Trend data.* Pew Research Center 2011 [cited May 13, 2011]. www.pewinternet.org/Trend-Data/Online-Activites-Total.aspx.

Pfaff, D.W. 2006. *Brain arousal and information theory: Neural and genetic mechanisms.* Cambridge, MA: Harvard University Press.

Phan, K.L., T. Wager, S.F. Taylor, and I. Liberzon. 2002. Functional neuroanatomy of emotion: A meta-analysis of emotion activation studies in PET and fMRI. *NeuroImage* 16 (2): 331-348.

Phillips, E.D. 1973. *Greek medicine: Philosophy and medicine from Alcmaeon to Alexandrians.* London: Thames and Hudson.

Phillips, K.A., G. Quinn, and R.L. Stout. 2008. Functional impairment in body dysmorphic disorder: A prospective, follow-up study. *Journal of Psychiatric Research* 42 (9): 701-707.

Phillips, K.A., R.L. O'Sullivan, and H.J. Pope. 1997. Muscle dysmorphia [letter]. *Journal of Clinical Psychiatry* 58 (Aug): 361.

Phillips, K.A., S. Wilhelm, L.M. Koran, et al. 2010. Body dysmorphic disorder: Some key issues for DSM-V. *Depression and Anxiety* 27 (6): 573-591.

Physical Activity Guidelines Advisory Committee. 2008. Physical Activity Guidelines Advisory Committee Report, pp. 1-58. Washington, DC: U.S. Department of Health and Human Services.

Pierce, T.W., D.J. Madden, W.C. Siegel, and J.A. Blumenthal. 1993. Effects of aerobic exercise on cognitive and psychosocial functioning in patients with mild hypertension. *Health Psychology* 12: 286-291.

Pinto, B.M., H. Lynn, B.H. Marcus, J. DePue, and M.G. Goldstein. 2001. Physician-based activity counseling: Intervention effects on mediators of motivational readiness for physical activity. *Annals of Behavioral Medicine* 23: 2-10.

Piters, K.M., A. Colombo, H.G. Olson, and S.M. Butman. 1985. Effect of coffee on exercise-induced angina pectoris due to coronary artery disease in habitual coffee drinkers. *American Journal of Cardiology* 55 (4): 277-280.

Pitts, F.J., and J.J. McClure. 1967. Lactate metabolism in anxiety neurosis. *New England Journal of Medicine* 277 (Dec 21): 1329-1336.

Plotnikoff, R.C., S.B. Hotz, N.J. Birkett, and K.S. Courneya. 2001. Exercise and the transtheoretical model: A longitudinal test of a population sample. *Preventive Medicine* 33 (5): 441-452.

Ployhart, R.E., and R.J. Vandenberg. 2010. Longitudinal research: The theory, design, and analysis of change. *Journal of Management* 36 (1): 94.

Plutchik, R. 1994. *The psychology and biology of emotion.* New York: HarperCollins College.

Polidori, M.C., G. Nelles, and L. Pientka. 2010. Prevention of dementia: Focus on lifestyle. *International Journal of Alzheimer's Disease.* 2010: Article ID 393579, 9 pages. doi: 10.4061/2010/393579.

Pollack, M.H., C. Allgulander, B. Bandelow, et al. 2003. WCA recommendations for the long-term treatment of panic disorder. *CNS Spectrums* 8 (8 Suppl. 1): 17-30.

Pollock, M.L., J.F. Carroll, J.E. Graves, et al. 1991. Injuries and adherence to walk/jog and resistance training programs in the elderly. *Medicine & Science in Sports & Exercise* 23 (10): 1194-1200.

Pontifex, M.B., and C.H. Hillman. 2007. Neuroelectric and behavioral indices of interference control during acute cycling. *Clinical Neurophysiology* 118: 570-580.

Poole, L., A. Steptoe, A.J. Wawrzyniak, S. Bostock, E.S. Mitchell, and M. Hamer. 2011. Associations of objectively measured physical activity with daily mood ratings and psychophysiological stress responses in women. *Psychophysiology* 48 (8): 1165-1172.

Pope, H.J., A.J. Gruber, P. Choi, R. Olivardia, and K.A. Phillips. 1997. Muscle dysmorphia. An underrecognized form of body dysmorphic disorder. *Psychosomatics* 38 (Nov-Dec): 548-557.

Pope, H.J., A.J. Gruber, B. Mangweth, B. Bureau, C. deCol, R. Jounent, and J.I. Hudson. 2000. Body perception among men in three countries. *American Journal of Psychiatry* 157: 1297-1231.

Porkka-Heiskanen, T., R.E. Strecker, M. Thakkar, A.A. Bjorkum, R.W. Greene, and R.W. McCarley. 1997. Adenosine: A mediator of the sleep-inducing effects of prolonged wakefulness. *Science* 276: 1265-1268.

Posadzki, P., E. Ernst, R. Terry, and M. Soo Lee. 2011. Is yoga effective for pain? A systematic review of randomized clinical trials. *Complementary Therapies in Medicine* 19 (5): 281-287.

Posner, M.I., and S. Dahaene. 1994. Attentional networks. *Trends in Neurosciences* 17: 75-79.

Posner, M.I., and M.E. Raichle. 1997. *Images of mind.* New York: Scientific American Library.

Poudevigne, M.S., and P.J. O'Connor. 2005. Physical activity and mood during pregnancy. *Medicine & Science in Sports & Exercise* 37 (8): 1374-1380.

Prakash, R.S., M.W. Voss, K.I. Erickson, J.M. Lewis, L. Chaddock, and E. Malkowski. 2011. Cardiorespiratory fitness and attentional control in the aging brain. *Frontiers in Human Neuroscience* 4: 1-12.

Price, D.D. 1999. *Psychological mechanisms of pain and analgesia.* Seattle: IASP Press.

Price, D.D. 2000. Psychological and Neural Mechanisms of the Affective Dimension of Pain. *Science* 288 (5472): 1769-1772.

Prince, S., K. Adamo, M. Hamel, J. Hardt, S. Gorber, and M. Tremblay. 2008. A comparison of direct versus self-report measures for assessing physical activity in adults: A systematic review. *International Journal of Behavioral Nutrition and Physical Activity* 5 (1): 56.

Prochaska, J.O. 1979. *Systems of psychotherapy: A transtheoretical analysis.* Homewood, IL: Dorsey Press.

Prochaska, J.O., and C.C. DiClemente. 1982. Transtheoretical therapy: Toward a more integrative model of change. *Psychotherapy: Theory, Research and Practice* 20: 161-173.

Prochaska, J.O., and C.C. DiClemente. 1983. Stages and processes of self-change of smoking: Toward an integrative model of change. *Journal of Consulting and Clinical Psychology* 51 (3): 390-395.

Prochaska, J.O., and W.F. Velicer. 1997. The Transtheoretical Model of behavior change. *American Journal of Health Promotion.* 12: 38-48.

Puetz, T.W. 2006. Physical activity and feelings of energy and fatigue: Epidemiological evidence. *Sports Medicine* 36 (9): 767-780.

Puetz, T.W., S.S. Flowers, and P.J. O'Connor. 2008. A randomized controlled trial of the effect of aerobic exercise training on feelings of energy and fatigue in sedentary young adults with persistent fatigue. *Psychotherapy and Psychosomatics* 77 (3): 167-174.

Puetz, T.W., and M.P. Herring. 2012. Differential effects of exercise on cancer-related fatigue during and following treatment. *American Journal of Preventive Medicine* 43(2): e1-e10.

Puetz, T.W., P.J. O'Connor, and R.K. Dishman. 2006. Effects of chronic exercise on feelings of energy and fatigue: A quantitative synthesis. *Psychological Bulletin* 132 (6): 866-876.

Pugliese, J., and B. Tinsley. 2007. Parental socialization of child and adolescent physical activity: A meta-analysis. *Journal of Family Psychology* 21 (3): 331-343.

Quan, S.F., G.T. O'Connor, J.S. Quan, et al. 2007. Association of physical activity with sleep-disordered breathing. *Sleep & Breathing [Schlaf & Atmung]* 11 (3): 149-157.

Radegran, G., and Y. Hellsten. 2000. Adenosine and nitric oxide in exercise-induced human skeletal muscle vasodilatation. *Acta Physiologica Scandinavica* 168 (Apr): 575-591.

Raglin, J.S. 1997. Anxiolytic effects of physical activity. In *Physical activity and mental health*, edited by W.P. Morgan. Washington, DC: Taylor & Francis.

Raglin, J. S., P.E. Turner, and F. Eksten. 1993. State anxiety and blood pressure following 30 min of leg ergometry or weight training. *Medicine & Science in Sports & Exercise* 25 (9): 1044-1048.

Raglin, J.S., and L. Moger. 1999. Adverse consequences of physical activity: When more is too much. In *Lifestyle medicine*, edited by J.M. Rippe. Malden, MA: Blackwell Science.

Raglin, J.S., and W.P. Morgan. 1985. Influence of vigorous exercise on mood state. *The Behavior Therapist* 8 (9): 179-183.

Raglin, J.S., and M. Wilson. 1996. State anxiety following 20 minutes of bicycle ergometer exercise at selected intensities. *International Journal of Sports Medicine* 17 (Aug): 467-471.

Raglin, J.S., and G.S. Wilson. 2000. Overtraining in athletes. In *Emotions in sport*, edited by Y.L. Hanin. Champaign, IL: Human Kinetics.

Ramachandran, V.S., and W. Hirstein. 1998. The perception of phantom limbs. The D.O. Hebb lecture. *Brain* 121 (Pt 9): 1603-1630.

Ramel, J., R. Bannuru, M. Griffith, and C. Wang. 2009. Exercise for fibromyalgia pain: A meta-analysis of randomized controlled trials. *Current Rheumatology Reviews* 5 (4): 188-193.

Rankinen, T., T. Rice, M. Teran-Garcia, D.C. Rao, and C. Bouchard. 2010. FTO genotype is associated with exercise training-induced changes in body composition. *Obesity* 18 (2): 322-326.

Rankinen, T., S.M. Roth, M.S. Bray, et al. 2010. Advances in exercise, fitness, and performance genomics. *Medicine & Science in Sports & Exercise* 42 (5): 835-846.

Rankinen, T., A. Zuberi, Y.C. Chagnon, et al. 2006. The human obesity gene map: The 2005 update. *Obesity* 14 (4): 529-644.

Rasch, G. 1960. *Studies in mathematical psychology: I. Probabilistic models for some intelligence and attainment tests.* Copenhagen, Denmark: Nielsen & Lydiche.

Rasmussen, K., D.A. Morilak, and B.L. Jacobs. 1986. Single unit activity of locus coeruleus neurons in the freely moving cat. I. During naturalistic behaviors and in response to simple and complex stimuli. *Brain Research* 371 (Apr 23): 324-334.

Rasmussen, P., P. Brassard, H. Adser, et al. 2009. Evidence for a release of brain-derived neurotrophic factor from the brain during exercise. *Experimental Physiology* 94 (10): 1062-1069.

Rathbone, J.L., F.L. Bacon, and C.H. Keene 1932 *Foundations of Health*. Boston: Houghton Mifflin.

Raudenbush, S.W., and A.S. Bryk. 2002. *Hierarchical linear models: Applications and data analysis methods*. Vol. 1. Thousand Oaks, CA: Sage.

Raynor, D.A., K.J. Coleman, and L.H. Epstein. 1998. Effects of proximity on the choice to be physically active or sedentary. *Research Quarterly for Exercise and Sport* 69: 99-103.

Rechel, J.A., Yard, E.E., Comstock, R.D. 2008. An epidemiological comparison of high school sports injuries sustained in practice and competition. *Journal of Athletic Training* 43 (2): 197-204.

Rector, N.A., and D. Roger. 1997. The stress buffering effects of self-esteem. *Personality & Individual Differences* 23 (5): 799-808.

Reed, J., and S. Buck. 2009. The effect of regular aerobic exercise on positive-activated affect: A meta-analysis. *Psychology of Sport and Exercise* 10 (6): 581-594.

Reed, J., and D.S. Ones. 2006. The effect of acute aerobic exercise on positive activated affect: A meta-analysis. *Psychology of Sport and Exercise* 7 (5): 477-514.

Reeves, W.C., T.W. Strine, L.A. Pratt, et al. 2011. Mental illness surveillance among adults in the United States. *Morbidity and Mortality Weekly Report Surveillance Summaries*. 60(Suppl. 3): 1-29.corrected

Reger, B., L. Cooper, S. Booth-Butterfield, et al. 2002. Wheeling Walks: A community campaign using paid media to encourage walking among sedentary older adults. *Preventive Medicine* 35 (3): 285-292.

Regier, D.A., R.M. Hirschfeld, F.K. Goodwin, J.D. Burke, Jr., J.B. Lazar, and L.L. Judd. 1988. The NIMH Depression Awareness, Recognition, and Treatment Program: Structure, aims, and scientific basis. *American Journal of Psychiatry*. 145 (11): 1351-7.

Reid, K.J., K.G. Baron, B. Lu, E. Naylor, L. Wolfe, and P.C. Zee. 2010. Aerobic exercise improves self-reported sleep and quality of life in older adults with insomnia. *Sleep Medicine* 11 (9): 934-940.

Reiman, E.M. 1997. The application of positron emission tomography to the study of normal and pathologic emotions. *Journal of Clinical Psychiatry* 58 (Suppl. 16): 4-12.

Reis, J.P., H.R. Bowels, B.E. Ainsworth, K.D. DuBose, S. Smith, and J.N. Laditka. 2004. Nonoccupational physical activity by degree of urbanization and U.S. geographic region. *Medicine & Science in Sports & Exercise* 36 (12): 2093-2098.

Rejeski, W.J. 1981. Perception of exertion: A social psychophysiological integration. *Journal of Sport Psychology* 3: 305-320.

Renner, B., S. Kwon, B.H. Yang, et al. 2008. Social-cognitive predictors of dietary behaviors in South Korean men and women. *International Journal of Behavioral Medicine* 15 (1): 4-13.

Rethorst, C.D., D.M. Landers, C.T. Nagoshi, and J.T. Ross. 2010. Efficacy of exercise in reducing depressive symptoms across 5-HTTLPR genotypes. *Medicine & Science in Sports & Exercise* 42 (11): 2141-2147.

Rethorst, C.D., D.M. Landers, C.T. Nagoshi, and J.T. Ross. 2011. The association of 5-HTTLPR genotype and depressive symptoms is moderated by physical activity. *Journal of Psychiatric Research* 45 (2): 185-189.

Rethorst, C.D., B.M. Wipfli, and D.M. Landers. 2009. The antidepressive effects of exercise: A meta-analysis of randomized trials. *Sports Medicine* 39 (6): 491-511.

Rhodes, J.S., S.C. Gammie, and T. Garland, Jr. 2005. Neurobiology of mice selected for high voluntary wheel-running activity. *Integrative and Comparative Biology* 45 (3): 438-455.

Rhodes, R.E., and K.S. Courneya. 2003. Investigating multiple components of attitude, subjective norm, and perceived control: An examination of the theory of planned behaviour in the exercise domain. *British Journal of Social Psychology* 42 (Pt 1): 129-146.

Rhodes, R.E., and G.-J. de Bruijn. 2010. Automatic and motivational correlates of physical activity: Does intensity moderate the relationship? *Behavioral Medicine* 36 (2): 44-52.

Rhodes, R.E., G.-J. de Bruijn, and D.H. Matheson. 2010. Habit in the physical activity domain: Integration with intention temporal stability and action control. *Journal of Sport & Exercise Psychology* 32 (1): 84-98.

Rhodes, R.E., B. Fiala, and M. Conner. 2009. A review and meta-analysis of affective judgments and physical activity in adult populations. *Annals of Behavioral Medicine* 38 (3): 180-204.

Rhodes, R.E., and C.R. Nigg. 2011. Advancing physical activity theory: A review and future directions. *Exercise and Sport Sciences Reviews* 39 (3): 113-119.

Rhodes, R.E., and L.A. Pfaeffli. 2010. Mediators of physical activity behaviour change among adult non-clinical populations: A review update. *International Journal of Behavioral Nutrition and Physical Activity* 7: 37.

Rhodes, R.E., D.E. Warburton, and H. Murray. 2009. Characteristics of physical activity guidelines and their effect on adherence: A review of randomized trials. *Sports Medicine* 39 (5): 355-375.

Rhyu, I.J., J.A. Bytheway, S.J. Kohler, et al. 2010. Effects of aerobic exercise training on cognitive function and cortical vascularity in monkeys. *Neuroscience* 167 (4): 1239-1248.

Rice, D.P., and L.S. Miller. 1998. Health implications and cost implications of anxiety and other mental disorders in the United States. *British Journal of Psychiatry* 34 (Suppl.): 4-9.

Richards, K.C., C. Lambert, C.K. Beck, et al. 2011. Strength training, walking, and social activity improve sleep in nursing home and assisted living residents: A randomized controlled trial. *Journal of the American Geriatrics Society* 59 (2): 214-223.

Richter, E.A., and J.R. Sutton. 1994. Hormonal adaptations to physical activity. In *Physical activity, fitness and health: International proceedings and consensus statement*, edited by C. Bouchard, R. Shephard, and T. Stephens. Champaign, IL: Human Kinetics.

Ridgers, N.D., G. Stratton, S.J. Fairclough, and J.W. Twisk. 2007. Long-term effects of playground markings and physical structures on children's recess physical activity levels. *Preventive Medicine* 44 (5): 393-397.

Riley, W.T., D.E. Rivera, A.A. Atienza, W. Nilsen, S.M. Allison, and R. Mermelstein. 2011. Health behavior models in the age of mobile interventions: Are our theories up to the task? *Translational Behavioral Medicine* 1 (1): 53-71.

Rimmer, J.H., M.D. Chen, J.A. McCubbin, C. Drum, and J. Peterson. 2010. Exercise intervention research on persons with disabilities: What we know and where we need to go. *American Journal of Physical Medicine & Rehabilitation* 89 (3): 249-263.

Rittweger, J., K. Just, K. Kautzsch, P. Reeg, and D. Felsenberg. 2002. Treatment of chronic lower back pain with lumbar extension and whole-body vibration exercise: A randomized controlled trial. *Spine* 27 (17): 1829-1834.

Robbins, T.W., M. Cador, J.R. Taylor, and B.J. Everitt. 1989. Limbic-striatal interactions in reward-related processes. *Neuroscience and Biobehavioral Reviews* 13 (2-3): 155-162.

Roberts, C.K., B. Freed, and W.J. McCarthy. 2010. Low aerobic fitness and obesity are associated with lower standardized test scores in children. *Journal of Pediatrics* 156: 711-718.

Robert, G., and J. Hockey. 1997. Compensatory control in the regulation of human performance under stress and high workload: A cognitive-energetical framework. *Biological Psychology* 45 (1-3): 73-93.

Roberts, W.R. (trans.). 1924. Rhetorica: The Works of Aristotle, Vol.11. Oxford: Clarendon Press. Rpt. 1954 in Aristotle, "Rhetoric" and "Poetics" (trans. Roberts & Ingram Bywater). New York: Modern Library.

Roberts, R.J. 1982. Central signals of perceived exertion during dynamic exercise. *Medicine and Science in Sport and Exercise* 14(5): 390-396..

Robertson, R.J., F.L. Goss, D.J. Aaron, et al. 2006. Observation of perceived exertion in children using the OMNI pictorial scale. *Medicine & Science in Sports & Exercise* 38 (1): 158-166.

Robertson, R.J., F.L. Goss, J.L. Andreacci, et al. 2005. Validation of the Children's OMNI-Resistance Exercise Scale of perceived exertion. *Medicine & Science in Sports & Exercise* 37 (5): 819-826.

Robertson, R.J., F.L. Goss, N.F. Boer, et al. 2000. Children's OMNI scale of perceived exertion: Mixed gender and race validation. *Medicine & Science in Sports & Exercise* 32 (2): 452-458.

Robertson, R.J., J.E. Falkel, A.L. Drash, et al. 1986. Effect of blood pH on peripheral and central signals of perceived exertion. *Medicine & Science in Sports & Exercise* 18 (Feb): 114-122.

Robertson, R.J., R.L. Gillespie, E. Hiatt, and K.D. Rose. 1977. Perceived exertion and stimulus intensity modulation. *Perceptual & Motor Skills* 45: 211-218.

Robertson, R.J., and B.J. Noble. 1997. Perception of physical exertion: Methods, mediators, and applications. *Exercise and Sport Sciences Reviews* 25: 407-452.

Rochester, C.L. 2003. Exercise training in chronic obstructive pulmonary disease. *Journal of Rehabilitation Research and Development* 40 (5): 59-80.

Rodgers, W.M., C.R. Hall, L.R. Duncan, E. Pearson, and M.I. Milne. 2010. Becoming a regular exerciser: Examining change in behavioural regulations among exercise initiates. *Psychology of Sport and Exercise* 11 (5): 378-386.

Roid, G.H., and W.H. Fitts. 1994. *Tennessee self-concept scale [revised manual]*. Los Angeles: Western Psychological Services.

Rollnick, S., W.R. Miller, and C. Butler. 2007. *Motivational interviewing in health care: Helping patients change behavior*. New York: Guilford Press.

Romberg, A., A. Virtanen, and J. Ruutiainen. 2005. Long–term exercise improves functional impairment but not quality of life in multiple sclerosis. *Journal of Neurology* 252 (7): 839-845.

Ronis, D.L., J.F. Yates, and J.P. Kirscht. 1989. Attitudes, decisions, and habits as determinants of repeated behavior. In *Attitude Structure and Function*. edited by A.R. Pratkanis, S.J. Breckler, and A.G. Greenwald. Hillsdale, NJ: Erlbaum.

Rooks, C.R., K.K. McCully, and R.K. Dishman. 2011. Acute exercise improves endothelial function despite increasing vascular resistance during stress in smokers and nonsmokers. *Psychophysiology* 48 (9): 1299-1308.

Rooks, C.R., N.J. Thom, K.K. McCully, and R.K. Dishman. 2010. Effects of incremental exercise on cerebral oxygenation measured by near-infrared spectroscopy: A systematic review. *Progress in Neurobiology* 92 (2): 134-150.

Rosekind, M.R., and K.B. Gregory. 2010. Insomnia risks and costs: Health, safety, and quality of life. *American Journal of Managed Care* 16 (8): 617-626.

Rosenberg, M. 1965. *Society and the adolescent self-image*. Princeton, NJ: University Press.

Rosenzweig, M.R., A.L. Leiman, and S.M. Breedlove. 1999a. *Biological psychology: An introduction to behavioral, cognitive, and clinical neuroscience*. 2nd ed. Sunderland, MA: Sinauer Associates.

Rosenzweig, M.R., A.L. Leiman, and S.M. Breedlove. 1999b. Emotions, aggression, and stress. In *Biologi-*

cal psychology: An introduction to behavioral, cognitive, and clinical neuroscience, edited by M.R. Rosenzweig, A.L. Leiman, and S.M. Breedlove. 2nd ed. Sunderland, MA: Sinauer Associates.

Rosner, F. 1965. The hygienic principles of Moses Maimonides. *The Journal of the American Medical Association* 194 (13); 1352-1354.

Roth, K.B., G. Borges, M.E. Medina-Mora, R. Orozco, C. Oueda, and H.C. Wilcox. 2011. Depressed mood and antisocial behavior problems as correlates for suicide-related behaviors in Mexico. *Journal of Psychiatric Research* 45 (5): 596-602.

Roth, T., S. Jaeger, R. Jin, A. Kalsekar, P.E. Stang, and R.C. Kessler. 2006. Sleep problems, comorbid mental disorders, and role functioning in the national comorbidity survey replication. *Biological Psychiatry* 60 (12): 1364-1371.

Rothwell, J.C., M.M. Traub, B.L. Day, J.A. Obeso, P.K. Thomas, and C.D. Marsden. 1982. Manual motor performance in a deafferented man. *Brain: A Journal of Neurology* 105 (Pt 3): 515-542.

Rowe, D.A., J. Benson, and T.A. Baumgartner. 1999. Development of the Body Self-Image Questionnaire. *Measurement in Physical Education and Exercise Science* 3 (4): 223-248.

Rowell, L.B. 1993. *Human cardiovascular control*. New York: Oxford University Press.

Rowland, T.W. 1998. The biological basis of physical activity. *Medicine & Science in Sports & Exercise* 30 (3): 392-399.

Roy, C.S., and C.S. Sherrington. 1890. On the regulation of the blood-supply of the brain. *Journal of Physiology* 11 (1-2): 85-158.

Rudolph, D. L. and J. G. Kim. 1996. Mood responses to recreational sport and exercise in a Korean sample. *Journal of Social Behavior & Personality* 11 (4): 841-849.

Rush, A.J., M.H. Trivedi, S.R. Wisniewski, et al. 2006. Bupropion-SR, sertraline, or venlafaxine-XR after failure of SSRIs for depression. *New England Journal of Medicine* 354 (12): 1231-1242.

Rushton, A., C. Wright, P. Goodwin, M. Calvert, and N. Freemantle. 2011. Physiotherapy rehabilitation post first lumbar discectomy: A systematic review and meta-analysis of randomized controlled trials. *Spine* 36 (14): E961-E972. doi: 10.1097/BRS.0b013e3181f0e8f8.

Rushton, J.L., M. Forcier, and R.M. Schectman. 2002. Epidemiology of depressive symptoms in the National Longitudinal Study of Adolescent Health. *Journal of the American Academy of Child and Adolescent Psychiatry* 41 (2): 199-205.

Russell, J.A. 1980. A circumplex model of affect. *Journal of Personality and Social Psychology*. 39 (6): 1161-1178.

Russell, J.A., M. Lewicka, and T. Niit. 1989. A cross-cultural study of a circumplex model of affect. *Journal of Personality & Social Psychology* 57 (5): 848-856.

Russell, J.A., and A. Mehrabian. 1977. Evidence for a 3-factor theory of emotions. *Journal of Research in Personality* 11 (3): 273-294.

Russell, J.A., A. Weiss, and G.A. Mendelsohn. 1989. Affect Grid: A single-item scale of pleasure and arousal. *Journal of Personality & Social Psychology* 57 (3): 493-502.

Russo-Neustadt, A. 2003. Brain-derived neurotrophic factor, behavior, and new directions for the treatment of mental disorders. *Seminars in Clinical Neuropsychiatry* 8 (2): 109-118.

Ryan, R.M., and E.L. Deci. 2001. On happiness and human potentials: A review of research on hedonic and eudaimonic well-being. *Annual Review of Psychology* 52: 141-166.

Ryan, R.M., and E.L. Deci. 2002. Overview of self-determination theory. In *Handbook of self-determination research*, edited by E.L. Deci and R.M. Ryan. Rochester, NY: University of Rochester Press.

Sabatinelli, D., E.E. Fortune, Q. Li, et al. 2011. Emotional perception: A meta-analyses of face and natural scene processing. *NeuroImage* 54 (3): 2524-2533.

Sacheck, J.M., J.F. Kuder, and C.D. Economos. 2010. Physical fitness, adiposity, and metabolic risk factors in young college students. *Medicine & Science in Sports & Exercise* 42 (6): 1039-1044.

Sacks, M.H., and M.L. Sachs. 1981. *Psychology of running*. Champaign, IL: Human Kinetics.

Saelens, B.E., and S.L. Handy. 2008. Built environment correlates of walking: A review. *Medicine & Science in Sports & Exercise* 40 (7 Suppl.): S550-S566.

Sagatun, A., A.J. Sogaard, E. Bjertness, R. Selmer, and S. Heyerdahl. 2007. The association between weekly hours of physical activity and mental health: A three-year follow-up study of 15-16-year-old students in the city of Oslo, Norway. *BMC Public Health* 7: 155.

Salam, J.N., J.H. Fox, E.M. Detroy, M.H. Guignon, D.F. Wohl, and W.A. Falls. 2009. Voluntary exercise in C57 mice is anxiolytic across several measures of anxiety. *Behavioural Brain Research* 197 (1): 31-40.

Salamone, J.D., M. Correa, A. Farrar, and S.M. Mingote. 2007. Effort-related functions of nucleus accumbens dopamine and associated forebrain circuits. *Psychopharmacology* 191 (3): 461-482.

Sallis, J.F., W.L. Haskell, S.P. Fortmann, K.M. Vranizan, C.B. Taylor, and D.S. Solomon. 1986. Predictions of adoption and maintenance of physical activity in a community sample. *Preventive Medicine* 15: 331-341.

Sallis, J.F., and M.F. Hovell. 1990. Determinants of exercise behavior. *Exercise and Sport Sciences Reviews* 11: 307-330.

Sallis, J.F., T.L. McKenzie, T.L. Conway, et al. 2003. Environmental interventions for eating and physical activity: A randomized controlled trial in middle schools. *American Journal of Preventive Medicine* 24 (3): 209-217.

Sallis, J.F., and N. Owen. 1999. *Physical activity and behavioral medicine.* Thousand Oaks, CA: Sage.

Sallis, J.F., N. Owen, and E.B. Fisher. 2008. Ecological models of health behavior. In *Health behavior and health education: Theory, research, and practice,* edited by K. Glanz, B.K. Rimer, and P. Viswanath. San Francisco: Jossey-Bass.

Sallis, J.F., J.J. Prochaska, and W.C. Taylor. 2000. A review of correlates of physical activity of children and adolescents. *Medicine & Science in Sports & Exercise* 32: 963-975.

Sallis, J.F., B.G. Simons-Morton, E.J. Stone, et al. 1992. Determinants of physical activity and interventions in youth. *Medicine & Science in Sports & Exercise* 24 (6): S248-S257.

Salthouse, T.A. 1988. The role of processing resources in cognitive aging. In *Cognitive development in adulthood: Progress in cognitive development research,* edited by M.L. Howe and C.J. Brainerd. New York: Springer-Verlag.

Sanchez-Villegas, A., I. Ara, F. Guillen-Grima, M. Bes-Rastrollo, J.J. Varo-Cenarruzabeitia, and M.A. Martinez-Gonzalez. 2008. Physical activity, sedentary index, and mental disorders in the SUN cohort study. *Medicine & Science in Sports & Exercise* 40 (5): 827-834.

Sanders, A.F. 1998. *Elements of human performance: Reaction processes and attention in human skill.* Mahwah, NJ: Lawrence Erlbaum.

Sanes, J.N., and R. Shadmehr. 1995. Sense of muscular effort and somesthetic afferent information in humans. *Canadian Journal of Physiology and Pharmacology* 73 (2): 223-233.

Santos, M.P., H. Gomes, and J. Mota. 2005. Physical activity and sedentary behaviors in adolescents. *Annals of Behavioral Medicine* 30 (1): 21-24.

Sapolsky, R.M. 1994. *Why zebras don't get ulcers: A guide to stress, stress-related diseases, and coping.* New York: W.H. Freeman.

Sarter, M., and J.P. Bruno. 1999. Abnormal regulation of corticopetal cholinergic neurons and impaired information processing in neuropsychiatric disorders. *Trends in Neurosciences* 22 (Feb): 67-74.

Sayers, S.P., P.M. Clarkson, P.A. Rouzier, and G. Kamen. 1999. Adverse events associated with eccentric exercise protocols: Six case studies. *Medicine & Science in Sports & Exercise* 31 (12): 1697.

Schaefer, E.S., and R. Plutchik. 1966. Interrelationships of emotions, traits, and diagnostic constructs. *Psychological Reports* 18: 399-410.

Schaefer, S., O. Huxhold, and U. Lindenberger. 2006. Healthy mind in healthy body? A review of sensorimotor-cognitive interdependencies in old age. *European Review of Aging and Physical Activity* 3: 45-54.

Schappert, S.M. 1998. Ambulatory care visits to physician offices, hospital outpatient departments, and emergency departments: United States, 1996. *Vital and Health Statistics.* 13 (134). Wahsington, DC: National Center for Health Statistics, Centers for Disease Control and Prevention.

Sciolino N.R., R.K. Dishman, and P.V. Holmes. 2012. Voluntary exercise offers anxiolytic potential and amplifies galanin gene expression in the locus coeruleus of the rat. *Behavioural Brain Research.* 233 (1): 191-200.

Sciolino N.R., P.V. Holmes. 2012. Exercise offers anxiolytic potential: A role for stress and brain noradrenergic-galaninergic mechanisms. *Neuroscience and Biobehaviol Reviews.* Jul 5. [Epub ahead of print].

Schechtman, K.B., and M.G. Ory. 2001. The effects of exercise on the quality of life of frail older adults: A preplanned meta-analysis of the FICSIT trials. *Annals of Behavioral Medicine* 23 (3): 186-197.

Scheier, M.F., and C.S. Carver. 1992. Effects of optimism on psychological and physical well-being: Theoretical overview and empirical update. *Cognitive Therapy and Research* 16 (2): 201-228.

Schlicht, W. 1994. Does physical exercise reduce anxious emotions? A meta-analysis. *Anxiety, Stress & Coping: An International Journal* 6 (4): 275-288.

Schmader, K.E. 2002. Epidemiology and impact on quality of life of postherpetic neuralgia and painful diabetic neuropathy. *Clinical Journal of Pain* 18 (6): 350-354.

Schmitz, K.H., K.S. Courneya, C. Matthews, et al. 2010. American College of Sports Medicine roundtable on exercise guidelines for cancer survivors. *Medicine & Science in Sports & Exercise* 42 (7): 1409-1426.

Schmitz, K., S.A. French, and R.W. Jeffery. 1997. Correlates of changes in leisure time physical activity over 2 years: The Healthy Worker Project. *Preventive Medicine* 26: 570-579.

Schmitz, K.H., J. Holtzman, K.S. Courneya, L.C. Mâsse, S. Duval, and R. Kane. 2005. Controlled physical activity trials in cancer survivors: A systematic review and meta-analysis. *Cancer Epidemiology Biomarkers & Prevention* 14 (7): 1588-1595.

Schneirla, T. 1959. An evolutionary and developmental theory of biphasic processes underlying approach and withdrawal. In *Nebraska Symposium on Motivation,* edited by M. Jones. Lincoln: University of Nebraska Press.

Scholz, U., B. Schuz, J.P. Ziegelmann, S. Lippke, and R. Schwarzer. 2008. Beyond behavioural intentions: Planning mediates between intentions and physical activity. *British Journal of Health Psychology* 13 (Pt 3): 479-494.

Schuz, B., F.F. Sniehotta, N. Mallach, A.U. Wiedemann, and R. Schwarzer. 2009. Predicting transitions from preintentional, intentional and actional stages of change. *Health Education Research* 24 (1): 64-75.

Schwarzer, R. 1992. *Self-efficacy in the adoption and maintenance of health behaviors: Theoretical approaches and a new model:* Washington, DC: Hemisphere.

Schwarzer, R. 2008. Modeling health behavior change: How to predict and modify the adoption and maintenance of health behaviors. *Applied Psychology—an International Review* 57 (1): 1-29.

Schwarzer, R., A. Luszczynska, J.P. Ziegelmann, U. Scholz, and S. Lippke. 2008. Social-cognitive predictors of physical exercise adherence: Three longitudinal studies in rehabilitation. *Health Psychology* 27 (1 Suppl.): S54-S63.

Schwarzer, R., B. Schüz, J.P. Ziegelmann, S. Lippke, A. Luszczynska, and U. Scholz. 2007. Adoption and maintenance of four health behaviors: Theory-guided longitudinal studies on dental flossing, seat belt use, dietary behavior, and physical activity. *Annals of Behavioral Medicine* 33 (2): 156-166.

Secher, N.H., T. Seifert, and J.J. Van Lieshout. 2008. Cerebral blood flow and metabolism during exercise: Implications for fatigue. *Journal of Applied Physiology* 104 (1): 306-314.

Secord, P.F., and S.M. Jourard. 1953. The appraisal of body-cathexis: Body-cathexis and the self. *Journal of Consulting Psychology* 17: 343-347.

Segal, R., W. Evans, D. Johnson, et al. 2001. Structured exercise improves physical functioning in women with stages I and II breast cancer: Results of a randomized controlled trial. *Journal of Clinical Oncology* 19 (3): 657-665.

Segar, M.L., V.L. Katch, R.S. Roth, et al. 1998. The effect of aerobic exercise on self-esteem and depressive and anxiety symptoms among breast cancer survivors [see comments]. *Oncology Nursing Forum* 25 (Jan-Feb): 107-113.

Sehested J., G. Reinicke, K. Ishino, et al. 1995. Blunted humoral responses to mental stress and physical exercise in cardiac transplant recipients. *European Heart Journal* 166: 852-858

Seip, R.L., D. Snead, E.F. Pierce, P. Stein, and A. Weltman. 1991. Perceptual responses and blood lactate concentration: Effect of training state. *Medicine & Science in Sports & Exercise* 23 (Jan): 80-87.

Seligman, M.E.P., and M. Csikszentmihalyi. 2000. Positive psychology: An introduction. *American Psychologist* 55 (1): 5-14.

Selye, H. 1936. A syndrome produced by diverse nocuous agents. *Nature* 138: 32.

Selye, H. 1950. *Stress.* Montreal: Acta.

Sexton, H., A. Maere, and N.H. Dahl. 1989. Exercise intensity and reduction in neurotic symptoms: A controlled follow-up study. *Acta Psychiatrica Scandinavica* 80 (3): 231-235.

Shankarappa, S.A., E.S. Piedras-Rentería, and E.B. Stubbs. 2011. Forced-exercise delays neuropathic pain in experimental diabetes: Effects on voltage-activated calcium channels. *Journal of Neurochemistry* 118 (2): 224-236.

Shaper, A.G., D.G. Cook, M. Walker, and P.W. Macfarlane. 1984. Prevalence of ischaemic heart disease in middle aged British men. *British Heart Journal* 51 (6): 595-605.

Shapiro, D., L.D. Jamner, J.D. Lane, et al. 1996. Blood pressure publication guidelines. *Psychophysiology* 33: 1-12.

Shapiro P.A., R.P. Sloan, E. Bagiella, J.T. Bigger, Jr., and J.M. Gorman. 1996. Heart rate reactivity and heart period variability throughout the first year after heart transplantation. *Psychophysiology* 331: 54-62

Shapiro, P.A., R.P. Sloan, J.T. Bigger, Jr., E. Bagiella, and J.M. Gorman. 1994. Cardiac denervation and cardiovascular reactivity to psychological stress. *American Journal of Psychiatry* 1518: 1140-1147.

Shavelson, R.J., J.J. Hubner, and G.C. Stanton. 1976. Self-concept: Validation of construct interpretations. *Review of Educational Research* 46 (3): 407-441.

Shaver, P., J. Schwartz, D. Kirson, and C. O'Connor. 1987. Emotion knowledge: further exploration of a prototype approach. *Journal of Personality and Social Psychology.* 52 (6): 1061-86.

Sherman, K.J., D.C. Cherkin, R.D. Wellman, et al. 2011. A randomized trial comparing yoga, stretching, and a self-care book for chronic low back pain. *Archives of Internal Medicine.* 171(22): 2019-2026.

Sherrill, D.L., K. Kotchou, and S.F. Quan. 1998. Association of physical activity and human sleep disorders. *Archives of Internal Medicine* 158: 1894-1898.

Sherrington, C.S. 1900. The muscular sense. In *Textbook of Physiology*, edited by E.A. Schafer, Vol 2: p. 1002-1025. Edinburgh & London: Pentland.

Sherrington, C.S. 1906. *The integrative action of the nervous system.* New Haven: Yale University.

Shields, M.R., C.L. Larson, A.M. Swartz, and J.C. Smith. 2011. Visual threat detection during moderate- and high-intensity exercise. *Emotion* 11 (3): 572.

Shilts, M.K., M. Horowitz, and M.S. Townsend. 2004. Goal setting as a strategy for dietary and physical activity behavior change: A review of the literature. *American Journal of Health Promotion* 19 (2): 81-93.

Shilts, M., Townsend, B., Dishman, RK. 2013. Using goal setting to promote health behavior change: Diet and physical activity. In *New developments in goal setting and task performance,* edited by E. Locke and G. Latham. London: Taylor & Francis.

Shippenberg, T.S., and W. Rea. 1997. Sensitization to the behavioral effects of cocaine: Modulation by dynorphin and kappa-opioid receptor agonists. *Pharmacology, Biochemistry, and Behavior* 57 (3): 449-455.

Sibley, B.A., and J.L. Etnier. 2003. The relationship between phys ical activity and cognition in children: A meta-analysis. *Pediatric Exercise Science* 15: 243-256.

Siegel, J.M. 2000. Brainstem mechanisms generating REM sleep. In *Principles and practice of sleep medicine,* edited by M.K. Kryger, T. Roth and W.O. Dement. New York: Saunders.

Silber, H.A., D.A. Bluemke, P. Ouyang, Y.P. Du, W.S. Post, and J.A. Lima. 2001. The relationship between vascular wall shear stress and flow-mediated dilation: Endothelial function assessed by phase-contrast magnetic resonance angiography. *Journal of the American College of Cardiology* 38 (7): 1859-1865.

Silva, M.N., D. Markland, E.V. Carraca, et al. 2011. Exercise autonomous motivation predicts 3-yr weight loss in women. *Medicine & Science in Sports & Exercise* 43 (4): 728-737.

Silverberg, A.B., S.D. Shah, M.W. Haymond, and P.E. Cryer. 1978. Norepinephrine: Hormone and neurotransmitter in man. *American Journal of Physiology* 234: E252-E256.

Simkin, L.R., and A.M. Gross. 1994. Assessment of coping with high-risk situations for exercise relapse among healthy women. *Health Psychology* 13 (3): 274-277.

Singer, J.D., and J.B. Willett. 2003. *Applied longitudinal data analysis: Modeling change and event occurrence.* New York: Oxford University Press.

Singh, N.A., K.M. Clements, and M.A. Fiatarone. 1997. A randomized controlled trial of the effect of exercise on sleep. *Sleep* 20 (2): 95-101.

Singh, N.A., T.M. Stavrinos, Y. Scarbek, G. Galambos, C. Liber, and M.A. Fiatarone Singh. 2005. A randomized controlled trial of high versus low intensity weight training versus general practitioner care for clinical depression in older adults. *Journals of Gerontology. Series A, Biological Sciences and Medical Sciences* 60 (6): 768-776.

Sinyor, D., S.G. Schwartz, F. Peronnet, G. Brisson, and P. Seraganian. 1983. Aerobic fitness level and reactivity to psychosocial stress: Physiological, biochemical, and subjective measures. *Psychosomatic Medicine* 45 (Jun): 205-217.

Sjogren, T., K.J. Nissinen, S.K. Jarvenpaa, M.T. Ojanen, H. Vanharanta, and E.A. Malkia. 2006. Effects of a physical exercise intervention on subjective physical well-being, psychosocial functioning and general well-being among office workers: A cluster randomized-controlled cross-over design. *Scandinavian Journal of Medicine & Science in Sports* 16 (6): 381-390.

Skapinakis, P., G. Lewis, and V. Mavreas. 2003. Cross-cultural differences in the epidemiology of unexplained fatigue syndromes in primary care. *British Journal of Psychiatry* 182: 205-209.

Skinner, B.F. 1938. *The behavior of organisms.* New York: Appleton-Century-Crofts.

Skinner, J.S., R. Hutsler, V. Bergsteinova, and E.R. Buskirk. 1973. The validity and reliability of a rating scale of perceived exertion. *Medicine and Science in Sports* 5 (2): 94-96.

Skrinar, G.S., S.P. Ingram, and K.B. Pandolf. 1983. Effect of endurance training on perceived exertion and stress hormones in women. *Perceptual & Motor Skills* 57 (Dec): 1239-1250.

Sloan, R.P., P.A. Shapiro, R.E. DeMeersman, et al. 2011. Impact of aerobic training on cardiovascular reactivity to and recovery from challenge. *Psychosomatic Medicine* 73 (2): 134-141.

Smith, J.C., and J.B. Crabbe. 2000. Emotion and exercise. *International Journal of Sport Psychology* 31 (2): 156-174.

Smith, J.C., K.A. Nielson, J.L. Woodard, et al. 2010. Interactive effects of physical activity and APOE-e4 on Bold semantic memory activation in healthy elders. *NeuroImage.* 54: 635-644. doi: 10.1016/j.neuroimage.2010.07.070.

Smith, J.C., and P.J. O'Connor. 2003. Physical activity does not disturb the measurement of startle and corrugator responses during affective picture viewing. *Biological Psychology* 63 (3): 293-310.

Smith, J.C., P.J. O'Connor, J.B. Crabbe, and R.K. Dishman. 2002. Emotional responsiveness after low- and moderate-intensity exercise and seated rest. *Medicine & Science in Sports & Exercise* 34 (7): 1158-1167.

Smith, J.C., E.S. Paulson, D.B. Cook, M.D. Verber, and Q. Tian. 2010. Detecting changes in human cerebral blood flow after acute exercise using arterial spin labeling: Implications for fMRI. *Journal of Neuroscience Methods* 191 (2): 258-262.

Smith, K.S., and K.C. Berridge. 2007. Opioid limbic circuit for reward: Interaction between hedonic hotspots of nucleus accumbens and ventral pallidum. *Journal of Neuroscience* 27 (7): 1594-1605.

Smith, L.L. 1991. Acute inflammation: The underlying mechanism in delayed onset muscle soreness? *Medicine & Science in Sports & Exercise* 23 (5): 542-551.

Smith, M.T., and J.A. Haythornthwaite. 2004. How do sleep disturbance and chronic pain inter-relate? Insights from the longitudinal and cognitive-behavioral clinical trials literature. *Sleep Medicine Reviews* 8 (2): 119-132.

Smith, P.J., J.A. Blumenthal, M.A. Babyak, et al. 2010. Effects of the dietary approaches to stop hypertension diet, exercise, and caloric restriction on neurocognition in overweight adults with high blood pressure. *Hypertension* 55 (6): 1331-1338.

Smith, T.L., K.H. Masaki, K. Fong, et al. 2010. Effect of walking distance on 8-year incident depressive symptoms in elderly men with and without chronic disease: The Honolulu-Asia Aging Study. *Journal of the American Geriatrics Society* 58 (8): 1447-1452.

Smits, J.A., A.C. Berry, D. Rosenfield, M.B. Powers, E. Behar, and M.W. Otto. 2008. Reducing anxiety sensitivity with exercise. *Depression and Anxiety* 25 (8): 689-699.

Smits, J.A., A.C. Berry, C.D. Tart, and M.B. Powers. 2008. The efficacy of cognitive-behavioral interventions for reducing anxiety sensitivity: A meta-analytic review. *Behaviour Research and Therapy* 46 (9): 1047-1054.

Snodgrass, J.G., G. Levy-Berger, and M. Hydon. 1985. *Human experimental psychology.* New York: Oxford University Press.

Soares, J., P.V. Holmes, K.J. Renner, G.L. Edwards, B.N. Bunnell, and R.K. Dishman. 1999. Brain noradrenergic responses to footshock after chronic activity-wheel running. *Behavioral Neuroscience* 113 (Jun): 558-566.

Sobocki P., B. Jönsson, J. Angst, and C. Rehnberg. 2006. Cost of depression in Europe. *Journal of Mental Health Policy and Economics.* 9(2): 87-98.

Sonstroem, R.J. 1978. Physical estimation and attraction scales: Rationale and research. *Medicine and Science in Sports* 10 (Summer): 97-102.

Sonstroem, R.J. 1998. Physical self-concept: Assessment and external validity. *Exercise and Sport Sciences Reviews* 26: 133-164.

Sonstroem, R.J. 1988. Psychological models. In *Exercise adherence: its impact on public health*, edited by R.K. Dishman. Champaign, IL: Human Kinetics.

Sonstroem, R.J., L.L. Harlow, and L. Josephs. 1994. Exercise and self-esteem: Validity of model expansion and exercise associations. *Journal of Sport & Exercise Psychology* 16 (1): 29-42.

Sonstroem, R.J., and W.P. Morgan. 1989. Exercise and self-esteem: Rationale and model. *Medicine & Science in Sports & Exercise* 21 (3): 329-337.

Sorabji, R. 2004. *Aristotle on memory*. 2nd ed. Chicago: University of Chicago Press.

Sothmann, M.S., J. Buckworth, R.P. Claytor, R.H. Cox, J.E. White-Welkley, and R.K. Dishman. 1996. Exercise training and the cross-stressor adaptation hypothesis. *Exercise and Sport Sciences Reviews* 24: 267-287.

Sothmann, M.S., A.B. Gustafson, T.L. Garthwaite, T.S. Horn, and B.A. Hart. 1988. Cardiovascular fitness and selected adrenal hormone responses to cognitive stress. *Endocrine Research* 14: 59-69.

Southall, J.P. C. 1924. *Helmholtz's treatise on physiological optics*. Translated from the third German edition, Vol. I: The Optical Society of America. Menasha, WI: Banta

Spalding, T.W., L.S. Jeffers, S.W. Porges, and B.D. Hatfield. 2000. Vagal and cardiac reactivity to psychological stressors in trained and untrained men. *Medicine and Science in Sports and Exercise.* 32 (3): 581-91.

Sparks, A.C. 1997. Reflections on the socially constructed physical self. In *The physical self: From motivation to well-being*, edited by K.R. Fox. Champaign, IL: Human Kinetics.

Sparling, P.B. 2003. College physical education: An unrecognized agent of change in combating inactivity-related diseases. *Perspectives in Biology and Medicine* 46 (4): 579-587.

Sparling, P.B., A. Giuffrida, D. Piomelli, L. Rosskopf, and A. Dietrich. 2003. Exercise activates the endocannabinoid system. *Neuroreport* 14 (17): 2209-2211.

Sparling, P.B., T.K. Snow, and B. Beavers. 1999. Serum cholesterol levels in college students: Opportunities for education and intervention. *Journal of American College Health Association* 48: 123-127.

Speck, R.M., K.S. Courneya, L.C. Masse, S. Duval, and K.H. Schmitz. 2010. An update of controlled physical activity trials in cancer survivors: A systematic review and meta-analysis. *Journal of Cancer Survivorship: Research and Practice* 4 (2): 87-100.

Spence, J.C., K.R. McGannon, and P. Poon. 2005. The effect of exercise on global self-esteem: A quantitative review. *Journal of Sport & Exercise Psychology* 27 (3): 311-334.

Sperry, R.W. 1950. Neural basis of the spontaneous optokinetic response produced by visual inversion. *Journal of Comparative and Physiological Psychology* 43 (6): 482-489.

Spielberger, C.D., R.L. Gorsuch, R. Lushene, P.R. Vagg, and G.A. Jacobs. 1983. *Manual for the State-Trait Anxiety Inventory*. Palo Alto, CA: Consulting Psychologists Press.

Spirduso, W.W. 1980. Physical fitness, aging, and psychomotor speed: A review. *Journal of Gerontology* 35: 850-865.

Spirduso, W.W., L.W. Poon, and W.J. Chodzko-Kajko. 2008. *Exercise and its mediating effects on cognition*. Edited by L.W. Poon, W.W. Spirduso, and W.J. Chodzko-Kajko. Vol. 2, *Aging, exercise, and cognition series*. Champaign, IL: Human Kinetics.

Stagg, N.J., H.P. Mata, M.M. Ibrahim, et al. 2011. Regular exercise reverses sensory hypersensitivity in a rat neuropathic pain model: Role of endogenous opioids. *Anesthesiology* 114 (4): 940-948. doi: 10.1097/ALN.0b013e318210f880.

Stahl, S.M. 2002. The psychopharmacology of energy and fatigue. *Journal of Clinical Psychiatry* 63 (1): 7-8.

Ståhl, T., A. Rutten, D. Nutbeam, et al. 2001. The importance of the social environment for physically active lifestyle: Results from an international study. *Social Science and Medicine* 52: 1-10.

Steele, T. 1972. *Treatise of man. Rene Descartes*. Cambridge, MA: Harvard University Press.

Stefoni, S., K. Midtved, E. Cole, et al. 2005. Efficacy and safety outcomes among de novo renal transplant recipients managed by C2 monitoring of cyclosporine a microemulsion: Results of a 12-month, randomized, multicenter study. *Transplantation* 79 (5): 577-583.

Steimer, T. 2002. The biology of fear-and anxiety-related behaviors. *Dialogues in Clinical Neuroscience* 4: 231-249.

Stein, P.N., and R.W. Motta. 1992. Effects of aerobic and nonaerobic exercise on depression and self-concept. *Perceptual & Motor Skills* 74 (1): 79-89.

Steinberg, H., B.R. Nicholls, E.A. Sykes, et al. 1998. Weekly exercise consistently reinstates positive mood. *European Psychologist* 3 (4): 271-280.

Steinhardt, M., and R.K. Dishman. 1989. Reliability and validity of expected outcomes and barriers for habitual physical activity. *Journal of Occupational Medicine* 31 (6): 536-546.

Stenson, P.D., M. Mort, E.V. Ball, et al. 2009. The Human Gene Mutation Database: 2008 update. *Genome Medicine* 1 (1): 13.

Stenström, C.H., and M.A. Minor. 2003. Evidence for the benefit of aerobic and strengthening exercise in rheumatoid arthritis. *Arthritis Care & Research* 49 (3): 428-434.

Stephens, T. 1988. Physical activity and mental health in the United States and Canada: Evidence from four population surveys. *Preventive Medicine* 17: 35-47.

Steptoe, A., J. Wardle, R. Fuller, et al. 1997. Leisure-time physical exercise: Prevalence, attitudinal correlates, and behavioral correlates among young Europeans from 21 countries. *Preventive Medicine* 26 (6): 845-854.

Sternberg, S. 1969. Memory-scanning: Mental processes revealed by reaction time experiments. *American Scientist* 57: 421-457.

Stetson, B.A., A.O. Beacham, S.J. Frommelt, et al. 2005. Exercise slips in high-risk situations and activity patterns in long-term exercisers: An application of the relapse prevention model. *Annals of Behavioral Medicine* 30 (1): 25-35.

Stevens, J.C. 1957. On the psychophysical law. *Psychological Review* 64 (3): 153-181.

Stevens, J.C., and E.H. Galanter. 1957. Ratio scales and category scales for a dozen perceptual continua. *Journal of Experimental Psychology* 54: 377-411.

Stevens, J.C., and J.D. Mack. 1959. Scales of apparent force. *Journal of Experimental Psychology* 58: 405-413.

Stewart, A.L., K.M. Mills, P.G. Sepsis, et al. 1997. Evaluation of CHAMPS, a physical activity promotion program for older adults. *Annals of Behavioral Medicine* 19 (4): 353-361.

Stewart, W.F., J.A. Ricci, E. Chee, D. Morganstein, and R. Lipton. 2003. Lost productive time and cost due to common pain conditions in the U.S. workforce. *Journal of the American Medical Association* 290 (18): 2443-2454.

Stone, E.J., T.L. McKenzie, G.J. Welk, and M. Booth. 1998. Effects of physical activity interventions in youth: Review and synthesis. *American Journal of Preventive Medicine* 15 (4): 298-315.

Stones, M.J., and A. Kozma. 1988. Physical activity, age, and cognitive/motor performance. In *Cognitive development in adulthood: Progress in cognitive development research*, edited by M.L. Howe and C.J. Branerd. New York: Springer-Verlag.

Strawbridge, W.J., S. Deleger, R.E. Roberts, and G.A. Kaplan. 2002. Physical activity reduces the risk of subsequent depression for older adults. *American Journal of Epidemiology* 156 (4): 328-334.

Strijk, J.E., K.I. Proper, L. Klaver, A.J. van der Beek, and W. van Mechelen. 2010. Associations between V̇O₂max and vitality in older workers: A cross-sectional study. *BMC Public Health* 10: 684.

Strine, T.W., A.H. Mokdad, L.S. Balluz, et al. 2008. Depression and anxiety in the United States: Findings from the 2006 Behavioral Risk Factor Surveillance System. *Psychiatric Services* 59 (12): 1383-1390.

Ströhle, A. 2009. Physical activity, exercise, depression and anxiety disorders. *Journal of Neural Transmission* 116 (6): 777-784.

Ströhle, A., C. Feller, M. Onken, F. Godemann, A. Heinz, and F. Dimeo. 2005. The acute antipanic activity of aerobic exercise. *American Journal of Psychiatry* 162 (12): 2376-2378.

Ströhle, A., B. Graetz, M. Scheel, et al. 2009. The acute antipanic and anxiolytic activity of aerobic exercise in patients with panic disorder and healthy control subjects. *Journal of Psychiatric Research* 43 (12): 1013-1017.

Ströhle, A., M. Hofler, H. Pfister, et al. 2007. Physical activity and prevalence and incidence of mental disorders in adolescents and young adults. *Psychological Medicine* 37 (11): 1657-1666.

Ströhle, A., M. Stoy, B. Graetz, et al. 2010. Acute exercise ameliorates reduced brain-derived neurotrophic factor in patients with panic disorder. *Psychoneuroendocrinology* 35 (3): 364-368.

Strong, W.B., R.M. Malina, C.J. Blimkie, et al. 2005. Evidence based physical activity for school-age youth. *Journal of Pediatrics* 146 (6): 732-737. doi: 10.1016/j.jpeds.2005.01.055

Stroth, S., K. Hille, M. Spitzer, and R. Reinhardt. 2009. Aerobic endurance exercise benefits memory and affect in young adults. *Neuropsychological Rehabilitation* 19 (2): 223-243.

Stubbe, J.H., D.I. Boomsma, J.M. Vink, et al. 2006. Genetic influences on exercise participation in 37,051 twin pairs from seven countries. *PLoS ONE* 1: e22.

Stuifbergen, A.K., H. Becker, S. Blozis, G. Timmerman, and V. Kullberg. 2003. A randomized clinical trial of a wellness intervention for women with multiple sclerosis. *Archives of Physical Medicine and Rehabilitation* 84 (4): 467-476.

Stunkard, A.J., M.S. Faith, and K.C. Allison. 2003. Depression and obesity. *Biological Psychiatry* 54 (3): 330-337.

Sturman, M.T., M.C. Morris, C.F. Mendes De Leon, R.S. Wilson, and D.A. Evans. 2005. Physical activity, cognitive activity, and cognitive decline in a biracial community population. *Archives of Neurology* 62: 1750-1754.

Sun, Y.-C., Y.-C. Hung, Y. Chang, and S.-C. Kuo. 2010. Effects of a prenatal yoga programme on the discomforts of pregnancy and maternal childbirth self-efficacy in Taiwan. *Midwifery* 26 (6): e31-e36.

Sundgot-Borgen, J. 1994. Risk and trigger factors for the development of eating disorders in female elite athletes. *Medicine & Science in Sports & Exercise* 26 (Apr): 414-419.

Sundgot-Borgen, J., and M.K. Torstveit. 2004. Prevalence of eating disorders in elite athletes is higher than in the general population. *Clinical Journal of Sport Medicine* 14 (1): 25-32.

Swallow, J.G., P.A. Carter, and T. Garland, Jr. 1998. Artificial selection for increased wheel-running behavior in house mice. *Behavior Genetics* 28 (3): 227-237.

Szabo, A., E. Billett, and J. Turner. 2001. Phenylethylamine, a possible link to the antidepressant effects of exercise? *British Journal of Sports Medicine* 35 (5): 342-343.

Tammelin, T. 2003. Adolescent participation in sports and adult physical activity. *American Journal of Preventive Medicine* 24 (1): 22.

Tanaka, K., A.C. de Quadros, R.F. Santos, F. Stella, L.T. Gobbi, and S. Gobbi. 2009. Benefits of physical exercise on executive functions in older people with Parkinson's disease. *Brain and Cognition* 69: 435-441.

Tancer, M.E., M.B. Stein, and T.W. Uhde. 1993. Growth hormone response to intravenous clonidine in social phobia: Comparison to patients with panic disorder and healthy volunteers. *Biological Psychiatry* 34 (Nov 1): 591-595.

Tanha, T., P Wollmer, O Thorsson, et al. 2011. Lack of physical activity in young children is related to higher composite risk factor score for cardiovascular disease. *Acta Paediatrica* 100 (5): 717-721.

Tantillo M, C.M. Kesick, G.W. Hynd, R.K. Dishman. 2002. The effects of exercise on children with attention-deficit hyperactivity disorder. *Medicine and Science in Sports and Exercise* 34(2): 203-212.

Task Force of the European Society of Cardiology and the North American Society of Pacing and Electrophysiology. 1996. Heart rate variability: Standards of measurement, physiological interpretation and clinical use. *Circulation* 93: 1043-1065.

Taylor, A.H., N.T. Cable, G. Faulkner, et al. 2004. Physical activity and older adults: A review of health benefits and the effectiveness of interventions. *Journal of Sports Sciences* 22 (8): 703-725.

Taylor, S.E. 1999. Health behaviors. In *Health psychology*, 4th ed. Boston: McGraw-Hill.

Tellegen, A. 1985. Structures of mood and personality their relevance to assessing anxiety, with emphasis on self-report. In *Anxiety and the Anxiety Disorders*, edited by A.H. Tuma, and J. Maser. Hillsdale, NJ: Erlbaum.

Tenebaum, G. 1999. The implementation of Thurstone's and Guttman's measurement ideas in Rasch analysis. *International Journal of Sport Psychology* 30: 3-16.

Thayer, J.F., B.H. Friedman, and T.D. Borkovec. 1996. Autonomic characteristics of generalized anxiety disorder and worry. *Biological Psychiatry* 39 (Feb 15): 255-266.

Thayer, R.E. 1987. Energy, tiredness, and tension effects as a function of a sugar snack vs. moderate exercise. *Journal of Personality & Social Psychology* 52: 119-125.

Thayer, R.E. 1989. *The biopsychology of mood and arousal*. New York: Oxford University Press.

Thayer, R.E., J.R. Newman, and T.M. McClain. 1994. Self-regulation of mood: Strategies for changing a bad mood, raising energy, and reducing tension. *Journal of Personality and Social Psychology* 67 (Nov): 910-925.

Thelen, E. 2004. The central role of action in typical and atypical development: A dynamical systems perspective. In *Movement and action in learning and development: Clinical implications for pervasive developmental disorders*, edited by I.J. Stockman. New York: Elsevier.

Thom, N.J., B.A. Clementz, O'Connor P.J., and R.K. Dishman. 2012. *The effects of an acute bout of moderate intensity exercise on anger*. Athens, GA: University of Georgia.

Thompson, J. 2004. The (mis)measurement of body image: Ten strategies to improve assessment for applied and research purposes. *Body Image* 1 (1): 7-14.

Thorndike, E.L. 1904. *An introduction to the theory of mental and social measurements*. New York: The Science Press.

Thorsen, L., W. Nystad, H. Stigum, et al. 2005. The association between self-reported physical activity and prevalence of depression and anxiety disorder in long-term survivors of testicular cancer and men in a general population sample. *Supportive Care in Cancer* 13 (8): 637-646.

Thurstone, L.L. 1926. The scoring of individual performance. *Journal of Educational Psychology* 17: 446-457.

Thurstone, L.L. 1927. A law of comparative judgment. *Psychological Review* 34: 273-286.

Thurstone, L.L. 1928. *Attitudes can be measured*. Vol. 33. Chicago: University of Chicago Press,.

Thurstone, L.L. 1931. The measurement of social attitudes. *Journal of Abnormal & Social Psychology* 26: 249-269.

Thurstone, L.L., and E.J. Chave. 1929. *The measurement of attitude*. Chicago: University of Chicago Press.

Tian, Q., and J.C. Smith. 2011. Attentional bias to emotional stimuli is altered during moderate- but not high-intensity exercise. *Emotion*. 11(6): 1415-1424. doi: 10.1037/a0023568.

Tieman, J.G., L.J. Peacock, K.J. Cureton, and R.K. Dishman. 2001. Acoustic startle eyeblink response after acute exercise. *International Journal of Neuroscience* 106: 21-33.

Tieman, J.G., L.J. Peacock, K.J. Cureton, and R.K. Dishman. 2002. The influence of exercise intensity and physical activity history on state anxiety after exercise. *International Journal of Sport Psychology* 33 (2): 155-166.

Tiger, L. 1979. *Optimism: The biology of hope.* New York: Simon and Schuster.

Tomarken, A.J., and D.H. Zald. 2009. Conceptual, methodological, and empirical ambiguities in the linkage between anger and approach: comment on Carver and Harmon-Jones (2009). *Psychological Bulletin.* 135 (2): 209-214; discussion 215-217. doi: 10.1037/a0014735.

Tomporowski, P.D. 1997. The effects of physical and mental training on the mental abilities of older adults. *Journal of Aging and Physical Activity* 5: 9-27.

Tomporowski, P.D. 2003. Effects of acute bouts of exercise on cognition. *Acta Psychologica* 112: 297-324.

Tomporowski, P.D., C.L. Davis, P.H. Miller, and J.A. Naglieri. 2008. Exercise and children's intelligence, cognition, and academic achievement. *Educational Psychology Review* 20 (2): 111-131.

Tomporowski, P.D., and N.R. Ellis. 1986. The effects of exercise on cognitive processes: A review. *Psychological Bulletin* 99: 338-346.

Tomporowski, P.D., K. Lambourne, and M.S. Okumura. 2011. Physical activity interventions and children's mental function: An introduction and overview. *Preventive Medicine* 52, S3-S9.

Tomporowski, P.D., B.A. McCullick, and M. Horvat. 2010. *Role of contextual interference and mental engagement on learning: Perspectives on cognitive psychology.* New York: Nova Science.

Tomporowski, P.D., J.A. Naglieri, and K. Lambourne. 2010. Exercise psychology and children's intelligence. In *Oxford Handbook of Exercise Psychology,* edited by E.O. Acevedo. New York: Oxford University Press.

Torregrossa, M.M., E.M. Jutkiewicz, H.I. Mosberg, G. Balboni, S.J. Watson, and J.H. Woods. 2006. Peptidic delta opioid receptor agonists produce antidepressant-like effects in the forced swim test and regulate BDNF mRNA expression in rats. *Brain Research* 1069 (1): 172-181.

Torrubia, R., C. Avila, J. Moltó, and X. Caseras. 2001. The Sensitivity to Punishment and Sensitivity to Reward Questionnaire (SPSRQ) as a measure of Gray's anxiety and impulsivity dimensions. *Personality and Individual Differences* 31 (6): 837-862.

Trivedi, M.H., M. Fava, S.R. Wisniewski, et al. 2006a. Medication augmentation after the failure of SSRIs for depression. *New England Journal of Medicine* 354 (12): 1243-1252.

Trivedi, M.H., T.L. Greer, B.D. Grannemann, H.O. Chambliss, and A.N. Jordan. 2006b. Exercise as an augmentation strategy for treatment of major depression. *Journal of Psychiatric Practice* 12 (4): 205-213.

Troiano, R.P., D. Berrigan, K.W. Dodd, L.C. Masse, T. Tilert, and M. McDowell. 2008. Physical activity in the United States measured by accelerometer. *Medicine & Science in Sports & Exercise* 40 (1): 181-188.

Troped, P.J., and R.P. Saunders. 1998. Gender differences in social influence on physical activity at different stages of exercise adoption. *American Journal of Health Promotion* 13: 112-115.

Trost, S.G., N. Owen, A.E. Bauman, J.F. Sallis, and W. Brown. 2002. Correlates of adults' participation in physical activity: Review and update. *Medicine & Science in Sports & Exercise* 34 (12): 1996-2001.

Trzesniewski, K.H., M.B. Donnellan, T.E. Moffitt, R.W. Robins, R. Poulton, and A. Caspi. 2006. Low self-esteem during adolescence predicts poor health, criminal behavior, and limited economic prospects during adulthood. *Developmental Psychology* 42 (2): 381-390.

Tsuji, H., M.G. Larson, F.J. J. Venditti, et al. 1996. Impact of reduced heart rate variability on risk for cardiac events: The Framingham Study. *Circulation* 94: 2850-2855.

Tsutsumi, T., B.M. Don, L.D. Zaichkowsky, K. Takenaka, K. Oka, and T. Ohno. 1998. Comparison of high and moderate intensity of strength training on mood and anxiety in older adults. *Perceptual & Motor Skills* 87 (3, Pt 1): 1003-1011.

Tucker, L.A. 1985. Effect of weight training on self-concept: A profile of those influenced most. *Research Quarterly for Exercise and Sport* 54: 389-397.

Turk, D.C., and R. Melzack. 2001. The measurement of pain and the assessment of people experiencing pain. In *Handbook of pain assessment,* edited by D.C. Turk and R. Melzack. New York: Guilford Press.

Tworoger, S.S., Y. Yasui, M.V. Vitiello, et al. 2003. Effects of a yearlong moderate-intensity exercise and a stretching intervention on sleep quality in postmenopausal women. *Sleep* 26 (7): 830-836.

Uhlenhuth, E.H., M.B. Balter, G.D. Mellinger, I.H. Cisin, and J. Clinthorne. 1983. Symptom checklist syndromes in the general population: Correlations with psychotherapeutic drug use. *Archives of General Psychiatry* 40: 1167-1173.

Umeda, M., L.W. Newcomb, L.D. Ellingson, and K.F. Koltyn. 2010. Examination of the dose–response relationship between pain perception and blood pressure elevations induced by isometric exercise in men and women. *Biological Psychology* 85 (1): 90-96.

Unlu, E., E. Eksioglu, E. Aydog, S. Tolga Aydoð, and G. Atay. 2007. The effect of exercise on hip muscle strength, gait speed and cadence in patients with total hip arthroplasty: A randomized controlled study. *Clinical Rehabilitation* 21 (8): 706-711.

Urponen, H., I. Vuori, J. Hasan, and M. Partinen. 1988. Self evaluations of factors promoting and disturbing sleep: An epidemiological survey in Finland. Social Science Medicine 26(4): 443-450.

U.S. Census Bureau. 2012. *Facts for features—Back to school: 2011-2012.* U.S. Department of Commerce,

June 27, 2011 www.census.gov/newsroom/releases/archives/facts_for_features_special_editions/cb11-ff15.html.

U.S. Department of Health and Human Services (USDHHS). 1996. *Physical activity and health: A report of the surgeon general.* Atlanta, GA: U.S. Department of Health and Human Services, Centers for Disease Control and Prevention, National Center for Chronic Disease Prevention and Health Promotion.

U.S. Department of Health and Human Services (USDHHS). 2000. *Healthy people 2010: Understanding and improving health.* Washington, DC: U.S. Government Printing Office.

U.S. Department of Health and Human Services (USDHHS). 2000. *Mental health: A report of the surgeon general.* Atlanta, GA: U.S. Department of Health and Human Services, Centers for Disease Control and Prevention, National Center for Chronic Disease Prevention and Health Promotion.

U.S. Department of Health and Human Services (USDHHS). 2010. *Healthy people 2020.* Washington, DC: U.S. Government Printing Office.

U.S. Public Health Services. 1990. *Promoting health/preventing disease: Year 2000 objectives for the nation.* Washington, DC: U.S. Government Printing Office.

Utter, A.C., R.J. Robertson, D.C. Nieman, and J. Kang. 2002. Children's OMNI Scale of Perceived Exertion: Walking/running evaluation. *Medicine & Science in Sports & Exercise* 34 (1): 139-144.

Valkeinen, H., M. Alen, P. Hannonen, A. Häkkinen, O. Airaksinen, and K. Häkkinen. 2004. Changes in knee extension and flexion force, EMG and functional capacity during strength training in older females with fibromyalgia and healthy controls. *Rheumatology* 43 (2): 225-228.

Van Ameringen, M., C. Allgulander, B. Bandelow, et al. 2003. WCA recommendations for the long-term treatment of social phobia. *CNS spectrums* 8 (8 Suppl. 1): 40-52.

Van Baar, M.E., W.J.J. Assendelft, J. Dekker, R.A.B. Oostendorp, and J.W.J. Bijlsma. 1999. Effectiveness of exercise therapy in patients with osteoarthritis of the hip or knee: A systematic review of randomized clinical trials. *Arthritis & Rheumatism* 42 (7): 1361-1369.

Van Cauwenberg, J., I. De Bourdeaudhuij, F. De Meester, et al. 2011. Relationship between the physical environment and physical activity in older adults: A systematic review. *Health and Place* 17 (2): 458-469.

Van Landuyt, L.M., P. Ekkekakis, E.E. Hall, and S.J. Petruzzello 2000. Throwing the mountains into the lakes: On the perils of nomothetic conceptions of the exercise-affect relationship. *Journal of Sport and Exercise Psychology*, 22 (2): 208-234.

van der Horst, K., A. Oenema, I. Ferreira, et al. 2007. A systematic review of environmental correlates of obesity-related dietary behaviors in youth. *Health Education Research* 22 (2): 203-226.

Van Der Horst, K., M.J.C.A. Paw, J.W.R. Twisk, and W. Van Mechelen. 2007. A brief review on correlates of physical activity and sedentariness in youth. *Medicine & Science in Sports & Exercise* 39 (8): 1241-1250. doi: 10.1249/mss.0b013e318059bf35.

Van der Linden, D. 2011. The urge to stop: The cognitive and biological nature of acute mental fatigue. In *Cognitive fatigue*, edited by P.L. Ackerman. Washington, DC: American Psychological Association.

van der Molen, M.W. 1996. Energetics and the reaction process: Running threads through experimental psychology. In *Handbook of perception and action*, edited by O. Neumann and A.F. Sanders. New York: Academic Press.

Van Dorsten, B. 2007. The use of motivational interviewing in weight loss. *Current Diabetes Reports* 7 (5): 386-390.

Van Hoomissen, J.D., H.O. Chambliss, P.V. Holmes, and R.K. Dishman. 2003. Effects of chronic exercise and imipramine on mRNA for BDNF after olfactory bulbectomy in rat. *Brain Research* 974 (1-2): 228-235.

Van Hoomissen, J., J. Kunrath, R. Dentlinger, A. Lafrenz, M. Krause, and A. Azar. 2011. Cognitive and locomotor/exploratory behavior after chronic exercise in the olfactory bulbectomy animal model of depression. *Behavioural Brain Research* 222 (1): 106-116.

Van Hoomissen, J.D., P.V. Holmes, A.S. Zellner, A. Poudevigne, and R.K. Dishman. 2004. Effects of beta-adrenoreceptor blockade during chronic exercise on contextual fear conditioning and mRNA for galanin and brain-derived neurotrophic factor. *Behavioral Neuroscience* 118 (6): 1378-1390.

Van Hoomissen, J.D., H.A. O'Neal, P.V. Holmes, and R.K. Dishman. 2001. Serotonin transporter mRNA in dorsal raphe is unchanged by treadmill exercise training. *Medicine and Science in Sports and Exercise*, 32(5): S42.

van Praag, H. 2009. Exercise and the brain: Something to chew on. *Trends in Neurosciences* 32 (5): 283-290.

van Praag, H., B.R. Christie, T.J. Sejnowski, and F.H. Gage. 1999. Running enhances neurogenesis, learning, and long-term potentiation in mice. *Proceedings of the National Academy of Sciences of the United States of America* 96 (23): 13427-13431.

Van Reeth, O., J. Sturis, M.M. Byrne, et al. 1994. Nocturnal exercise phase delays circadian rhythms of melatonin and thyrotropin secretion in normal men. *American Journal of Physiology* 266 (6 Pt 1): E964-E974.

van Uffelen, J.G.Z., M.J.M. Chinapaw, W. van Mechelen, and M. Hopman-Rock. 2011. Walking or vitamin B for cognition in older adults with mild cognitive impairment? A randomized controlled trial. *British Journal of Sports Medicine* 42: 344-351.

Van Vorst, J.G., J. Buckworth, and C. Mattern. 2002. Physical self-concept and strength changes in college weight training classes. *Research Quarterly for Exercise and Sport* 73 (1): 113-117.

Varkey, E, Å. Cider, J. Carlsson, and M. Linde. 2011. Exercise as migraine prophylaxis: A randomized study using relaxation and topiramate as controls. *Cephalalgia* 31 (14): 1428-1438.

Varrassi, G., C. Bazzano, and W.T. Edwards. 1989. Effects of physical activity on maternal plasma beta-endorphin levels and perception of labor pain. *American Journal of Obstetrics and Gynecology* 160 (3): 707-712.

Vaux, C.L. 1926. A discussion of physical exercise and recreation. *Occupational Therapy & Rehabilitation* 5: 329-333.

Vaynman, S., and F. Gomez-Pinilla. 2006. Revenge of the "Sit": How lifestyle impacts neuronal and cognitive health through molecular systems that interface energy metabolism with neuronal plasticity. *Journal of Neuroscience Research* 84: 699-715.

Vaynman, S., Z. Ying, and F. Gomez-Pinilla. 2004. Hippocampal BDNF mediates the efficacy of exercise on synaptic plasticity and cognition. *European Journal of Neuroscience* 20 (10): 2580-2590.

Veasey, S.C., C.A. Fornal, C.W. Metzler, and B.L. Jacobs. 1995. Response of serotonergic caudal raphe neurons in relation to specific motor activities in freely moving cats. *Journal of Neuroscience* 15 (Jul): 5346-5359.

Velikonja, O., K. Curic, A. Ozura, and S.S. Jazbec. 2010. Influence of sports climbing and yoga on spasticity, cognitive function, mood and fatigue in patients with multiple sclerosis. *Clinical Neurology and Neurosurgery* 112 (7): 597-601.

Verplanken, B., and O. Melkevik. 2008. Predicting habit: The case of physical exercise. *Psychology of Sport and Exercise* 9 (1): 15-26.

Verplanken, B., and S. Orbell. 2003. Reflections on past behavior: A self report index of habit strength. *Journal of Applied Social Psychology* 33 (6): 1313-1330.

Viner, R.M., C. Clark, S.J. Taylor, et al. 2008. Longitudinal risk factors for persistent fatigue in adolescents. *Archives of Pediatrics & Adolescent Medicine* 162 (5): 469-475.

Vitiello, M.V. 2008. Exercise, sleep, and cognition. In *Exercise and its mediating effects on cognition*, edited by W.W. Spirduso, L.W. Poon, and W.J. Chodzko-Zajko. Champaign, IL: Human Kinetics.

Volinn, E. 1997. The epidemiology of low back pain in the rest of the world: A review of surveys in low- and middle-income countries. *Spine* 22 (15): 1747-1754.

von Holst, E., and H. Mittelstaedt. 1950. Das reafferenzprinzip: Wechselwirkungen zwischen Zentralnervensystem und Peripherie [The re-afference principle: Mutual effects between the central nervous system and the periphery]. *Naturwissenschaften* 37: 464-476.

Von Korff, M., P. Crane, M. Lane, et al. 2005. Chronic spinal pain and physical–mental comorbidity in the United States: Results from the national comorbidity survey replication. *Pain* 113 (3): 331-339.

Vytal, K., and S. Hamann. 2010. Neuroimaging support for discrete neural correlates of basic emotions: A voxel-based meta-analysis. *Journal of Cognitive Neuroscience* 22 (12): 2864-2885.

Wallace, L.S., J. Buckworth, T.E. Kirby, and W.M. Sherman. 2000. Characteristics of exercise behavior among college students: Application of social cognitive theory to predicting stage of change. *Preventive Medicine* 31 (5): 494-505.

Waller, B., J. Lambeck, and D. Daly. 2009. Therapeutic aquatic exercise in the treatment of low back pain: A systematic review. *Clinical Rehabilitation* 23 (1): 3-14.

Walters, S.T., and J.E. Martin. 2000. Does aerobic exercise really enhance self-esteem in children? A prospective evaluation in 3rd-5th graders. *Journal of sport behavior* 23 (1): 53-62.

Wang, G., C.A. Macera, B. Scudder-Soucie, T. Schmid, M. Pratt, and D. Buchner. 2004. Cost effectiveness of a bicycle/pedestrian trail development in health promotion. *Preventive Medicine* 38 (2): 237-242.

Wang, G.J., N.D. Volkow, J.S. Fowler, et al. 2000. PET studies of the effects of aerobic exercise on human striatal dopamine release. *Journal of Nuclear Medicine* 41 (Aug): 1352-1356.

Wankel, L.M., and J.M. Sefton. 1989. A season-long investigation of fun in youth sports. *Journal of Sport & Exercise Psychology* 11 (4): 355-366.

Wasserman, J.D., and D.S. Tulsky. 2005. A history of intelligence assessment. In *Contemporary intellectual assessment: Theories, tests, and issues*, edited by D.P. Flanagan and P.L. Harrison. New York: Guilford Press.

Watanabe, Y., B. Evengard, B.H. Natelson, L.A. Jason, and H. Kuratsune. 2010. *Fatigue science for human health*. Japan: Springer.

Waters, R.P., K.J. Renner, R.B. Pringle, et al. 2008. Selection for aerobic capacity affects corticosterone, monoamines and wheel-running activity. *Physiology & Behavior* 93 (4-5): 1044-1054.

Waters, R.P., K.J. Renner, C.H. Summers, et al. 2010. Selection for intrinsic endurance modifies endocrine stress responsiveness. *Brain Research* 1357: 53-61.

Watson, D. 2009. Locating anger in the hierarchical structure of affect: Comment on Carver and Harmon-Jones (2009). *Psychological Bulletin* 135 (2): 205-208; discussion 215-217.

Watson, D., and L.A. Clark. 1994. The vicissitudes of mood: A schematic model. In *The nature of emotion: Fundamental questions*, edited by P. Ekman and R.J. Davidson. New York: Oxford University Press.

Watson, D., L.A. Clark, and A. Tellegen. 1988. Development and validation of brief measures of positive and negative affect: The PANAS scales. *Journal of Personality & Social Psychology* 54 (6): 1063-1070.

Watson, D., and A. Tellegen. 1985. Toward a consensual structure of mood. *Psychological Bulletin* 98 (2): 219-235.

Watson, J.B. 1919. *Psychology from the standpoint of a behaviorist*. Philadelphia: Lippincott.

Watson L., B. Ellis, and G.C. Leng. 2008. Exercise for intermittent claudication. *Cochrane Database System Review* 8 (4): CD000990.

Weber, E.H., 1834. *De pulsu, resorptione et tactu*. Annotationes Anatomicae et Physiologicae, Leipzig, Germany: Koehler.

Webber, L.S., D.J. Catellier, L.A. Lytle, et al. 2008. Promoting physical activity in middle school girls: Trial of activity for adolescent girls. *American Journal of Preventive Medicine* 34 (3): 173-184.

Wedekind, D., A. Broocks, N. Weiss, K. Engel, K. Neubert, and B. Bandelow. 2010. A randomized, controlled trial of aerobic exercise in combination with paroxetine in the treatment of panic disorder. *World Journal of Biological Psychiatry* 11 (7): 904-913.

Weir, L.T., and A.S. Jackson. 1992. % $\dot{V}O_2$max and %HRmax reserve are not equal methods of assessing exercise intensity. *Medicine & Science in Sports & Exercise* 24 (5 Suppl.): 1057.

Weir, P.T., G.A. Harlan, F.L. Nkoy, et al. 2006. The incidence of fibromyalgia and its associated comorbidities: A population-based retrospective cohort study based on international classification of diseases, 9th revision codes. *Journal of Clinical Rheumatology* 12 (3): 124-128. doi: 10.1097/01.rhu.0000221817.46231.18.

Weisberg, R.B. 2009. Overview of generalized anxiety disorder: Epidemiology, presentation, and course. *Journal of Clinical Psychiatry* 70 (Suppl. 2): 4-9.

Weiser, P.C., R.A. Kinsman, and D.A. Stamper. 1973. Task-specific symptomatology changes resulting from prolonged submaximal bicycle riding. *Medicine & Science in Sports & Exercise* 5: 79-85.

Weiser, P.C., and D.A. Stamper. 1977. Psychophysiological interactions leading to increased effort, leg fatigue, and respiratory distress during prolonged strenuous bicycle riding. In *Physical work and effort*, edited by G.A. Borg. New York: Pergamon Press.

Weissman, M. M., R. C. Bland, G. J. Canino, C. Faravelli, S. Greenwald, H. G. Hwu, P. R. Joyce, E. G. Karam, C. K. Lee, J. Lellouch, J. P. Lepine, S. C. Newman, M. Rubio-Stipec, J. E. Wells, P. J. Wickramaratne, H. Wittchen, and E. K. Yeh. 1996. Cross-national epidemiology of major depression and bipolar disorder. *Journal of the American Medical Association*. 276 (Jul 24-31): 293-299.

Weissman, M. M., R. C. Bland, G. J. Canino, C. Faravelli, S. Greenwald, H. G. Hwu, P. R. Joyce, E. G. Karam, C. K. Lee, J. Leeouch, S. C. Newman, M. A. Oakley-Browne, M. Rubio-Stipec, J. E. Wells, P. J. Wickramaratne, H. Wittchen, and E. K. Yeh. 1997. The cross-national epidemiology of panic disorder. *Archives of General Psychiatry* 54: 305-309.

Weissman, M.M., J.S. Markowitz, R. Ouellette, S. Greenwald, and J.P. Kahn. 1990. Panic disorder and cardiovascular/cerebrovascular problems: Results from a community survey. *American Journal of Psychiatry* 147: 1504-1508.

Wendel-Vos, W., M. Droomers, S. Kremers, J. Brug, and F. van Lenthe. 2007. Potential environmental determinants of physical activity in adults: A systematic review. *Obesity Reviews* 8 (5): 425-440.

Werme, M., C. Messer, L. Olson, et al. 2002. Delta FosB regulates wheel running. *Journal of Neuroscience* 22 (18): 8133-8138.

Wessel, J. 2004. The effectiveness of hand exercises for persons with rheumatoid arthritis: A systematic review. *Journal of Hand Therapy* 17 (2): 174-180.

West, R.L. 1996. An application of prefrontal cortex function theory to cognitive aging. *Psychological Bulletin* 120: 272-292.

Weyerer, S. 1992. Physical inactivity and depression in the community: Evidence from the Upper Bavarian Field Study. *International Journal of Sports Medicine* 136: 492-496.

Whaley, M.H., P.H. Brubaker, L.A. Kaminsky, and C.R. Miller. 1997. Validity of rating of perceived exertion during graded exercise testing in apparently healthy adults and cardiac patients. *Journal of Cardiopulmonary Research* 17 (Jul-Aug): 261-267.

White, L.J., and V. Castellano. 2008a. Exercise and brain health: Implications for multiple sclerosis: Part 1—neuronal growth factors. *Sports Medicine* 38 (2): 91-100.

White, L.J., and V. Castellano. 2008b. Exercise and brain health: Implications for multiple sclerosis. Part II—immune factors and stress hormones. *Sports Medicine* 38 (3): 179-186.

White, P.D., K.A. Goldsmith, A.L. Johnson, et al. 2011. Comparison of adaptive pacing therapy, cognitive behaviour therapy, graded exercise therapy, and specialist medical care for chronic fatigue syndrome (PACE): A randomised trial. *Lancet* 377 (9768): 823-836.

White-Welkley, J.E., B.N. Bunnell, E.H. Mougey, J.L. Meyerhoff, and R.K. Dishman. 1995. Treadmill training and estradiol moderate hypothalamic-pituitary-adrenal cortical responses to acute running and immobilization. *Physiology and Behavior* 57: 533-540.

White-Welkley, J.E., G.L. Warren, B.N. Bunnell, E.H. Mougey, J.L. Meyerhoff, and R.K. Dishman. 1996. Treadmill exercise training and estradiol increase plasma ACTH and prolactin after novel footshock. *Journal of Applied Physiology* 80 (Mar): 931-939.

Whitt-Glover, M.C., W.C. Taylor, M.F. Floyd, M.M. Yore, A.K. Yancey, and C.E. Matthews. 2009. Disparities in physical activity and sedentary behaviors among U.S. children and adolescents: Prevalence, correlates, and intervention implications. *Journal of Public Health Policy* 30 (Suppl. 1): S309-S334.

Whybrow, P.C., H.S. Akiskal, and W.T. McKinney. 1984. *Mood disorders: Toward a new psychobiology*. New York: Plenum.

Wiedemann, A.U., S. Lippke, T. Reuter, B. Schuz, J.P. Ziegelmann, and R. Schwarzer. 2009. Prediction of stage transitions in fruit and vegetable intake. *Health Education Research* 24 (4): 596-607.

Wiggins, J.S., P. Trapnell, and N. Phillips. 1988. Psychometric and geometric characteristics of the Revised Interpersonal Adjective Scales (IAS6R). *Multivariate Behavioral Research* 23: 517-530.

Wilfley, D., and J.T. Kunce. 1986. Differential physical and psychological effects of exercise. *Journal of Counseling Psychology*. 33 (3): 337.

Williams, D.M., S. Dunsiger, J.T. Ciccolo, B.A. Lewis, A.E. Albrecht, and B.H. Marcus. 2008. Acute affective response to a moderate-intensity exercise stimulus predicts physical activity participation 6 and 12 months later. *Psychology of Sport and Exercise* 9 (3): 231-245.

Williams, D.M., C.E. Matthews, C. Rutt, M.A. Napolitano, and B.H. Marcus. 2008. Interventions to increase walking behavior. *Medicine & Science in Sports & Exercise* 40 (7 Suppl.): S567-S573.

Williams, D.S., J.A. Detre, J.S. Leigh, and A.P. Koretsky. 1992. Magnetic resonance imaging of perfusion using spin inversion of arterial water. *Proceedings of the National Academy of Sciences of the United States of America* 89 (1): 212-216.

Williams, G.C., M. Gagne, R.M. Ryan, and E.L. Deci. 2002. Facilitating autonomous motivation for smoking cessation. *Health Psychology* 21 (1): 40-50.

Williams, G.C., D.S. Minicucci, R.W. Kouides, et al. 2002. Self-determination, smoking, diet and health. *Health Education Research* 17 (5): 512-521.

Williams, J.W., Jr., C.D. Mulrow, E. Chiquette, P.H. Noel, C. Aguilar, and J. Cornell. 2000. A systematic review of newer pharmacotherapies for depression in adults: evidence report summary. *Annals of Internal Medicine*. 132 (9): 743-56.

Williams, J.W., B.L. Plassman, J. Burke, T. Holsinger, and S. Benjamin. 2010. Preventing Alzheimer's disease and cognitive decline. Edited by AHRQ. Rockville, MD: Agency for Healthcare Research and Quality.

Williams, M.A., P.A. Ades, L.F. Hamm, et al. 2006. Clinical evidence for a health benefit from cardiac rehabilitation: An update. *American Heart Journal* 152 (5): 835-841.

Williams, S.L., and D.P. French. 2011. What are the most effective intervention techniques for changing physical activity self-efficacy and physical activity behaviour—and are they the same? *Health Education Research* 26 (2): 308-322.

Williamson, J.W., P.J. Fadel, and J.H. Mitchell. 2006. New insights into central cardiovascular control during exercise in humans: A central command update. *Experimental Physiology* 91 (1): 51-58.

Williamson, J.W., D.B. Friedman, J.H. Mitchell, N.H. Secher, and L. Friberg. 1996. Mechanisms regulating regional cerebral activation during dynamic handgrip in humans. *Journal of Applied Physiology* 81 (5): 1884-1890.

Williamson, J.W., R. McColl, and D. Mathews. 2003. Evidence for central command activation of the human insular cortex during exercise. *Journal of Applied Physiology* 94 (5): 1726-1734.

Willner, P. 1995. Animal models of depression: Validity and applications. In *Depression and mania: From neurobiology to treatment*, edited by G. Gessa, W. Fratta, L. Pani, and G. Serra. New York: Raven Press.

Wilmore, J.H., and D.L. Costill. 1994. *Physiology of sport and exercise*. Champaign, IL: Human Kinetics.

Wilmore, J.H., A.S. Leon, D.C. Rao, J.S. Skinner, J. Gagnon, and C. Bouchard. 1997. Genetics, response to exercise, and risk factors: the HERITAGE Family Study. *World Review of Nutrition & Dietetics* 81: 72-83.

Wilson, C.A., J.R. Pearson, A.J. Hunter, P.A. Tuohy, and A.P. Payne. 1986. The effect of neonatal manipulation of hypothalamic serotonin levels on sexual activity in the adult rat. *Pharmacology, Biochemistry, and Behavior* 24 (May): 1175-1183.

Wilson, G.F., J.A. Caldwell, and C.A. Russell. 2007. Performance and psychophysiological measures of fatigue effects on aviation related tasks of varying difficulty. *International Journal of Aviation Psychology* 17 (2): 219-247.

Wilson, P.M., D.E. Mack, and K.P. Grattan. 2008. Understanding motivation for exercise: A self-determination theory perspective. *Canadian Psychology* 49 (3): 250-256.

Winchester, P.K., J.W. Williamson, and J.H. Mitchell. 2000. Cardiovascular responses to static exercise in patients with Brown-Sequard syndrome. *Journal of Physiology* 527 Pt 1: 193-202.

Winters, E., ed. 1951. *The collected works of Adolf Meyer*. Baltimore: Johns Hopkins Press.

Wipfli, B.M., C.D. Rethorst, and D.M. Landers. 2008. The anxiolytic effects of exercise: A meta-analysis of randomized trials and dose-response analysis. *Journal of Sport & Exercise Psychology* 30 (4): 392-410.

Wise, L.A., L.L. Adams-Campbell, J.R. Palmer, and L. Rosenberg. 2006. Leisure time physical activity in relation to depressive symptoms in the Black Women's Health Study. *Annals of Behavioral Medicine*. 32 (1): 68-76. doi: 10.1207/s15324796abm3201_8.

Wise, R.A. 2004. Dopamine, learning and motivation. *Nature reviews. Neuroscience* 5 (6): 483-494.

Wise, R.A. 2008. Dopamine and reward: The anhedonia hypothesis 30 years on. *Neurotoxicity Research* 14 (2-3): 169-183.

Wolf, M., M. Ferrari, and V. Quaresima. 2007. Progress of near-infrared spectroscopy and topography for brain and muscle clinical applications. *Journal of Biomedical Optics* 12: 062104. doi: 10.1117/1.2804899.

Wolf, P.A., A. Beiser, M.F. Elias, A. Rhoda, R.S. Vasan, and S. Seshadri. 2007. Relation of obesity to cognitive function: Importance of central obesity and synergistic influence of concomitant hypertension. The Framingham Heart Study. *Current Alzheimer Research* 4: 111-116.

Wolfe, F., K. Ross, J. Anderson, I.J. Russell, and L. Hebert. 1995. The prevalence and characteristics of fibromyalgia in the general population. *Arthritis & Rheumatism* 38 (1): 19-28.

Wolff, E., and A. Ströhle. 2010. Causal associations of physical activity/exercise and symptoms of depression and anxiety. *Archives of General Psychiatry* 67 (5): 540-541.

Wolin, K.Y., R.J. Glynn, G.A. Colditz, I.M. Lee, and I. Kawachi. 2007. Long-term physical activity patterns and health-related quality of life in U.S. women. *American Journal of Preventive Medicine* 32 (6): 490-499.

Woo, M., S. Kim, J. Kim, S.J. Petruzzello, and B.D. Hatfield. 2009. Examining the exercise-affect dose-response relationship: Does duration influence frontal EEG asymmetry? *International Journal of Psychophysiology* 72 (2): 166-172.

Woolf, C.J., and R.J. Mannion. 1999. Neuropathic pain: Aetiology, symptoms, mechanisms, and management. *The Lancet* 353 (9168): 1959-1964.

World Health Organization. 1992. *International classification of diseases.* 10th ed. Geneva: World Health Organization.

World Health Organization. 2008. *Global burden of disease: 2004 update.* Geneva: World Health Organization.

World Health Organization. 2011a. *Global recommendations on physical activity for health.* Geneva: World Health Organization.

World Health Organization. 2011b. mHealth: New horizons for health through mobile technologies. In *Global observatory for eHealth series.* Geneva: World Health Organization.

Wozniak, R.H. 1992. *Mind and body: Rene Descartes to William James.* Bethesda, MD, and Washington, DC: National Library of Medicine and American Psychological Association.

Wylie, R.C. 1989. *Measures of self-concept.* Lincoln: University of Nebraska Press.

Yagi, Y., K.L. Coburn, K.N. Estes, and J.E. Arruda. 1999. Effects of aerobic exercise and gender on visual and auditory P300, reaction time, and accuracy. *Journal of Applied Physiology and Occupational Physiology* 80: 402-408.

Yamamoto, U., M. Mohri, K. Shimada, et al. 2007. Six-month aerobic exercise training ameliorates central sleep apnea in patients with chronic heart failure. *Journal of Cardiac Failure* 13 (10): 825-829.

Yancey, A.K., W.J. McCarthy, W.C. Taylor, et al. 2004. The Los Angeles Lift Off: A sociocultural environmental change intervention to integrate physical activity into the workplace. *Preventive Medicine* 38 (6): 848-856.

Yang, C.Y., J.C. Tsai, Y.C. Huang, and C.C. Lin. 2011. Effects of a home-based walking program on perceived symptom and mood status in postoperative breast cancer women receiving adjuvant chemotherapy. *Journal of Advanced Nursing* 67 (1): 158-168.

Yates, A., K. Leehey, and C.M. Shisslak. 1983. Running—an analogue of anorexia? *New England Journal of Medicine* 308 (Feb 3): 251-255.

Yeung, R.R. 1996. The acute effects of exercise on mood state. *Journal of Psychosomatic Research* 40 (2): 123-141.

Yeung, R.R., and D.R. Hemsley. 1996. Effects of personality and acute exercise on mood states. *Personality & Individual Differences* 20 (5): 545-550.

Yoo, H.S., B.N. Bunnell, J.B. Crabbe, L.R. Kalish, and R.K. Dishman. 2000. Failure of neonatal clomipramine treatment to alter forced swim immobility: Chronic treadmill or activity-wheel running and imipramine. *Physiology & Behavior* 70 (3-4): 407-411.

Yoo, H., H.A. O'Neal, S. Hong, R.L. Tackett, and R.K. Dishman. 1999. Brain β-adrenergic responses to footshock after wheel running. *Medicine & Science in Sports & Exercise* 31 (5) (Suppl.): S109, 647.

Yoo, H., R.L. Tackett, and R.K. Dishman. 1996. Brain β-adrenergic responses to wheel running. *Medicine & Science in Sports & Exercise* 28 (5) (Suppl.): S109, 647.

Yorio, J.M., R.K. Dishman, W.R. Forbus, and K.J. Cureton. 1992. Breathlessness predicts perceived exertion in young women with mild asthma. *Medicine & Science in Sports & Exercise* 24 (8): 860-867.

Young, D.R., W.L. Haskell, C.B. Taylor, and S.P. Fortmann. 1996. Effect of community health education on physical activity knowledge, attitudes, and behavior. The Stanford Five-City Project. *American Journal of Epidemiology* 144 (3): 264-274.

Youngstedt, S.D. 1997. Does exercise truly enhance sleep? *Physician and Sportsmedicine* 25 (10): 73-82.

Youngstedt, S.D. 2000. The exercise-sleep mystery. *International Journal of Sport Psychology* 31 (2): 241-255.

Youngstedt, S.D. 2005. Effects of exercise on sleep. *Clinics in Sports Medicine* 24 (2): 355-365, xi.

Youngstedt, S.D., R.K. Dishman, K.J. Cureton, and L.J. Peacock. 1993. Does body temperature mediate anxiolytic effects of acute exercise? *Journal of Applied Physiology* 74 (Feb): 825-831.

Youngstedt, S.D., and C.E. Kline. 2006. Epidemiology of exercise and sleep. *Sleep and Biological Rhythms* 4 (3): 215-221.

Youngstedt, S.D., D.F. Kripke, and J.A. Elliott. 1999. Is sleep disturbed by vigorous late-night exercise?

Medicine and Science in Sports and Exercise 31 (6): 864-869.

Youngstedt, S.D., P.J. O'Connor, J.B. Crabbe, and R.K. Dishman. 1998. Acute exercise reduces caffeine-induced anxiogenesis. *Medicine & Science in Sports & Exercise* 30 (5): 740-745.

Youngstedt, S.D., P.J. O'Connor, J.B. Crabbe, and R.K. Dishman. 2000. The influence of acute exercise on sleep following high caffeine intake. *Physiology & Behavior* 68 (4): 563-570.

Youngstedt, S.D., P.J. O'Connor, and R.K. Dishman. 1997. The effects of acute exercise on sleep: A quantitative synthesis. *Sleep* 20 (3): 203-214.

Yurtkuran, M., A. Alp, and K. Dilek. 2007. A modified yoga-based exercise program in hemodialysis patients: A randomized controlled study. *Complementary Therapies in Medicine* 15 (3): 164-171.

Zago, S., R. Ferrucci, S. Marceglia, and A. Priori. 2009. The Mosso method for recording brain pulsation: The forerunner of functional neuroimaging. *NeuroImage* 48 (4): 652-656.

Zagrodnik, J.A., and M. Horvat. 2009. Chronic exercise and developmental disabilities. In *Exercise and cognitive function*, edited by T. McMorris, P.D. Tomporowski, and M. Audiffren. Chichester, UK: Wiley.

Zajonc, R.B. 1985. Emotions and facial expression. *Science* 230 (4726): 608-687.

Zajonc, R.B., and D.N. McIntosh. 1992. Emotions research: Some promising questions and some questionable promises. *Psychological Science* 3 (1): 70-74.

Zhang, H.N., and M.C. Ko. 2009. Seizure activity involved in the up-regulation of BDNF mRNA expression by activation of central mu opioid receptors. *Neuroscience* 161 (1): 301-310.

Zhao, G., X. Zhang, X. Xu, M. Ochoa, and T.H. Hintze. 1997. Short-term exercise training enhances reflex cholinergic nitric oxide-dependent coronary vasodilation in conscious dogs. *Circulation Research* 80 (Jun): 868-876.

Zmijewski, C.F., and M.O. Howard. 2003. Exercise dependence and attitudes toward eating among young adults. *Eating Behaviors* 4 (2): 181-196.

Index

Note: The italicized f and t following page numbers refer to figures and tables, respectively.

About the Authors

Janet Buckworth, PhD, is an associate professor of exercise science at Ohio State University in Columbus, where she teaches upper-level undergraduate and graduate courses on behavior change in exercise. She has written and presented extensively on exercise psychology and behavior change.

Respected for her expertise in the field, Buckworth has been invited as a keynote presenter for several conferences on exercise psychology and exercise and depression. She is also the recipient of an NIH grant for her research in exercise adherence.

Buckworth is a member of the Society of Behavioral Medicine and the American Alliance for Health, Physical Education, Recreation and Dance. She is also a fellow of the American College of Sports Medicine.

She and her husband, Chuck Moody, reside in Dublin, Ohio. Buckworth enjoys running with her dog, cooking, and reading science fiction and mystery novels.

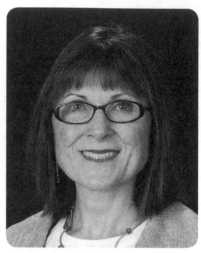

Janet Buckworth

Rod K. Dishman, PhD, is a professor of exercise science, adjunct professor of psychology, and codirector of the Exercise Psychology Laboratory at the University of Georgia at Athens. He has served as a consultant on exercise to government agencies in the United States, Canada, and Europe. His research has been funded by the NIH, the Centers for Disease Control and Prevention (CDC), the American Heart Association, and the United States Olympic Committee (USOC).

Dishman is a fellow of the American College of Sports Medicine and the National Academy of Kinesiology and was one of 22 founding members of the International Olympic Committee's Olympic Academy of Sport Sciences. He was a member of the Scientific Advisory Committee for the 2008 Physical Activity Guidelines for Americans.

He resides in Athens, Georgia, and enjoys cycling and resistance exercise.

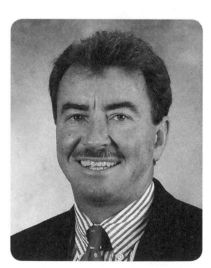

Rod K. Dishman

Patrick J. O'Connor, PhD, is a professor of kinesiology and the codirector of the Exercise Psychology Laboratory at the University of Georgia at Athens. He has served as a consultant to the U.S. Department of Health and Human Services on their 2008 Physical Activity Guidelines for Americans.

He has presented original research at 80 conferences, written numerous journal articles, and contributed to several books. O'Connor is fellow of the National Academy of Kinesiology and the American College of Sports Medicine.

He resides in Athens, Georgia, with his wife, Sarah Covert, and twins, Aydan and Siena. O'Connor enjoys training for and competing in various running events from 5Ks to the Boston Marathon.

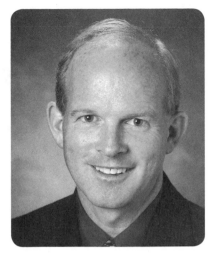

Patrick J. O'Connor

Phillip D. Tomporowski, PhD, is a professor of kinesiology and director of the Cognition and Skill Acquisition Laboratory at the University of Georgia at Athens. He has coauthored three books, coedited two texts, and authored numerous book chapters and journal articles. He has served as a consultant to university extension programs, international programs, local community service programs, and governmental and nongovernmental agencies in the United States and the United Kingdom. Tomporowski is a fellow of the American College of Sports Medicine.

He resides in Athens, Georgia. Tomporowski is a martial arts instructor and practitioner. He also enjoys competing in triathlons and obstacle course races.

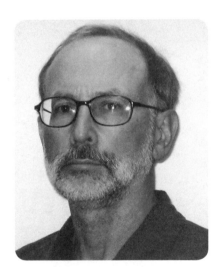

Phillip D. Tomporowski

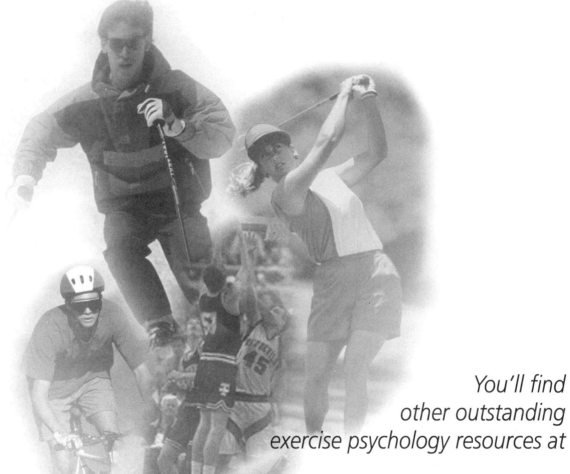